CHONDROITIN SULFATE: STRUCTURE, ROLE AND PHARMACOLOGICAL ACTIVITY

CHONDROITIN SULFATE: STRUCTURE, ROLE AND PHARMACOLOGICAL ACTIVITY

Edited by

Nicola Volpi

University of Modena & Reggio Emilia
Modena, Italy

ADVANCES IN
PHARMACOLOGY

VOLUME 53

ELSEVIER

AMSTERDAM • BOSTON • HEIDELBERG • LONDON
NEW YORK • OXFORD • PARIS • SAN DIEGO
SAN FRANCISCO • SINGAPORE • SYDNEY • TOKYO
Academic Press is an imprint of Elsevier

Academic Press is an imprint of Elsevier
525 B Street, Suite 1900, San Diego, California 92101-4495, USA
84 Theobald's Road, London WC1X 8RR, UK

For information on all Academic Press publications
visit our Web site at www.books.elsevier.com

ISBN-13: 978-012-032955-7
ISBN-10: 0-12-032955-7

PRINTED IN THE UNITED STATES OF AMERICA
06 07 08 09 9 8 7 6 5 4 3 2 1

Contents

PART I   Structure

Isolation, Purification, and Analysis of Chondroitin Sulfate Proteoglycans

Fumiko Matsui and Atsuhiko Oohira

Isolation and Purification of Chondroitin Sulfate

Luiz-Claudio F. Silva

Structure of Chondroitin Sulfate

Fotini N. Lamari and Nikos K. Karamanos

Progress in the Structural Biology of Chondroitin Sulfate

Barbara Mulloy

The Biosynthesis and Catabolism of Galactosaminoglycans

Vikas Prabhakar and Ram Sasisekharan

Biosynthesis of Chondroitin Sulfate: From the Early, Precursor Discoveries to Nowadays, Genetics Approaches

Mauro S. G. Pavão, Ana Cristina Vilela-Silva, and Paulo A. S. Mourão

Advances in the Analysis of Chondroitin/ Dermatan Sulfate

M. Stylianou, I.-E. Triantaphyllidou, and D. H. Vynios

Chondroitin Sulfate Lyases: Applications in Analysis and Glycobiology

Emmanuel Petit, Cedric Delattre, Dulce Papy-Garcia, and Philippe Michaud

CS Lyases: Structure, Activity, and Applications in Analysis and the Treatment of Diseases

Robert J. Linhardt, Fikri Y. Avci, Toshihiko Toida, Yeong Shik Kim, and Miroslaw Cygler

PART II · Biological Role of Chondroitin Sulfate

Structure, Metabolism, and Tissue Roles of Chondroitin Sulfate Proteoglycans

Christopher J. Handley, Tom Samiric, and Mirna Z. Ilic

Chondroitin Sulfate Proteoglycans in Tumor Progression

Yanusz Wegrowski and François-Xavier Maquart

Chondroitin Sulfate Proteoglycans in the Brain

Sachiko Aono and Atsuhiko Oohira

Chondroitin/Dermatan Sulfates in the Central Nervous System: Their Structures and Functions in Health and Disease

Uwe Rauch and Joachim Kappler

Chondroitin Sulfate Proteoglycan and its Degradation Products in CNS Repair

Asya Rolls and Michal Schwartz

Role of Chondroitin-4-Sulfate in Pregnancy-Associated Malaria

D. Channe Gowda

PART III   Pharmacological Activities of Chondroitin Sulfate

In Vitro Effects of Chondroitin Sulfate

A. Fioravanti and G. Collodel

Effect of Chondroitin Sulfate as Nutraceutical in Dogs with Arthropathies

Britta Dobenecker

Chondroitin Sulfate as a Structure-Modifying Agent

Daniel Uebelhart, Ruud Knols, Eling D de Bruin, and Gust Verbruggen

PART IV Clinical Efficacy and Trials

Chondroitin Sulfate in the Management of Erosive Osteoarthritis of the Interphalangeal Finger Joints

Gust Verbruggen

Chondroitin Sulfate in the Management of Hip and Knee Osteoarthritis: An Overview

Géraldine Bana, Bénédicte Jamard, Evelyne Verrouil, and Bernard Mazières

Treatment of Knee Osteoarthritis with Oral Chondroitin Sulfate

Daniel Uebelhart, Ruud Knols, Eling D de Bruin, and Gust Verbruggen

Abbreviations

2-AMAC:	2-Aminoacridone
AAP:	Anatomical phase progression
C4S:	Chondroitin-4-sulfate
C6S:	Chondroitin-6-sulfate
CA:	Carbonic anhydrase
CAT:	Catalase
CE:	Capillary electrophoresis
ChPF:	Chondroitin polymerizing factor
CIA:	Collagen-induced autoimmune arthritis
CNS:	Central nervous system
CPS:	Chemically polysulfated chondroitin sulfate
CRMP:	Collapsin response mediator proteins
CRP:	Complement regulatory protein
CS:	Chondroitin sulfate
CS-A:	Chondroitin-4-sulfate
CS-B or DS:	Dermatan sulfate
CS-C:	Chondroitin-6-sulfate
CS-H:	Hagfish notochord CS
CSPG:	Chondroitin sulfate proteoglycan
CSS:	CS synthase
CTSMA:	Connective tissue structure-modifying agents
CZE:	Capillary zone electrophoresis
DIP:	Distal interphalangeal joints
DJD:	Degenerative joint disease
DMOAD:	Disease modifying osteoarthritis drugs

DSPG:	Dermatan sulfate proteoglycan
ECM:	Extracellular matrix
EGF:	Epidermal growth factor
ELISA:	Enzyme-linked immunosorbent assay
EOF:	Electroosmotic flow
FACE:	Fluorophore-assisted carbohydrate electrophoresis
FGF:	Fibroblast growth factor
Fuc:	Fucose
GAG:	Glycosaminoglycan
Gal:	D-Galactose
GalAG:	Galactosaminoglycan
GalN:	D-Galactosamine
GalNAc:	N-Acetyl-D-galactosamine
GalpNAc:	2-Deoxy, 2-acetamido-D-galactopyranose
GlcA:	Glucuronic acid
GlcAp:	D-Glucopyranosyl uronic acid
GlcN:	D-Glucosamine
GlcNAc:	N-Acetyl D-glucosamine
Gly:	Glycine
GPx:	Glutathione peroxidase
HA:	Hyaluronan or Hyaluronic acid
HAS:	Hyaluronan synthases
HCII:	Heparin cofactor II
Hep:	Heparin
HPLC:	High performance liquid chromatography
HS:	Heparan sulfate
HSPG:	Heparan sulfate proteoglycan
IdoA:	Iduronic acid
IdoAp:	L-Idopyranosyl uronic acid
IP:	Interphalangeal
IRBCs:	Infected red blood cells
KS:	Keratan sulfate
LDL:	Low-density lipoprotein
LTP:	Long term potentiation
Mab:	Monoclonal antibody
MCP:	Carpometacarpal joints
MECC:	Micellar electrokinetic capillary chromatography
MEEKC:	Microemulsion electrokinetic capillary chromatography
MMPs:	Matrix metalloproteinases
MPS:	Mucopolysaccharidosis
M_r:	Molecular mass
MS:	Mass spectroscopy
NGC:	Neuroglycan C
NO:	Nitric oxide

OA:	Osteoarthritis
PAP:	3′-Phosphoadenosine-5′phosphate
PBS:	Phosphate buffered saline
PG:	Proteoglycan
PIP:	Proximal interphalangeal joints
PNNs:	Perineuronal nets
ROS:	Reactive oxygen species
RPTPβ:	Receptor-type protein tyrosine phosphatase β
S:	O-sulfate
SADOA:	Slow-acting drugs for osteoarthritis
SDS:	Sodium dodecyl sulfate
SEM:	Scanning electron microscopy
Ser:	Serine
SLRP:	Small leucine-rich proteoglycan
SMOAD:	Symptom-modifying osteoarthritis drug
SOD:	Superoxide dismutase
SYSADOA:	Symptomatic slow acting drugs for treating osteoarthritis
TEM:	Transmission electron microscopy
TGFβ:	Transforming growth factor beta
TIMPs:	Tissue inhibitors of metalloproteinases
Xyl:	Xylose

Contributors

Numbers in parentheses indicate the pages on which the authors' contributions begin.

Hiroshi Akiyama (403) National Institute of Health Sciences, Tokyo 158-8501, Japan

Sachiko Aono (323) Department of Perinatology, Institute for Developmental Research, Aichi Human Service Center, Aichi 480-0392, Japan

Fikri Y. Avci (187) Department of Chemistry and Chemical Biology, Biology and Chemical and Biological Engineering, Rensselaer Polytechnic Institute, Troy, New York 12180

A. Avenoso (417) Department of Biochemical, Physiological and Nutritional Sciences, School of Medicine, University of Messina, Policlinico Universitario, I-98125 Messina, Italy

Géraldine Bana (507) Paul-Sabatier University, Faculty of Pharmacy, Toulouse, France

N. Brandl (433) Medical University Vienna, Center Physiology and Pathophysiology, 1090 Vienna, Währingerstrasse 10 Austria

A. Calatroni (417) Department of Biochemical, Physiological and Nutritional Sciences, School of Medicine, University of Messina, Policlinico Universitario, I-98125 Messina, Italy

G. M. Campo (417) Department of Biochemical, Physiological and Nutritional Sciences, School of Medicine, University of Messina, Policlinico Universitario, I-98125 Messina, Italy

S. Campo (417) Department of Biochemical, Physiological and Nutritional Sciences, School of Medicine, University of Messina, Policlinico Universitario, I-98125 Messina, Italy

G. Collodel (449) Department of Pediatrics, Obstetrics and Reproductive Medicine, Biology Section, University of Siena, Siena, Italy

Miroslaw Cygler (187) Biotechnology Research Institute, NRC, Montreal, Quebec H4P2R2, Canada

Eling D de Bruin (475,523) Department of Rheumatology and Institute of Physical Medicine, University Hospital Zurich, Switzerland; Institute for Human Movement Sciences, ETH Zurich, Switzerland

Cedric Delattre (167) Laboratoire Des Glucides-EPMV CNRS FRE 2779, IUT/GB, UPJV Avenue Des Facultés, Le Bailly, 80025 Amiens Cedex, France

Britta Dobenecker (467) Institute of Physiology, Physiological Chemistry and Animal Nutrition, Ludwig-Maximilians University Munich, Germany

A. M. Ferlazzo (417) Department of Biochemical, Physiological and Nutritional Sciences, School of Medicine, University of Messina, Policlinico Universitario, I-98125 Messina, Italy

A. Fioravanti (449) Rheumatology Unit, Department of Clinical Medicine and Immunological Sciences, University of Siena, Siena, Italy

D. Channe Gowda (375) Department of Biochemistry and Molecular Biology, Pennsylvania State University College of Medicine, Hershey, Pennsylvania 17033

Christopher J. Handley (219) School of Human Biosciences, La Trobe University, Melbourne, Victoria 3086, Australia

J. Holzmann (433) Medical University Vienna, Center Physiology and Pathophysiology, 1090 Vienna, Währingerstrasse 10 Austria

M. Huettinger (433) Medical University Vienna, Center Physiology and Pathophysiology, 1090 Vienna, Währingerstrasse 10 Austria

Mirna Z. Ilic (219) School of Human Biosciences, La Trobe University, Melbourne, Victoria 3086, Australia

Bénédicte Jamard (507) Rangueil University Hospital, Toulouse, France

Joachim Kappler (337) Physiologisch-Chemisches Institut, Rheinische Friedrich-Wilhelms-Universität Bonn 53115 Bonn, Germany

Nikos K. Karamanos (33,281) Laboratory of Biochemistry, Department of Chemistry, University of Patras, 26500 Patras, Greece

Yeong Shik Kim (187) Natural Products Research Institute, College of Pharmacy, Seoul National University, Seoul 110-460, Korea

Ruud Knols (475,523) Department of Rheumatology and Institute of Physical Medicine, University Hospital Zurich, Switzerland

Fotini N. Lamari (33) Laboratory of Pharmacognosy and Chemistry of Natural Products, Department of Pharmacy, University of Patras, 26500 Patras, Greece

Robert J. Linhardt (187,403) Department of Chemistry and Chemical Biology, Biology and Chemical and Biological Engineering, Rensselaer Polytechnic Institute, Troy, New York 12180

François-Xavier Maquart (297) CNRS UMR 6198, Faculty of Medicine, IFR-53, 51095 Reims Cedex, France

Fumiko Matsui (1) Department of Perinatology, Institute for Developmental Research, Aichi Human Service Center, Kasugai, Aichi 480-0392, Japan

Bernard Mazières (507) Paul-Sabatier University, Faculty of Medicine and Rangueil University Hospital, Toulouse, France

Philippe Michaud (167) Laboratoire de Génie Chimique et Biochimique, Université Blaise Pascal CUST, 63174 Aubière, France

Paulo A. S. Mourão (117) Laboratório de Tecido Conjuntivo, Hospital Universitário Clementino Fraga Filho, Instituto de Bioquímica Médica and Instituto de Ciências Biomédicas, Universidade Federal do Rio de Janeiro, RJ 21941-590, Brazil

Barbara Mulloy (49) National Institute for Biological Standards and Control, Herts. EN6 3QG, United Kingdom

Helena B. Nader (233) Disciplina de Biologia Molecular, Departamento de Bioquímica, Universidade Federal de São Paulo, Rua Três de Maio, 100 04044-020 São Paulo, São Paulo, Brazil

*Chilkunda D. Nandini** (253) Department of Biochemistry, Kobe Pharmaceutical University, Kobe 658–8558, Japan

Atsuhiko Oohira (1,323) Department of Perinatology, Institute for Developmental Research, Aichi Human Service Center, Aichi 480-0392, Japan

Dulce Papy-Garcia (167) Laboratoire de Recherche sur la Croissance, la Réparation et la Régénération Tissulaires (CRRET), CNRS FRE-2412, Université Paris 12-Val de Marne, 94010 Créteil cedex, France

Mauro S. G. Pavão (117) Laboratório de Tecido Conjuntivo, Hospital Universitário Clementino Fraga Filho, Instituto de Bioquímica Médica and Instituto de Ciências Biomédicas, Universidade Federal do Rio de Janeiro, RJ 21941-590, Brazil

---

*Present address: Department of Pathology and Laboratory Medicine, University of Wisconsin, Madison, WI 53792–8550, USA.

Emmanuel Petit (167) Société OTR³ SAS, 75001 Paris, France

Vikas Prabhakar (69) Division of Biological Engineering, Massachusetts Institute of Technology, Cambridge, Massachusetts 02139

Uwe Rauch (337) Department of Experimental Pathology, Universitet Lund, Lund, Sweden

Asya Rolls (357) Department of Neurobiology, The Weizmann Institute of Science, 76100 Rehovot, Israel

Shinobu Sakai (403) Graduate School of Pharmaceutical Sciences, Chiba University, Chiba 263-8522, Japan

Tom Samiric (219) School of Human Biosciences, La Trobe University, Melbourne, Victoria 3086, Australia

Lucia O. Sampaio (233) Disciplina de Biologia Molecular, Departamento de Bioquímica, Universidade Federal de São Paulo, Rua Três de Maio, 100 04044-020 São Paulo, São Paulo, Brazil

Ram Sasisekharan (69) Division of Biological Engineering, Massachusetts Institute of Technology, Cambridge, Massachusetts 02139

R. Schabus (433) Department of Traumatology, University Hospital, 1090 Vienna, Währinger Gürtel 18–20, Austria

Michal Schwartz (357) Department of Neurobiology, The Weizmann Institute of Science, 76100 Rehovot, Israel

Luiz-Claudio F. Silva (21) Laboratório de Tecido Conjuntivo, Hospital Universitário Clementino Fraga Filho and Instituto de Bioquímica Médica, Programa de Glicobiologia, Centro de Ciências da Saúde, Universidade Federal do Rio de Janeiro 21941–590, Rio de Janeiro, Brazil

M. Stylianou (141) Laboratory of Biochemistry, Department of Chemistry, University of Patras, 26500 Patras, Greece

Kazuyuki Sugahara† (253) Department of Biochemistry, Kobe Pharmaceutical University, Kobe 658–8558, Japan

A. D. Theocharis (281) Laboratory of Biochemistry, Department of Chemistry, University of Patras, 26500 Patras, Greece

Toshihiko Toida (187,403) Graduate School of Pharmaceutical Sciences, Chiba University, Chiba 263-8522, Japan

I.-E. Triantaphyllidou (141) Laboratory of Biochemistry, Department of Chemistry, University of Patras, 26500 Patras, Greece

---

†Present address: Graduate School of Life Science, Faculty of Advanced Life Science, Hokkaido University, Sapporo 001–0021, Japan.

I. Tsolakis (281) Department of Surgery, School of Medicine, University of Patras, 26500 Patras, Greece

G. N. Tzanakakis (281) Department of Histology, School of Medicine, University of Crete, 71110 Heraklion, Greece

Daniel Uebelhart (475,523) Department of Rheumatology and Institute of Physical Medicine, University Hospital Zurich, Switzerland; Department of Biochemistry, Rush Presbyterian-St. Luke's Medical Center, Chicago, Illinois

Gust Verbruggen (475,491,523) Department of Rheumatology, Ghent University Hospital, Gent, Belgium

Evelyne Verrouil (507) Rangueil University Hospital, Toulouse, France

Ana Cristina Vilela-Silva (117) Laboratório de Tecido Conjuntivo, Hospital Universitário Clementino Fraga Filho, Instituto de Bioquímica Médica and Instituto de Ciências Biomédicas, Universidade Federal do Rio de Janeiro, RJ 21941-590, Brazil

D. H. Vynios (141) Laboratory of Biochemistry, Department of Chemistry, University of Patras, 26500 Patras, Greece

Yanusz Wegrowski (297) CNRS UMR 6198, Faculty of Medicine, IFR-53, 51095 Reims Cedex, France

Preface

Chondroitin sulfate, a complex glycosaminoglycan extracted and purified from various tissues, is a ubiquitous component of all connective tissue extracellular matrices, where it serves a number of functions mainly covalently attached to proteins in the form of proteoglycans. Furthermore, chondroitin sulfate represents a highly heterogeneous family of polysaccharides, in terms of degree of sulfatation, molecular mass, and relative amounts of iduronic acid and glucuronate, depending on the tissue of origin.

During the past few years, a dramatic shift in the isolation, characterization, and investigation of the biological actions of this glycosaminoglycan has become evident. Furthermore, it is now apparent that chondroitin sulfate derived drugs may exhibit marked physiological activity, such as anti-inflammatory, chondroprotective, and antirheumatic effects. The source material, manufacturing processes, molecular structure, presence of contaminants, chemical modifications during manufacturing, and many other factors contribute to the overall biological and pharmacological actions of chondroitin sulfate. The chemical industry has begun to exploit its isolation, purification, and modification. Furthermore, synthetic and biotechnological routes have been developed to produce unnatural sugars and to prepare a broad range of carbohydrate derivatives and biologically active intermediates. This area of research is rapidly expanding and is expected to have a major impact on future therapeutic regimens.

This special issue of Advances in Pharmacology is dedicated to chondroitin sulfate with emphasis on the recent developments in its structure, biological role and pharmacological activity. It consists of four chapters written by outstanding scientists across the world carrying out research at the cutting edge of their disciplines. The topics dealt with in this book include: (1) structure of chondroitin sulfate and the most advanced preparative and analytical techniques to determine its structure and properties, (2) biological role of chondroitin sulfate, (3) its pharmacological activities, and (4) clinical efficacy and trials. I would like to thank all the authors for generously contributing their time and expertise in the preparation of this publication. Acknowledgement is due to Elsevier Publishers for their assistance in bringing this issue to publication. Finally, I would like to express my gratitude to the contributors and consider myself to have been abundantly rewarded by the opportunity to further my knowledge in the field during the reading and editing process.

Professor Nicola Volpi
Associate Professor of Biochemistry
Department of Biologia Animale
University of Modena and Reggio Emilia
Italy

PART I

Structure

Fumiko Matsui and Atsuhiko Oohira

Department of Perinatology
Institute for Developmental Research
Aichi Human Service Center
Kasugai, Aichi 480-0392, Japan

Isolation, Purification, and Analysis of Chondroitin Sulfate Proteoglycans

I. Chapter Overview

Chondroitin sulfate proteoglycans (CSPGs) are glycoproteins that carry at least one chondroitin sulfate (CS) chain. In the early studies, CSPGs isolated from the cartilage were widely analyzed because the cartilage contains a large amount of CSPGs, mainly aggrecan. In subsequent studies, over 10 species of CSPG have been isolated from various tissues such as vascular tissues, muscles, skins, and nervous tissues. Proteoglycans (PGs) are extracted from tissues with a saline usually containing denaturing agents and/or detergents, then they are separated from other proteins by a combination of separation methods including ultracentrifugation, ion-exchange chromatography, and gel chromatography. Antibodies are also useful tools to purify the corresponding PGs. Many antibodies are now available for particular domains of CS and core proteins of individual CSPGs. There are some CS lyases with different specificities. These CSPG-related antibodies

Advances in Pharmacology, Volume 53
Copyright 2006, Elsevier Inc. All rights reserved.

1054-3589/06 $35.00
DOI: 10.1016/S1054-3589(05)53001-1

and CS lyases are both powerful tools for identification, structural characterization, and quantification of CS/CSPGs. In addition, since CSPGs usually attach N- and O-linked oligosaccharides, lectins are used to characterize the oligosaccharide moiety. In this chapter, we explain widely applicable procedures for purification and characterization of CSPGs, using several typical CSPG species as examples.

II. Introduction

CSPGs have been isolated from various tissues such as connective tissues, nervous tissues, and vascular tissues. Using those CSPGs, it has been shown that CS chains exert important biological activities. For example, the affinities of some brain CSPGs to their binding partners become less after removal of their CS side chains (Maeda *et al.*, 1996; Milev *et al.*, 1998a,b). Further, the structural differences of their CS chains often correlate well with functional difference of CSPGs (Maeda and Noda, 1998). Although modern molecular biology technologies have made it possible for *E. coli* and animal cells to express CSPG-core proteins in a large amount (Iozzo, 2001), the core protein expressed in *E. coli* does not attach CS chains. Even though it is expressed in animal cells, the structure of CS chains is not necessarily the same as that of a native PG isolated from tissues. Therefore, to examine the structure and function of CS chains of native CSPGs, it is necessary to purify them from tissues. In this chapter, we describe several typical examples to isolate, purify, and characterize CSPGs.

III. Preparation of Tissues for CSPGs Extraction

To extract CSPGs in an intact form, inhibition of core protein degradation is essential. Therefore, tissues should be excised on ice and should be quickly frozen and kept in a deep freezer or in liquid nitrogen. However, in the case of extraction of CSPGs associated with membranes, usually membrane fractions are prepared from the freshly excised tissues because freezing and thawing disrupt cell membranes. In some cases, tissue-specific pretreatments should be done before extraction of PGs. For example, mineralized tissues need to be frozen and grinded (Fedarko, 2001). To extract CSPGs from hard tissues, an efficient method to smash the tissue should be determined beforehand.

We often encounter a problem of the starting materials being limited. To trace a small amount of PG through purification steps, metabolic radiolabeling is useful (Hascall *et al.*, 1994). However, a facility to deal with radioisotopes is necessary for radiolabeling of CSPGs. Another option to detect a small amount of sample is immunological detection using specific antibodies. Various methods that amplify a weak immunological signal have been developed, and some of them are described in Section VI. Because dealing with a small amount of material often makes the recovery rate smaller and amplification of a weak signal tends to result in a higher background, collecting a sufficient amount of material is the best solution.

IV. Extraction of CSPGs

CSPGs are roughly divided into two groups; secretory CSPGs that exist in the extracellular matrix (ECM) and membrane-bound CSPGs that are intercalated into the cell membrane or tightly associated with the surface of cell membrane. Secretory CSPGs are easily extracted from soft tissues, such as the brain, with phosphate buffered saline (PBS). However, for relatively hard tissues, such as cartilage, solutions containing protein-denaturing reagents are usually used to solubilize CSPG effectively, even though the target CSPG itself is soluble with PBS. To extract membrane-bound CSPGs from membrane fractions or tissues, solutions need to contain detergents. A mixture of protease inhibitors should be included in extraction buffers to minimize proteolysis of CSPG core proteins during the solu-bilization procedure. In this section, we describe three examples of proto-cols to extract CSPGs; brain secretory CSPGs, cartilage CSPGs, and brain membrane-bound CSPGs.

A. Extraction of Brain CSPGs with PBS Solution

We first describe a protocol to extract secretory CSPGs from rat brains with a PBS solution (Oohira et al., 1988). About 0.1 mg protein of a soluble CSPG mixture (= about 1 μmol uronic acid) is obtained from 10 brains (about 10 g wet weight) of a postnatal-day-10 rat.

1. Stock solutions
   a. 10× PBS: Store at room temperature.
   b. 0.2 M neutralized ethylenediaminetetraacetic acid (EDTA) as a metalloprotease inhibitor: dissolve EDTA with deionized water, neutralize with NaOH, and add deionized water to make 0.2 M EDTA. Store at room temperature.
   c. 0.2 M phenylmethylsulfonyl fluoride (PMSF)–1 M N-ethylma-leimide (NEM) as inhibitors for serine- and SH-proteases: dissolve PMSF and NEM with ethanol. Store at −20°C.
2. Chill a tight-fitting glass-Teflon homogenizer and tubes on ice.
3. Mix 5 ml of 10× PBS, 5 ml of 0.2 M neutralized EDTA, and 0.5 ml of 0.2 M PMSF–1 M NEM to make 50 ml of PBS–20 mM EDTA–10 mM NEM–2 mM PMSF (PBS-inhibitors).
4. Pour 40 ml of PBS-inhibitors into the homogenizer.

5. Homogenize 10 fresh or frozen brains of the postnatal-day-10 rat. If the frozen brain is too big and hard, cut with a blade before homogenization.
6. Pour the homogenate into tubes.
7. Wash the homogenizer with 10 ml of PBS-inhibitors, and combine with the homogenate.
8. Centrifuge at $27,000 \times g$ for 1 h at $4 \, ^\circ$C.
9. Transfer a supernatant to a new tube, and rehomogenize the pellet in 20 ml of PBS-inhibitors.
10. Centrifuge the second homogenate at $27,000 \times g$ for 1 h at $4 \, ^\circ$C.
11. Combine the first and second supernatants. Store at $-80 \, ^\circ$C.

B. Extraction of Cartilage CSPGs with 4 M Guanidine-HCl

Here, we describe a protocol to extract CSPGs from the cartilage with 4 M guanidine-HCl, a protein-denaturing reagent (Hascall and Kimura, 1982; Hascall *et al.*, 1994; Matsui *et al.*, 1989).

1. Stock solutions
   a. 1 M Tris-HCl, pH 7.5: Store at room temperature.
   b. 4 M guanidine-HCl–50 mM Tris-HCl, pH 7.5–20 mM EDTA (Guanidine-HCl–EDTA): Dissolve solid guanidine-HCl in ca.1/2 vol. of deionized water. Add 1/20 vol. of 1 M Tris-HCl, pH 7.5, 1/10 vol. of 0.2 M neutralized EDTA (Section IV.A), and then add deionized water to a guanidine HCl-concentration of 4 M. Store at $4 \, ^\circ$C.
   c. 1 M NEM–1 M 6-aminohexanoic acid–0.5 M benzamidine HCl–0.2 M PMSF (Inhibitor mixture): dissolve NEM, 6-amino-hexanoic acid, benzamidine HCl, and PMSF in methanol. Store at $-20 \, ^\circ$C.
2. Chill a glass homogenizer and tubes on ice.
3. Mix 4 ml of Guanidine-HCl–EDTA and 40 µl of inhibitor mixture (4 M guanidine-HCl solution). The mixed solution should be used immediately since most of the protease inhibitors are unstable in an aqueous solution.
4. Pour 2 ml of 4 M guanidine-HCl solution into the homogenizer.
5. Homogenize the newborn rat costal cartilage (about 100 mg wet weight). Cut the cartilage into small pieces before homogenization.
6. Pour the homogenate into a tube.
7. Wash the homogenizer with 2 ml of 4 M guanidine-HCl solution, and combine with the homogenate.
8. Stir gently with a magnetic bar for 24 h at $4 \, ^\circ$C.
9. Centrifuge at $27,000 \times g$ for 1 h at $4 \, ^\circ$C.

10. Transfer the supernatant to a tube, and add 2 ml of 4 M guanidine-HCl solution to the pellet.
11. Stir again for 24 h at 4°C.
12. Centrifuge at 27,000× g for 1 h at 4°C.
13. Combine the first and second supernatants. Store at −80°C.

C. Extraction of Membrane-Bound CSPGs

We explain here the methods to prepare brain membrane fractions and extract CSPGs from the membrane fraction (Nishiwaki *et al.*, 1998). About 8 mg protein of a membrane-bound CSPG mixture is obtained from 25 brains (about 20 g wet weight) of the postnatal-day-7 rat.

1. Stock solutions
   a. 10% 3-[(3-cholamidopropyl)dimethylammonio]propanesulfonic acid (CHAPS): dissolve 5 g of CHAPS in deionized water to make 50 ml of 10% CHAPS. Store at −20°C.
   b. 0.2 M neutralized EDTA (Section IV.A).
   c. 1 M Tris-HCl, pH 7.5 and 1 M NaCl: Store at room temperature.
   d. 1 M sucrose. Store at 4°C.
   e. 1 M NEM–0.1 M benzamidine HCl–1 µM pepstatin–1 µM leupeptin–10 mM PMSF (inhibitor-mixture): dissolve NEM, benzamidine HCl, pepstatin, leupeptin, and PMSF with methanol. Store at −20°C.
2. Working solutions
   a. 0.32 M sucrose solution: mix stock solutions to make 0.32 M sucrose–50 mM Tris-HCl, pH 7.5 containing 5 mM EDTA, 10 mM NEM, 1 mM benzamidine HCl, 10 µM pepstatin, 10 µM leupeptin, and 0.1 mM PMSF, and chill on ice.
   b. 0.1 M sucrose solution: mix stock solutions to make 0.1 M sucrose–50 mM Tris-HCl, pH 7.5 containing 5 mM EDTA, 10 mM NEM, 1 mM benzamidine HCl, 10 µM pepstatin, 10 µM leupeptin, and 0.1 mM PMSF.
   c. 0.1 M NaCl solution: mix stock solutions to make 0.1 M NaCl–50 mM Tris-HCl, pH 7.5 containing 5 mM EDTA, 10 mM NEM, 1 mM benzamidine HCl, 10 µM pepstatin, 10 µM leupeptin, and 0.1 mM PMSF.

The mixed solutions should be used immediately because most of the protease inhibitors are unstable in an aqueous solution.

3. Chill a glass-Teflon homogenizer and tubes on ice.
4. Pour 100–200 ml (5–10 vol. of wet weight) of 0.32 M sucrose solution into the homogenizer.
5. Remove brains from skulls and homogenize immediately.
6. Pour the homogenate into tubes.

7. Centrifuge at $1000 \times g$ for 10 min at $4 \,^{\circ}$C.
8. Transfer the supernatant to a tube, and rehomogenize the pellet using 40 ml of 0.32 M sucrose solution.
9. Pour the homogenate into a new tube.
10. Centrifuge at $1000 \times g$ for 10 min at $4 \,^{\circ}$C.
11. Combine the first and second supernatants.
12. Centrifuge at $100,000 \times g$ for 1 h at $2 \,^{\circ}$C.
13. Discard the supernatant.
14. Homogenize the pellet (membrane fraction P2/P3) (Rodriguez de Lores *et al.*, 1967) with 50 ml of 0.1 M sucrose solution.
15. Centrifuge at $100,000 \times g$ for 1 h at $2 \,^{\circ}$C.
16. Discard the supernatant.
17. Homogenize the pellet with 90 ml of 0.1 M NaCl solution.
18. Pour the homogenized pellet into a new tube.
19. Add 10 ml of 10% CHAPS.
20. Stir for 30 min on ice to solubilize CSPGs.
21. Centrifuge at $17,000 \times g$ for 1 h at $2 \,^{\circ}$C.
22. Subsequently subject the supernatant to purification steps for CSPGs, for example, a DEAE-Sephacel column chromatography.

The buffer of the final extract should be replaced depending on the subsequent purification processes. Several methods to exchange buffers have been utilized (e.g., dialysis and molecular sieve). Solubilization of CSPGs, after being precipitated from a buffer with ethanol (see the following section), in another buffer is sometimes a useful buffer-exchange method, especially for secretory CSPGs. However, it is usually very hard to dissolve crude membrane-bound proteins precipitated with ethanol even in a detergent-containing buffer. Therefore, ethanol precipitation should be avoided especially at early purification steps of membrane-bound CSPGs.

V. Isolation and Purification of CSPGs

We take advantage of distinct physicochemical properties of CS side chains to isolate and purify CSPGs. The highly polyanionic property of CS chains makes CSPGs bind more tightly to an anion exchanger, such as DEAE-Sephacel, in comparison to many other proteins. The CS chains also give CSPGs a high buoyant density and, therefore, give them a faster sedimentation rate in a CsCl equilibrium density gradient. In addition, if a CSPG bears a number of CS chains, the molecular weight of the whole molecule is extraordinarily large compared with those of average proteins. This property makes gel filtration a useful tool to separate large CSPGs from ordinary sized molecules. In contrast, we sometimes need more specified methods to purify small CSPGs with only a few short CS chains.

In such a case, immunoaffinity purification using antibodies specific to their core proteins is promising. In this section, several useful and, therefore, frequently used methods to isolate and purify CSPGs are described.

A. Anion-Exchange Chromatography

To isolate PGs from other proteins, anion-exchangers are useful tools. With a linear salt gradient usually from 0.15 to 1.0 M NaCl, PGs are separated into a lower-charged group and a higher-charged group in many cases (Fig. 1). In order to obtain a fine resolution and a good recovery of PGs, a buffer containing nonionic chaotropic reagents, such as urea, is preferable for anion-exchange column chromatography. If extraction is carried out with PBS, adding solid urea to the extract is sufficient. The following is an example using DEAE-Sephacel (Amersham Biosciences Corp., NJ, USA) as an anion-exchanger.

1. To a PBS extract, add 128 mg/ml of solid urea, 0.134 mg/ml of solid NEM, and 1 µl/ml of 0.2 M PMSF to make PBS–2 M urea–1 mM NEM–0.2 mM PMSF. If the PBS extract has been freshly prepared as described in Section IV.A , addition of the protease inhibitors is not needed.

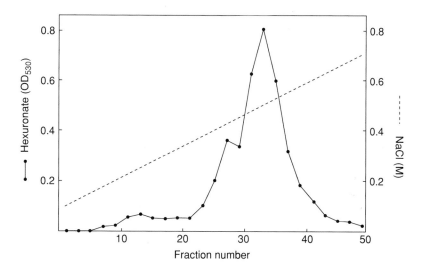

FIGURE I   An elution profile of PGs from a DEAE-Sephacel column. An extract of 26 adult rat brains (about 26 g wet weight) was chromatographed on a column (1.6 × 15 cm) of DEAE-Sephacel equilibrated with 2 M urea–50 mM Tris-HCl, pH 7.5 containing protease inhibitors. Proteoglycans were eluted with a linear gradient of NaCl from 0.1 to 0.7 M in 250 ml of the urea buffer. Fractions of 5 ml were collected. The amount of uronic acid was determined using an aliquot (250 µl) of each fraction as described in Section VI.D.

2. Stir with a magnetic stirrer for 1 h at 4°C.
3. Centrifuge at $27,000 \times g$ for 1 h at 4°C, and transfer the supernatant to tubes.
4. To the supernatant, add DEAE-Sephacel. For a solution derived from 1 g wet weight of the brain, 1.5–2 ml of DEAE-Sephacel is sufficient.
5. Stir gently with a magnetic stirrer for 2 h at 4°C.
6. Centrifuge at $4000 \times g$ for 10 min, and discard the supernatant.
7. Add 2 M urea–0.25 M NaCl–50 mM Tris-HCl, pH 7.5–2 mM EDTA–1 mM NEM–0.2 mM PMSF (urea–0.25 M NaCl) to the resin, and stir gently with a magnetic stirrer for 15–30 min at 4°C. Prepare urea solutions before use because urea breaks down into cyanide, which disrupts a particular peptide bond.
8. Centrifuge at $4000 \times g$ for 10 min, and discard the supernatant.
9. Add 5 vol. of urea–0.25 M NaCl, and pour the slurry to a column.
10. Wash the column with additional 5 vol. of urea–0.25 M NaCl.
11. Elute bound materials with 5 vol. of urea–0.7 M NaCl. Fractionate the eluate into 10–20 tubes.
12. Elute residual materials with 5 vol. of urea–2 M NaCl.
13. Monitor or measure OD_{280} of each fraction and collect peak fractions.
14. Concentrate the collected fractions with an adequate molecular sieve apparatus at 4°C.
15. Dialyze against PBS or 1 M guanidine-HCl–50 mM Tris-HCl, pH 7.5–2 mM EDTA–1 mM NEM–0.2 mM PMSF (1 M guanidine-HCl solution). Avoid leaving PGs for a long time in urea solutions. Purified PGs are stable in a PBS solution or in a 1 M guanidine-HCl solution and can be stored at −80°C.

B. CsCl Density Gradient Ultracentrifugation

Glycosaminoglycan (GAG) chains give PGs a high-buoyant density, and therefore, CsCl density gradient ultracentrifugation is useful to separate PGs from many other proteins. An adequate initial concentration of CsCl varies depending on the buoyant density of each PG. The following is an example of separating soluble CSPGs obtained from a rat brain (Fig. 2; Oohira *et al.*, 1988).

1. Add CsCl (0.55 g/ml) to the sample in 1 M guanidine-HCl solution (Section V.A), and invert several times to dissolve CsCl (an initial density = 1.38 g/ml).
2. Ultracentrifuge at $150,000 \times g$ for 40 h at 10°C.
3. Fractionate into six to eight fractions.
4. To examine the density of each fraction, weigh a small amount of sample (e.g., 30 µl) taken from each fraction.

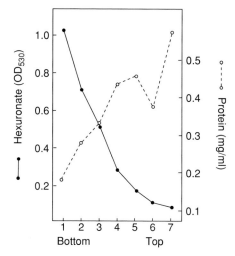

FIGURE 2 An example of ultracentrifugation of PGs in a CsCl density gradient. A PG mixture partially purified from 16 brains of the postnatal-day-10 rats by DEAE-Sephacel column chromatography was subjected to ultracentrifugation in a CsCl density gradient by the method described in Section V.B. After centrifugation, the sample (4.5 ml) was divided into seven fractions. The amounts of uronic acid and protein were determined using an aliquot (10 μl) of each fraction.

5. To the weighed samples, add 3 vol. of 95% ethanol containing 1.3% potassium acetate (95% ethanol–1.3% KOAc), and leave 1 h on ice (or overnight at 4°C).
6. Centrifuge at 10,000× g for 20 min at 4°C to precipitate PGs.
7. Dissolve the precipitate in the original volume of deionized water, add 3 vol. of 95% ethanol–1.3% KOAc, and leave 1 h on ice (or overnight at 4°C).
8. Centrifuge at 10,000× g for 20 min at 4°C to ensure salt removal and to precipitate proteins.
9. Determine uronic acid and protein amounts in the precipitates (for the determination of uronic acid, see Section VI.D).
10. Collect peak fractions.

C. Gel Filtration Column Chromatography

Gel filtration column chromatography is also used frequently to purify PGs. One should be aware that a PG is usually eluted as a very broad peak from a gel filtration column mainly due to the heterogeneity in the number and length of its GAG side chains.

There are various gel filtration media with a different fractionation range of molecular sizes, so it is essential to choose the media with the size range adequate for one's own sample. Figure 3 shows an example of separating PGs of fetal rat limb buds using a Sepharose CL-2B column. The PG sample (0.3 ml) labeled with [^{35}S]sulfate was chromatographed on a column (1.0 × 48 cm) of Sepharose CL-2B (Amersham Biosciences Corp.) equilibrated with 2 M guanidine HCl–50 mM Tris-HCl, pH 7.5 containing 0.4% nonanoyl-N-methyl-glucamide, 2 mM EDTA, 1 mM NEM, and 0.2 mM PMSF at a flow rate of 6 ml/h (Matsui *et al.*, 1989). To determine the void volume (V_0) and total volume (V_t), another sample containing 2% blue dextran (for V_0) and 30,000 cpm of Na$_2$[^{35}S]O$_4$ (for V_t) was chromatographed under the same conditions.

D. Hydrophobic Column Chromatography

PGs with hydrophobic domains including transmembrane PGs can be separated using hydrophobic interaction chromatography (Hascall *et al.*, 1994). A linear detergent gradient elutes molecules from hydrophobic resins according to their hydrophobicity. The following is an example of separating membrane-bound PGs of the young rat brain (Watanabe *et al.*, 1995). A PG sample dissolved in 10 ml of 4 M guanidine-HCl–50 mM Tris-HCl, pH 7.5 was applied to a column (1.6 × 5 cm) of Octyl-Sepharose (Amersham Biosciences Corp.). Elution was performed with a linear gradient of Nonidet P-40 from 0% to 0.8% (v/v) in 100 ml of the 4 M guanidine HCl–50 mM Tris-HCl, pH 7.5 at a flow rate of 10 ml/h. Peak fractions containing PGs were obtained at a detergent concentration from 0.3% to 0.6%.

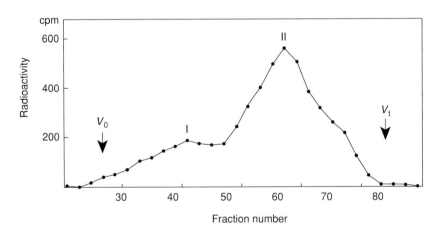

FIGURE 3   Sepharose CL-2B column chromatography of the ^{35}S-labeled materials in the PBS extract of the limb buds of embryonic day-13 fetal rats. Elution was performed under the conditions described in detail in Section V.C. Two broad peaks were obtained; peak I mainly contained CSPGs, and peak II mainly contained HSPGs. V_0, void volume; V_t, total volume.

E. Immunoaffinity Purification with Proteoglycan-Specific Antibodies

Affinity chromatography with a specific antibody is a useful tool to purify a particular PG. The disadvantage of this method is that only a small amount of the antigen is obtained. For example, using 2.1 mg of anti-neurocan antibody conjugated to 2 ml of Affi-Gel Hz gel (Bio-Rad Laboratories, Inc., CA, USA), 90 nmol uronic acid (= 9 μg protein) of neurocan was obtained after applying 800 nmol uronic acid of a brain CSPG mixture probably containing 400 nmol uronic acid (= 40 μg protein) of neurocan (Matsui *et al.*, 1994). This method is extremely efficacious when isolating a target PG from a mixture of PGs with similar physico-chemical parameters. Figure 4 shows an example of purifying neurocan, a nervous tissue CSPG, from a mixture of brain soluble CSPGs using an antibody-conjugated column.

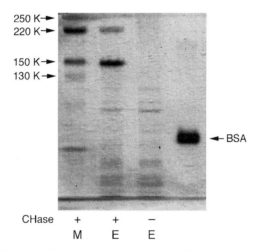

FIGURE 4   Purification of neurocan, a nervous-tissue CSPG, using an immunoadsorption column. A PBS-soluble CSPG mixture isolated from 10-day-old rat brains was applied to a column conjugated with a monoclonal anti-neurocan antibody 1G2 (MAb-1G2), and materials adsorbed to the column were eluted with 3 M KSCN–0.1% CHAPS as described previously (Matsui *et al.*, 1994). The original CSPG mixture (M) and the eluate (E) were separated by SDS-PAGE before (−) and after (+) chondroitinase ABC (CHase) digestion. The CSPG mixture contains phosphacan (another nervous-tissue CSPG; the molecular mass of its core glycoprotein is 250 K), neurocan (220 K), and two proteolytic fragments of neurocan (150 K and 130 K). Since MAb-1G2 recognizes the C-terminal half of neurocan, the eluate from the column contains both intact neurocan (220 K) and its C-terminal half fragment (150 K). Protein bands were stained with Coomassie brilliant blue R-250. BSA, bovine serum albumin.

VI. Structural Analyses of CSPGs _____

A. Analysis of Core Proteins

1. Removal of CS Chains from Core Proteins by CS Lyases

To prepare core proteins of PGs, GAG side chains are removed by digestion with GAG lyases in the presence of protease inhibitors. In this section, we describe a protocol to digest CS chains with protease-free chondroitinase ABC. Other GAG lyases are also needed to examine whether the PG also attaches other types of GAG such as heparan sulfate or keratan sulfate.

Chondroitinase ABC (EC 4.2.2.4, Seikagaku Kogyo Co., Tokyo) digests CS, dermatan sulfate, and hyaluronic acid. Although the presence of protease inhibitors in the enzymatic reaction mixture is necessary to block proteolytic degradation of core proteins, high concentrations of the inhibitors may disturb the chondroitinase ABC activity. In addition, a high concentration of ethanol also disturbs the enzyme activity. Therefore, if a sample is precipitated with ethanol, residual ethanol should be dried up before the enzymatic digestion. The following is an example of a reaction mixture for chondroitinase ABC.

CSPG (50 nmol uronic acid) in deionized water	43 μl
10× buffer (1 M Tris-HCl, pH 7.5–0.3 M sodium acetate)	5 μl
100× inhibitor mixture (20 mM PMSF–7.2 mM pepstatin–0.2 M NEM in ethanol)	0.5 μl
0.2 M neutralized EDTA (Section IV.A)	0.5 μl
Protease-free chondroitinase ABC (10 mU/μl)	1 μl

Stock solutions (the 10× buffer and the 100× inhibitor mixture) are stored at −20°C. The final reaction mixture contains 100 mM Tris-HCl, pH 7.5, 30 mM NaOAc, 0.2 mM PMSF, 0.072 mM pepstatin, 2 mM NEM, and 2 mM EDTA in addition to CSPGs and chondroitinase ABC. After the reaction mixture is incubated for 1 h at 37°C, the core protein is precipitated by adding 3 vol. (150 μl) of 95% ethanol–1.3% KOAc.

2. Removal of O- and N-Linked Oligosaccharide Chains by Various Glycosidases

Since many PGs bear O- and N-linked oligosaccharide chains as well as GAG chains, elimination of the oligosaccharides from a core protein is sometimes needed. Sequential digestion of a PG with various glycosidases provides information about the species of oligosaccharides attaching the core protein and about a molecular mass of the core protein without carbohydrate chains. An example of sequential digestion using neuraminidase, endo-β-galactosidase, O-glycosidase, and N-glycosidase F was described by Oohira et al. (1994).

3. SDS-PAGE and Western Blotting

As explained in Section V.C, heterogeneity in number and length of the GAG chains is characteristic of PGs, thus a PG is generally recovered as a very broad band or a smear, upon SDS-PAGE. The broad band is converted to a low molecular weight, narrow band representing the core protein by digestion with GAG lyases, and this property is utilized to confirm that the target molecule is actually a PG. Hydrophilicity is another characteristic of PGs mainly due to the high content of the carbohydrate moiety as described earlier. Therefore, PGs are not efficiently electrotransferred onto a hydrophobic transfer membrane such as a PVDF membrane or a nitrocellulose membrane. The conditions of the wet electrotransfer that we use for Western blot analyses of PGs are described later in this section. This and some other points to be considered are as follows:

a. In our experience, several brain CSPGs were efficiently transferred to those membranes with a Bio-Rad Minitransblot apparatus (Bio-Rad Laboratories) at 60 V overnight in 25 mM Tris, 192 mM glycine (pH 8.3), which contained 20% (v/v) methanol at 4 °C. It is likely that this condition may let small molecules pass through a membrane, and an optimized condition should be employed for each protein.

b. Many PG core proteins tend to migrate much slower upon SDS-PAGE than expectation from their molecular weights deduced from their amino acid sequence.

c. Various kits to amplify weak immunosignals on transfer membranes have been developed, for example, the Vectastain ABC Kit (Vector Lab., Burlingame, CA). Amplification of a signal developed with a naphtol-derivative reagent system (e.g., Immunostain HRP-1000; Konica Minolta Medical & Graphic, Inc., Tokyo, Japan) is also convenient because it does not require specific equipment. Chemiluminescence reagent systems are widely used because they are powerful methods to amplify weak immunosignals and because reprobing with different antibodies is possible. The problem is that amplification of weak signals sometimes brings a higher background of immunostaining. Lower antibody concentration or higher blocking buffer concentration could reduce the background. In addition, blocking of artificial protein binding to membrane with a skim milk (or nonfat dry milk) solution is not recommended to use in a biotin-avidin system because skim milk itself contains biotin.

d. Using biotinylated lectins and anticarbohydrate antibodies, such as an HNK-1 antibody, various oligosaccharides bound to core proteins can be detected. Combination of glycosidases, lectins, and anticarbohydrate antibodies may provide more information about the structure of oligosacchride chains (Shuo et al., 2004).

B. Analysis of CSPGs in Crude Samples

Many antibodies have been raised specific to core proteins of individual CSPGs. Using these antibodies, one can identify a particular PG and demonstrate the developmental or pathological change in the amount of a PG with Western blotting of tissue homogenates or extracts without purification of the PG. This analytical procedure consists of preparation of tissue homogenates or extracts, chondroitinase ABC-digestion of the crude samples, and Western blotting using antibodies specific to CSPG-core proteins. The following is an example to process the cerebrum for Western blotting to identify brain specific CSPGs in cerebral tissue homogenates.

1. Excise cerebral tissues on ice (about 150 mg wet weight).
2. Homogenize in 0.6 ml of ice-cold PBS containing 20 mM EDTA, 10 mM NEM, and 2 mM PMSF as protease inhibitors with a tight-fitting glass-Teflon homogenizer.
3. Mix an aliquot (50 μl) of the homogenate with 200 μl of 2% SDS–50 mM Tris-HCl, pH 7.5 containing the protease inhibitors.
4. Boil immediately for 5 min. The cerebral tissues can be solubilized completely by this method.
5. Determine the protein concentration using 1–3 μl of the solution.
6. Take two aliquots of the sample (~200 μg protein); one is to be treated with chondroitinase ABC, and the other is to be processed as a control without the enzyme.
7. Add 2–3 vol. of deionized water to dilute the SDS solution.
8. Add 95% ethanol–1.3% KOAc to precipitate proteins from the solution and to remove SDS as described in Section V.B.
10. Dry the precipitated proteins for 5 min to remove ethanol.
11. Digest with protease-free chondroitinase ABC as described in Section VI.A.1. It is very hard to dissolve the precipitate in the chondroitinase reaction buffer, especially in the case of tissue homogenate. Therefore, it is often necessary to smash the precipitate with a small spatula. Thus, the reaction mixture becomes opaque, and the mixture should be stirred with a Vortex mixer at 15–20 min intervals.
12. Stop the enzyme reaction, and precipitate proteins by adding 3 vol. of 95% ethanol–1.3% KOAc at 0°C.
13. Dissove the proteins with the SDS-PAGE sample buffer without dithiothreitol (DTT), and store it at −80°C until use.
14. For SDS-PAGE, mix an aliquot of the dissolved sample with the same volume of the sample buffer containing DTT (15 mg/ml) and boil it for 3 min.
15. Separate proteins with SDS-PAGE, and proceed to Western blot analysis.

C. Preparation of the CS Chains from a Purified CSPG

Various sensitive methods have been developed to analyze the structure of CS chains. Some of the updated methods are described in other chapters of this book. In this section, we describe methods to process purified (or isolated) CSPGs for structural analysis of the CS side chains.

To release CS chains from the core protein, treatment with a weak alkaline solution is commonly performed. The following is an example of alkaline treatment of CSPGs to prepare the CS side chains.

1. Dissolve CSPG(s) with deionized water.
2. Add 2 M NaOH solution to a final concentration of 0.1–0.5 M.
3. Mix and store at 4 °C for overnight.
4. Neutralize with 2 M HCl on ice.
5. Add 50% trichloroacetic acid to a final concentration of 5%, and leave on ice for 10 min to precipitate proteins. Avoid leaving a longer time in the acidic solution because trichloroacetic acid may break CS chains.
6. Centrifuge at 10,000× g for 20 min at 4 °C, transfer the supernatant to another tube on ice, and neutralize immediately with NaOH.
7. Precipitate CS chains from the neutralized supernatant by adding 3 vol. of 95% ethanol–1.3% KOAc.

To remove nucleic acids that are occasionally copurified with CSPGs, treatments with DNase and RNase are required. Samples precipitated with 95% ethanol–1.3% KOAc are dried up, dissolved with a buffer appropriate for each enzyme (refer to the manufacture's instruction for each enzyme), and incubated with deoxyribonuclease I (EC 3.1.4.5) or ribonuclease T1 (EC 3.1.27.3). Then, CS chains are precipitated from the reaction mixture by adding 3 vol. of 95% ethanol–1.3% KOAc.

D. Determination of the Amount of CS

The amount of CS is estimated by determination of the amount of uronic acid, a component of the CS disaccharides. Following is an example of a method for uronic acid determination reported originally by Bitter and Muir (1962).

1. Stock solutions
   a. Standard solution (10 μmol/ml glucuronolactone): dissolve 3.88 mg of D-glucuronic acid to 2 ml of 0.01 M NaOH, and boil for 5 min. Store at −20 °C.
   b. Borate solution: dissolve 2.6 g of sodium tetraborate ($Na_2B_4O_7 \cdot 10H_2O$) with 500 g of conc. H_2SO_4 (gr. 1.84) to make 0.025 M $Na_2B_4O_7$. Store at room temperature.

   c. Carbazole solution: dissolve 12.5 mg of carbazole with 10 ml of ethanol. Store at 4°C.
2. Precipitate CS from a sample solution as described in Section V.B to remove salts in the sample that may interfere the carbazole reaction.
3. Dissolve the precipitate (0–50 nmol of uronic acid) in 100 μl of deionized water on ice.
4. Add 0.5 ml of the borate solution, stir, and heat at 100°C for 10 min.
5. Chill on ice.
6. Add 20 μl of carbazole, stir, and heat at 100°C for 15 min.
7. Chill on ice to room temperature.
8. Measure the optical density at 530 nm in a cuvette with a path length of 10 mm.

A smaller amount of sample (e.g., 1–5 nmol uronic acid corresponding to about 0.5–2.5 μg of CS) can be measured with a smaller cuvette. In addition, dot-blot assays (Gaffen *et al.*, 1994; Jortikka *et al.*, 1993; Lammi and Tammi, 1988) and a direct dye-binding method (Thuy and Nyhan, 1992) have also been reported to estimate CS amounts. One can determine nanogram quantities (10–300 ng) of GAGs with these methods. One of these methods using Safranin O (Lammi and Tammi, 1988) is recommended by Hascall *et al.* (1994) as a method giving good sensitivity and low backgrounds.

E. Preparation of CSPGs for Functional Analyses

To determine a biological function of CSPGs, purified CSPGs are often used in culture systems or administered to animals. Before use, a CSPG solution may be concentrated with an adequate molecular sieve apparatus at 4°C. The solution containing CSPGs should be replaced with an atoxic and isotonic solution such as PBS by dialysis or molecular sieve apparatuses. After adjusting the CSPG concentration to an appropriate value, the sample is sterilized by filtration through a filter with a 0.22 μm pore size and is stored at −80°C.

VII. Conclusions _____

Purification of CSPGs is an essential step to determine the structure and function of CSPGs. The number, length, and extent of sulfation of CS side chains of an individual CSPG vary in general depending on the developmental or pathological stages of tissues from which the CSPG is isolated, and biological function of a CSPG is believed to be modulated by the modification or variation of its CS side chains. Although a CSPG can be expressed in mammalian cell lines by transfection of its core protein gene, the expressed CSPG does not always have CS side chains with structural parameters identical to those of the CSPG in animal tissues. Therefore, to reveal the exact function of a CSPG in the development, maintenance, or pathogenesis of a tissue, it is ideal to isolate the CSPG from the corresponding tissue and to apply it to an experimental system of the functional analyses.

In this chapter, we explained several typical methods to purify CSPGs with different principles; anionic charge, molecular size, buoyant density, and hydrophobicity. A successful purification of a target PG from tissues could be accomplished by the best combination of these methods. Immunoaffinity purification of a target PG using the antibody to its core protein is a potent method, especially when the source of the PG is very limited and small or contains PGs with physicochemical properties very similar to that of the target molecule. A number of works have been reported to purify a particular PG from various tissues with a combination of biochemical and immunochemical procedures, and many of them are introduced in a review by Hascall *et al.* (1994) and a book edited by Iozzo (2001). Readers may refer to these extensive works as well.

Acknowledgments

We thank all of our colleagues and collaborators who have contributed so much dedicated effort and thought to our work. Research conducted at the authors' laboratory was supported in part by Grants-in-Aid for Scientific Research from the Ministry of Education, Science, Culture, and Sports of Japan and from the Japan Society for the Promotion of Science.

References

Bitter, T., and Muir, H. M. (1962). A modified uronic acid carbazole reaction. *Anal. Biochem.* **4**, 330–334.

Fedarko, N. S. (2001). Purification of proteoglycan from mineralized tissues. *In* "Proteoglycan Protocols" (R. V. Iozzo, Ed.), Vol. 171, pp. 19–25. Humana Press, Totowa, NJ.

Gaffen, J. D., Price, F. M., Bayliss, M. T., and Mason, R. M. (1994). A ruthenium-103 red dot blot assay specific for nanogram quantities of sulfated glycosaminoglycans. *Anal. Biochem.* **218**, 124–130.

Hascall, V. C., and Kimura, J. H. (1982). Proteoglycans: Isolation and characterization. *Methods Enzymol.* **82**(Pt A), 769–800.

Hascall, V. C., Calabro, A., Midura, R. J., and Yanagishita, M. (1994). Isolation and characterization of proteoglycans. *Methods Enzymol.* **230**, 390–417.

Iozzo, R. V. (2001). "Proteoglycan Protocols." Humana Press, Totowa, NJ.

Jortikka, M., Lammi, M. J., Parkkinen, J. J., Lahtinen, R., and Tammi, M. I. (1993). A high sensitivity dot-blot assay for proteoglycans by cuprolinic blue precipitation. *Connect. Tissue Res.* **29**, 263–272.

Lammi, M., and Tammi, M. (1988). Densitometric assay of nanogram quantities of proteoglycans precipitated on nitrocellulose membrane with Safranin O. *Anal. Biochem.* **168**, 352–357.

Maeda, N., and Noda, M. (1998). Involvement of receptor-like protein tyrosine phosphatase ζ/RPTPβ and its ligand pleiotrophin/heparin-binding growth-associated molecule (HB-GAM) in neuronal migration. *J. Cell Biol.* **142**, 203–216.

Maeda, N., Nishiwaki, T., Shintani, T., Hamanaka, H., and Noda, M. (1996). 6B4 proteoglycan/phosphacan, an extracellular variant of receptor-like protein-tyrosine phosphatase ζ/RPTPβ, binds pleiotrophin/heparin-binding growth-associated molecule (HB-GAM). *J. Biol. Chem.* **271**, 21446–21452.

Matsui, F., Oohira, A., Shoji, R., and Nogami, H. (1989). Three distinct molecular species of proteoglycan synthesized by the rat limb bud at the prechondrogenic stage. *Arch. Biochem. Biophys.* **275**, 192–201.

Matsui, F., Watanabe, E., and Oohira, A. (1994). Immunological identification of two proteoglycan fragments derived from neurocan, a brain-specific chondroitin sulfate proteoglycan. *Neurochem. Int.* **25**, 425–431.

Milev, P., Chiba, A., Häring, M., Rauvala, H., Schachner, M., Ranscht, B., Margolis, R. K., and Margolis, R. U. (1998a). High affinity binding and overlapping localization of neurocan and phosphacan protein-tyrosine phosphatase-ζ/β with tenascin-R, amphoterin, and the heparin-binding growth-associated molecule. *J. Biol. Chem.* **273**, 6998–7005.

Milev, P., Monnerie, H., Popp, S., Margolis, R. K., and Margolis, R. U. (1998b). The core protein of the chondroitin sulfate proteoglycan phosphacan is a high-affinity ligand of fibroblast growth factor-2 and potentiates its mitogenic activity. *J. Biol. Chem.* **273**, 21439–21442.

Nishiwaki, T., Maeda, N., and Noda, M. (1998). Characterization and developmental regulation of proteoglycan-type protein tyrosine phosphatase ζ/RPTPβ isoforms. *J. Biochem. (Tokyo)* **123**, 458–467.

Oohira, A., Matsui, F., Matsuda, M., Takida, Y., and Kuboki, Y. (1988). Occurrence of three distinct molecular species of chondroitin sulfate proteoglycan in the developing rat brain. *J. Biol. Chem.* **263**, 10240–10246.

Oohira, A., Matsui, F., Watanabe, E., Kushima, Y., and Maeda, N. (1994). Developmentally regulated expression of a brain specific species of chondroitin sulfate proteoglycan, neurocan, identified with a monoclonal antibody 1G2 in the rat cerebrum. *Neuroscience* **60**, 145–157.

Rodriguez de Lores, A., Alberici, M., and De Robertis, E. (1967). Ultrastructural and enzymic studies of cholinergic and non-cholinergic synaptic membranes isolated from brain cortex. *J. Neurochem.* **14**, 215–225.

Shuo, T., Aono, S., Matsui, F., Tokita, Y., Maeda, H., Shimada, K., and Oohira, A. (2004). Developmental changes in the biochemical and immunological characters of the carbohydrate moiety of neuroglycan C, a brain-specific chondroitin sulfate proteoglycan. *Glycoconjugate J.* **20**, 267–278.

Thuy, L. P., and Nyhan, W. L. (1992). A new quantitative assay for glycosaminoglycans. *Clin. Chim. Acta* **212**, 17–26.

Watanabe, E., Maeda, N., Matsui, F., Kushima, Y., Noda, M., and Oohira, A. (1995). Neuroglycan C, a novel membrane-spanning chondroitin sulfate proteoglycan that is restricted to the brain. *J. Biol. Chem.* **270**, 26876–26882.

Luiz-Claudio F. Silva

Laboratório de Tecido Conjuntivo
Hospital Universitário Clementino Fraga Filho and
Instituto de Bioquímica Médica
Programa de Glicobiologia
Centro de Ciências da Saúde
Universidade Federal do Rio de Janeiro 21941–590
Rio de Janeiro, Brazil

Isolation and Purification of Chondroitin Sulfate

I. Chapter Overview

This short chapter focuses on current methods for the isolation and purification of chondroitin sulfate (CS). This molecule is a sulfated glycosaminoglycan (GAG) composed of a linear polysaccharide chain with repeating disaccharides of defined structures that usually contain one hexosamine and one hexuronic acid and a sulfate ester. The tissue CS can be extracted along with other GAG by proteolytic digestion. Once extracted, CS can be purified from other contaminant GAG by precipitation with organic solvents or enzymatic degradation of contaminant GAG species or also by column chromatography techniques. The most frequently assays for tracking CS isolation typically utilize uronic acid content as a marker.

Advances in Pharmacology, Volume 53
Copyright 2006, Elsevier Inc. All rights reserved.

1054-3589/06 $35.00
DOI: 10.1016/S1054-3589(05)53002-3

II. Introduction

This short chapter summarizes the methods for extraction and isolation of the sulfated GAG CS. Methods for isolation and characterization of other GAG species can be found elsewhere (Rodén *et al.*, 1972; Silva, 2002). Although a great number of methods are available for the isolation and purification of GAGs, there is no single set of procedures that permit single-step purification process, but different preparative approaches are required to purify a single species of GAG from tissue extracts. Thus, the techniques outlined later in this chapter can be used as guidelines for those researchers interested in the specific isolation of CS.

III. General Characteristics of CS

To discuss methods of CS isolation efficiently, a brief overview of CS structure needs to be given, since the various techniques take advantage of CS structure. CS consists of hexosamine (D-galactosamine) and hexuronic acid (D-glucuronic acid) units that are arranged in alternating unbranched sequence and carry sulfate substituents in various positions. The other sulfated GAG species are composed of dermatan sulfate (DS), heparan sulfate (HS), heparin, and keratan sulfate (Conrad, 1998; Coombe and Kett, 2005; Funderburgh, 2000; Nader *et al.*, 2004; Sugahara *et al.*, 2003; Trowbridge and Gallo, 2002). Hyaluronic acid (HA) is also a GAG species, but it is not sulfated (Toole, 2004). Owing to the variability in sulfate substitution, CS displays some sequence heterogeneity. However, the most common (and commercial) form of CS presents sulfated groups at position C-4 or C-6 of the hexosamine in the disaccharide unit [corresponding to chondroitin-4-sulfate (C4S) and chondroitin-6-sulfate (C6S), respectively]. CS with highly sulfated structures presenting different types of disulfated disaccharides has been described in marine organisms such as in squid cartilage (Kinoshita-Toyoda *et al.*, 2004) and shark skin (Nandini *et al.*, 2005). The general composition of the characteristic disaccharides for the most common types of CS is described in Table I.

In the tissue, CS is covalently bound to a protein core forming a structure known as proteoglycan (PG). Comprehensive reviews on the biochemistry and structure of PGs can be found elsewhere (Iozzo, 1998; Kresse and Schonnherr, 2001; Lindahl *et al.*, 1998; Prydz and Dalen, 2000). Information regarding PG isolation and purification can be found in three recent reviews (Fedarko, 1993; Hascall *et al.*, 1994; Savolainen, 1999).

Several glycobiology studies have suggested fundamental biological functions for CS. These molecules have intriguing functions in central nervous system, wound repair, as receptors for various pathogens, growth factor signaling, morphogenesis, and cell division (Sugahara *et al.*, 2003).

TABLE I   **Structural Features of CS from Different Sources**

| CS source | Disaccharide composition (%) | | | Reference |
	$^a\Delta di\text{-}0S^b$	$\Delta di\text{-}4S^c$	$\Delta di\text{-}6S^d$	
Beef trachea	10	57	33	Volpi (2004)
Chicken trachea	12	70	18	Volpi (2004)
Porcine trachea	4	80	16	Volpi (2004)
Human placenta	92	8	0	Muthusamy et al., 2004
Shark cartilage	4	14	82	Nadkarni et al., 1996

$^a\alpha\text{-}\Delta di$, $\alpha\text{-}\Delta^{4,5}$-unsaturated disaccharide.
$^b\alpha\text{-}\Delta diUA\text{-}1\rightarrow3\text{-}GalNAc$; UA, hexuronic acid; GalNAc, N-acetylated galactosamine.
$^c\alpha\text{-}\Delta UA\text{-}1\rightarrow3\text{-}GalNAc(4SO_4)$; UA, hexuronic acid; GalNAc, N-acetylated galactosamine bearing a sulfate ester at position 4.
$^d\alpha\text{-}\Delta UA\text{-}1\rightarrow3\text{-}GalNAc(6SO_4)$; UA, hexuronic acid; GalNAc, N-acetylated galactosamine bearing a sulfate ester at position 6.

In addition, CS has been suggested to be beneficial in the treatment of osteoarthritis (Hungerford and Jones, 2003; Uebelhart et al., 2004) by acting as a chondroprotector. Sim et al. (2005) have developed an interesting method for the quantitative analysis of CS in raw materials and CS-containing pharmaceutical preparations.

IV. Sources and Structure of Commercial Forms of CS _____

CS is an integral component of articular cartilage and is important to the physiology and mechanical properties of this tissue. The main source of commercial CS is cartilage from marine organisms. These CS preparations can be found with different grades of purity. Commercial C6S is prepared from shark cartilage, while C4S is obtained from whale cartilage. Alternatively, CS can be prepared from tissues obtained from land animals such as bovine or porcine.

V. General Preparative Procedures to Extract CS from Tissues

CS is often firmly associated with other tissue components. The procedure used for quantitative isolation of CS from a tissue involves the proteolytic digestion of proteins with nonspecific proteases. Solubilized CS can be further purified from other macromolecules present in the proteinase-digest by precipitation with ethanol or quaternary ammonium ions or adsorption on by ion-exchange resins. A few tissues contain only CS, and the isolation procedure may then be relatively simple, but the recovered CS is generally mixed with other GAG species, and further fractionation steps are necessary to the preparation of pure CS fractions. Different preparative approaches are performed to prepare CS such as organic solvents fractionation, ion-exchange chromatography, and degradation of single species of GAGs by highly specific enzymes followed by gel-permeation chromatography. General procedures for CS purification are illustrated in the Fig. 1. Because of the diversity of GAG contaminants in CS preparations, no single set of procedures will be suitable for the specific isolation of CS. Thus, the techniques outlined in a later section illustrate general principles that can be modified and used in different combination for preparation of this particular GAG.

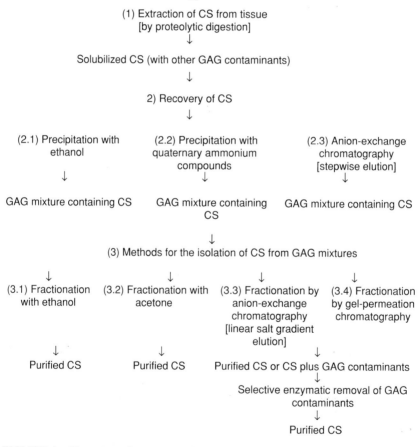

FIGURE I Illustration of some general procedures for isolation and purification of CS. These methods can be used with different combination to purify and fractionate CS obtained from tissues.

VI. Extraction from Tissues

The CS extraction procedure involves a preliminary treatment of tissues with organic solvents to remove as much lipid as possible. A common procedure is to extract the ground tissue with several changes of acetone at room temperature over a period of several days. After drying, the defatted powder is subjected to proteolytic digestion for the extraction of CS. Extraction by digestion with proteolytic enzymes is the most common procedure for releasing CS from tissues. Usually, extensive proteolysis with a protease of broad specificity is desirable, and treatment with papain or pronase yields single CS chains with only small residual peptide (the author has some preference for the use of papain, since this enzyme is generally very effective in achieving complete solubilization of various tissues). Details of digestion procedures can be found elsewhere (Medeiros *et al.*, 2000; Rocha *et al.*, 2000).

VII. Recovery of CS from Proteinase Extracts

After proteolysis, it is generally advantageous to remove low-molecular weight digestion products prior to purification of CS from GAG contaminants. This is accomplished by dialysis of the supernatant liquid (that contains the solubilized CS contaminated with other GAG species). Alternatively, the GAGs may be precipitated directly, usually with ethanol or a quaternary ammonium salt, or recovered by anion-exchange chromatography, as described in a later section.

A. Precipitation with Ethanol

Precipitation with ethanol is used as a simple means of recovering CS quantitatively from solutions. A sufficient concentration of salt is necessary for complete precipitation. This is seldom a problem with tissue digests that generally contain buffer salts. Any of the tissue GAGs will be precipitated completely by four to five volumes of ethanol, provided that the GAG concentration is high enough and sufficient salt is present. In the course of purification of crude proteolytic digests, however, it is preferable not to exceed about two volumes so as to avoid simultaneous precipitation of unwanted digestion products.

B. Precipitation with Quaternary Ammonium Compounds

Polyanions form water-insoluble salts with certain detergent cations such as cetylpyrydinium and cetyltrimethylammonium. The complexes are dissociated and dissolved by inorganic salts at high concentration. The quaternary ammonium compounds are used for the recovery of GAGs in bulk from tissue digests or other solutions. The low solubility of the complexes makes it possible to precipitate GAGs even from solutions as diluted as 0.01% or less (Rodén *et al.*, 1972). Cetylpyridinium complexes are converted to sodium salts by dissolving the precipitate in 2 M NaCl–ethanol (100:15, v/v), and the GAG is precipitated by addition of two volumes of ethanol (Cardoso and Mourão, 1994).

C. Ion-Exchange Chromatography

Because of the high-negative charge density of the GAGs, isolation based upon anion-exchange chromatography can be employed. The general techniques for ion-exchange chromatography are well known and need no further comment. A number of different ion-exchange materials are available, including Dowex 1-X2, ECTEOLA-cellulose, DEAE-cellulose, and DEAE-Sephacel. The author has some preference for the use of DEAE-cellulose or DEAE-Sephacel. GAGs elute from anion-exchange columns with high salt. A typical protocol involves the application of the proteinase-digest into an ion-exchange column equilibrated with a buffer solution. The column is washed with the same buffer and then eluted stepwise with 1.0 M NaCl in the same buffer. The GAGs eluted from the column are exhaustively dialyzed against distilled water, lyophilized, and dissolved in distilled water.

D. Comments

Several different criteria are generally applied to the evaluation of the purity of GAG preparations. The colorimetric carbazole–sulfuric acid assay as modified by Bitter and Muir (1962), which involves the reaction of unstable acid hydrolyzed dehydrated derivatives of hexuronic acid with carbazole, is frequently used to quantify the content of GAGs in solutions. This is a degradative assay, so aliquots from extractions and/or chromatographic separations are analyzed. Alternatively, assays that take advantage of metachromatic shifts upon binding of GAG to dyes, such as alcian blue (Gold, 1979), or 1,9-dimethylmethylene blue (Farndale *et al.*, 1986) can also be used. Electrophoresis is generally utilized for qualitative and quantitative analyses of mixtures of GAGs or single species. Cellulose acetate (Sunwoo *et al.*, 1998), polyacrylamide gel (Cavari and Vannucchi, 1996), and agarose gel (Medeiros *et al.*, 2000; Rocha *et al.*, 2000; Volpi, 1999) electrophoresis are routine in many laboratories.

If a sample contains nucleic acids, they may copurify with GAG fractions recovered by the above-mentioned procedures. These highly negative charged polymers containing sugar may interfere on colorimetric assays for the detection of GAGs. In addition, they will comigrate with GAGs on agarose gel electrophoresis, interfering on the step of staining of GAGs by toluidine blue. These compounds usually show an intense blue color under the staining conditions that overlaps the purple staining (metachromasia) of GAGs in this system. Therefore, if necessary, enzyme digestion (e.g., DNAse) may be required to remove these compounds (Rocha *et al.*, 2000).

VIII. Fractionation Methods

Several procedures can be used to isolate CS from other GAG species present in a mixture after tissue extraction, such as sequential precipitation with organic solvents, fractionation by using anion-exchange chromatography, and degradation of single species of GAGs by highly specific enzymes followed by gel-permeation chromatography, as described in a later section.

A. Ethanol Fractionation

Fractional precipitation with ethanol is one of the classical methods for the separation of GAG mixtures. In favorable situations, the method can be applied directly to a tissue digest. Fractionation with ethanol is most successfully carried out in the presence of divalent metal ions such as calcium, barium, or zinc. Briefly, NaCl (2%) is added to the mixture, and the GAGs are fractionated by increasing volumes of ethanol (from 0.1 to 2.0 volumes). For each 0.1 volume of ethanol, the mixture is allowed to equilibrate at 4°C for 24 h. Afterward, the precipitate is collected by centrifugation and dried. Another 0.1 volume of ethanol is added to the supernatants, and the procedure is repeated up to a maximum of 2.0 volumes of ethanol.

In an article, Volpi (1996) has reported the fractionation of mixtures of GAGs by sequential precipitation in the presence of methanol, ethanol, or propanol. The same behavior was obtained with the three different solvents. In particular, heparin was the first GAG species to precipitate, followed by DS and lastly by CS. It was also noted that as the hydrophobic chains of the solvents increase (from methyl to propyl), there was a greater capacity to precipitate GAGs with lower amounts of solvent.

B. Fractionation with Acetone

Fractionation of a GAG mixture by acetone at different percentages, as reported by Volpi (1994), is a rapid and useful method for purifying a single species of GAG. In addition, bivalent cations are not required, and this permits a further purification without further need for cation-exchange resins to remove contaminant ions. At low percentage of acetone, heparin is the first GAG precipitated. DS is precipitated by acetone over a narrow range (0.6–0.7 volumes). CS is the most soluble GAG in mixed acetone/water.

C. Fractionation by Anion-Exchange Chromatography

Different GAGs differ in their average negative charge density, which allows purification based upon anion-exchange chromatography. The stepwise ion-exchange process, described earlier (Section VII.C), normally achieves a reasonably high level of purification of GAGs from other types of macromolecules. However, a second ion-exchange step with a continuous salt gradient often achieves better purity and can separate different classes of GAGs. In anion-exchange chromatography, the most common resin employed is a diethylaminoethyl (DEAE) resin, and a NaCl salt gradient is used to elute bound GAGs. Residual glycoproteins, which elute from DEAE-cellulose columns in low salt, are completely separated from GAGs, which elute with high salt. GAGs with different charge densities can resolve, at least particularly, into separated peaks, as often occurs when both HS and CS/DS GAGs are present. However, the different types of GAGs may be difficult to separate by this method, even with quite shallow gradients. Thus, additional approaches may be required such as the removal of a specific species of GAG by enzymatic digestion with commercially available enzymes that can degrade one or more classes of GAG. We have used such approach to obtain CS chains that were isolated from thymic epithelial cells and could not be separated from HS chains by anion-exchange chromatography. Thus, enzymatic degradation of HS by the action of HS lyases allowed the isolation of pure CS chains to structural characterization (Werneck *et al.*, 2000). Many different types of ion exchangers are now available in fast performance liquid chromatography (FPLC), which can offer advantages in analysis time, capacity recoveries, and separation properties.

D. Gel-Permeation Chromatography

Molecular sieve chromatography can also be employed to separate and purify single species of GAG from mixtures. The choice of support matrix, porosity, and elution solvents depends on the properties of the particular GAGs being studied. HA, which has the highest molecular mass among the different types of GAGs, is easily separated from the other classes of GAGs by this method (Martins *et al.*, 2003). However, generally the fractionation among the different sulfated GAG classes may be more difficult, as often occur when CS and DS, that have similar size, are present (Martins *et al.*, 2003). Thus, additional approaches may be required such as the removal of a specific species of GAG by enzymatic digestion with commercially available enzymes that can degrade one or more classes of GAG. When dealing with CS/DS mixture the researcher can use an approach in which DS chains present in the mixture are degraded by the action of chondroitinase B, an enzyme that specific degrades this type of GAG, allowing the isolation of pure CS fractions, which can be separated from DS degradative products and recovered by gel filtration chromatography (Theocharis *et al.*, 2001).

IX. Conclusions

Current analytical techniques allow the isolation of CS in sufficient quantity and purity for their chemical analysis. The identification and primary structure determination of CS have significantly contributed to elucidate its possible function on mechanisms modulating cell–cell and cell–matrix interactions.

Acknowledgments

Work in the author's laboratory was supported by grants from Conselho Nacional de Desenvolvimento Científico e Tecnológico (CNPq: PADCT and PRONEX) and Fundação de Amparo à Pesquisa do Estado do Rio de Janeiro (FAPERJ).

References

Bitter, T., and Muir, H. M. (1962). A modified uronic acid carbazole reaction. *Anal. Biochem.* **4**, 330–334.

Cardoso, L. E. M., and Mourão, P. A. S. (1994). Glycosaminoglycan fractions from human arteries presenting diverse susceptibilities to atherosclerosis have different affinities to plasma LDL. *Arterioscler. Thromb.* **14**, 115–124.

Cavari, S., and Vannucchi, S. (1996). Detection of heparin-like glycosaminoglycans in normal human plasma by polyacrylamide-gel electrophoresis. *Clin. Chim. Acta* **252**, 159–170.

Conrad, H. E. (1998). "Heparin-binding proteins." Academic Press, San Diego.

Coombe, D. R., and Kett, W. C. (2005). Heparan sulfate-protein interactions: Therapeutic potential through structure-function insights. *Cell. Mol. Life Sci.* **62**, 410–424.

Farndale, R. W., Buttle, D. J., and Barret, A. J. (1986). Improved quantitation and discrimination of sulfated glycosaminoglycans by use of dimethylmethylene blue. *Biochim. Biophys. Acta* **883**, 173–177.

Fedarko, N. S. (1993). Isolation and purification of proteoglycans. *Experientia* **49**, 369–383.

Funderburgh, J. L. (2000). Keratan sulfate: Structure, biosynthesis, and function. *Glycobiology* **10**, 951–958.

Gold, E. W. (1979). A simple spectrophotometric method for estimating glycosaminoglycan concentrations. *Anal. Biochem.* **99**, 183–188.

Hascall, V. C., Calabro, A., Midura, R. J., and Yanagishita, M. (1994). Isolation and characterization of proteoglycans. *Methods Enzymol.* **230**, 390–417.

Hungerford, D. S., and Jones, L. C. (2003). Glucosamine and chondroitin sulfate are effective in the management of osteoarthritis. *J. Arthroplasty* **18**, 5–9.

Iozzo, R. V. (1998). Matrix proteoglycans: From molecular design to cellular functions. *Annu. Rev. Biochem.* **67**, 609–652.

Kinoshita-Toyoda, A., Yamada, S., Haslam, S. M., Khoo, K. H., Sugiura, M., Morris, H. R., Dell, A., and Sugahara, K. (2004). Structural determination of five tetrasaccharides containing 3-O-sulfated D-glucuronic acid and two rare oligosaccharides containing a β-D-glucose branch isolated from squid cartilage chondroitin sulfate E. *Biochemistry* **43**, 11063–11074.

Kresse, H., and Schonnherr, E. (2001). Proteoglycans of the extracellular matrix and growth control. *J. Cell. Physiol.* **189**, 266–274.

Lindahl, U., Kusche-Gullberg, M., and Kjellén, L. (1998). Regulated diversity of heparan sulfate. *J. Biol. Chem.* **273**, 24979–24982.

Martins, R. C. L., Werneck, C. C., Rocha, L. A. G., Feres-Filho, E. J., and Silva, L. C. F. (2003). Molecular size distribution analysis of human gingival glycosaminoglycans in cyclosporin- and nifedipine-induced overgrowths. *J. Periodont. Res.* **38**, 182–189.

Medeiros, G. F., Mendes, A., Castro, R. A. B., Baú, E. C., Nader, H. B., and Dietrich, C. P. (2000). Distribution of sulfated glycosaminoglycans in the animal kingdom: Widespread occurrence of heparin-like compounds in invertebrates. *Biochim. Byophys. Acta* **1475**, 287–294.

Muthusamy, A., Archur, R. N., Valiyaveettil, M., and Gowda, D. C. (2004). *Plasmodium falciparum*: Adherence of the parasite-infected erythrocytes to chondroitin sulfate proteoglycans bearing structurally distinc chondroitin sulfate chains. *Exp. Parasitol.* **107**, 183–188.

Nader, H. B., Lopes, C. C., Rocha, H. A. O., Santos, E. A., and Dietrich, C. P. (2004). Heparins and heparinoids: Occurrence, structure and mechanism of antithrombotic and hemorrhagic activities. *Curr. Pharm. Des.* **10**, 951–966.

Nadkarni, V. D., Toida, T., Van Gorp, C. L., Schubert, R. L., Weiler, J. M., Hansen, K. P., Caldwell, E. E. O., and Linhardt, R. J. (1996). Preparation and biological activity of N-sulfonated chondroitin sulfate and dermatan sulfate derivatives. *Carbohyd. Res.* **290**, 87–96.

Nandini, C. D., Itoh, N., and Sugahara, K. (2005). Novel 70 kDa chondroitin sulfate/dermatan sulfate hybrid chains with a unique heterogeneous sulfation pattern from shark skin, which exhibit neuritogenic activity and binding activities for growth factors and neurothrophic factors. *J. Biol. Chem.* **280**, 4058–4069.

Prydz, K., and Dalen, K. T. (2000). Synthesis and sorting of proteoglycans. *J. Cell Sci.* **113**, 193–205.

Rocha, L. A. G., Martins, R. C. L., Werneck, C. C., Feres-Filho, E. J., and Silva, L. C. F. (2000). Human gingival glycosaminoglycans in cyclosporin-induced overgrowth. *J. Periodont. Res.* **35**, 158–164.

Rodén, L., Baker, J. R., Cifonelli, J. A., and Mathews, M. B. (1972). Isolation and characterization of connective tissue polysaccharides. *Methods Enzymol.* **28**, 73–140.

Savolainen, H. (1999). Isolation and separation of proteoglycans. *J. Chromatogr. B* **722**, 255–262.

Silva, L. C. F. (2002). Isolation and purification of glycosaminoglycans. In "Analytical Techniques to Evaluate the Structure and Functions of Natural Polysaccharides, Glycosaminoglycans" (N. Volpi, Ed.), pp. 1–14. Research Signpost, Trivandrum.

Sim, J. S., Jun, G., Toida, T., Cho, S. Y., Choi, D. W., Chang, S. Y., Linhardt, R. J., and Kim, Y. S. (2005). Quantitative analysis of chondroitin sulfate in raw materials, ophtalmic solutions, soft capsules and liquid preparations. *J. Chromatogr. B* **818**, 133–139.

Sugahara, K., Mikami, T., Uyama, T., Mizuguchi, S., Nomura, K., and Kitagawa, H. (2003). Recent advances in the structural biology of chondroitin sulfate and dermatan sulfated. *Curr. Opin. Struc. Biol.* **13**, 612–620.

Sunwoo, H. H., Nakano, T., Hudson, R. J., and Sim, J. S. (1998). Isolation, characterization and localization of glycosaminoglycans in growing antlers of wapiti (*Cervus elaphus*). *Comp. Biochem. Physiol. B* **120**, 273–283.

Theocharis, D. A., Papageorgecopoulou, N., Vynios, D. H., Anagnostides, S. Th., and Tsiganos, C. P. (2001). Determination and structural characterisation of dermatan sulfate in the presence of other galactosaminoglycans. *J. Chromatogr. B* **754**, 297–309.

Toole, B. P. (2004). Hyaluronan: From extracellular glue to pericellular cue. *Nat. Rev. Cancer* **4**, 528–539.

Trowbridge, J. M., and Gallo, R. L. (2002). Dermatan sulfate: New functions from an old glycosaminoglycan. *Glycobiology* **12**, 117R–125R.

Uebelhart, D., Malaise, M., Marcolongo, R., DeVathaire, F., Piperno, M., Mailleux, E., Fioravanti, A., Matoso, L., and Vignon, E. (2004). Intermittent treatment of knee osteoarthritis with oral chondroitin sulfate: A one-year, randomized, double-blind, multicenter study versus placebo. *Osteoarthritis Cartilage* **12**, 269–276.

Volpi, N. (1994). Fractionation of heparin, dermatan sulfate, and chondroitin sulfate by sequential precipitation: A method to purify a single glycosaminoglycan species from a mixture. *Anal. Biochem.* **218**, 382–391.

Volpi, N. (1996). Purification of heparin, dermatan sulfate and chondroitin sulfate from mixtures by sequential precipitation with various organic solvents. *J. Chromatogr. B* **685**, 27–34.

Volpi, N. (1999). Disaccharide analysis and molecular mass determination to microgram level of single sulfated glycosaminoglycan species in mixtures following agarose-gel electophoresis. *Anal. Biochem.* **273**, 229–239.

Volpi, N. (2004). Disaccharide mapping of chondroitin sulfate of different origins by high-performance capillary electrophoresis and high-performance liquid chromatography. *Carbohyd. Polym.* **55**, 273–281.

Werneck, C. C., Oliveira-dos-Santos, A. J., Silva, L. C. F., Villa-Verde, D. M. S., Savino, W., and Mourão, P. A. S. (2000). Is there a glycosaminoglycan-related heterogeneity of the thymic epithelium? *J. Cell. Physiol.* **185**, 68–79.

Fotini N. Lamari* and Nikos K. Karamanos[†]

*Laboratory of Pharmacognosy and
Chemistry of Natural Products
Department of Pharmacy
University of Patras
26500 Patras, Greece

[†]Laboratory of Biochemistry
Department of Chemistry
University of Patras
26500 Patras, Greece

Structure of Chondroitin Sulfate

I. Chapter Overview

Chondroitin sulfate (CS) is an anionic linear polysaccharide, which is synthesized as part of proteoglycan (PG) molecules in vertebrates and invertebrates. Chondroitin sulfate consists of alternating disaccharide units of glucuronic acid and galactosamine and is attached to serine (Ser) residues of the protein cores via a tetrasaccharide linkage. Despite the simplicity of the backbone structure, the CS molecule is complex enough to carry biologic information and thus determine many biologic functions. A highly modified CS chain at least at the level of uronic acid is called dermatan sulfate (DS). Complexity of CS/DS is brought about by structural features, such as sulfonylation at hydroxyl groups of galactosamine and glucuronic acid residues, epimerization of certain glucuronic residues to iduronic acid, and distribution of these uronic acid residues through the polymeric chain. This chapter presents the up-to-date information on the structure of CS and DS.

Advances in Pharmacology, Volume 53
1054-3589/06 $35.00
DOI: 10.1016/S1054-3589(05)53003-5

II. Introduction ————————————————————————

A. Chondroitin Sulfate: Basic Structure and Isomeric Forms

Chondroitin sulfate is a glycosaminoglycan (GAG) covalently linked to proteins forming PGs. GAGs are all anionic linear heteropolysaccharide chains of repeating disaccharide units. According to the monosaccharide types and the glycosidic bonds between them, GAGs are divided into: (1) hyaluronan, (2) CS and DS, (3) heparan sulfate (HS) and heparin, and (4) keratan sulfate. CS had been isolated from cartilage in 1884, but the nature of its monosaccharides and structure were first described by P. Levene in 1925; Levene showed that the constituents were D-glucuronic acid (GlcA), D-galactosamine (GalN), and acetic and sulfuric acid in equimolar ratios (Roseman, 2001). The correct structure for CS was shown later; CS is composed of the repeating unit [→4GlcAβ1→3GalNAcβ1→], which in mammals is commonly sulfated at the C-4 and/or C-6 of N-acetyl-D-galactosamine (GalNAc).

The term CS-A has been used to describe CS rich in [GlcA-GalNAc(4S)] (A unit) and CS-C, CS rich in [GlcA-GalNAc(6S)] (C unit) (Fig. 1). The DS chain (formerly known as CS-B) has a hybrid copolymeric structure consisting of low modified (CS) and highly modified (DS) domains (Fransson *et al.*, 1990). The modifications involve C-5 epimerization of GlcA to L-iduronic acid (IdoA) and O-sulfation at C-4 and C-6 of GalNAc and C-2 of IdoA. IdoA imparts conformational flexibility to DS and alters the shape and spatial orientation of sulfate residues, endowing the chain with higher negative charge content than GlcA (Casu *et al.*, 1998). The content of IdoA ranges from 0% in CS to 80–90% in various DS chains; the highest percentages have been observed in skin PGs (Choi *et al.*, 1989; Karamanos *et al.*, 1995). The disulfated disaccharide D [GlcA(2S)-GalNAc (6S)] and E [GlcA-GalNAc(4S, 6S)] units are characteristic components in shark cartilage CS-D (∼20%) and squid cartilage CS-E (∼60%), respectively, but are also found in DS chains from mammalian sources (Table I) (Sugahara and Yamada, 2000; Suzuki *et al.*, 1968). The oversulfated CS-H, isolated from the hagfish notochord, contains a high proportion (68%) of the disaccharide H (or iE) unit [IdoA-GalNAc(4S, 6S)], which is also found in other DS chains (Anno *et al.*, 1971; Sugahara and Yamada, 2000; Ueoka *et al.*, 1999).

3-O-sulfation of GlcA is a noncommon structural modification, which has been identified in polysaccharides from marine invertebrate sources (Section IV.B), leading to some rare disaccharide units such as the K, L, and M units (Fig. 1). The only occurrence of 3-O-sulfation of IdoA has been reported for DS from the skin of *Anguilla japonica* (Sakai *et al.*, 2003); these authors also show the existence of IdoA(2S, 3S) residues, which was earlier shown for DS from skin of *Raja clavata* (Chatziioannidis *et al.*, 1999).

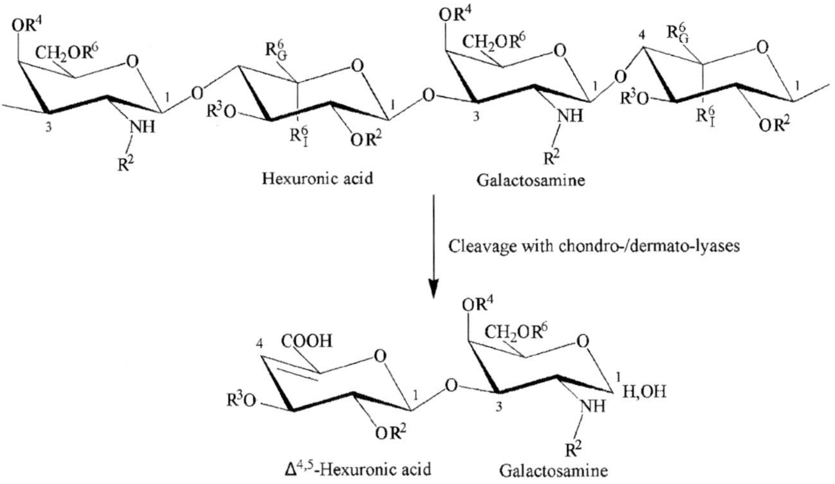

$\Delta^{4,5}$-Hexuronic acid   Galactosamine

No	Name	Other names	Hexuronic acid				Galactosamine		
			R^2	R^3	R_G^6	R_I^6	R^2	R^4	R^6
1	ΔDi-nonS$_{GlcA}$	ΔDi-0S$_{CS}$	H	H	COOH	H	Ac	H	H
2	ΔDi-nonS$_{IdoA}$		H	H	H	COOH	Ac	H	H
3	ΔDi-mono4S$_{GlcA}$	ΔDi-4S/ A unit	H	H	COOH	H	Ac	SO$_3$H	H
4	ΔDi-mono4S$_{IdoA}$		H	H	H	COOH	Ac	SO$_3$H	H
5	ΔDi-mono6S$_{GlcA}$	ΔDi-6S/ C unit	H	H	COOH	H	Ac	H	SO$_3$H
6	ΔDi-mono6S$_{IdoA}$		H	H	H	COOH	Ac	H	SO$_3$H
7	ΔDi-mono2S$_{GlcA}$		SO$_3$H	H	COOH	H	Ac	H	H
8	ΔDi-mono2S$_{IdoA}$		SO$_3$H	H	H	COOH	Ac	H	H
9	ΔDi-mono3S$_{GlcA}$		H	SO$_3$H	COOH	H	Ac	H	H
10	ΔDi-mono3S$_{IdoA}$		H	SO$_3$H	H	COOH	Ac	H	H
11	ΔDi-monoNS$_{IdoA}$		H	H	H	COOH	SO$_3$H	H	H
12	ΔDi-di(2,6)S$_{GlcA}$	ΔDi-diS$_D$/ D unit	SO$_3$H	H	COOH	H	Ac	H	SO$_3$H
13	ΔDi-di(2,6)S$_{IdoA}$		SO$_3$H	H	H	COOH	Ac	H	SO$_3$H
14	ΔDi-di(2,4)S$_{GlcA}$		SO$_3$H	H	COOH	H	Ac	SO$_3$H	H
15	ΔDi-di(2,4)S$_{IdoA}$	ΔDi-diS$_B$ / B unit	SO$_3$H	H	H	COOH	Ac	SO$_3$H	H
16	ΔDi-di(4,6)S$_{GlcA}$	ΔDi-diS$_E$ / E unit	H	H	COOH	H	Ac	SO$_3$H	SO$_3$H
17	ΔDi-di(4,6)S$_{IdoA}$	ΔDi-diS$_H$ / iE unit	H	H	H	COOH	Ac	SO$_3$H	SO$_3$H
18	ΔDi-di(3,6)S$_{GlcA}$	ΔDi-diS$_L$ / L unit	H	SO$_3$H	COOH	H	Ac	H	SO$_3$H
19	ΔDi-di(2,3)S$_{IdoA}$		SO$_3$H	SO$_3$H	H	COOH	Ac	H	H
20	ΔDi-di(3,4)S$_{GlcA}$	ΔDi-diS$_K$ / K unit	H	SO$_3$H	COOH	H	Ac	SO$_3$H	H
21	ΔDi-di(2,N)S$_{IdoA}$		SO$_3$H	H	H	COOH	SO$_3$H	H	H
22	ΔDi-tri(2,4,6)S$_{GlcA}$	ΔDi-triS	SO$_3$H	H	COOH	H	Ac	SO$_3$H	SO$_3$H
23	ΔDi-tri(2,4,6)S$_{IdoA}$	ΔDi-triS$_{IT}$ / iT unit	SO$_3$H	H	H	COOH	Ac	SO$_3$H	SO$_3$H
24	ΔDi-tri(3,4,6)S$_{GlcA}$	ΔDi-triS$_M$ / M unit	H	SO$_3$H	COOH	H	Ac	SO$_3$H	SO$_3$H
25	ΔDi-tri(2,6,N)S$_{IdoA}$		SO$_3$H	H	H	COOH	SO$_3$H	H	SO$_3$H

FIGURE I Structures of Δ-disaccharides derived from CS/DS by chondroitinase digestions and their common names. Subscripts G and I show the GlcA and IdoA origins of Δ-disaccharide, respectively. The IdoA- or GlcA-derived disaccharides obtain the same structure at C-5 after digestion with chondro-/dermatolyases. The commonest disaccharides are those in bold. The others have been determined only in CS/DS chains from marine invertebrates. Adapted from Karamanos *et al.* (1994a).

TABLE I   Composition of Disaccharides (% of Total) of Galactosaminoglycans from Various Mammals as Determined by Karamanos et al. (1994a)

Type of disaccharide	Whale cartilage CS-A	Porcine rib cartilage CS-A	Porcine skin CS-B
ΔDi-nonS$_{GlcA}$	9.0	3.8	0.4
ΔDi-nonS$_{IdoA}$	–	–	1.6
ΔDi-mono4S$_{GlcA}$	64.8	35.2	2.4
ΔDi-mono4S$_{IdoA}$	–	43.4	69.0
ΔDi-mono6S$_{GlcA}$	18.4	11.4	1.0
ΔDi-mono6S$_{IdoA}$	–	–	–
ΔDi-di(2,6)S$_{GlcA}$	4.9	3.5	–
ΔDi-di(2,6)S$_{IdoA}$	–	–	1.5
ΔDi-di(2,4)S$_{GlcA}$	–	0.8	–
ΔDi-di(2,4)S$_{IdoA}$	–	–	24.1
ΔDi-di(4,6)S$_{GlcA}$	3.9	1.1	–
ΔDi-tri(2,4, 6)S	–	0.8	–

N-sulfonylation of GalN is a unique feature, which has only been reported for DS from sea urchin shell (Manouras *et al.*, 1991). According to the extent of modifications, 25 different non-, mono-, di-, and trisulfated galactosaminoglycan (GalAG) disaccharides have been described (Chatziioannidis *et al.*, 1999; Karamanos *et al.*, 1994a; Sakai *et al.*, 2003). The structures and common names of these 25 GalAG disaccharides are shown in Fig. 1. With the exception of oversulfated CS/DS from marine organisms, non-, di-, and trisulfated disaccharides are generally minor components of CS molecules, and the great majority are monosulfated units. Completely nonsulfated chondroitin chains have only been found in squid skin, *Caenorhabditis elegans*, and some bacteria (Karamanos *et al.*, 1988, 1990; Yamada *et al.*, 2002).

B. Biosynthesis, Localization, and Function of CS

GalAGs are present as part of PGs in intracellular granules of certain cells (i.e., mast cells in mammals), at the cell membrane and the extracellular matrix (ECM) of invertebrate and vertebrate organisms. In a thorough study of the distribution of sulfated mucopolysaccharides, it has been showed that GAGs are present in life forms that exhibit some cell organization (Cassaro and Dietrich, 1977). Interestingly, some bacterial strains (*Escherichia coli* K4 and *Pasteurella multosida*) produce extracellular chondroitin chains with no sulfation or epimerization, which are not covalently linked to protein cores and seem to enhance the ability of bacteria to infect or colonize the host (De Angelis, 2002).

The function of GalAGs is closely related to their localization; GalAGs in matrix contribute to the organization of the ECM and tissues, and GalAGs at the cell membrane usually function as receptors/coreceptors and participate in several structure-specific interactions regulating a wide range of cellular events (Trowbridge and Gallo, 2002). Generally, these interactions depend on specific oligomeric GAG domains; that is, sequences of five to eight monosaccharides. For instance, CS binding to type V collagen is mediated via oligosaccharides of at least eight monosaccharides, which contain a continuous sequence of three GlcA-GalNAc(4S, 6S) units (Takagaki *et al.*, 2002). However, studies in *C. elegans* have shown that even nonsulfated chondroitin is required for embryonic cytokinesis and cell division (Mizuguchi *et al.*, 2003).

CS chains are composed of the linkage region to the proteins (reducing end), the main chain composed of repeating disaccharides and the nonreducing terminal (Fig. 2A). The linkage region for CS/DS is synthesized on the core proteins by enzymes in the endoplasmic reticulum and Golgi apparatus. Chain elongation occurs by sequential transfer of the appropriate UDP-monosaccharides to the nonreducing terminal of the growing nascent PG acceptor (Prydz and Dalen, 2000; Silbert and Sugumaran, 2002). Addition of sulfate groups from 3′-phosphoadenosine 5′-phosphosulfate to the

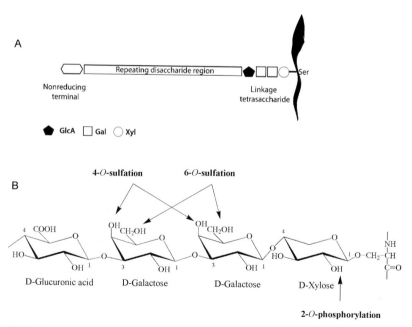

FIGURE 2   (A) CS chains are linear heteropolysaccharides of repeating disaccharide units, which are attached to the protein core of a PG through a linkage tetrasaccharide at the reducing end. At the nonreducing end, multiple "capping" residues have been identified. (B) Structure of the linkage tetrasaccharide and common modifications.

growing chondroitin chain takes place in the Golgi apparatus by appropriate sulfotransferases. DS is formed as a CS chain, during which process the glucuronate C-5 epimerase converts a varying number of the GlcA residues to IdoA. Results suggest that the core protein is responsible for routing PGs to subcellular compartments with or without sufficient access to glucuronate 5-epimerase and, thus, determines the content of IdoA residues (Seidler *et al.*, 2002).

III. Linkage Region

GalAGs and heparin/heparan sulfate are covalently linked to Ser residues in Gly-Ser-Gly sequences in the protein cores of PGs via the linkage tetrasaccharide region: GlcAβ1→3Galβ1→3Galβ1→4Xylβ1-O-Ser (Fig. 2B) (Lindahl and Roden, 1966; Stern *et al.*, 1971). The presence of IdoA instead of GlcA has been reported only for the linkage region of DSPGs of bovine aorta (Sugahara *et al.*, 1995). This linkage tetrasaccharide has been identified in many organisms, even in *C. elegans* chondroitin and *Drosophila melanogaster* HS and CS, and seems to have been conserved during evolution (Yamada *et al.*, 2002).

Linkage regions with respect to the repeating disaccharides have been shown undersulfated in comparison to the main repeat region (Lauder *et al.*, 2000a, 2001). In particular, in linkage region oligosaccharides derived from bovine articular cartilage aggrecan there is a decreased incidence of GalNAc (6S) and a concomitant increase in the abundance of nonsulfated and 4-sulfated residues in comparison to the main repeat region (Lauder *et al.*, 2000a). Karamanos *et al.* (1995) showed that in porcine skin DS-18, which is rich in IdoA (~80%), two GlcA-containing disaccharides are next to the linkage tetrasaccharide; the one linked to the tetrasaccharide is a C unit as the rest GlcA-containing disaccharides, and the next one is nonsulfated (Fig. 3).

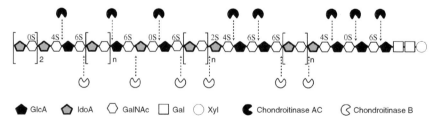

FIGURE 3   Structure of DS-18 from pig skin proposed by Karamanos *et al.* (1995). The sites of enzymic action are indicated. The number of disaccharide units *n* is equal to or larger than 4.

Common modifications of the linkage region are phosphorylation of xylose (Xyl) and 4- or 6-O-sulfation of Gal residues. In the CS linkage region, the Gal sulfation and Xyl phosphorylation have not been found on the same chain (de Waard *et al.*, 1992; Ueno *et al.*, 2001) (Fig. 2B). None of the linkage region oligosaccharides examined so far had any uronic acid sulfation.

2-O-phosphorylation of Xyl has been found in CS from D. *melanogaster*, shark cartilage, rat and mouse tumors, CS/DS from rat fibroblast cell line, and CS chains of syndecan-1 from normal murine mammary gland epithelial cells. Fransson *et al.* (2000) have reported that the phosphorylation of Xyl in decorin (a small CSPG) is a transient phenomenon; in the early steps of the CS biosynthesis of decorin the degree of phosphorylation increases to ~90% until the linkage region grows into the Gal-Gal-Xyl trisaccharide, and then dephosphorylation takes place extensively accompanied by glucuronidation. The transient 2-phosphorylation of Xyl may be involved in intracellular transport and/or in the control of modifications of the glycan chain.

Gal 4-O-sulfation has been reported for CS from rat chondrosarcoma, whale and bovine cartilage, human trypsin inhibitors, and appican (a brain CSPG) and DS from bovine aorta. In addition, Gal 6-O-sulfation has also been revealed for CS from shark (de Waard *et al.*, 1992) and bovine articular cartilage (Lauder *et al.*, 2000b). So far, sulfated Gal residues of the linkage region have been demonstrated for GalAGs but not for HS/heparin even when they are on the same syndecan-1 core protein (Ueno *et al.*, 2001). The sulfate groups on the Gal residues might be biosynthetic sorting signals for CS/DS or key elements that control the glycosyltransferases involved in the formation of the linkage region controlling the maturation of part-time PGs (Gulberti *et al.*, 2005; Sugahara and Kitagawa, 2000). Interestingly, 6-O-sulfation of the first GalNAc residue next to the linkage region and Gal 6-O-sulfation have been identified on the same chain in bovine articular cartilage aggrecan (Lauder *et al.*, 2000b), and 4-O-sulfation of the first GalNAc residue next to the linkage region has been colocalized with Gal 4-O-sulfation in appican (Tsuchida *et al.*, 2001), but not vice versa.

IV. Repeating Disaccharide Region

A. CS from Vertebrate Organisms

Structural studies of CS chains from vertebrate and especially mammalian species have shown the great heterogeneity of structural organization. In a study of CS chains of the vitreous gel, Noulas *et al.* (2004) showed species-specific variation in the content, length, and sulfation pattern; in human-derived CS chains, the 6-sulfated disaccharide was dominant, whereas in CS chains from other mammalian species (pig, sheep, and goat) the predominant disaccharide type was the 4-sulfated one. In a study of the CS/DS chains from the same PG of various bovine tissues, tissue-specific modifications were observed; scleral decorin contained 6-O-sulfated GlcA-rich domains, decorin from bovine dermis cartilage and bone contained 4-O-sulfated GlcA-rich domains, and decorin from bovine tendon contained 6-O-sulfated GlcA domains near the linkage region and 4-O-sulfated in more distal domains (Cheng et al., 1994). CS chains on the syndecan-1 and syndecan-4 synthesized from normal murine mammary gland epithelial cells are structurally distinct, unlike the HS chains; CS chains from syndecan-4 have a higher degree of sulfation and different functionality (Deepa et al., 2004). Furthermore, CS/DS hybrid chains from embryonic pig brain contain a higher proportion of IdoA and different sulfation pattern than those from adult pig brain, showing age-related structural variability (Bao et al., 2004). Thus, mounting evidence shows that the structure of CS depends on the animal species, tissue, physiological or pathological stimuli, and PG source.

Sequence analysis of entire CS/DS chains or oligosaccharides has been performed only by a few research groups via carefully controlled enzymic reactions. The sequence analysis of porcine skin DS-18 by Karamanos et al. (1995) showed that mono- and disulfated IdoA-containing saccharides form clusters larger than four disaccharides ("blocks") (Fig. 3). GlcA residues are located periodically and not randomly in the DS chain (Fig. 3). Separate treatments of human myometrium and uterine leiomyoma GalAGs with chondroitinase ABC and chondroitinase B have also shown that both GalAGs are hybrid polymer structures composed of at least five oligomeric domains (Mitropoulou et al., 2001). Desaire et al. (2001) showed that CS-A from bovine trachea has randomly distributed 4-sulfated and 6-sulfated disaccharides throughout the repeat region of the polysaccharide, but in CS-C from shark cartilage the 6-sulfated disaccharides form "blocks" of repeating disaccharides with the same sulfation pattern.

Sequence analysis of porcine skin DS-18 also showed that the sulfation pattern of DS has a specificity with the uronic acid, that is, the Δdi-mono6S is associated with GlcA, whereas both the Δdi-mono4S and Δdi-di(2,4)S are associated with IdoA (Fig. 3). In support, other research groups have also shown GalNAc(4S) residues in the IdoA-containing regions and GalNAc(6S) and/or GalNAc(4S) residues in the GlcA-containing segments of the polysaccharides (Cheng et al., 1994; Coster et al., 1991; Silbert, 1996). In GalAGs from normal human myometrium and uterine leiomyoma, IdoA-containing oligosaccharide domains contain not only IdoA-GalNAc(4S) residues but also the disulfated Δdi-di(2,4)S and Δdi-di(2,6)S, and the trisulfated Δdi-tri(2,4,6)S, whereas in GlcA-containing domains, disaccharides are mainly sulfated at either C-6 or C-4 of GalNAc (Mitropoulou et al., 2001). Eklund et al. (2000) showed that IdoA, formed during biosynthesis, enhances 4-O-sulfation of their adjacent GalNAc residues, and thus back epimerization to GlcA is prevented. Dermatan-specific *N*-acetylgalactosamine 4- and 6-*O*-sulfotransferases have been characterized, supporting the suggestion that sulfation of GalNAc follows GlcA epimerization (Evers *et al.*, 2001; Nadanaka *et al.*, 1999). Enzymological studies are now providing information on the specificities of the chondroitin 4- and 6-sulfotransferases and thus on the structural organization (Mikami *et al.*, 2003; Yamada *et al.*, 2004). Furthermore, GlcA sulfation seems to occur only between GalNAc(4S) residue on a nonreducing side and a GalNAc(6S) residue on the reducing side (Lauder *et al.*, 2000b; Nadanaka and Sugahara, 1997).

B. CS from Invertebrate Organisms

Studies on CS from various invertebrate species (usually marine) have revealed CS chains with neutral sugar branches and/or unusual sulfation patterns. 3-*O*-sulfation of GlcA and neutral sugar branches rich in glucose was shown for squid skin CS (Aletras *et al.*, 1991; Karamanos *et al.*, 1990, 1992, 1994b). Neutral sugar branches have also been found in corneal CS from *Illex illecebrocus coidentii* (Karamanos *et al.*, 1991) and the case of squid pen (*Sepia officinalis*) (Theocharis *et al.*, 1999). Skin and head cartilage CS of *Nototodarus gouldi* also has branches of neutral sugars, particularly glucose (Falshaw *et al.*, 2000). Squid cartilage CS contains small amounts of glucose branches linked to C-6 of the GalNAc moieties and has 3-*O*-sulfated GlcA residues (Habuchi *et al.*, 1977; Kinoshita-Toyoda *et al.*, 2004). GlcA(3S) residues in squid cartilage CS-E are usually found in di- or trisulfated disaccharide units (Fig. 4) (Kinoshita *et al.*, 1997; Kinoshita-Toyoda *et al.*, 2004). Squid ink from *Illex argentinus* contains a branched polysaccharide with the repeating unit GlcA-GalNAc(1→4) a-D-fucopyranose (Takaya *et al.*, 1996). The molecular weight (M$_r$) of the CS species isolated from squid has generally been higher than those from

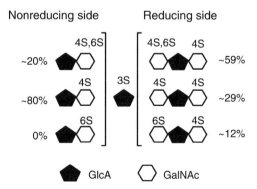

FIGURE 4   Frequencies of sequences found on the reducing and nonreducing sides of GlcA (3S) in squid cartilage CS-E. Adapted from Kinoshita-Toyoda *et al.* (2004, Fig. 6, p. 11072).

mammalian sources. CS species with M_r of 110 and 43 kDa have been isolated from squid skin PGs and with 73 kDa from squid cornea (Karamanos, 1992; Karamanos et al., 1991). Mammalian CS lies in the molecular weight range of 10–50 kDa with the typical bovine tracheal CS having an average M_r of 26 kDa.

A unique fucose (Fuc)-branched CS occurs in the body wall of a sea cucumber (*Ludwigothurea grisea*, Echinodermata-Holothuroidea) (Vieira and Mourão, 1988). The GalNAc residues may be sulfated at C-6 or C-4, whereas C-3 of GlcA residues may carry sulfate groups or sulfated Fuc residues (Mourão et al., 1996). 3-O-fucosylation on GlcA residues has also been reported in king crab cartilage CS-K (Kitagawa et al., 1997a). Thus, king crab cartilage CS-K and squid cartilage CS-E share in common not only the presence of sugar branches but also 3-O-sulfation of GlcA; the relation between these two uncommon structural characteristics remains to be investigated.

Unusually low-sulfated or nonsulfated CS chains and oversulfated DS chains have been isolated from many invertebrate species. A CS of high M_r, containing 42% nonsulfated disaccharides and 48% A units, was isolated from the body of *Viviparus ater* (Mollusca, Gastropoda) (Volpi and Mucci, 1998). Interestingly, the percentage of nonsulfated units significantly increased after lead exposure (Volpi and Mucci, 1998). An oversulfated DS with unique structure and neutral sugars has been isolated from sea urchin shell; DS was composed of disulfated (87%) and trisulfated (12%) disaccharide units, a significant proportion (23%) of which were sulfonylated at the amino group of GalN (Manouras et al., 1991). The trisulfated disaccharide units were Δdi-tri(2,6,N)S and the disulfated units were mainly Δdi-di(2,4)S and Δdi-di(2,N)S (Karamanos et al., 1994a). A DS rich in IdoA (68% of total uronic acid) and composed mainly of monosulfated A (62%) or C units (4%) and disulfated (32%) units with the peculiar disulfation at C-2 and C-3 of IdoA residues has been isolated from ray skin (*Raja clavata*) (Chatziioannidis et al., 1999).

V. Nonreducing Terminal

Multiple studies have shown that CS chains do not contain a single distinct terminal "capping residue" (Midura et al., 1995; Otsu et al., 1985; Plaas et al., 1997). The predominant terminal structures in human cartilage aggrecan are GalNAc(4S) and GalNAc (4S, 6S); the remaining chains terminated with the disaccharides: GlcA-GalNAc(4S) and GlcA-GalNAc(6S) (Plaas et al., 1997). GalNAc(4S, 6S) has also been found at the nonreducing terminus of CS in the *in vitro* culture of chick and rat embryo cartilage (Otsu et al., 1985), in chick chondrocytes and swarm rat chondrosarcoma (Kim and Conrad, 1982; Midura et al., 1995) and in rabbit thrombomodulin

CS (Bourin *et al.*, 1990) much more abundantly than in the repeating disaccharide chain and is suggested as the possible termination signal in CS biosynthesis. In support to this hypothesis, sulfated CS tetra- or hexasaccharides with GlcA-GalNAc(4S, 6S) or GlcA(3S)-GalNAc(4S) at the nonreducing ends did not serve as acceptors for chondroitin GalNAc transferase (Kitagawa *et al.*, 1997b), supporting the notion of the termination signal. Ohtake *et al.* (2003) have reported that a specific enzyme, *N*-acetylgalactosamine 4-sulfate 6-*O*-sulfotransferase, seems to be involved in the generation of this terminal modification.

In human aggrecan CS, nonreducing terminal GalNAc(4S) or GalNAc (4S, 6S) can be linked to either a 4- or 6-sulfated disaccharide, showing no preferential activity of CS terminal GalNAc sulfotransferases (West *et al.*, 1999). In rabbit thrombomodulin CS, nonreducing terminal GalNAc(4S, 6S) is linked to a GlcA-GalNAc(4S, 6S) disaccharide, which does not occur in the repeating disaccharide region (Bourin *et al.*, 1990). Studies on the substrate specificity of the isolated *N*-acetylgalactosamine 4-sulfate 6-*O*-sulfotransferase have shown that the 2-*O*-sulfation of the penultimate GlcA residue adjacent to GalNAc(6S) appears to stimulate 6-*O*-sulfation of the nonreducing terminal GalNAc(4S) (Ohtake *et al.*, 2003).

VI. Future Perspectives

CS is present in all organisms from worms to humans (not in plants) and serves multiple important biological roles. Despite the simple nature of the backbone polysaccharide, a great heterogeneity exists regarding degree of sulfation, distribution of sulfate groups, and of the two epimeric uronic acids within the chain. Fine structure determines the specificity of functions and interactions of CS/DS. Although there are many methods for analysis of constituent disaccharides, methodologies for complete structure elucidation are not so mature yet and thus hinder knowledge on sequence. Progress in this field and in identification of the enzymes involved in CS biosynthesis, determination of their specificities, and regulation mechanisms will undoubtedly allow the elucidation of CS structural organization according to the PG, tissue, organism, and developmental status.

References

Aletras, A. J., Karamanos, N. K., and Hjerpe, A. (1991). Presence of the HNK-1 epitope (3-sulfoglucuronic acid) on oligosaccharides from squid skin chondroitin proteoglycans and degradation of proteoglycans by proteolytic enzymes. *Biochem. Int.* **25**(2), 331–338.

Anno, K., Seno, N., Mathews, M. B., Yamagata, T., and Suzuki, S. (1971). A new dermatan polysulfate, chondroitin sulfate H, from hagfish notochord. *Biochim. Biophys. Acta* **237**(1), 173–177.

Bao, X., Nushimura, S., Mikami, T., Yamada, S., Itoh, N., and Sugahara, K. (2004). Chondroitin sulfate/dermatan sulfate hybrib chains from embryonic pig brain, which contain a higher proportion of L-iduronic acid than those from adult pig brain, exhibit neuritogenic and growth factor binding activities. *J. Biol. Chem.* **279**(11), 9765–9776.

Bourin, M. C., Lundgren-Akerlund, E., and Lindahl, U. (1990). Isolation and characterization of the glycosaminoglycan component of rabbit thrombomodulin proteoglycan. *J. Biol. Chem.* **265**, 15424–15431.

Cassaro, C. M. F., and Dietrich, C. P. (1977). Distribution of sulfated mucopolysaccharides in invertebrates. *J. Biol. Chem.* **252**(7), 2254–2261.

Casu, B., Petitou, M., Provasoli, M., and Sinay, P. (1998). Conformational flexibility: A new concept for explaining binding and biological properties of iduronic acid-containing glycosaminoglycans. *Trends Biochem. Sci.* **13**, 221–225.

Chatziioannidis, C. C., Karamanos, N. K., and Tsegenidis, T. (1999). Isolation and characterization of a small dermatan sulfate proteoglycan from ray skin (*Raja clavata*). *Comp. Biochem. Physiol. B* **124**, 15–24.

Cheng, F., Heinegard, D., Malmstrom, A., Schmidtchen, A., Yoshida, K., and Fransson, L. A. (1994). Patterns of uronosyl epimerization and 4-/6-O-sulphation in chondroitin/dermatan sulphate from decorin and biglycan of various bovine tissues. *Glycobiology* **4**(5), 685–696.

Choi, H. U., Johnson, T. L., Pal, S., Tang, L. H., Rosenberg, L., and Neame, P. J. (1989). Characterization of the dermatan sulfate proteoglycans, DS-PGI and DS-PGII, from bovine articular cartilage and skin isolated by octyl-sepharose chromatography. *J. Biol. Chem.* **264**(5), 2876–2884.

Coster, L., Hernnas, J., and Malmstrom, A. (1991). Biosynthesis of dermatan sulphate proteoglycans. *Biochem. J.* **276**, 533–539.

De Angelis, P. (2002). Microbial glycosaminoglycan glycosyltransferases. *Glycobiology* **12**(1), 9R–16R.

de Waard, P., Vliegenthart, J. F. G., Harada, T., and Sugahara, K. (1992). Structural studies on sulfated oligosaccharides derived from the carbohydrate-protein linkage region of chondroitin 6-sulfate proteoglycans of shark cartilage. II. *J. Biol. Chem.* **267**, 6036–6043.

Deepa, S. S., Yamada, S., Zako, M., Goldberger, O., and Sugahara, K. (2004). Chondroitin sulfate chains on syndecan-1 and syndecan-4 from normal murine gland epithelial cells are structurally and functionally distinct and cooperate with heparan sulfate chains to bind growth factors. *J. Biol. Chem.* **279**(36), 37368–37376.

Desaire, H., Sirich, T. L., and Leary, J. A. (2001). Evidence of block and randomly sequenced chondroitin polysaccharides: Sequential enzymatic digestion and quantification using on trap tandem mass spectrometry. *Anal. Chem.* **73**(15), 3513–3520.

Eklund, E., Roden, L., Malmstrom, M., and Malmstrom, A. (2000). Dermatan is a better substrate for 4-O-sulfation than chondroitin: Implications in the generation of 4-O-sulfated, L-iduronate-rich galactosaminoglycans. *Arch. Biochem. Biophys.* **383**(2), 171–177.

Evers, M. R., Xia, G., Kang, H.-G., Schachner, M., and Baenziger, J. U. (2001). Molecular cloning and characterization of a dermatan-specific N-acetylgalactosamine 4-O-sulfotransferase. *J. Biol. Chem.* **276**(39), 36344–36353.

Falshaw, R., Hubl, U., Ofman, D., Slim, G. C., Amjad Tariq, M., Watt, D. K., and Yorke, S. C. (2000). Comparison of the glycosaminoglycans isolated from the skin and head cartilage of Gould's arrow squid (*Nototodarus gouldi*). *Carbohyd. Polym.* **41**, 357–364.

Fransson, L. A., Havsmark, B., and Silverberg, I. (1990). A method for the sequence analysis of dermatan sulphate. *Biochem. J.* **269**(2), 381–388.

Fransson, L. A., Belting, M., Jonsson, M., Mani, K., Moses, J., and Oldberg, A. (2000). Biosynthesis of decorin and glypican. *Matrix Biol.* **19**, 367–376.

Gulberti, S., Lattard, V., Fondeur, M., Jacquinet, J.-C., Mulliert, G., Netter, P., Magdalou, J., Ouzzine, M., and Fournel-Gigleux, S. (2005). Phosphorylation and sulfation of oligosaccharide substrates critically influence the activity of human 1,4-galactosyltransferase 7 (GalT-I) and 1,3-glucuronosyltransferase I (GlcAT-I) involved in the biosynthesis of the glycosaminoglycan-protein linkage region of proteoglycans. *J. Biol. Chem.* **280**(2), 1417–1425.

Habuchi, O., Sugiura, K., and Kawai, N. (1977). Glucose branches in chondroitin sulfates from squid cartilage. *J. Biol. Chem.* **252**, 4570–4576.

Karamanos, N. K. (1992). Two squid skin proteoglycans each containing chondroitin sulfates with different sulfation patterns. *Biochem. Cell Biol.* **70**(8), 629–635.

Karamanos, N. K., Aletras, A. J., Antonopoulos, C. A., Tsegenidis, T., Tsiganos, C. P., and Vynios, D. H. (1988). Extraction and fractionation of proteoglycans from squid skin. *Biochim. Biophys. Acta* **966**(1), 36–43.

Karamanos, N. K., Aletras, A. J., Antonopoulos, C. A., Hjerpe, A., and Tsiganos, C. P. (1990). Chondroitin proteoglycans from squid skin. Isolation, characterization and immunological studies. *Eur. J. Biochem.* **192**(1), 33–38.

Karamanos, N. K., Manouras, A., Tsegenidis, T., and Antonopoulos, C. A. (1991). Isolation and chemical study of the glycosaminoglycans from squid cornea. *Int. J. Biochem.* **23**(1), 67–72.

Karamanos, N. K., Aletras, A. J., Tsegenidis, T., Tsiganos, C. P., and Antonopoulos, C. A. (1992). Isolation, characterization and properties of the oversulphated chondroitin sulphate proteoglycan from squid skin with peculiar glycosaminoglycan sulphation pattern. *Eur. J. Biochem.* **204**(2), 553–560.

Karamanos, N. K., Syrokou, A., Vanky, P., Nurminen, M., and Hjerpe, A. (1994a). Determination of 24 variously sulfated galactosaminoglycan- and hyaluronan-derived disaccharides by high-performance liquid chromatography. *Anal. Biochem.* **221**, 189–199.

Karamanos, N. K., Aletras, A. J., Antonopoulos, C. A., and Hjerpe, A. (1994b). Determination of the HNK-1 epitope (3-sulphated glucuronic acid) in intact chondroitin sulphates by ELISA. *Biochimie* **76**, 79–82.

Karamanos, N. K., Vanky, P., Syrokou, A., and Hjerpe, A. (1995). Identity of dermatan and chondroitin sequences in dermatan sulfate chains determined by using fragmentation with chondroitinases and ion-pair high-performance liquid chromatography. *Anal. Biochem.* **225**(2), 220–230.

Kim, J. J., and Conrad, H. E. (1982). Proteochondroitin sulfate synthesis in subcultured chick embryo tibial chondrocytes. *J. Biol. Chem.* **257**, 1670–1675.

Kinoshita, A., Yamada, S., Haslam, S. M., Morris, H. R., Dell, A., and Sugahara, K. (1997). Novel tetrasaccharides isolated from squid cartilage chondroitin sulfate E contain unusual sulfated disaccharide units GlcA(3-O-sulfate)beta1–3GalNAc(6-O-sulfate) or GlcA(3-O-sulfate)beta1–3GalNAc. *J. Biol. Chem.* **272**(32), 19656–19665.

Kinoshita-Toyoda, A., Yamada, S., Haslam, S. M., Khoo, K.-H., Sugiura, M., Morris, H. R., Dell, A., and Sugahara, K. (2004). Structural determination of five novel tetrasaccharides containing 3-O-sulfated D-glucuronic acid and two rare oligosaccharides containing a β-D-glucose branch isolated from squid cartilage chondroitin sulfate E. *Biochemistry* **43**, 11063–11074.

Kitagawa, H., Tanaka, Y., Yamada, S., Seno, N., Haslam, S. M., Morris, H. R., Dell, A., and Sugahara, K. (1997a). A novel pentasaccharide sequence GlcA(3-sulfate)(beta1–3)GalNAc(4-sulfate)(beta1–4)(Fuc alpha1–3)GlcA(beta1–3)GalNAc(4-sulfate) in the oligosaccharides isolated from king crab cartilage chondroitin sulfate K and its differential susceptibility to chondroitinases and hyaluronidase. *Biochemistry* **36**(13), 3998–4008.

Kitagawa, H., Tsutsumi, K., Ujikawa, M., Goto, F., Tamura, J., Neumann, K. W., Ogawa, T., and Sugahara, K. (1997b). Regulation of chondroitin sulfate biosynthesis by specific sulfation: Acceptor specificity of serum beta-GalNAc transferase revealed by structurally defined oligosaccharides. *Glycobiology* 7, 531–537.

Lauder, R. M., Huckerby, T. N., and Nieduzynski, I. A. (2000a). Increased incidence of unsulfated and 4-sulfated residues in the chondroitin sulfate linkage region observed by high pH anion-exchange chromatography. *Biochem. J.* 347, 339–348.

Lauder, R. M., Huckerby, T. N., and Nieduszynski, I. A. (2000b). A fingerprinting method for chondroitin/dermatan sulfate and hyaluronan oligosaccharides. *Glycobiology* 10(4), 393–401.

Lauder, R. M., Huckerby, T. N., Brown, G. M., Bayliss, M. T., and Nieduszynski, I. A. (2001). Age-related changes in the sulfation of the chondroitin sulphate linkage region from human articular cartilage aggrecan. *Biochem. J.* 358, 523–528.

Lindahl, U., and Roden, L. (1966). The chondroitin 4-sulfate-protein linkage. *J. Biol. Chem.* 241(9), 2113–2119.

Manouras, A., Karamanos, N. K., Tsegenidis, T., and Antonopoulos, A. (1991). Isolation and chemical characterization of two acid carbohydrates from the sea urchin shell, extraction and fractionation of their protein complexes. *Comp. Biochem. Physiol. B* 99(1), 119–124.

Midura, R. J., Calabro, A., Yanagishita, M., and Hascall, V. C. (1995). Nonreducing end structures of chondroitin sulfate chains on aggrecan isolated from swarm rat chondrosarcoma cultures. *J. Biol. Chem.* 270, 8009–8015.

Mikami, T., Mizumoto, S., Kago, N., Kitagawa, H., and Sugahara, K. (2003). Specificities of three distinct human chondoritin/dermatan N-acetylgalactosamine 4-O-sulfotransferases demonstrated using partially desulfated dermatan sulfate as an acceptor. *J. Biol. Chem.* 278(38), 36115–36127.

Mitropoulou, T. N., Lamari, F., Syrokou, A., Hjerpe, A., and Karamanos, N. K. (2001). Identification of oligomeric domains within dermatan sulfate chains using differential enzymic treatments, derivatization with 2-aminoacridone and capillary electrophoresis. *Electrophoresis* 22(12), 2458–2463.

Mizuguchi, S., Uyama, T., Kitagawa, H., Nomura, K. H., Dejima, K., Gengyo-Ando, K., Mitani, S., Sugahara, K., and Nomura, K. (2003). Chondroitin proteoglycans are involved in cell division of *Caenorhabditis elegans. Nature* 423(6938), 443–448.

Mourão, P. A. S., Pereira, M. S., Pavão, M. S., Mulloy, B., Tollefsen, D. M., Mowinckel, M. C., and Abilgaard, U. (1996). Structure and anticoagulant activity of a fucosylated chondroitin sulfate from echinoderm. *J. Biol. Chem.* 271(39), 23973–23984.

Nadanaka, S., and Sugahara, K. (1997). The unusual tetrasaccharide sequence GlcAβ1–3GalNAc (4-sulfate)β1–4GlcA(2-sulfate)β1–3GalNAc (6-sulfate) found in the hexasaccharides prepared by testicular hyaluronidase digestion of shark cartilage chondroitin sulfate D. *Glycobiology* 7, 253–263.

Nadanaka, S., Fujita, M., and Sugahara, K. (1999). Demonstration of a novel sulfotransferase in fetal bovine serum, which transfers sulfate to the C6 position of the GalNAc residue in the sequence iduronic acid alpha1–3GalNAc beta1–4iduronic acid in dermatan sulfate. *FEBS Lett.* 452(3), 185–189.

Noulas, A. V., Skandalis, S. S., Feretis, E., Theocharis, D. A., and Karamanos, N. K. (2004). Variations in content and structure of glycosaminoglycans of the vitreous gel from different mammalian species. *Biomed. Chromatogr.* 18, 457–461.

Ohtake, S., Kimata, K., and Habuchi, O. (2003). A unique nonreducing terminal modification of chondroitin sulfate by N-acetylgalactosamine 4-sulfate 6-O-sulfotransferase. *J. Biol. Chem.* 278(40), 38443–38452.

Otsu, K., Inoue, H., Tsuzuki, Y., Yonekura, H., Nakanishi, Y., and Suzuki, S. (1985). A distinct terminal structure in newly synthesized chondroitin sulphate chains. *Biochem. J.* 227, 37–48.

Plaas, A. H. K., Wong-Palms, S., Roughley, P. J., Midura, R. J., and Hascall, V. C. (1997). Chemical and immunological assay of the nonreducing terminal residues of chondroitin sulfate from human aggrecan. *J. Biol. Chem.* **272**(33), 20603–20610.

Prydz, K., and Dalen, K. T. (2000). Synthesis and sorting of proteoglycans. *J. Cell Science* **113**, 193–205.

Roseman, S. (2001). Reflections on glycobiology. *J. Biol. Chem.* **276**(45), 41527–41542.

Sakai, S., Kim, W. S., Lee, I. S., Kim, Y. S., Nakamura, A., Toida, T., and Imanari, T. (2003). Purification and characterization of dermatan sulfate from the skin of the eel, *Anguilla japonica*. *Carbohydr. Res.* **338**, 263–269.

Seidler, D. G., Breuer, E., Grande-Allen, K. J., Hascall, V. C., and Kresse, H. (2002). Core protein dependence of epimerization of glucuronosyl residues in galactosaminoglycans. *J. Biol. Chem.* **277**(44), 42409–42416.

Silbert, J. E. (1996). Organization of glycosaminoglycan sulfation in the biosynthesis of proteochondroitin sulfate and proteodermatan sulfate. *Glycoconj. J.* **13**, 907–912.

Silbert, J. E., and Sugumaran, G. (2002). Biosynthesis of chondroitin/dermatan sulfate. *IUBMB Life* **54**, 177–186.

Stern, E. L., Lindahl, B., and Roden, L. (1971). The linkage of dermatan sulfate to protein. II. Monosaccharide sequence of the linkage region. *J. Biol. Chem.* **246**(18), 5707–5715.

Sugahara, K., Ohkita, Y., Shibata, Y., Yoshida, K., and Ikegami, A. (1995). Structural studies on the hexasaccharide alditols from the carbohydrate-protein linkage region of dermatan sulfate proteoglycans of bovine aorta. *J. Biol. Chem.* **270**(13), 7204–7212.

Sugahara, K., and Kitagawa, H. (2000). Recent advances in the study of the biosynthesis and functions of sulfated glycosaminoglycans. *Curr. Opin. Struct. Biol.* **10**(5), 518–527.

Sugahara, K., and Yamada, S. (2000). Structure and function of oversulfated chondroitin sulfate variants: Unique sulfation patterns and neuroregulatory activities. *Trends Glycosci. Glycotechnol.* **12**, 321–349.

Suzuki, S., Saito, H., Yamagata, T., Anno, K., Seno, N., Kawai, Y., and Furuhashi, T. (1968). Formation of three types of disulfated disaccharides from chondroitin sulfates by chondroitinase digestion. *J. Biol. Chem.* **243**(7), 1543–1550.

Takagaki, K., Munakata, H., Kakizaki, I., Iwafune, M., Itabashi, T., and Endo, M. (2002). Domain structure of chondroitin sulfate E octasaccharides binding to type V collagen. *J. Biol. Chem.* **277**(11), 8882–8889.

Takaya, Y., Uchisawa, H., Narumi, F., and Matsue, H. (1996). Illexins A, B and C from squid ink should have a branched structure. *Biochem. Biophys. Res. Commun.* **226**, 335–338.

Theocharis, A. D., Karamanos, N. K., and Tsegenidis, T. (1999). Isolation and analysis of a novel acidic polysaccharide from the case of squid pen. *Int. J. Biol. Macromol.* **26**(1), 83–88.

Trowbridge, J. M., and Gallo, R. L. (2002). Dermatan sulfate: New functions from an old glycosaminoglycan. *Glycobiology* **12**(9), 117R–125R.

Tsuchida, K., Shioi, J., Yamada, S., Boghosian, G., Wu, A., Cai, H., Sugahara, K., and Robakis, N. K. (2001). Appican, the proteoglycan form of the amyloid precursor protein, contains chondroitin sulfate E in the repeating disaccharide region and 4-O-sulfated galactose in the linkage region. *J. Biol. Chem.* **276**(40), 37155–37160.

Ueno, M., Yamada, A., Zako, M., Bernfield, M., and Sugahara, K. (2001). Structural characterization of syndecan-1 purified from normal murine mammary gland epithelial cells. *J. Biol. Chem.* **276**(31), 29134–29140.

Ueoka, C., Nadanaka, S., Seno, N., Khoo, K.-H., and Sugahara, K. (1999). Structural determination of novel tetra- and hexasaccharide sequences isolated from chondroitin sulfate H (oversulfated dermatan sulfate) of hagfish notochord. *Glycoconj. J.* **16**, 291–305.

Vieira, R. P., and Mourao, P. A. S. (1988). Occurrence of a unique fucose-branched chondroitin sulfate in the body wall of a sea cucumber. *J. Biol. Chem.* **263**(34), 18176–18183.

Volpi, N., and Mucci, A. (1998). Characterization of a low-sulfated chondroitin sulfate from the body of *Viviparus ater* (mollusca gastropoda). Modification of its structure by lead pollution. *Glycoconj. J.* **15**, 1071–1078.

West, L. A., Roughley, P., Nelson, F. R. T., and Plaas, A. H. K. (1999). Sulphation heterogeneity in the trisaccharide (GalNAcSb1,4GlcAb1,3GalNAcS) isolated from the non-reducing terminal of human aggrecan chondroitin sulphate. *Biochem. J.* **342**, 223–229.

Yamada, S., Okada, Y., Ueno, M., Iwata, S., Deepa, S. S., Nishimura, S., Fujita, M., Van Die, I., Hirabayashi, Y., and Sugahara, K. (2002). Determination of the glycosaminoglycan-protein linkage region oligosaccharide structures of proteoglycans from *Drosophila melanogaster* and *Caenorhabditis elegans*. *J. Biol. Chem.* **277**(35), 31877–31886.

Yamada, T., Ohtake, S., Sato, M., and Habuchi, O. (2004). Chondroitin 4-sulfotransferase-1 and chondroitin 6-sulfotransferase-1 are affected by uronic acid residues neighbouring the acceptor GalNAc residues. *Biochem. J.* **384**(Pt 3), 567–575.

Barbara Mulloy

National Institute for Biological Standards and Control
Herts. EN6 3QG
United Kingdom

Progress in the Structural Biology of Chondroitin Sulfate

I. Chapter Overview

The chondroitin sulfates (CSs) are, like most other glycosaminoglycans (GAGs), linear polysaccharides in which a simple disaccharide repeating unit has been modified postpolymerization to give a more complex and heterogeneous set of structures. The significance of CS to the structural integrity of extracellular matrix has long been recognized, and in that context the three-dimensional structures of CS and whole proteoglycans (PGs) of which they are a part have been the subject of classic studies. CS has been recognized in more diverse structural roles, and it has been shown to link two proteins together. However, CS may also take part in specific interactions with proteins through specific oligosaccharide sequences, some of which are highly sulfated, and the significance of these interactions for growth and development of tissues has inspired structural determinations for these active structures. Experimental studies of protein–CS complex structures are now appearing, and theoretical as well as experimental approaches have been applied to CS with interesting results.

Advances in Pharmacology, Volume 53
Copyright 2006, Elsevier Inc. All rights reserved.

1054-3589/06 $35.00
DOI: 10.1016/S1054-3589(05)53004-7

II. Introduction

The CSs are three galactosaminoglycans (GalAGs); that is, they are polysaccharides made up of alternating galactosamine and uronic acid monosaccharide residues. They are the GAG side chains of PGs, either alone or with other GAGs, such as heparan sulfate (HS) or keratan sulfate (KS), and are found throughout the animal kingdom. There are three main structural categories of CS, traditionally known as CS-A, CS-B, and CS-C. The predominant structures of these categories are shown in Fig. 1. CS-A is also known as chondroitin-4-sulfate (C4S), CS-C as chondroitin-6-sulfate (C6S), and CS-B as dermatan sulfate (DS); these are the names used in this chapter. In all chondroitins, the galactosamine is N-acetylated (in contrast

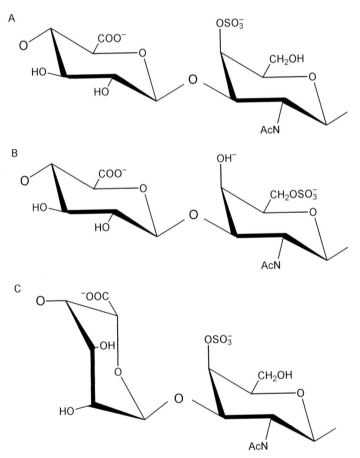

FIGURE I   The major repeating disaccharides in the structure of: (A) chondroitin-4-sulfate [4]-β-D-GlcA-(1→3)-β-D-GalNAc4SO$_3^-$(1→], (B) chondroitin-6-sulfate [4]-β-D-GlcA-(1→3)-β-D-GalNAc6SO$_3^-$(1→], and (C) dermatan sulfate [4]-α-L-IdoA-(1→3)-β-D-GalNAc4SO$_3^-$ (1→].

with the occurrence of N-sulfated and unsubstituted glucosamine found in HS). In C4S and C6S, the uronic acid is β-D-glucuronic acid; in DS it is α-L-iduronic acid, formed from glucuronic acid by epimerization at C5 during biosynthesis. The region of linkage to the protein core has a different and specific structure, and the nonreducing ends are capped with sequences displaying specific substitution patterns.

Very few existing chondroitins have the simple structures implied in Fig. 1. To a greater or lesser extent they are all mixtures of the structures shown, named according to whichever structure predominates. Variants of these structures are found in invertebrates, differing from the mammalian forms in their substitution with extra sulfates or even bearing sulfated fucose side chains (Vieira et al., 1991). In addition, there exist sequences within mammalian chondroitins, which bear extra sulfate substitution, and some such sequences appear to have specific functions (Sugahara et al., 2003).

Chondroitins are major constituents of the extracellular matrix (ECM), in the context of densely glycosylated PGs such as aggrecan. Their role has been seen as primarily structural, depending on bulk properties of the hydrated, negatively charged polysaccharide chains in association with aggrecan protein core, collagen, and hyaluronan. However, it has been recognized that chondroitin, like HS, can play a part in growth and development of tissues by means of specific interactions with functional proteins. In this respect the smaller PGs, bearing only one or two GAG chains, may be important.

The structural biology of chondroitins, as isolated polysaccharides, as components of PGs, and in their interactions with protein ligands, has a long and varied history. The chondroitins are particularly intractable to standard experimental methods; native PGs will not crystallize and are too large and heterogeneous for solution structural analysis by NMR. The isolated polysaccharide chains are also heterogeneous and polydisperse, and the proton NMR spectra of chondroitins are not sufficiently well dispersed to allow analysis of structure and dynamics in solution in the way that has been done for other polysaccharides, including the GAG heparin (a highly sulfated HS used widely in medicine as an anticoagulant and antithrombotic).

The following sections of this chapter discuss first, the conformational analysis of isolated CS chains; second, some of the methods that have been used to determine and visualize the structures of chondroitin PGs; and finally, some studies of specific chondroitin–protein interactions.

III. Experimental Structures of CS Chains

Coordinates for the three-dimensional structures of glycans are found in the protein database (PDB) (http://www.rcsb.org/pdb/), for free polysaccharides as well as for glycoconjugates and glycan–protein complexes. Two x-ray structures for C4S have been in the database for many years, both based on fiber diffraction patterns; one of them [PDB code 1C4S (Winter et al., 1978)] for the sodium salt of pure C4S and the other [PDB code 2C4S (Cael *et al.*, 1978)] for the calcium salt; the data on which this structure was based was obtained from an oriented sample of PG. The two C4S structures are illustrated in Fig. 2. They are both fairly extended; the sodium salt adopts a regular

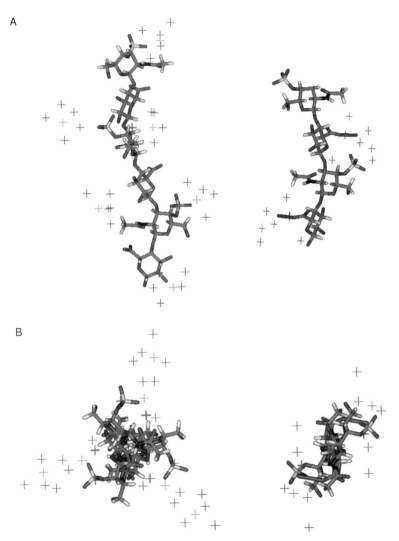

FIGURE 2   X-ray diffraction structures of C4S, in (A) side and (B) end views, shown in stick representation with carbon in green, oxygen in red, nitrogen in blue, and cation in purple. Water in the crystal structure and sodium ions are shown as star shapes. On the left of each panel is the structure 1C4S (in which the cation is sodium) and on the right is 2C4S (in which the cation is closely coordinated calcium). In 1C4S the helix makes a complete turn every three disaccharides, whereas in 2C4S the polysaccharide is more extended, making a complete turn every two disaccharides. (See Color Insert.)

threefold helix and the calcium salt a more extended twofold helix. Intramolecular hydrogen bonds stabilize the structures, and the closely packed polysaccharide chains also interact by means of intermolecular hydrogen bonds.

It is only recently that additional solid-state chondroitin coordinates have been added to the database, in the form of oligosaccharide structures in complex with some of the enzymes of chondroitin degradation. The overall shapes of polysaccharides in solution are determined by the torsional angles around the two bonds between each monosaccharide residue (Fig. 3A), and these angles, ϕ and ψ, provide a convenient way to compare all the published experimental three-dimensional structures. The top section of Table I lists these values, and Fig. 3B shows a plot of ϕ vs. ψ for each of the experimental structures of C4S, which demonstrates good agreement between the classic structure for the isolated polysaccharide and the more recent structures of protein-bound oligosaccharides. Conformations of the oligosaccharides bound to chondroitinase AC are close to those found in the calcium structure (2C4S) (Huang *et al.*, 2001; Lunin *et al.*, 2004); the 1–4 linkage of the C4S tetramer bound to chondroitinase B (Michel *et al.*, 2004) is, however, somewhat distorted.

An x-ray structure for DS has been published (Mitra *et al.*, 1983), but the coordinates have not been deposited in the PDB. Torsional angles ϕ and ψ are however given for three allomorphs; an eightfold, a threefold, and a twofold helix; these are listed in Table I. One crystal structure of chondroitinase AC bound to a dermatan tetrasaccharide also provides torsional angle data (Table I) (Huang *et al.*, 2001). Chondroitin B lyase retains activity in the crystal, so only disaccharides are seen in the crystal structure of the complex of a dermatan hexasaccharide bound to this enzyme (Michel *et al.*, 2004). The conformation of a bound tetrasaccharide has been estimated by modeling the docked complex, and the oligosaccharide is predicted to be distorted away from the helical solid-state structure of DS.

Experimental data for C6S (listed in the lower portion of Table I) are limited to one linkage in a mixed tetrasaccharide bound to the hyaluronate lyase of *S. pneumoniae* (Rigden and Jedrzejas, 2003).

IV. Theoretical Studies

There are no experimental data to indicate that the structures identified in the solid state are dominant, or even present, in solution: NMR spectroscopic techniques useful for other GAGs, such as heparin (Mulloy *et al.*, 1993), are problematic in the case of the GalAGs, which, fortuitously, have inconvenient overlaps in their proton NMR spectra even at high field. In any case, it is not clear whether the close-packed solid-state structures or the dilute solution structures with no interactions between solute molecules are the most suitable model of CS within ECM. In this situation, molecular

A   Residue *i*   Residue (*i*-1)

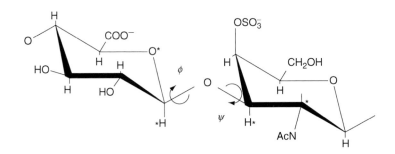

B

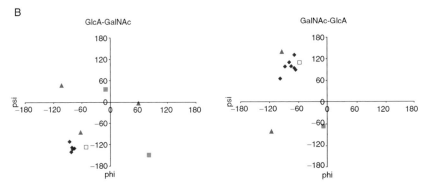

FIGURE 3   (A) The angles ϕ and ψ illustrated for the GlcA 1→3 GalNAc linkage of C4S. Atoms used to define torsional angles around the two glycosidic bonds are marked with an asterisk. The symbols ϕ and ψ conventionally represent the torsional angles at the glycosidic linkage between residue *i* and residue (*i*−1). According to current recommendations from the IUPAC-IUBMB [IUPAC-IUB Joint Commission on Biochemical Nomenclature (JCBN). Symbols for specifying the conformation of polysaccharide chains. Recommendations 1981. *Eur. J. Biochem.* 1983, 131:5–7], these are defined from heavy atoms in the structure as follows: "The angle ϕ about the bond from the anomeric carbon to the oxygen that joins the two residues is specified using the ring oxygen as a reference atom. The torsion angle ψ about the bond from the glycosylated oxygen of the (*i*−1)th residue to a carbon of this residue uses the carbon atom one lower in numbering as a reference atom." This is the convention used in this article; care must be taken in comparison with values given in publications in which the angle ψ is defined using the carbon atom one higher in numbering. The values ϕ_H and ψ_H are defined using the hydrogen atoms at C1 of residue *i* and at the linked carbon of residue (*i*−1). (B) Plots of observed and predicted glycosidic torsional angles ϕ and ψ for the β–1→3 and β–1→4 glycosidic linkages in A: C4S, ◆ experimentally determined values; ■ predicted values from Kaufmann *et al.* (1999); ▲ predicted values from Bayraktar *et al.* (2004); □ predicted values from Bathe *et al.* (2005).

TABLE I Glycosidic Linkage Torsional Angles for GlcA-GlcNAc (1→3) and GlcNAc-GlcA (1→4) Linkages in (A) C4S and (B) C6S and DS Conformations

(A) Experimental and Theoretical C4S Conformations

Chondroitin-4-sulfate

				GlcA-GalNAc (1→3 linkage)		GalNAc-GlcA (1→4 linkage)	
				φ	ψ	φ	ψ
Experimental			Helix				
1C4S (Winter et al., 1978)	Polymer	Fiber	3-fold	−86	−111	−80	110
2C4S (Cael et al., 1978)			2-fold	−80	−132	−98	66
1OFM[a]	Tetramer	Crystal		−83	−141	−69	131
1RWF[b]				−76	−130	−66	90
1RWG[b]				−81	−127	−69	94
1RWH[b]				−78	−131	−76	100
1HMW[c]	Mixed tetramer					−88	99
			Minimum				
Kaufmann et al. (1999)	Tetramer	Molecular dynamics	1	−10	154	−10	169
			2	80	−149		
Bayraktar et al. (2004)			1	59	−124	−95	139
			2	−103	46	−118	−83
			3	−63	−85		
Bathe et al. (2005a)	Polymer	Coarse-grained calcs		−58	−124	−58	108
Almond and Sheehan (2000)		Molecular dynamics		−71	−149	−71	120

(continues)

TABLE I (continued)

			GlcA-GalNAc ($1\rightarrow3$ linkage)		GalNAc-GlcA ($1\rightarrow4$ linkage)	
			ϕ	ψ	ϕ	ψ
(B) Experimental and Theoretical C6S and DS Conformations						
Dermatan sulfate						
Experimental		Helix				
Mitra et al. (1983)	Polymer	Fiber	8-fold	−160	−133	−103	92
			3-fold	−64	−116	−87	97
			2-fold	−106	−102	−98	55
			−108	−159	−64	83
1HM2[c]	Tetramer	Crystal				
Theoretical						
Almond and Sheehan (2000)		Molecular dynamics	−69	−164	−68	162
		Proposed solid state	−59	−169	−72	117
Chondroitin-6-sulfate						
Experimental						
1HMW[c]	Mixed Tetramer	Crystal	Minimum	−90	−151		
Theoretical						
Bayraktar et al. (2004)			1	98	−131	−103	156
			2	−119	51	−121	−62
			3	−78	−91		
Bathe et al. (2005)	Polymer	Coarse-grained calcs	−51	−126	−55	102

[a]In complex with the chondroitin B lyase of *Pedobacter heparinus* (Michel et al., 2004).
[b]In complex with the chondroitin AC lyase of *Arthrobacter aurescens* (Lunin et al., 2004).
[c]In complex with the chondroitin AC lyase of *Pedobacter heparinus* (Huang et al., 2001).
Note: Experimental values from x-ray structures and oligosaccharide–enzyme cocrystals, excluding linkages between nonreducing terminal uronic acid and GalNAc. Predictions from theoretical calculations are also included for comparison. The glycosidic torsional angles ϕ and ψ (expressed in degrees) are defined as described for Figure 3.

modeling can at least predict which conformations of chondroitin are energetically preferred, both in a vacuum and in aqueous solution.

Kaufmann *et al.* (1999) have studied a C4S tetrasaccharide in aqueous solution by molecular dynamics; an example of a study using the molecular mechanics type of conformational energy calculation. The low-energy conformations identified by this method (square symbols in Fig. 3B) do not include the experimentally determined solid-state structures, although the starting structure was taken directly from it. Bayraktar *et al.* (2004) have used semiempirical methods to map the conformational space round the two linkages in C4S and C6S; in some respects, this is more a rigorous type of calculation than molecular mechanics, but it does not take account of solvation. The approach identifies the solid-state conformations of both linkages as one minimum in the energy map. The coarse-grained approach of Bathe *et al.* (2005a) with lower resolution (at the residue level rather than the atomic level) has energy minima in the ϕ/ψ map, which approximate the solid-state structures quite well.

Simulation of large PGs and their complexes in ECM cannot be achieved at atomic resolution, and this more coarsely grained type of molecular model is being developed to cope with huge macromolecular systems (Bathe *et al.*, 2005a). The approach is well suited to GAGs in which a limited number of residue and linkage types are arranged in a linear fashion.

V. NMR Studies of CS and DS Polysaccharides

Both ^{1}H and ^{13}C NMR spectroscopy are extensively used in the characterization of CS structures, both for oligosaccharides and for heterogeneous polysaccharide preparations (Mucci *et al.*, 2000). No detailed solution structure based on NMR spectroscopic data is available for any of the chondroitins; this is partly because of overlap of signals even in high-field spectra, and partly because, in contrast to the glucosaminoglycan heparin (Mulloy *et al.*, 1993), there are no strong inter-residue nuclear Overhauser effects with which to define a well-determined solution conformation (author's unpublished observations).

Analysis of proton spectra has been useful in examining dynamic aspects of CS and DS structure (Huster *et al.*, 2004; Naji *et al.*, 2000). Both the glucuronic and galactosamine residues in C4S and C6S adopt the $^4C_1$ chair conformation typical of D-hexopyranoses. However, the uronic acid in DS, α-L-iduronic acid, has been for many years a source of conformational controversy, in two respects: the conformation of the iduronate pyranose ring in the solid state and its conformational equilibrium in solution. The original refinement of the x-ray structure of DS was performed with alpha-L-iduronic acid (IdoA) in the $^4C_1$ conformation (Mitra *et al.*, 1983); the $^1C_4$ chair, which might be expected for an L-hexopyranose, is incompatible with the height per residue and number of residues per turn measured from the diffraction data (Almond and Sheehan, 2000; Mitra *et al.*, 1983; Venkataraman *et al.*, 1994). Almond and Sheehan (2000), using a molecular dynamics approach (and giving a thorough account of the previous three decades of the controversy), come to the conclusion that the diffraction data can best be interpreted with the iduronate residues in the $^2S_0$ skew-boat conformation, giving a left-handed helix similar to those of the other GAG solid-state structures.

Early solid-state NMR studies (Winter *et al.*, 1986) had indicated that the conformation of the iduronate pyranose ring is similar in the solid and solution states. Solution NMR data available at that date clearly ruled out the $^4C_1$ chair form and seemed to indicate a distorted $^1C_4$ chair (Gatti *et al.*, 1979). This conclusion was not, however, supported by the ease with which DS is oxidized by periodate, which prefers adjacent equatorial hydroxyls such as are found in the $^4C_1$ chair. A more detailed examination of the proton–proton coupling constants of iduronate residues in GAGs indicated a conformational equilibrium between the $^1C_4$ chair and a $^2S_0$ skew-boat form at least; possibly also with small proportions of $^4C_1$ chair in the mix (Ferro *et al.*, 1990; Inuoe *et al.*, 1990). Both the $^2S_0$ skew boat and the $^4C_1$ chair are susceptible to periodate oxidation; in spite of this the controversy continued. Some authors find this equilibrium explanation convincing (Scott *et al.*, 1995) and other prefer the idea of a single, distorted $^1C_4$ chair (Rao *et al.*, 1995). Molecular dynamics studies, interpreted together with NMR data, have indicated that the $^2S_0$ skew-boat form may itself be a simplification of a rapidly interchanging group of related boat and skew-boat conformations (Forster and Mulloy, 1993). Modeling of a DS oligosaccharide into the active site of chondroitinase B has indicated a $^{2,5}B$ boat form for one of the iduronate rings, a conformation closely related to the $^2S_0$ skew boat by pseudorotation through a low-energy barrier (Michel *et al.*, 2004). This additional source of internal mobility may have functional significance; the iduronate-containing sequences of HS bear patterns of sulfate substitution conferring differential specificity for protein ligands such as growth factors and their receptors, and DS also has affinity for some of the same proteins (Penc *et al.*, 1998).

VI. Structures of CS Proteoglycans

The many and varied structures of PGs have been well reviewed elsewhere (Hardingham and Fosang, 1992; Iozzo, 1998; Knudson and Knudson, 2001). As they are by definition glycosylated and are sometimes very large, neither x-ray crystallography nor NMR spectroscopy has been able to provide structural information at atomic resolution. The structural biology of whole PGs is put together piecemeal from several techniques, and when dealing with the structural PGs of cartilage the subject overlaps heavily with the areas of biomechanics and materials science. Two PGs will here serve as illustrations: the large matrix PG aggrecan and the small, leucine rich PG decorin.

Aggrecan is the main structural PG of articular cartilage and has been the subject of structural studies by a variety of physicochemical methods. Each core protein bears many CS chains, closely spaced along its central extended CS1 and CS2 domains. Aggrecan associates (through its globular G1 domain) with hyaluronate and link protein, forming a supramolecular complex with collagen, which produces the exceptional biomechanical properties of cartilage. Figure 4 shows an atomic force microscopy (AFM) image (Ng *et al.*, 2003) that illustrates the "mop-like" structure of this PG; the polysaccharides, however flexible they may be in theory, are so close to their neighbors (the GAG–GAG spacing is about 4 nm) that they have little freedom to do other than adopt an extended conformation such as the x-ray structures shown in Fig. 4. Incidentally, these images also give the impression that all or most of the chondroitin side chains are similar in length; the "mop" looks quite tidy, especially in the case of fetal epiphyseal cartilage (Fig. 4). These closely packed, negatively charged polysaccharides, with their counterions and solvation shells, are well designed for a space-filling role in cartilage, providing an elastic cushion effect under conditions of load. It has been estimated by a theoretical biomechanics study that CS intermolecular electrostatic repulsive forces are responsible for about 50% of the equilibrium compressive modulus of articular cartilage (Dean *et al.*, 2003); this figure was in reasonable agreement with the results from a nanomechanics study in which the repulsive force between two chondroitin substituted surfaces, a probe tip and a planar substrate, was measured (Seog *et al.*, 2005). The coarse-grained molecular modeling system of Bathe *et al.* (2005a) has been used to predict the effects of CS structure on osmotic pressure in aqueous solution (Bathe *et al.*, 2005b); neither the position nor the extent of sulfation of CS chains is predicted to affect osmotic pressure at physiological ionic strength. The fine structure of chondroitin chains and differences in 4- and 6-sulfation in different circumstances do not affect such bulk properties; simple charge-density models of CS as a polyelectrolyte are adequate. The observed variations of chondroitin fine structure with changes in tissue environment have more complex explanations, which may involve sequence specific interactions with proteins. For example, Sauerland *et al.* (2003) have investigated changes in CS sequence in response to mechanical loading in cartilage explants and found that the 4,6 disulfated nonreducing caps of CS decrease in abundance. These terminal sequences, in heavily glycosylated PGs, are those that most accessible for such interactions.

The mobility of the various components of cartilage may be investigated by ^{13}C NMR relaxation times. Comparison of isolated chondroitin and its monosaccharides with whole cartilage samples has shown that the carbohydrate component of cartilage retains mobility, whereas the protein components remain relatively rigid (Huster *et al.*, 2002; Naji *et al.*, 2000).

A   Fetal epiphyseal   B   Mature nasal

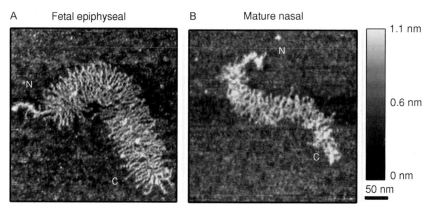

FIGURE 4   Atomic force microscopy images: (A) Fetal epiphyseal aggrecan; (B): Adult nasal aggrecan. The N-terminal globular domains, as well as the heavily glycosylated CS domains, can clearly be seen. The closely packed chondroitin side-chains are shorter and perhaps have a wider length distribution, in the adult PG. Reproduced with permission from Ng *et al.* (2003). (See Color Insert.)

The case for aggregation between GAG molecules in the ECM has been summarized by Scott (1992), based on a variety of theoretical and experimental methods including besides the NMR and x-ray work already mentioned, additional studies using electron microscopy, by which method aggregation into a mesh was demonstrated particularly clearly for C6S (Scott *et al.*, 1992).

A structurally and functionally different group of PGs are known as small leucine-rich proteoglycans (SLRPs), of which decorin will serve as an example. The SLRPs bear only a few sidechains and clearly cannot perform the same type of structural role as aggrecan, for example. Decorin, which bears a single CS or DS sidechain, has been associated with collagen assembly; electron micrographic studies have visualized single extended GAG chains orthogonal to the direction of collagen fibrils (Scott, 1992). Theoretical studies (Redaelli *et al.*, 2003) have indicated that the GAG chains may be able to cross-link collagen fibrils by noncovalent interactions, transferring forces from one to the other without rupture under moderate strain, but there is at present a dearth of experimental evidence for the nature of the fibril–PG interactions.

VII. Chondroitin as a Covalent Cross-Link Between Two or More Proteins

The small PG bikunin is a component of the inter-alpha-trypsin inhibitor (ITI) protein complexes (Zhuo *et al.*, 2002). Its single chondroitin chain has the unusual property of acting as a covalent link between the three protein components of the complex (bikunin) and heavy chains 1 (HC1) and 2 (HC2). HC1 and HC2 are attached via ester linkages near the nonreducing end of the CS chain. This is more than a merely unusual structure; the side proteins are transferred from the CS linker to hyaluronan (Rugg *et al.*, 2005), forming a complex that is essential for ECM formation in some critical tissues such as the cumulus oophorus. Without the presentation of HC1 and HC2 by CS-bikunin this complex cannot form, resulting in infertility. So far, no examples of covalent CS cross-linking outside the ITI family have been described.

VIII. Crystal Structures of Complexes Between Chondroitin Degrading Enzymes and Oligosaccharides _____

Experimentally determined structures of complexes between chondroitin and proteins are limited to a few bacterial enzymes that degrade chondroitin. These have, however, provided a good deal of interesting information concerning the structures of the enzymes, their mechanisms, and the structures of the oligosaccharides bound in their active sites (Section III). The enzymes for which structures of complexes have so far been published are the chondroitin AC lyases of *Pedobacter heparinus* (formerly known as *Flavobacterium heparinum*) (Huang *et al.*, 2001) and of *Arthrobacter aurescens* (Lunin *et al.*, 2004); the chondroitin B lyase of *P. heparinus* (Michel *et al.*, 2004) and the hyaluronate lyase of *Streptococcus pneumoniae* (Rigden and Jedrzejas, 2003). Both of the chondroitin AC lyases belong to the same fold family (in the SCOP system: http://scop.mrc-lmb.cam.ac.uk) as the hyaluronate lyase, an α/α toroid in which several α-hairpins are arranged in a circle (Fig. 5A). The chondroitinase B has a quite different structure, a right-handed β-helix, and its mode of binding with its substrate and lytic mechanism are distinct from the other enzymes, although all of them cleave the $1 \rightarrow 4$ linkage, leaving an unsaturated uronic acid at the nonreducing end of one of the oligosaccharide products by a β-elimination reaction. This uronic acid has the same structure regardless of whether it originated as a glucuronate or iduronate residue.

The structures of the cocrystals have been deposited in the PDB (http://www.rcsb.org/pdb/). Some of them are listed in Table I, but these do not include the disaccharide complexes such as those reported by Huang *et al.* (2003). The hyaluronate lyase and the chondroitinase AC lyases bind to the oligosaccharides by a mixture of ring stacking, between the pyranose rings of the sugars and tryptophan residues in the protein, and ionic interactions between basic amino acid side-chains and the sulfate and carboxylate groups on the oligosaccharide. Their mechanisms of action are also similar. Differences between these closely related enzymes are subtle but account for the differences in activity between them. For example, the detailed amino acid

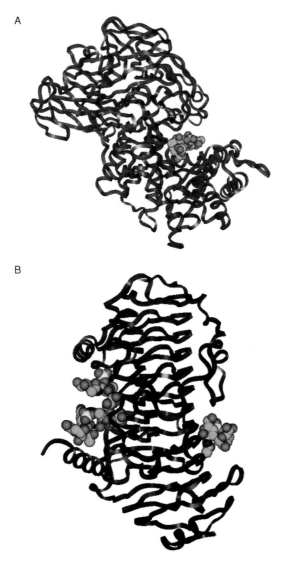

FIGURE 5 Crystal structures of chondroitin-degrading enzymes in complex with oligosaccharides. The proteins are shown as ribbons that follow the backbone atoms, and the oligosaccharides are shown in a space-filling representation colored as in Fig. 2. (A) Chondroitin AC lyase, with a C4S tetrasaccharide in the active site (Huang *et al.*, 2001). (B) Chondroitin B lyase, with a DS hexasaccharide degraded into three disaccharides in the binding site (on the left of the image) (Michel *et al.*, 2004). These two enzymes are unrelated in structure, in the way they bind to the substrate and in their mechanism of action. Chondroitin B lyase displays a dermatan binding site distant from the active site, occupied in this structure by a DS disaccharide (on the right of the image). (See Color Insert.)

sequence at the active site of the *Arthrobacter* enzyme causes one of the glucuronate residues to adopt a distorted pyranose ring form; this may explain why it acts as an exolyase (clipping successive disaccharides from the nonreducing end of a chondroitin chain), whereas the *Pedobacter* enzyme, which can accommodate the glucuronic acid without strain, is an endolyase, cutting at random points within the polysaccharide chain. The hyaluronate lyase of *S. pneumoniae* can cleave both hyaluronate and C6S but cannot cleave at the reducing side of a 4-sulfated GalNAc, so leaving a uniform C4S chain intact. It is surmised that hyaluronate lyase evolved from a chondroitin lyase ancestor, its specificity having shifted but retaining some activity toward chondroitins (Rigden and Jedrzejas, 2003).

Chondroitinase B is the only enzyme that cleaves DS as its only substrate. Besides its different protein fold, this enzyme forms a completely distinct type of complex with its substrate and acts by a different mechanism. Interactions between the protein and oligosaccharides are principally electrostatic in nature, including ionic interactions and hydrogen bonding. There are no ring-stacking interactions. Unlike the other enzymes discussed, chondroitin B lyase requires calcium for its activity. The calcium ion is coordinated with the carboxyl of iduronate, which may determine the selectivity of the enzyme for iduronate rather than glucuronate (Michel *et al.*, 2004).

Another factor of considerable interest in these enzymes is the presence of additional carbohydrate binding sites, separate from the active sites of the enzymes. Such a site may exist in the N-terminal part of the *S. pneumoniae* hyaluronate lyase not included in the crystal structure (Rigden and Jedrzejas, 2003). For the *P. heparinus* chondroitinase B, a positively charged site on the opposite side of the protein from the active site is occupied by a DS disaccharide in the crystal structure (Michel *et al.*, 2004) (Fig. 5B). The function of such a site is a matter for speculation, but it has been suggested that it may help in the disruption by the enzyme of charge-based aggregates in the matrix, allowing the presentation of a single DS chain to the active site for processing.

Chondroitin ABC lyase I, a useful enzyme with wide specificity, has been crystallized alone, but no cocrystal with a chondroitin oligosaccharide has been published to date. Its close structural relationship to the other α/α toroidal chondroitinases has, however, been used to model such a complex, based on the coordinates for the ABC lyase (Huang *et al.*, 2003) and those for the AC lyase/oligosaccharide complexes (Huang *et al.*, 2001). Mutagenesis and other biochemical data have allowed the mapping of individual residues in the active site and their roles in the catalytic mechanism (Prabhakar *et al.*, 2005).

A

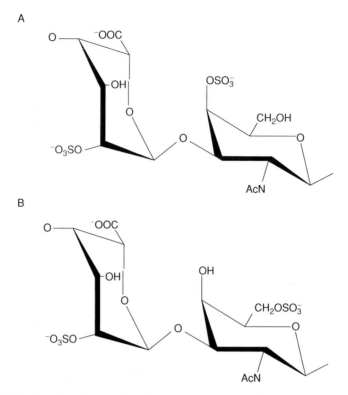

B

FIGURE 6   Repeating disaccharides of (A) sequence in mammalian DS with high affinity for heparin cofactor II; at least a hexasaccharide length of this structure is necessary within the DS polysaccharide, most of which has the structure depicted in Fig. 1(B), and (B) a DS like polysaccharide from *Ascidia nigra*, with negligible affinity for heparin cofactor II. This polysaccharide is almost fully sulfated at the 2-position of iduronate.

IX. Specificity of Interactions Between Chondroitin Sequences and Proteins

Chondroitin in its context as a component of ECM has been regarded as a bulk polysaccharide, acting as a hydrated, negatively charged space-filler. However, recent findings implicating chondroitin as a modulator of growth, development, and infection require a more detailed account of individual protein–GAG interactions (Sugahara *et al.*, 2003). This is not the place for a detailed account of progress in structural determination of CS structures with specific affinities for particular proteins, but the question of chondroitin binding sites on proteins, and the specificity with which they recognize their ligands, is an important consideration in their structural biology.

Evidence in this area is sparse, compared with the analogous case for the GAG HS; the "heparin binding proteins" are generally supposed to have less highly sulfated HS sequences as their native ligands. The best studied example of a protein that binds to both heparin and to a member of the CS family is heparin cofactor II (HCII), a plasma serine protease that inhibits thrombin, the coagulation enzyme that converts fibrinogen to fibrin, causing blood to clot. Unlike the more abundant plasma serpin, antithrombin, HCII can be activated either by heparin or by DS; the sequence in DS with high affinity for HCII is known and consists of a sequence with both 4-sulfation of the galactosamine and 2-sulfation of the iduronic acid residue (Maimone and Tollefsen, 1991) (Fig. 6). This sequence forms only a small proportion of mammalian DS. The heparin and dermatan binding sites on HCII overlap, but interestingly, they are not identical (Tollefsen, 1994). These two highly anionic glycans are not simply binding to a nonspecific basic patch on the protein surface. Further evidence for specificity has been provided by DS-like compounds from marine invertebrates. One such compound, from the sea squirt *Ascidia nigra*, consists almost entirely of alternating 2-sulfated iduronate and 6-sulfated *N*-acetyl galactosamine (Pavao *et al.*, 1995) (Fig. 6). This compound, although highly sulfated, does not bind to or activate HCII. The difference in activity due to this altered substitution, from the 4-sulfation of mammalian DS to the 6-sulfation of the ascidian DS, demonstrates clear structural specificity. It is reasonable to expect similar cases of specific interactions to be demonstrated in the future also for the glucuronate-containing chondroitins in their interactions with, for example, selectins, growth factors, and pathogens (Sugahara *et al.*, 2003).

References

IUPAC-IUB Joint Commission on Biochemical Nomenclature (JCBN) (1983). Symbols for specifying the conformation of polysaccharide chains: Recommendations 1981. *Eur. J. Biochem.* **131**, 5–7.

Almond, A., and Sheehan, J. K. (2000). Glycosaminoglycan conformation: Do aqueous molecular dynamics simulations agree with x-ray fiber diffraction? *Glycobiology* **10**, 329–338.

Bathe, M., Rutledge, G. C., Grodzinsky, A. J., and Tidor, B. (2005a). A coarse-grained molecular model for glycosaminoglycans: Application to chondroitin, chondroitin sulfate, and hyaluronic acid. *Biophys. J.* **88**, 3870–3887.

Bathe, M., Rutledge, G. C., Grodzinsky, A. J., and Tidor, B. (2005b). Osmotic pressure of aqueous chondroitin sulfate solution: A molecular modeling investigation. *Biophys. J.* **89**, 2357–2371.

Bayraktar, H., Akal, E., Sarper, O., and Varnali, T. (2004). Modeling glycosaminoglycans: Hyaluronan, chondroitin, chondroitin sulfate A, chondroitin sulfate C and keratan sulfate. *J. Mol. Struct.: THEOCHEM* **683**, 121–132.

Cael, J. J., Winter, W. T., and Arnott, S. (1978). Calcium chondroitin 4-sulfate: Molecular conformation and organization of polysaccharide chains in a proteoglycan. *J. Mol. Biol.* **125**, 21–42.

Dean, D., Seog, J., Ortiz, C., and Grodzinsky, A. J. (2003). Molecular-level theoretical model for electrostatic interactions within polyelectrolyte brushes: Applications to charged glycosaminoglycans. *Langmuir* **19**, 5526–5539.

Ferro, D. R., Provasoli, A., Ragazzi, M., Casu, B., Torri, G., Bossennec, V., Perly, B., Sinay, P., Petitou, M., and Choay, J. (1990). Conformer populations of L-iduronic acid residues in glycosaminoglycan sequences. *Carbohydr. Res.* **195,** 157–167.

Forster, M. J., and Mulloy, B. (1993). Molecular-dynamics study of iduronate ring conformation. *Biopolymers* **33,** 575–588.

Gatti, G., Casu, B., Torri, G., and Vercellotti, J. R. (1979). Resolution-enhanced 1H-NMR spectra of dermatan sulfate and chondroitin sulfates: Conformation of the uronic acid residues. *Carbohydr. Res.* **68,** C3–C7.

Hardingham, T. E., and Fosang, A. J. (1992). Proteoglycans: Many forms and many functions. *FASEB J.* **6,** 861–870.

Huang, W., Boju, L., Tkalec, L., Su, H., Yang, H. O., Gunay, N. S., Linhardt, R. J., Yeong, S. K., Matte, A., and Cygler, M. (2001). Active site of chondroitin AC lyase revealed by the structure of enzyme: Oligosaccharide complexes and mutagenesis. *Biochemistry* **40,** 2359–2372.

Huang, W., Lunin, V., Li, Y., Suzuki, S., Sugiura, N., Miyazono, H., and Cygler, M. (2003). Crystal structure of *Proteus vulgaris* chondroitin sulfate ABC lyase I at 1.9 Å resolution. *J. Mol. Biol.* **328,** 623–634.

Huster, D., Schiller, J., and Arnold, K. (2002). Comparison of collagen dynamics in articular cartilage and isolated fibrils by solid-state NMR spectroscopy. *Magn. Reson. Med.* **48,** 624–632.

Huster, D., Naji, L., Schiller, J., and Arnold, K. (2004). Dynamics of the biopolymers in articular cartilage studied by magic angle spinning NMR. *Appl. Magn. Reson.* **27,** 471–487.

Inuoe, Y., Inouye, Y., and Nagasawa, K. (1990). Conformational equilibria of the L-iduronate residue in non-sulphated di-, tetra- and hexa-saccharides and their alditols derived from dermatan sulphate. *Biochem. J.* **265,** 533–538.

Iozzo, R. V. (1998). Matrix proteoglycans: From molecular design to cellular function. *Annu. Rev. Biochem.* **67,** 609–652.

Kaufmann, J., Mohle, K., Hofmann, H. J., and Arnold, K. (1999). Molecular dynamics of a tetrasaccharide subunit of chondroitin 4-sulfate in water. *Carbohydr. Res.* **318,** 1–9.

Knudson, C. B., and Knudson, W. (2001). Cartilage proteoglycans. *Semin. Cell Dev. Biol.* **12,** 69–78.

Lunin, V. V., Li, Y., Linhardt, R. J., Miyazono, H., Kyogashima, M., Kaneko, T., Bell, A. W., and Cygler, M. (2004). High-resolution crystal structure of *Arthrobacter aurescens* chondroitin AC lyase: An enzyme-substrate complex defines the catalytic mechanism. *J. Mol. Biol.* **337,** 367–386.

Maimone, M. M., and Tollefsen, D. M. (1991). Structure of a dermatan sulfate hexasaccharide that binds to heparin cofactor II with high affinity. *J. Biol. Chem.* **266,** 14830.

Michel, G., Pojasek, K., Li, Y., Sulea, T., Linhardt, R. J., Raman, R., Prabhakar, V., Sasisekharan, R., and Cygler, M. (2004). The structure of chondroitin B lyase complexed with glycosaminoglycan oligosaccharides unravels a calcium-dependent catalytic machinery. *J. Biol. Chem.* **279,** 32882–32896.

Mitra, A. K., Arnott, S., Atkins, E. D. T., and Isaac, D. H. (1983). Dermatan sulfate: Molecular conformations and interactions in the condensed state. *J. Mol. Biol.* **169,** 873–901.

Mucci, A., Schenetti, L., and Volpi, N. (2000). ^{1}H and ^{13}C nuclear magnetic resonance identification and characterization of components of chondroitin sulfates of various origin. *Carbohyd. Polym.* **41,** 37–45.

Mulloy, B., Forster, M. J., Jones, C., and Davies, D. B. (1993). NMR and molecular-modelling studies of the solution conformation of heparin. *Biochem. J.* **293,** 849–858.

Naji, L., Kaufmann, J., Huster, D., Schiller, J., and Arnold, K. (2000). ^{13}C NMR relaxation studies on cartilage and cartilage components. *Carbohydr. Res.* **327,** 439–446.

Ng, L., Grodzinsky, A. J., Patwari, P., Ortiz, C., Sandy, J., and Plaas, A. (2003). Individual cartilage aggrecan macromolecules and their constituent glycosaminoglycans visualized via atomic force microscopy. *J. Struct. Biol.* **143,** 242–257.

Pavao, M. S. G., Mourao, P. A. S., Mulloy, B., and Tollefsen, D. M. (1995). A unique dermatan sulfate-like glycosaminoglycan from ascidian: Its structure and the effect of its unusual sulfation pattern on anticoagulant activity. *Blood* **86**, 3523.

Penc, S. F., Pomahac, B., Winkler, T., Dorschner, R. A., Eriksson, E., Herndon, M., and Gallo, R. L. (1998). Dermatan sulfate released after injury is a potent promoter of fibroblast growth factor-2 function. *J. Biol. Chem.* **273**, 28116–28121.

Prabhakar, V., Raman, R., Capila, I., Bosques, C. J., Pojasek, K., and Sasisekharan, R. (2005). Biochemical characterization of the chondroitinase ABC I active site. *Biochem. J.* **390**, 395–405.

Rao, V. S., Balaji, P. V., and Qasba, P. K. (1995). Controversial iduronate ring conformation in dermatan sulphate. *Glycobiology* **5**, 273–279.

Redaelli, A., Vesentini, S., Soncini, M., Vena, P., Mantero, S., and Montevecchi, F. M. (2003). Possible role of decorin glycosaminoglycans in fibril to fibril force transfer in relative mature tendons—a computational study from molecular to microstructural level. *J. Biomech.* **36**, 1555–1569.

Rigden, D. J., and Jedrzejas, M. J. (2003). Structures of *Streptococcus pneumoniae* hyaluronate lyase in complex with chondroitin and chondroitin sulfate disaccharides: Insights into specificity and mechanism of action. *J. Biol. Chem.* **278**, 50596–50606.

Rugg, M. S., Willis, A. C., Mukhopadhyay, D., Hascall, V. C., Fries, E., Fulop, C., Milner, C. M., and Day, A. J. (2005). Characterization of complexes formed between TSG-6 and Inter-alpha-inhibitor that act as intermediates in the covalent transfer of heavy chains onto hyaluronan. *J. Biol. Chem.* **280**, 25674–25686.

Sauerland, K., Plaas, A. H., Raiss, R. X., and Steinmeyer, J. (2003). The sulfation pattern of chondroitin sulfate from articular cartilage explants in response to mechanical loading. *Biochim. Biophys. Acta* **1638**, 241–248.

Scott, J. E. (1992). Supramolecular organization of extracellular matrix glycosaminoglycans, *in vitro* and in the tissues. *FASEB J.* **6**, 2639–2645.

Scott, J. E., Chen, Y., and Brass, A. (1992). Secondary and tertiary structures involving chondroitin and chondroitin sulphates in solution, investigated by rotary shadowing/electron microscopy and computer simulation. *Eur. J. Biochem.* **209**, 675–680.

Scott, J. E., Heatley, F., and Wood, B. (1995). Comparison of secondary structures in water of chondroitin-4-sulfate and dermatan sulfate: Implications in the formation of tertiary structures. *Biochemistry* **34**, 15467–15474.

Seog, J., Dean, D., Rolauffs, B., Wu, T., Genzer, J., Plaas, A. H. K., Grodzinsky, A. J., and Ortiz, C. (2005). Nanomechanics of opposing glycosaminoglycan macromolecules. *J. Biomech.* **38**, 1789–1797.

Sugahara, K., Mikami, T., Uyama, T., Mizuguchi, S., Nomura, K., and Kitagawa, H. (2003). Recent advances in the structural biology of chondroitin sulfate and dermatan sulfate. *Curr. Opin. Struct. Biol.* **13**, 612–620.

Tollefsen, D. M. (1994). The interaction of glycosaminoglycans with heparin cofactor II. *Ann. N. Y. Acad. Sci.* **714**, 21–31.

Venkataraman, G., Sasisekharan, V., Cooney, C. L., Langer, R., and Sasisekharan, R. (1994). A stereochemical approach to pyranose ring flexibility: Its implications for the conformation of dermatan sulfate. *Proc. Natl. Acad. Sci. USA* **91**, 6171–6175.

Vieira, R. P., Mulloy, B., and Mourao, P. A. (1991). Structure of a fucose-branched chondroitin sulfate from sea cucumber: Evidence for the presence of 3-O-sulfo-beta-D-glucuronosyl residues. *J. Biol. Chem.* **266**, 13530–13536.

Winter, W. T., Arnott, S., Isaac, D. H., and Atkins, E. D. (1978). Chondroitin 4-sulfate: The structure of a sulfated glycosaminoglycan. *J. Mol. Biol.* **125**, 1–19.

Winter, W. T., Taylor, M. G., and Stevens, E. S. (1986). Solid-state 13C NMR and X-ray diffraction of dermatan sulfate. *Biochem. Biophys. Res. Commun.* **137**, 87–93.

Zhuo, L., Salustri, A., and Kimata, K. (2002). A physiological function of serum proteoglycan bikunin: The chondroitin sulfate moiety plays a central role. *Glycoconj. J.* **19**, 241–247.

Vikas Prabhakar and Ram Sasisekharan

Division of Biological Engineering
Massachusetts Institute of Technology
Cambridge, Massachusetts 02139

The Biosynthesis and Catabolism of Galactosaminoglycans

I. GalAG Biopolymers

A. Introduction

The glycosaminoglycan (GAG) family of structurally complex linear polysaccharides is composed of four chemically distinct subsets: the heparin and heparan sulfate (HS) GAGs, the chondroitin and dermatan sulfate (CS and DS, respectively) GAGs, keratan sulfate (KS), and hyaluronic acid (Ernst *et al.*, 1995). The following material focuses on GAGs of the CS and DS type, also known as galactosaminoglycans (GalAGs). Covered herein are the most prominent details concerning GalAG structure, their roles in biology and medicine, GalAG biosynthesis, their *in vivo* cellular degradation, and analytical biotechnologies pertinent to the study of GalAGs (Fig. 1).

The study of biological phenomena, from the molecular to the tissue level, has evolved substantially as scientists have focused on the emerging

Advances in Pharmacology, Volume 53
Copyright 2006, Elsevier Inc. All rights reserved.

1054-3589/06 $35.00
DOI: 10.1016/S1054-3589(06)53005-9

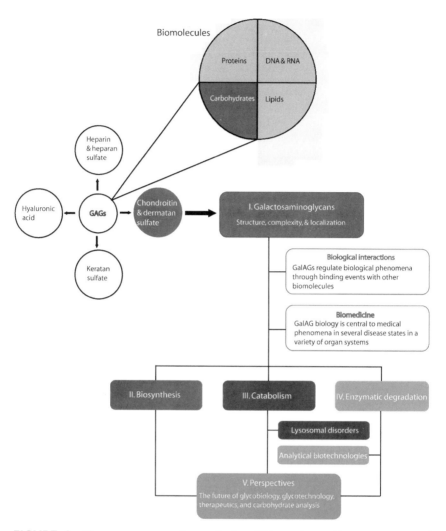

FIGURE I Chapter contents and organization. This work provides an overview of chondroitin and dermatan sulfate GAGs, including their structure, roles in biology and pathogenesis, biosynthesis, cellular degradation, and enzymatic degradation.

paradigm of extracellular regulation of cell function. GAG polysaccharides are attached to a protein core and are impelled to the cell surface and into the extracellular space. The cell surface machinery at the cell–extracellular matrix (ECM) interface acts as a complex battery of regulators that dynamically modulates outside cues from diverse signaling molecules. Specifically, GAGs govern signaling molecules by controlling their effective concentration and state at the cell surface.

B. Composition and Chemical Complexity

GalAGs are composed of a disaccharide repeat unit of uronic acid [α-L-iduronic acid (IdoA) or β-D-glucuronic acid (GlcA)] (1→3) linked to N-acetyl-D-galactosamine (GalNAc). These basic disaccharide units are linearly associated via β(1→4) linkages to form GalAG polymers (Fig. 2). In CS, all of the uronic acid moieties are GlcA. In DS, epimerization at the C-5 position of the uronic acid moiety during biosynthesis results in a mixture of IdoA and GlcA epimers. Biosynthesis of CS and DS also involves chemical modification of the sugar backbone at various positions, generating diversity in oligosaccharide sequences. CS is commonly O-sulfated at the C-4 of the galactosamine (chondroitin-4-sulfate, C4S, also known as CS-A) or the C6 of the galactosamine (chondroitin-6-sulfate, C6S, also known as CS-C). Less common modifications in CS, such as 2-O- or 3-O-sulfation of the GlcA moiety, have also been reported (Nadanaka and Sugahara, 1997; Sugahara *et al.*, 1996). DS (also known as CS-B) is commonly O-sulfated at C-4 of GalNAc; O-sulfation at C-6 of GalNAc and C-2 of IdoA also occasionally occur.

The various backbone modifications in GAG biopolymers confer infinitely more chemical complexity when compared to DNA and proteins. Theoretically, the five different modifications possible for each disaccharide unit give rise to $2^5 = 32$ chemical combinations. In comparison, DNA is composed of only four basic building blocks, and proteins are made up of 20 amino acids. This vast complexity makes these biopolymers among the most information-rich in nature.

C. Structural Features

GAGs are distinguished from other polysaccharides as a distinct class by their related backbone moieties. Modification of these backbone elements confers great diversity among GAGs. The heterogeneity of GAG sequences is notable, especially when compared to other biopolymers like DNA and proteins. The template-based biosynthesis of these molecules has greatly facilitated their study; in contrast, the nontemplate-driven biosynthesis of complex polysaccharides has largely suppressed attempts at their analysis. DS is predominantly 4-O-sulfated. Iduronic acid content of DS is variable and has been reported as low as 7% and as high as 93%, depending on tissue origin and the method of compositional analysis (Linhardt *et al.*, 1991; Maimone and Tollefsen, 1990; Poole, 1986). In CS, copolymers with both 4-O- and 6-O-sulfation in the same chain occur often (Ernst *et al.*, 1995). Individual CS residues sometimes are sulfated at both the 4-O- and 6-O-positions (Linhardt *et al.*, 1991). Two levels of organization have been described for GalAGs. Macroscopically, clustering of residues in DS results in regions with IdoA and a high degree of sulfation interspersed with regions

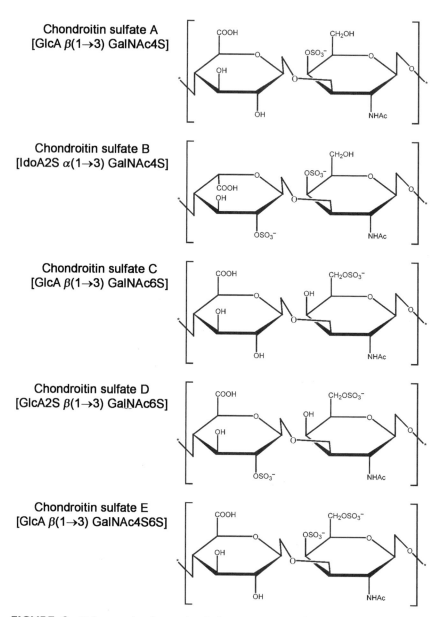

Chondroitin sulfate A
[GlcA β(1→3) GalNAc4S]

Chondroitin sulfate B
[IdoA2S α(1→3) GalNAc4S]

Chondroitin sulfate C
[GlcA β(1→3) GalNAc6S]

Chondroitin sulfate D
[GlcA2S β(1→3) GalNAc6S]

Chondroitin sulfate E
[GlcA β(1→3) GalNAc4S6S]

FIGURE 2 Galactosaminoglycan chemical structure. Biopolymers of the chondroitin sulfate and dermatan sulfate type are composed of a basic building block, a disaccharide consisting of an uronic acid β(1→3) linked to GalNAc. These disaccharide units are linearly associated via β(1→4) linkages. In the case of CS, all of the uronic acid moieties correspond to the glucuronic acid epimerization state. For DS, modification of the uronic acid C5 position during biosynthesis leads to a mixture of epimers within the chain. Common sulfation patterns within the oligosaccharide backbones are indicated for each GalAG form. Additionally, CS-A and CS-C are sometimes sulfated at the 2-O- or 3-O-positions of GlcA. The CS-B form is also known as DS. DS occasionally incorporates O-sulfation at GalNAc C6.

with GlcA and a lower degree of sulfation (Fransson *et al.*, 1990). Sulfation at the 6-O-position of CS often seems to be clustered near the chain termina (Cheng *et al.*, 1992). Microscopically, specific sequences of GAGs are functionally relevant. Rare residues can, in fact, have critical physiological functions. A specific DS hexasaccharide, for instance, has a specific affinity for heparin cofactor II (Maimone and Tollefsen, 1990). These two levels of organization, therefore, are important in modulating the physical form of GAGs and in regulating the specific interaction between a GAG and another biomolecule. Form is also a function of the ionic environment, which can shield repulsive ionic forces between charged chains.

In solution, CS seems to exist in defined spatial orientations; DS has a flexible conformation (Casu *et al.*, 1988; Venkataraman *et al.*, 1994). A central issue, a controversial one, regarding the structural diversity of GAGs is the conformational flexibility of the iduronate residue (Ferro *et al.*, 1990; Mitra *et al.*, 1983; Venkataraman *et al.*, 1994; Winter *et al.*, 1986). The four main conformers of IdoA are $^1C_4$, $^4C_1$, $^2T_0$, and $^0T_2$. These conformers for IdoA are stereochemically satisfactory and are consistent with the available physico-chemical data. Interconversion between IdoA puckers may generate chain conformational flexibility, facilitating interaction with proteins (Casu *et al.*, 1986).

Rotary shadowing/electron microscopy studies have revealed that C6S is capable of forming aggregates of two or more chains (Scott *et al.*, 1992). The charge distribution of the twofold helix of C6S is near the periphery, creating regions of hydrophobicity. Such hydrophobic zones from separate chains can interact with each other. Chondroitin-4-sulfate is incapable of such network formation, as sulfate groups are clustered close to the helical axis, minimizing aggregation behavior. Although C4S cannot self-aggregate, it is capable of association with DS. Alternating IdoA and GlcA in DS can self-associate in the absence of divalent cations under physiological conditions (Fransson and Coster, 1979). Chemical modification of the sugar backbone, hydrogen bonding, and cation chelation are critical determinants of self-aggregation potential and solid-state structural conformation, necessary for conferring the biological information inherent in GAG biomolecules.

D. GalAG Proteoglycans

GalAGs' chains, as with all other members of the GAG family with the exception of hyaluronic acid, occur as constituents of proteoglycans (PGs) (Table I) (Iozzo, 1998). As such, they are attached, via a glycosidic linkage, to a serine residue in a core protein through a tetrasaccharide composed of glucuronic acid-galactose-galactose-xylose. Core proteins can range in size from 10 to 500 kDa. CS is usually found in large aggregating PGs with 20–100 sidechains; DS occurs primarily in smaller PGs with 2–8 sidechains (Poole, 1986). Overall PG size ranges from 80 to 3500 kDa

TABLE I Galactosaminoglycan Proteoglycans

Core protein	Expression	References
Bamacan	Basement membranes	Ghiselli and Iozzo, 2000
Decorin	Connective tissue, cornea	Reed et al., 2005
Biglycan	Bone, cartilage, skin	Kinsella et al., 2004; Wadhwa et al., 2004
Thrombomodulin	Endothelia, cornea	Sadler, 1997
Astrochondrin	Glia	Streit et al., 1993
Collagen IX	Cartilage	Bishop, 2000
Endocan	Endothelia	Bechard et al., 2001
Epiphycan	Cartilage	Knudson and Knudson, 2001
Serglycin	Myeloid cells, granules	Valiyaveettil et al., 2004
Versican	Fibroblasts, connective tissue	Kinsella et al., 2004; Sheng et al., 2005
NG2	Glia	Blakemore et al., 2002
Neurocan	Glia, retinal and embryonic vasculature	Mishima and Hoffman, 2003; Zhang et al., 2003
CALEB	Glia, neurons	Schumacher et al., 1997
Aggrecan	Neurons, cartilage	Johnson et al., 2005
Brevican	Glia, neurons	Beggah et al., 2005
Phosphacan	Glia, neurons	Hayashi et al., 2005; Popp et al., 2003
Te38	Chick embryo brain	Monnier et al., 2003
Neuroglycan C	Cerebellum	Oohira et al., 2004
TAP-1	Nervous tissue	Iwata and Carlson, 1991
Testican-1, -2, -3	Neurons, glia	Edgell et al., 2004; Oohira et al., 2000
CD44	Lymphocytes	Lesley et al., 1997
Perlecan	Vasculature	Knudson and Knudson, 2001
APP	Glia	Umehara et al., 2004
Somatoglycan-S	Nervous tissue	Williams et al., 1994
Glypican-5	Neurons	Saunders et al., 1997
Syndecan-1	Nervous tissue	Deepa et al., 2004; Lee et al., 2004
CAT301, CAT315	Neurons	Lander et al., 1997

Adapted with permission from Trowbridge and Gallo (2002) and Hartmann and Maurer (2001).

(Ghiselli and Iozzo, 2000; Sadler, 1997; Silbert and Sugumaran, 2002; Streit et al., 1993).

E. GalAGs in Biology

Long thought of as inert structural components, GAGs have in recent years come to the forefront in the thinking of bioscientists as important modulators of biological phenomena. Polysaccharide structure governs myriad interactions between powerful biological players, imparting effects on cell function in both normal and aberrant pathophysiological states. Interactions between proteins and heparin/HS GAGs, and more recently GalAG polymers, have shed considerable light on basic biological functions. Further, the implications of these biomolecular interactions reverberate in importance through the entire cascade of biomedical events, from fundamental biological phenomena to clinical biomedicine.

II. GalAGs in the Extracellular Matrix

The ECM is a highly heterogeneous mixture of proteins, saccharides, and other biomolecules that surrounds cells. The ECM is instrumental in providing the physical support necessary for macromolecular organization into tissues and organs. Traditionally, the ECM was considered to be solely an inert scaffold providing structure. This conventional view has been overturned, and it has become apparent that the ECM is in fact a fundamental player in orchestrating cellular responses, both in normal and disease states.

GAGs are among the most important constituents of the ECM, as they interact with transient ECM molecules, such as growth factors, often resulting in a cascade of bioregulatory events including signal transduction and nuclear transcriptional phenomena (Kovanen and Pentikainen, 1999; Olsson *et al.*, 1999). These interactions impart profound implications on the type and strength of signaling in gene expression. The specialized functions elicited by GAG activity *in vivo* emphasize the importance of structural (and sequence) diversity among GAGs. In addition to binding heparin cofactor II (Tovar *et al.*, 2005), GalAGs also appear to be involved in a variety of processes, including the covalent crosslinking of the blood protein pre-α-inhibitor (Enghild *et al.*, 1991), infectivity mechanisms (Achur *et al.*, 2000; Alkhalil *et al.*, 2000; Schmidtchen *et al.*, 2001), and tenascin-X binding (Elefteriou *et al.*, 2001). GAGs are found in the ECM bound to structural proteins (including collagen, laminin, and fibronectin), aggregated with other PGs, or as constituents of integral membrane PGs (Hardingham and Fosang, 1992).

III. GalAG–Protein Interactions

GAGs bind a wide variety of ECM, intracellular, and plasma proteins (Table II) (Cardin and Weintraub, 1989; Frevert *et al.*, 2003; Garcia-Olivas *et al.*, 2003; Jackson *et al.*, 1991; Marino *et al.*, 2003; Murai *et al.*, 2004; Priglinger *et al.*, 1994; Proudfoot *et al.*, 2001; Schmidtchen *et al.*, 2001). Requirements for GAG–protein binding include sequence specificity within the oligosaccharide chain and, in many cases, a region of enriched basic amino acids for the protein (Cardin and Weintraub, 1989; Prabhakar *et al.*,

TABLE II Galactosaminoglycan–Protein Binding Interactions

Protein	GAGs bound	Physiologic effect	References
HC II	DS [IdoA2S-GalNAc4S]$_3$, Hep	Heparin inactivation	Liaw et al., 2001; Tovar et al., 2005
Thrombin	DS, Hep	Anticoagulation	Casu et al., 2004; Liaw et al., 2001
KGF	DS (oversulfated), HS	Wound healing	Trowbridge et al., 2002
Activ. Prot. C	DS, Hep	Anticoagulation	Fernandez et al., 1999
Protein C inhibitor	DS, HS, Hep	Stimulates serpin activity	Priglinger et al., 1994
Platelet factor 4	DS, Hep	Anticoagulation	Petersen et al., 1999
Collagen	DS	ECM stability	Iozzo, 1997
Fibronectin	DS, HS	ECM stability	Tumova et al., 2000
Tenascin-X	DS, HS	Collagen matrix stability	Elefteriou et al., 2001
α-defensin	DS	Increased infectivity	Schmidtchen et al., 2001
RANTES	DS, Hep, CS, HS	Inflammatory response	Proudfoot et al., 2001
Midkine	CS, HS	Neuronal development	Deepa et al., 2004
Interferon-γ	Hep, HS, DS	Receptor for IFN-γ	Brooks et al., 2000
TGF-β	DS	Growth regulation	Hildebrand et al., 1994
FGF-1 and -2	DS, Hep, HS (highly sulfated)	Cell proliferation	Tumova et al., 2000
HGF/SF	DS [IdoAGalNAc4S]$_4$, HS	Cell proliferation/cancer	Catlow et al., 2003
Pleiotrophin	CS	Morphogenesis in developing cerebellum	Tanaka et al., 2003
TSG-6	CS, HA	Inflammatory response; female fertility	Wisniewski et al., 2005
CD-44	CS, HA	Lymphocyte trafficking, tumorigenesis	Murai et al., 2004
Thyroglobulin	CS, DS, HA	Pathogenesis of thyroid-associated ophtalmopathy	Marino et al., 2003
PDGF	HS, CS	Cellular proliferation	Garcia-Olivas et al., 2003
EMR2	CS	Myeloid trafficking	Stacey et al., 2003
Interleukin-8	HS, CS	Pulmonary inflammation	Frevert et al., 2003
LDL	CS, HS, DS	Lipoprotein metabolism	Kovanen and Pentikainen, 1999; Olsson et al., 1999

Adapted with permission (Trowbridge and Gallo, 2002).

2005; Schreuder *et al.*, 1994). The spatial conformation of the GAG chain must be geometrically complementary to the protein's binding pocket. Since the protein is more rigid than the saccharide, it is likely that a given GAG molecule imparts some level of conformational flexibility that facilitates the interaction (Grootenhuis *et al.*, 1994; Ornitz *et al.*, 1995; Thompson *et al.*, 1994; Venkataraman *et al.*, 1994).

IV. GalAGs in Biomedicine

A. Cell Signaling and Cancer

Although there has long been a dedicated exploration of HS involvement in signaling, only recently have GalAGs emerged as central players. The GalAG constituents of PGs are critical regulators of growth factor and cytokine signaling (Table II) (Brooks *et al.*, 2000; Hildebrand *et al.*, 1994; Stacey *et al.*, 2003; Wisniewski *et al.*, 2005). Further, GalAG chains are central to a variety of interactions modulating ECM-mediated cell-to-cell signaling. For example, chondroitin sulfate proteoglycans (CSPGs) on neutrophils specifically bind to platelet factor 4 and are responsible for cellular activation (Petersen *et al.*, 1998, 1999). Interactions of DS chains with fibroblast growth factor-2 (FGF-2) and keratinocyte growth factor have been characterized with respect to cellular proliferation and wound repair (Trowbridge and Gallo, 2002; Trowbridge *et al.*, 2002). DS is additionally capable of activating the hepatocyte growth factor/scatter factor signaling pathway through the c-met receptor (Catlow *et al.*, 2003; Lyon *et al.*, 1998, 2002). The same signaling cascade can promote cell proliferation through endocan, a PG composed of both CS and DS sidechains (Bechard *et al.*, 2001). CS and DS chains found in the PG versican bind L-selectin, P-selectin, and chemokines, significant in leukocyte trafficking and inflammatory disease (Kawashima *et al.*, 2002; Kinsella *et al.*, 2004; Lesley *et al.*, 1997; Sheng *et al.*, 2005; Sugahara *et al.*, 2003).

Dermatan sulfate proteoglycans (DSPGs) play an active role both in modulating ECM integrity and cellular signaling processes, and it therefore follows that DS has also been implicated in oncogenesis and angiogenesis (Nelimarkka *et al.*, 2001). GAG-degrading enzymes led to a decrease in cell proliferation and invasion of melanoma or endothelial cells (Denholm *et al.*, 2001) and to a reduction in FGF-2 responsiveness (a known regulator of tumor cell proliferation) in human dermal fibroblasts (Denholm *et al.*, 2000; Liu *et al.*, 2002). GAG modulation of tumor growth and dissemination has revealed a regulatory layer of tumorigenesis governed by GAG crosstalk with various oncogenic agents (Sanderson *et al.*, 2004; Yang *et al.*, 2005).

B. Coagulation

DS selectively activates heparin cofactor II, an important member of the serpin family of proteins, resulting in the inactivation of thrombin without an accompanying interaction with antithrombin III (Liaw et al., 1999, 2001; Maimone and Tollefsen, 1990, 1991; Mascellani et al., 1993; Nenci, 2002; Tollefsen et al., 1989). An oversulfated DS hexasaccharide, (IdoA2S-GalNAc4S)$_3$, binds heparin cofactor II with high affinity, producing as much as a 100-fold increase in heparin cofactor II-mediated inhibition of thrombin (Casu et al., 2004; Maimone and Tollefsen, 1991; Mascellani et al., 1993). Sequence specificity of the DS oligosaccharide is critical, as a DS hexasaccharide with two repeats of the disaccharide sequence, IdoA-GalNAc4S, 6S, can also mediate heparin cofactor II activation but a hexasaccharide with the sequence IdoA2S-GalNAc6S cannot (Denti et al., 1995; Ernst et al., 1995; Trowbridge and Gallo, 2002). Thus, it is plausible that heparin cofactor II activation through a GalAG polymer requires a specific epimerization state (IdoA) and a precise sulfation pattern (GalNAc4S).

Heparin also activates heparin cofactor II through a chain length-dependent mechanism (Liaw et al., 1999), resulting in a far higher increase (1000-fold) in antithrombin activity when compared to DS-mediated phenomena. The action of DS regarding coagulation is distinct from heparin, as DS behaves as a selective thrombin inhibitor. Heparin acts on the coagulation system through a template-based mechanism, involving complex formation with the simultaneous binding of heparin to thrombin and the GAG-binding domain of heparin cofactor II. Interaction of DS with heparin cofactor II is capable of inactivating thrombin bound to fibrin on the surface of an injured vessel (Bendayan et al., 1994). This outcome cannot be achieved through heparan sulfate glycosaminoglycans (HSGAGs).

A variety of DS-based anticoagulant therapies have been developed. These include GAG mixtures, including mesoglycan, danaparoid, and sulodexide, which contain both DS and HSGAGs, and intimitan, a semisynthetic oversulfated DS. Intimitan contains an increased content of the IdoA-GalNAc4S,6S disaccharide and more effectively inhibits clot-bound thrombin than standard heparin or DS therapies (Buchanan and Brister, 2000; Buchanan et al., 2001; Coccheri et al., 2002a,b; Harenberg, 1998; Nenci, 2002; Nenci et al., 2001; Ofosu, 1998). DS-based therapeutics are being developed for heparin-induced thrombocytopenia, a disorder resulting from an autoimmune response to a complex of heparin and platelet factor 4 in which heparin treatment must be discontinued (Imberti et al., 2003; Taliani et al., 1999). Novel anticoagulants composed of complexes of GAGs, and heparin cofactor II are also under investigation (Fernandez et al., 1999; Monagle et al., 1998).

C. Cartilage Function and Osteoarthritis

Degenerative joint disease or osteoarthritis is characterized by the breakdown of cartilage. Cartilage, composed of up to 90% ECM, serves to essentially cushion the ends of bones. The disease affects more than 20 million Americans and becomes more prevalent on aging. CS is the predominant GAG present in cartilage ECM (Hardingham and Fosang, 1992; Iozzo, 1997; Tumova *et al.*, 2000). The high overall charge of the chemical groups present on CS chains in cartilage PGs are believed to provide the necessary electrostatic forces to promote high-water content, enabling joints to withstand dynamic mechanical compression (Ragan *et al.*, 2000). PG core proteins also interact with the collagen fibrils present in cartilage, thus imparting additional mechanical integrity. These and other biological roles are achieved through a variety of CS-containing PGs, including aggrecan (Plaas *et al.*, 2001; Watanabe *et al.*, 1998), decorin, biglycan, and perlecan (Table I) (Kinsella *et al.*, 2004; Knudson and Knudson, 2001; Reed *et al.*, 2005; Wadhwa *et al.*, 2004). Cartilage degradation in osteoarthritis proceeds both through mechanical forces at play in the joint and with the enzymatic degradation of critical cartilage ECM components. Chondrocytes are largely responsible for regulating ECM molecules, and the aberrant behavior of these cells results in pathogenesis (Ragan *et al.*, 2000). Arthritic tissues have been observed to carry GAG pattern profiles, most notably a decrease in the abundance of 6-O-sulfated disaccharides accompanying an increase in 4-O-sulfated CS disaccharides (Plaas *et al.*, 1998). The development of nutraceuticals (including chondroitin, glucosamine, and mannosamine) to treat osteoarthritis has been controversial.

D. Neurobiology

The neurons and glia of the central nervous system express a wide variety of PGs that impinge upon diverse processes, including the migration of neural precursor cells, control of neuronal tracking, the regulation of neuronal cell adhesion molecules, and the formation of synapses (Edgell *et al.*, 2004; Hartmann and Maurer, 2001; Iwata and Carlson, 1991; Monnier *et al.*, 2003; Oohira *et al.*, 2000, 2004). Through these processes, PGs of nervous system origin play an essential role during neural development (Deepa *et al.*, 2004; Lander *et al.*, 1997; Lee *et al.*, 2004; Saunders *et al.*, 1997; Umehara *et al.*, 2004; Williams *et al.*, 1994). CSPGs are particularly abundant in brain tissue. The signal transducing receptor-type protein tyrosine phosphatase (PTPξ) and phosphacan are CSPGs involved in neuron–glial cell interaction, gliogenesis, neuronal migration, and neurite outgrowth (Table II) (Holland *et al.*, 1998; Margolis and Margolis, 1993). Maintenance of long-term potentiation is repressed in mice deficient in the CSPGs neurocan and brevican (Beggah *et al.*, 2005; Blakemore *et al.*, 2002; Hayashi *et al.*, 2005; Johnson *et al.*, 2005; Mishima and Hoffman, 2003; Popp *et al.*, 2003; Schumacher *et al.*, 1997; Zhang *et al.*, 2003). The absence of CSPGs is in some notable cases (as with PTPζ, neurocan, and brevican) compensated for by other lecticans (Brakebusch *et al.*, 2002; Harroch *et al.*, 2000; Rauch *et al.*, 2005; Zhou *et al.*, 2001). The PTPζ signaling pathway has been examined, and several characterizations have been postulated (Garwood *et al.*, 2001; Margolis and Margolis, 1993; Sugahara *et al.*, 2003; Tanaka *et al.*, 2003). Pleiotrophin and midkine are growth factors that can bind PTPζ on cell surfaces through CS chains. Receptor dimerization and subsequent phosphatase inactivity could manifest, altering G protein-coupled receptor kinase interactor 1 (GIT1) tyrosine phosphorylation levels resulting in cytoskeleton modulation. Binding by pleitrophin and midkine can be thoroughly ablated by free CS-D and CS-E saccharides and partially inhibited via DS and C6S chains (but not through C4S) (Kawachi *et al.*, 2001; Sugahara *et al.*, 2003). Phosphacan is a secreted variant of PTPζ present in the ECM. Phosphacan CS chains can interact with pleitrophin and midkine as well, and it has been proposed that this interaction results in the presentation of these two ligands to PTPζ on the cell surface (Sugahara *et al.*, 2003).

Perhaps the most provocative evidence for the role of GalAGs in neural development is the findings that these sugars are critical in cytokinesis and morphogenesis during the early embryonic stages of the nematode, *Caenorhabditis elegans* (Hwang *et al.*, 2003; Mizuguchi *et al.*, 2003). Investigations of GalAG biosynthesis have led to a unique human chondroitin synthase gene family.

Although GAG chains are essential for the proper development and functioning of the central nervous system, CS chains in particular have also been implicated as a major deterrent to the regeneration of axons following traumatic injury to brain and spinal cord (Fawcett and Asher, 1999; Moon *et al.*, 2001; Morgenstern *et al.*, 2002; Properzi *et al.*, 2003; Zuo *et al.*, 1998, 2002). Such injuries result in paralysis, and the prognosis for recovery is bleak. One strategy in development for neural regeneration makes use of enzymes that prune away inhibitory CS chains present in the glial scar, allowing regrowth of axons and some functional locomotor recovery in animal models (Bradbury *et al.*, 2002).

E. Pathogen Receptors

Various pathogens, including viruses and bacteria, use CS and DS on cell surfaces as the point of attachment to host tissues (Menozzi *et al.*, 2002; Sugahara *et al.*, 2003; Trowbridge and Gallo, 2002). The role of glycoprotein C for the binding of herpes simplex virus type 1 to cell surface CS has been established (Mardberg *et al.*, 2002). By interfering with glycoprotein C–GAG interaction, a CS chain with the sequence GlcAβ1–3GalNAc4S6S can inhibit herpes simplex virus' infectivity (Nyberg *et al.*, 2004; Sugahara *et al.*, 2003). Undersulfated C4S dodecasaccharides (minimum length) are required for the adhesion of malaria-infected erythrocytes to placenta (Achur *et al.*, 2003; Gamain *et al.*, 2002; Valiyaveettil *et al.*, 2004); 6-O-sulfation inhibits this process (Chai *et al.*, 2002). The causative agent of Lyme disease, *Borrelia burgdorferi*, has strain-specific interactions with GAG chains, as some strains bind both HS and DS, and some recognize only DS (Parveen *et al.*, 2003). *Streptococcus pyogenes* expresses a variety of surface adhesins including M protein, an important virulence factor that binds heparin, HS, and DS (Frick *et al.*, 2003).

V. The Biosynthesis of GalAGs

GalAGs play such a central role in biology that it is worthwhile to consider just how the structural diversity that governs their function actually comes about. The chemical complexity that allows these biopolymers to control so many essential life functions is the result of a system of intricate molecular machines each of which put in place a particular structural element of the polymer chain. Unlike DNA or proteins, the biosynthesis of polysaccharides does not proceed through a template-based mechanism.

A. Overview

The extensive variation in GalAG composition based on core protein or tissue localization is so pronounced that one must closely examine GalAG production processes in order to further develop a context for their bioregulatory roles. It has become clear that cells apply exquisite control over GalAG composition and sequence. This supervision is governed by tissue-specific expression of only certain isoforms of GalAG biosynthetic enzymes (Table III). Since the polymer modification reactions colocalize to a specific area within the Golgi apparatus, it has been postulated that these enzymes form a larger supramolecular complex that coordinates polymer modification (Sasisekharan and Venkataraman, 2000). Such a situation may provide for enzyme "crosstalk" to supplement further control over the GalAG's structural milieu.

Figures 3 and 4 summarize the biosynthetic steps in the formation of CS and DS. Following synthesis of the core protein, xylosylation of specific serine residues sets in motion GAG formation (Esko, 1999). Addition of two galactose residues and a GlcA residue completes the linker tetrasaccharide common to both HSGAGs and GalAGs. Subsequent addition of GalNAc to the linker commits the chain to GalAG lineage. Then, the alternate addition of GlcA and GalNAc residues results in chain elongation. There is also variable modification of the chain through epimerization and sulfation reactions. Following synthesis of the GalAG chain within the PG context,

TABLE III   Galactosaminoglycan Biosynthetic Enzymes

Enzyme	Reaction	Accession
Linkage region		
Xyl transferase[a]	Xylosylation of specific core protein serines	AJ277442
Gal transferase I[b]	Addition of 1st Gal moiety in linkage region	AB028600 AF155582 AX092340
Gal transferase II[c]	Addition of 2nd Gal moiety to linkage region	Y15014
GlcA transferase I[d]	Transfers GlcA to complete linker tetrasaccharide	AB009598
GalNAc transferase I[e]	Transfer of GalNAc to linkage oligosaccharide, 1st GalAG specific step	AB071403
Chain elongation		
GlcA transferase II[f]	Transfer of GlcA to growing oligosaccharide chain	AB037823
GalNAc transferase II[g]	Transfer of GalNAc to growing oligosaccharide chain	AB024434 BC030268
Chondroitin synthase[h]	Polymerization: alternate addition of GlcA & GalNAc	AB023207
Chondroitin synthase 2[i]	Polymerization: alternate addition of GlcA & GalNAc	AB086063
Chondroitin synthase 3[j]	Polymerization: alternate addition of GlcA & GalNAc	AB086062
Chain modification		
Chondroitin 4-O-ST-1[k]	Sulfates GalNAc in CS at 4-O-position	AF239820
Chondroitin 4-O-ST-2[l]	Sulfates GalNAc in CS at 4-O-position	AF239822
Chondroitin 4-O-ST-3[m]	Sulfates GalNAc in CS at 4-O-position	AY120869
Dermatan 4-O-ST-1[n]	Sulfates GalNAc in DS at 4-O-position	AF401222
Chondroitin 6-O-ST[o]	Sulfates GalNAc in CS at 6-O-position	AB017915 U65637
Chondroitin 6-O-ST-2[p]	Sulfates GalNAc in CS at 6-O-position	AB037187
GalNAc4S 6-O-ST[q]	Sulfates GalNAc4S in CS	NM_015892
Galactosaminyl uronyl 2-O-ST[r]	Sulfates GlcA in [GlcA-GalNAc6S] or IdoA in [IdoA-GalNAc] or [IdoA-GalNAc4S]	NM_005715
Epimerase	Epimerization of GlcA to IdoA	None

[a]Gotting et al., 2000.
[b]Ju et al., 2002; Okajima et al., 1999; Uyama et al., 2003.
[c]Bai et al., 2001; Kolbinger et al., 1998.
[d]Kitagawa et al., 1998; Wei et al., 1999.
[e]Kitagawa et al., 2001; Uyama et al., 2003.
[f]Gotoh et al., 2002.
[g]Guo et al., 2001; Uyama et al., 2003.
[h]Kitagawa et al., 2001.
[i]Yada et al., 2003a.
[j]Yada et al., 2003b.

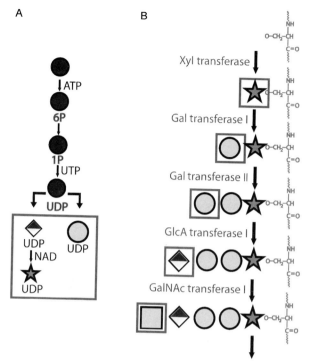

FIGURE 3 GalAG biosynthesis: precursor configuration and linkage region synthesis. (A) The formation of the sugars necessary for the biosynthesis of CS and DS. Glucose is the main source of all GalAG precursors. Galactose, derived predominantly from lactose, can be processed to UDP-Gal, UDP-GlcA, and UDP-Xyl. (B) The synthesis of the linkage region. GalAG chains are linked to specific serine residues in core proteins by the same tetrasaccharide sequence as HSGAGs (GlcA-Gal-Gal-Xyl). The first step that commits the nascent chain to GalAG formation rather than HSGAG formation is catalyzed by GalNAc transferase I. The pertinent chemistry outlined in each step in the GalAG biosynthesis pathway is highlighted in red. The nomenclature for the monosaccharides is as follows: glucose (blue circles), galactose (yellow circles), xylose (orange stars), galactose (yellow circles), glucuronic acid (diamond in blue), N-acetyl-D-galactosamine (yellow square), core protein with linkage serine (green), and iduronic acid (diamond in brown). Enzymes are indicated in purple.

[k]Hiraoka et al., 2000; Yamauchi et al., 2000.
[l]Hiraoka et al., 2000.
[m]Kang et al., 2002.
[n]Evers et al., 2001.
[o]Fukuta et al., 1998; Uchimura et al., 2002.
[p]Kitagawa et al., 2000.
[q]Ohtake et al., 2001.
[r]Kobayashi et al., 1999.
ST, sulfotransferase.

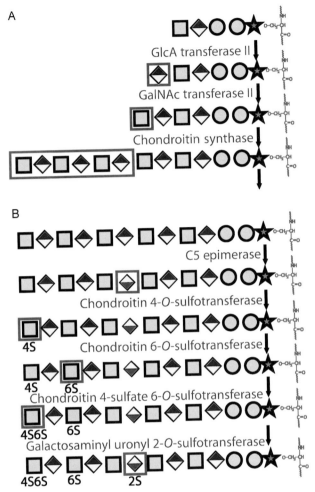

FIGURE 4 GalAG biosynthesis: chain polymerization and chain modification. (A) Chain polymerization is mediated by a variety of enzymes (Table III) that have alternating GlcA transferase II and GalNAc transferase II activities. (B) Modification of the polymer chain. GalAG biosynthesis ensues with a series of modification reactions that may alter the sulfation pattern of the oligosaccharide backbone or switch the epimerization state of uronic acid moieties. The pertinent chemistry of each step in the GalAG biosynthesis pathway is indicated in red. The nomenclature is as described in Fig. 3.

the PG is transported, using specific recognition, sorting, and delivery mechanisms, from the Golgi apparatus to the ECM, the cell surface, or intracellular organelles (Prydz and Dalen, 2000).

B. Core Protein Synthesis and Precursor Formation

It is unclear how a protein is committed to a particular PG lineage. No single consensus sequence has been determined for chain initiation, although generally a substituted serine and glycine pair (following several acidic amino acids) is required. Biosynthesis of the core protein is initiated with translation in the cytosol. Translocation of the nascent polypeptide into the lumen of the endoplasmic reticulum through the translocon follows via a signal sequence-mediated process. Then, N-linked oligosaccharides are added to asparagine residues from dolichol phosphate intermediates. Prior to exit from the endoplasmic reticulum, the core protein undergoes chaperone-mediated folding and the formation of disulfide bonds (Silbert and Sugumaran, 2002).

Cells active in GAG synthesis contain all of the necessary enzymes for precursor formation (Fig. 3A). This is critical as sugar nucleotides do not normally enter cells (Silbert and Sugumaran, 2002). Glucose is the chief source of sugar nucleotides for GalAG biosynthesis. To a lesser extent, galactose (from lactose or other sources) and glucosamine are also capable of contributing to precursor formation. ATP sulfurylase and APS kinase catalyze the formation of 3'-phosphoadenosine 5'-phosphosulfate (PAPS), important for backbone sulfation (Lyle et al., 1994). After cytosol-based activation of the sugars and sulfation, an antiport mechanism transports the nucleotides and PAPS into the lumen of the endoplasmic reticulum or Golgi apparatus (Abeijon et al., 1997).

C. The Linker Tetrasaccharide

Both GalAG and heparin/heparan chains are linked to core protein serine residues by the same tetrasaccharide sequence: GlcA-Gal-Gal-Xyl (Fig. 3B) (Silbert and Sugumaran, 2002; Sugahara and Kitagawa, 2002). Many of the enzymes that catalyze the addition of the linkage sugars in GalAG biosynthesis are the same for heparin/HS formation, including Xyl transferase and Gal transferase I (Esko and Zhang, 1996; Gotting et al., 2000; Prydz and Dalen, 2000; Silbert and Sugumaran, 2002; Sugahara and Kitagawa, 2002). Xylosylation is initiated in the endoplasmic reticulum and continues in the early Golgi apparatus (Kearns et al., 1993; Vertel et al., 1993). The interaction of the Xyl transferase first with the core protein and subsequently with Gal transferase I likely serves a docking purpose, delivering the xylosylated core protein to the Gal I transferase in the early Golgi apparatus (Ju et al., 2002; Okajima et al., 1999; Silbert and Sugumaran, 2002; Uyama et al., 2003). Gal transferase II mediates the transfer of another galatose residue (Bai et al., 2001; Kolbinger et al., 1998). The addition of GlcA to Gal in the linkage region proceeds in the medial/trans Golgi, distal to the position of Gal addition (Kitagawa et al., 1998;

Wei *et al.*, 1999). The next step in the pathway is a point of divergence, where addition of GalNAc to the linker tetrasaccharide commits to GalAG (rather than HSGAG) formation. This step is catalyzed by GalNAc transferase I (Kitagawa *et al.*, 2001; Uyama *et al.*, 2003). A cloned and expressed enzyme, human chondroitin N-acetylgalactosaminyltransferase, was shown to both add the initial GalNAc residue and synthesize the polymer chain. This suggests that there may exist several GalNAc I transferases, each differing in their polymerization capacity (Silbert and Sugumaran, 2002; Uyama *et al.*, 2003).

D. Polymer Biosynthesis

The GalAG chain undergoes polymerization in the Golgi (Gotoh *et al.*, 2002; Guo *et al.*, 2001; Kitagawa *et al.*, 2001; Silbert and DeLuca, 1969; Silbert and Freilich, 1980; Yada *et al.*, 2003a,b) with the alternate transfer of GlcA and GalNAc residues from activated precursors (Fig. 4A). The GalNAc and GlcA transferases add individual sugars to the nonreducing end of the PG acceptor (Prydz and Dalen, 2000).

The addition of each unit (GlcA and GalNAc) is independent (Silbert and Reppucci, 1976). That is, the addition of the next sugar does not proceed until the concentration of the chain with the first sugar in place is substantial. This suggests that the chemical machinery facilitating GlcA and GalNAc addition occurs on discrete proteins or at least through separate sets of catalytic machinery at distinct sites on the same protein. Several human and bacterial chondroitin synthases (DeAngelis and Padgett-McCue, 2000; Kitagawa *et al.*, 2001; Ninomiya *et al.*, 2002) have been identified that have both GlcA and GalNAc transferase activities (the ability to influence linkage region chemistry varies).

E. Chemical Modification

The linkage region of the GalAG chain can itself be chemically modified. The C-2 of xylose can be phosphorylated in a variety of PGs (Oegema *et al.*, 1984; Sugahara *et al.*, 1992a,b,c). Often, xylose is phosphorylated subsequent to the addition of the two Gal linker residues and dephosphorylated on addition of the linker GlcA (Moses *et al.*, 1997, 1999). Linkage region sulfation occurs in GalAGs but not in HSGAGs. CS and DS can be 4-O-sulfated at the second linker Gal and 4-O-sulfated or 6-O-sulfated in the first GalNAc distal to the linkage region (Sugahara *et al.*, 1988, 1991). Epimerization of the final moiety of the linker tetrasaccharide also occurs.

Studies with GAG-degrading enzymes (Ernst *et al.*, 1995; Saito *et al.*, 1968) have revealed that GalAG sulfation patterns are highly heterogeneous *in vivo* (Kusche-Gullberg and Kjellen, 2003). CS polymers can comprise only GalNAc4S; only GalNAc6S; both GalNAc4S and GalNAc6S in the same chain; GalNAc4S,6S; 2- or 3-sulfated GlcA; or unsulfated GalNAc. DS most commonly contains GalNAc4S, 2-sulfated IdoA, unsulfated GalNAc, and unsulfated IdoA. GalNAc6S also has been reported (Evers *et al.*, 2001; Hiraoka *et al.*, 2000; Kang *et al.*, 2002). GalAG 6-O-sulfation occurs in the medial/trans Golgi apparatus, and 4-O-sulfation takes place later in the trans Golgi (Silbert and Sugumaran, 2002). Polymer sulfation seems to occur as the chain grows (Sugumaran and Silbert, 1990) and not after chain termination. A number of chondroitin 6-O-sulfotransferases have been characterized (Table III) (Fukuta *et al.*, 1998; Kitagawa *et al.*, 2000; Uchimura *et al.*, 2002). These generally catalyze the sulfation of KS Gal residues and chondroitin GalNAc (Fukuta *et al.*, 1995; Habuchi *et al.*, 1993, 2000; Sugumaran *et al.*, 1995). Another 6-O-sulfotransferase, purified from squid cartilage and related to the human B-cell recombination activating gene-associated gene, transfers sulfate to the nonreducing terminal GalNAc4S residue of CS (Ohtake *et al.*, 2001). An additional 6-O-sulfotransferase (Nadanaka *et al.*, 1999) acts only on GalNAc residues adjacent to dermatan IdoA. Sulfation at the 4-O-position of GalNAc proceeds via specific 4-O-sulfotransferases that modify either chondroitin (Yamauchi *et al.*, 2000) or dermatan (Evers *et al.*, 2001), exclusively. Sulfation at the 2-O-position, prevalent in DS but relatively rare in CS, is mediated by a 2-O-sulfotransferase (Kobayashi *et al.*, 1999) that sulfates IdoA adjacent to GalNAc4S. Although 3-O-sulfated GlcA chondroitin has been observed from nonmammalian sources (Kitagawa *et al.*, 1997), no 3-O-sulfotransferase has been characterized to date.

Chemical modification at C5 of the uronic acid moiety of a GalAG disaccharide offers two possible epimerization states, resulting in CS (GlcA) or DS (IdoA). This process of transforming GlcA to IdoA likely takes place in the early Golgi apparatus, during or shortly after chondroitin formation and concomitant with sulfation at the 4-O-position (Silbert and Sugumaran, 2002). The C5-epimerase responsible has not been cloned.

F. Chain Termination

CS chains terminate in unsulfated GlcA or GalNAc with any of the usual sulfation states (Silbert, 1978). Although the addition of GlcA to terminal GalNAc6S is facile, the further addition of GlcA is blocked with GalNAc4S at the nonreducing end (Silbert and Freilich, 1980). Further, GalNAc addition is inhibited with a GalNAc4S residue preterminal to GlcA at the nonreducing end (Cogburn and Silbert, 1986; Silbert and Sugumaran, 2002). A process has been postulated whereby action with a 6-O-sulfotransferase specific for terminal GalNAc4S and desulfation at the 4-O-position results in terminal GalNAc6S (Nakanishi *et al.*, 1981; Otsu *et al.*, 1984), allowing further chain elongation.

VI. The Catabolism of GalAGs _____

Just as polysaccharides are synthesized by intricate biological and chemical processes, they must also be degraded as a part of the normal turnover of biomolecules. The cellular degradation of polysaccharides represents a cluster of critical biological pathways, essential for the continued proper functioning of the organism as a whole.

A. Cellular Degradation of GalAGs

GalAG polymers are degraded in lysosomes to liberated monosaccharide moieties, many of which are shuffled back into biosynthetic pathways. Aberrant degradation of GalAG polymers results in one of a group of lysosomal storage diseases. These genetic disorders are rare, yet their study has led to the elucidation of catabolic pathways for complex polysaccharides.

GalAG degradation *in vivo* is a highly ordered process dependent upon the action of specific hydrolases. These hydrolases are substrate specific according to: (1) sugar stereoconfiguration, (2) glycosidic linkage, (3) substitution pattern of backbone hydroxyl groups, (4) pH of the subcellular compartment, and (5) the sugar residues adjacent to the site of cleavage.

The first class of glycoprotein hydrolases is the exoglycosidases (Table IV), which catalyze the release of specific monosaccharides that terminate the nonreducing end of the oligosaccharide chain. Because they generally recognize only one nonreducing end monosaccharide, they are

TABLE IV   Enzymes of Galactosaminoglycan Cellular Degradation

Enzyme (EC number)	Reaction	References
Iduronate-2-sulfatase (3.1.6.13)	Hydrolysis of 2-sulfate groups of L-iduronate of DS and heparin/HS	Bielicki *et al.*, 1993; Wilson *et al.*, 1993
α-Iduronidase (3.2.1.76)	Hydrolysis of unsulfated α-L-iduronosidic linkages in DS	Scott *et al.*, 1991; Unger *et al.*, 1994
GalNAc-4-sulfatase (3.1.6.12)	Hydrolysis of 4-sulfate groups of GalNAc4S of GalAGs	Litjens *et al.*, 1996
GalNAc-6-sulfatase (3.1.6.4)	Hydrolysis of 6-sulfate groups of GalNAc6S of CS (and D-galactose of KS)	Masuno *et al.*, 1993; Morris *et al.*, 1994; Sukegawa *et al.*, 2000
β-N-acetylhexosaminidase (3.2.1.52)	Removal of terminal nonreducing GalNAc4S moiety	Keyhani and Roseman, 1996; Pennybacker *et al.*, 1996
β-Glucuronidase (3.2.1.31)	Cleavage of β-GlcA residue	Oshima *et al.*, 1987; Shipley *et al.*, 1993

often broadly specific, barely receptive to other sugar moieties in the chain. The endoglycosidases hydrolyze specific sugar sequences within the biopolymer (Jourdian, 1996). One should note that there are no highly conserved glycosidase domains. Oligosaccharide chains are therefore partially cleaved by enzymes at a few specific internal sites, generating fragments on the order of 10 kDa. This endoglycosidase action results in multiple terminal residues, which can be catalytically released through the action of various sulfatases (Table IV) and exoglycosidases, obviating the time-consuming and tedious scenario of exoglycosidase-only digestion. Since exoglycosidases do not degrade substituted sugars, such chemical groups must first be removed.

B. Pathological Catabolism

The loss of GAG-catabolizing lysosomal enzymes leads to the accumulation of undegraded oligosaccharide in cells and tissue, and the subsequent secretion of this material. Most diseases of GAG catabolic pathways share a variety of common symptoms (Table V). Specific diagnosis usually requires an experienced and expert clinician to pinpoint specific symptomatic features of the given disorder. Defects in glycan degradation generally manifest with a range of severities. The mucopolysaccharidoses are lysosomal disorders that share many clinical features. These involve mulitsystem involvement, organomegaly, dysostosis multiplex, and abnormal facies. Respiration, vision, and cardiovascular function may be impaired. Joint mobility and skeletal abnormalities are common (Neufeld and Muenzer, 2001). Onset in youth is usually the most severe; onset during adulthood is often more mild (Freeze, 1999; Jourdian, 1996; Michalski, 1996).

C. Catabolism of DS and CS

Figure 5 summarizes the important events in the cellular degradation of GalAG polymers. Following hyaluronidase-mediated slicing of an oligosaccharide chain, DS is degraded initially with iduronate-2-sulfatase (EC 3.1.6.13), a hydrolase of lysosomal origin (Bielicki *et al.*, 1993; Wilson *et al.*, 1993). The 24 kb gene for iduronate-2-sulfatase has been localized to Xq27/28. The protein is synthesized as two precursor forms of 76 and 90 kDa. Subsequent modification of N-linked sugar residues follows. Posttranslational processing to incorporate phosphorylated mannose-6-phosphate allows targeting of the protein to the lysosome. In humans, an inherited deficiency of this enzyme results in a congential storage disorder known as mucopolysaccharidosis type II (Hunter syndrome). Afflicted individuals accumulate undegraded DS (and HS) in the lysosome. Accumulation of these GAG chains leads to a spectrum of clinical phenotypes, including progressive neurological dysfunction and mental retardation. Preliminary

TABLE V   Summary of Lysosomal Disorders

Disorder	Enzyme deficiency	Substrate	Life expectancy (years)
Hunter syndrome (MPS Type II)	Iduronate-2-sulfatase	DS, HS	20–60
Hurler syndrome (MPS Type I H)	α-Iduronidase	DS, HS	5–10
Morquio syndrome			
MPS Type IV A	GalNAc-6-sulfatase	C6S, KS	20–40
MPS Type IV B	β-Galactosidase	KS	20–40
Sanfilippo syndrome			
MPS Type III A	Heparan N-sulfatase	HS	20–30
MPS Type III B	α-N-acetylglucosaminidase	HS	20–30
MPS Type III C	Acetyl CoA:α-glucosaminide N-acetyltransferase	HS	20–30
MPS Type III D	GalNAc-6-sulfatase	HS	20–30
Maroteaux-Lamy (MPS Type VI)	GalNAc-4-sulfatase	DS	10–30
Sly syndrome (MPS Type VII)	β-Glucuronidase	DS, HS, C6S, C4S	4–20
G$_{M2}$ gangliosidoses			
Tay-Sachs disease	β-Hexosaminidase A	Sphingolipid, oligosaccharides	5
Sandhoff disease	β-Hexosaminidase A and B	Sphingolipid, oligosaccharides	3
MPS Type IX	Hyaluronidase	Hyaluronan	Unknown

Adapted from Neufeld and Muenzer (2001), with permission.

approaches for therapy include the delivery of recombinant iduronate-2-sulfatase to neuronal and glial cells (Daniele *et al.*, 2002).

α-Iduronidase (EC 3.2.1.76) is a hydrolase that follows the action of iduronate-2-sulfatase in the lysosome (Scott *et al.*, 1991; Unger *et al.*, 1994). It cleaves terminal nonreducing IdoA from DS (and HS). A deficiency in this enzyme results in a failure to degrade GAGs, manifesting in mucopolysaccharidosis type I patients who present with a range of clinical phenotypes, including Hurler and Scheie syndromes. Enzyme replacement therapy has been shown to have some benefit (Brooks, 2002). The enzyme has been purified from a variety of mammalian tissues (Table IV). It has been proposed that α-iduronidase acts in concert with other GAG-degrading enzymes as a multienzyme complex near the lysosomal membrane (Jourdian, 1996).

Terminal GalNAc4S can be removed via multiple pathways. The first possibility is the sequential action of GalNAc-4-sulfatase (also known as arylsulfatase B) to remove sulfate at the 4-O-position followed by β-N-acetylhexosaminidase A or B to remove the hexosamine moiety. Alternatively, β-N-acetylhexosaminidase A can first clip the GalNAc4S moiety, and then

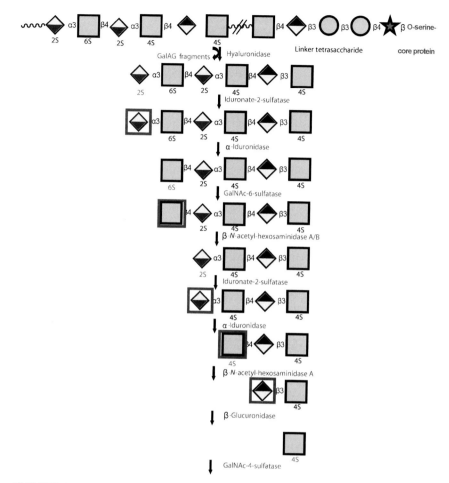

FIGURE 5 Cellular degradation of galactosaminoglycans.. The degradation *in vivo* of GalAG polymers proceeds sequentially via the action of a combination of endoglycosidases, sulfatases, and exoglycosidases. Degradation is initiated by the endolytic cleavage of the long oligosaccharide chain into smaller fragments. Then, removal of sulfatases and exoglycosidase action mediates further degradation. The pertinent target for degradation at each step is indicated in red. The nomenclature is as described in Fig. 3.

sulfatase cleavage occurs. *β*-*N*-acetylhexosaminidase A is one of the very few exoglycosidases that can cleave sulfated amino sugars at low pH (Keyhani and Roseman, 1996; Litjens *et al.*, 1996; Pennybacker *et al.*, 1996).

Absence of GalNAc-4-sulfatase affects DS catabolism and manifests in mucopolysaccharidosis type VI (Maroteaux-Lamy syndrome). Clinically, growth retardation starts at the age of two or three, with coarsening of facial features, corneal clouding, joint stiffness, and abnormalities in the hands and spine. Tay-Sachs disease is a disorder in glycolipid degradation resulting from deficiency in β-N-acetylhexosaminidase A. In its most severe form, neurodegeneration leads to death within 4 years. At its mildest, there is a somewhat slower onset of neurological symptoms. β-N-acetylhexosaminidase A and B deficiencies lead to Sandhoff disease with excreted glucosaminyl oligosaccharides. Clinical symptoms of Sandhoff disease closely resemble Tay-Sachs disease.

β-Glucuronidase cleaves the β-GlcA residue (Oshima *et al.*, 1987; Shipley *et al.*, 1993). This process is continuously cycled until the oligosaccharides are reduced to free monosaccharide derivatives and sulfate ions. Deficiency in β-glucuronidase activity results in mucopolysaccharidosis type VII, affecting the catabolism of DS, HS, and CS. Clinical features of this syndrome vary from patient to patient, but all patients have growth retardation with resultant short stature, some bone abnormalities, and mental retardation. Osteoarthritis is also prevalent. Survival into adulthood is common with milder forms of the pathology.

Hyaluronidase sets the stage for CS degradation at the cellular level. Lysosomal CS catabolism proceeds in analogous fashion to DS, with GalNAc-4-sulfatase and GalNAc-6-sulfatase (Masuno *et al.*, 1993; Morris *et al.*, 1994; Sukegawa *et al.*, 2000) leading the way for β-N-acetylhexosaminidase A or B and β-glucuronidase.

No mammalian endoglycosidases specific for GalAGs have been reported, although a variety of bacterial chondroitinases has been isolated and characterized. Hyaluronidase deficiency (MPS Type IX) has been reported in only one case in which it clinically manifested in periarticular soft tissue masses, episodic painful swelling, and short stature (Natowicz *et al.*, 1996).

VII. The Enzymatic Degradation of GalAGs _____

A. Mechanisms of GAG Depolymerization

We have seen that *in vivo*, GAGs are degraded by a variety of enzymes of predominantly lysosomal origin—the hydrolases and various exoglycosidases. Another class of GAG-degrading enzymes includes the bacterial lyases (Table VI). These come in three categories, classified according to substrate: hyaluronidases, heparinases, and chondroitinases. Many lyases have been purified and employed in a variety of analytical and industrial applications. The following describes the depolymerizing action of lyases that act on GalAGs, the chondroitinases, and the hyaluronidases.

There are two chemical mechanisms whereby GAGs undergo cleavage. With eliminative cleavage, the proton off of C5 of the uronic acid moiety is first abstracted. This results in an unsaturated bond between C4 and C5 of

TABLE VI   Overview of GalAG-Depolymerizing Lyases

Enzyme	Organism	Mode of action	Cleavable linkage	MW (kDa)
Chondroitinase ABC	Proteus (Type I)	Endolytic	$-GalNAc_{4X6X}(\beta1,4)U_{2X}-$	>100
	Proteus (Type II)	Exolytic	$GalNAc_{4X6X}(\beta1,4)U_{2X}-$	>100
	Pedobacter	Exolytic	$GalNAc_{4X6X}(\beta1,4)U_{2X}-$	>70
	Bacillus			53
	Beta (Type I)			104
	Beta (Type II)			108
Chondroitinase AC	Arthrobacter	Exolytic	$GalNAc_{4X6X}(\beta1,4)-$ $GlcA_{2X}-$	76
	Aurebacterium			>80
	Aeromonas			X
	Pedobacter	Endolytic	$GalNAc_{4X6X}(\beta1,4)-$ $GlcA_{2X}-$	75
	Serritia			70
Chondroitinase B	Pedobacter	Endolytic	$-GalNAc_{4X6X}(\beta1,4)-$ $IdoA_{2X}-$	54
Chondroitinase C	Pedobacter		$-GalNAc_{6S}(\beta1,4)GlcA_{2X}-$	<70
Hyaluronate lyase	Staphylococcus	Endolytic	$-GalNAc(\beta1,4)GlcA_{2X}-$	84
	Streptococcus	Endolytic		120
	Apis	Endolytic		40

X, sulfated or unsubstituted. U, uronic acid of either C5 epimerization state.

the uronic acid. Protonation of the anomeric oxygen completes the reaction with the breaking of the glycosidic bond. At its simplest, it can be visualized as a proton acceptance and donation mechanism (Jedrzejas, 2000). Hydrolytic cleavage proceeds slightly differently, first with proton donation to the glycosidic bond. This breaks away the glycosidic oxygen, creating an O5 oxonium ion. Water addition neutralizes the oxonium ion and saturates all carbons (Linhardt *et al.*, 1986). One should note that although lyases can only cleave linkages on the nonreducing side of uronic acid, the hydrolases have no such limitation and can cleave either bond.

B. GalAG Lyase-Mediated Degradation of GAGs

Chondroitinases (Table VI) are produced in soil and intestinal bacteria. Polysaccharides trafficked to the intestinal lumen with epithelial cells provide these bacteria with their nutrient source. Chondroitin lyases have been isolated and characterized from a variety genera, most notably *Pedobacter* (Fethiere *et al.*, 1999; Huang *et al.*, 1999; Michelacci *et al.*, 1987; Pojasek *et al.*, 2001, 2002; Yamagata *et al.*, 1968) and *Proteus* (Hamai *et al.*, 1997; Huang *et al.*, 2003; Michel *et al.*, 2004; Ryan *et al.*, 1994; Sato *et al.*, 1994; Yamagata *et al.*, 1968). Chondroitinases have also been isolated from *Arthrobacter* (Lunin *et al.*, 2004), *Aeromonas* (Kitamikado and Lee,

1975), *Bacillus* (Ernst *et al.*, 1995), and *Bacteroides* (Guthrie *et al.*, 1985; Hwa and Salyers, 1992a,b; Linn *et al.*, 1983).

C. Chondroitinases from *Pedobacter heparinus*

Chondroitinase ABC from *P. heparinus* is a broad substrate specificity lyase that acts on a variety of GAGs, including C4S, C6S, DS, chondroitin, chondroitin D and E. The enzyme is unable to catalyze the depolymerization of hyaluronate, heparin and HS, or KS. It has a molecular weight in excess of 70 kDa and an optimal activity temperature of 30°C. The enzyme is fully active against DS, which is unusual for cABC lyases generally. Other cABC lyases have DS activities under 40% of their C4S activity (Ernst *et al.*, 1995). Chondroitinase ABC causes the weight average molecular weight of a GalAG substrate to decrease slowly. The enzyme acts exclusively on the reducing end of the oligosaccharide chain, suggesting a wholly exolytic activity (Michelacci *et al.*, 1987). The enzyme does not seem amenable to modeling by Michaelis-Menten kinetics, and thus some other mechanism may be in force. The reaction is inhibited by its product (UA-GalNAc4S), by excess substrate (Michelacci *et al.*, 1987), Ca^{2+}, PO_4^{3-}, Fe^{3+}, and Mn^{2+}.

Chondroitinase AC (EC 4.2.2.5) from *P. heparinus* is a 75-kDa enzyme that acts on C4S, C6S, chondroitin, and hyaluronate (Fig. 6) (Huang *et al.*, 2001). It is completely incapable of DS cleavage. At the onset of reaction, the substrate's molecular weight drops dramatically, producing intermediate hexasaccharide and tetrasaccharide, with further degradation over time (Rye and Withers, 2002b). This suggests a predominantly endolytic mode of action. Heparin and DS are notable inhibitors of enzyme activity (Pojasek *et al.*, 2001; Rye and Withers, 2002a,b,c).

Chondroitinase B from *P. heparinus* has been characterized extensively (Fig. 7) (Huang *et al.*, 1999; Michel *et al.*, 2004; Pojasek *et al.*, 2001, 2002). It is the only known lyase that cleaves DS as its sole substrate. Chondroitinase B can cleave DS $\beta(1,4)$ bonds that contain the commonly occurring 4-O-sulfate but also linkages with sulfation at the 2-O-position, 6-O-position, or both. X-ray crystallography (Huang *et al.*, 1999), site-directed mutagenesis (Michel *et al.*, 2004; Pojasek *et al.*, 2002), and modeling studies (Pojasek *et al.*, 2002) have identified critical amino acids involved in substrate binding and catalytic activity. Chondroitinase B's activity is nonrandom, nonprocessive, and endolytic, preferring longer substrate to shorter ones. It works primarily by cutting internal bonds proximal to the reducing end, although other cleavage sites are also susceptible. An Arg364Ala mutant has been shown to have an altered mode of action yielding an altered product profile. This phenomenon is most likely explained through the differentiated binding between this mutant and DS. Additionally, a complex between Ca^{2+}, chondroitinase B, and DS is required for substrate cleavage. It has been proposed that the Ca^{2+} ion neutralizes the IdoA carboxylate in

A

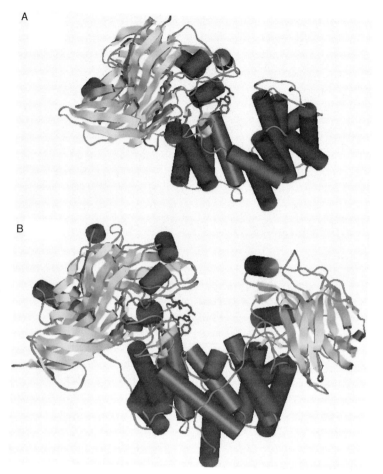

B

FIGURE 6   Structural comparision of cAC and cABC I. (A) Structure of chondroitinase AC from *Pedobacter heparinus* based on the crystal structure of Fethière *et al.* (1999) and Huang *et al.* (2001). (B) Structure of chondroitinase ABC I from *Proteus vulgaris* based on the crystal structure by Huang *et al.* (2003). The similarities in the domains of both enzymes are evident. On a closer inspection, the middle domain of cABC I has very little sequence identity with the catalytic domain of cAC (and bacterial hyaluronidases). However, the residues that are implicated to play important roles in catalysis are conserved in both enzymes (Prabhakar *et al.,* 2005). These catalytic residues are shown in full (purple). The more open cleft of cABC I is possibly suggestive of this enzyme's ability to accommodate a variety of oligosaccharide geometries and thus its wider substrate specificity. (See Color Insert.)

the catalytic groove, and two residues, Lys250 and Arg271, act as Bronsted base and acid, respectively (Michel *et al.,* 2004). This strategy makes use of the flexibility of the IdoA moiety.

Very little is known about chondroitinase C from *P. heparinus,* an enzyme specific for 6-O-sulfated CS linkages. Cross-reactivity with C4S is

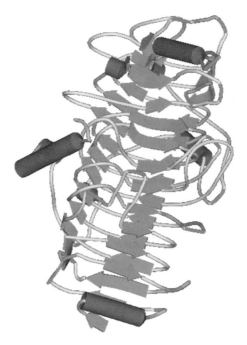

FIGURE 7   Chondroitinase B from *Pedobacter heparinus*. Structure of chondroitinase B based on the crystal structure of Huang *et al.* (1999) and Michel *et al.* (2004). Chondroitinase B is the only known enzyme that cleaves dermatan sulfate as its sole substrate. The structure shows the right-handed parallel β-helix fold representative in chondroitinase B and pectate lyases. The authors thank Dr Rahul Raman for support in preparing this schematic. (See Color Insert.)

the result of the general heterogeneity of GAG polymers in which oligosaccharides that may contain predominantly C6S actually exist as copolymers with C4S.

D. Chondroitinases from *Proteus vulgaris*

The conventional broad substrate specificity enzyme from *P. vulgaris* (Ernst *et al.*, 1995; Sato *et al.*, 1994; Yamagata *et al.*, 1968) has actually been found to comprise two distinct lyases, chondroitinases ABC I and II. Both enzymes cleave a wide variety of GalAGs and hyaluronan. Chondroitinase ABC I has been recombinantly expressed and characterized (Hamai *et al.*, 1997; Michel *et al.*, 2004), and its structure has been elucidated (Fig. 7) (Huang *et al.*, 2003). It has a molecular weight of 105 kDa and optimally processes CS and DS substrates at 37°C. CS substrates are processed at greater rates than DS: 40% greater activity with C6S and more than a twofold increase with C4S. Activity is maximal for CS substrates at a pH of 7.9; for hyaluronan, the optimal pH is 6.1. Chondroitinase ABC I activity is inhibited by Zn^{2+} and heparin. The products of an exhaustive digestion of CS or DS comprise a mixture of unsaturated tetrasaccharides and disaccharides (Prabhakar *et al.*, 2005). Putative catalytic residues of cABC I include His501, Tyr508, Arg560, and Glu653 (Prabhakar *et al.*, 2005). Arginine-500 may also be involved in substrate catalysis (Huang *et al.*, 2003). The lyase acts using the proton acceptance and donation mechanism described earlier. Chondroitinase ABC I is commercially available.

The cABC II lyase from *P. vulgaris* has been scrutinized far less thoroughly (Hamai *et al.*, 1997; Ryan *et al.*, 1994). Chondroitinase ABC II is 100 kDa in size and optimally processes GalAG substrates at pH 7.9 at 40°C. Although cABC II is just as broad as cABC I in terms of substrate profile, it is a far less efficient enzyme regarding catalytic activity. In fact, cABC II processes C4S 16-fold less effectively than cABC I and DS 8-fold less (Hamai *et al.*, 1997; Ryan *et al.*, 1994). The product profile for cABC II is similar to that of cABC I.

E. Chondroitinase AC from *Arthrobacter aurescens*

Chondroitinase AC from *A. aurescens* (Hiyama and Okada, 1976, 1977) is a 76-kDa enzyme that processes C4S, C6S, chondroitin, and hyaluronan. It is inhibited by DS. The enzyme processes these substrates exolytically, producing almost exclusively disaccharide products (Jandik *et al.*, 1994). Chondroitinase AC will cleave CS/DS copolymers but only at linkages containing glucuronic acid (Gu *et al.*, 1993; Linhardt *et al.*, 1991).

F. Bacterial Hyaluronidases

Hyaluronidases have been purified from the bacterial genera *Propionibacterium*, *Peptostreptococcus*, *Staphylococcus*, *Streptococcus*, and *Streptomyces* (Linhardt *et al.*, 1986). Specific activities of hyaluronidases vary widely. The lyase from *Peptostreptococcus* has a remarkably high turnover number, with an activity of 600,000 IU/mg (Tam and Chan, 1985). Hyaluronidase from *Staphylococcus* has a specific activity of 15 IU/mg (Rautela and Abramson, 1973; Vesterberg, 1968). Though hyaluronate is the major substrate, C4S and C6S can also be cleaved by many hyaluronidases, albeit at lower rates. Because of the great variation in catalytic rates among hyaluronidases and the relative inconsequentiality of pH for activity, it has been suggested that these enzymes may employ a mechanism fundamentally distinct from other GAG lyases.

VIII. Perspectives

The limited availability and vast heterogeneity of tissue-derived GalAGs (and other GAGs) has hampered efforts to characterize their sequence-specific influences on proteins and other signaling molecules. Their complex nontemplate-driven biosynthesis precludes the possibility of amplification, unlike DNA and proteins, further complicating glycobiological study. Novel synthetic strategies for the fabrication of complex polysaccharides are still in their infancy. These limitations have forced investigators to cultivate sensitive analytical systems to examine GAG properties.

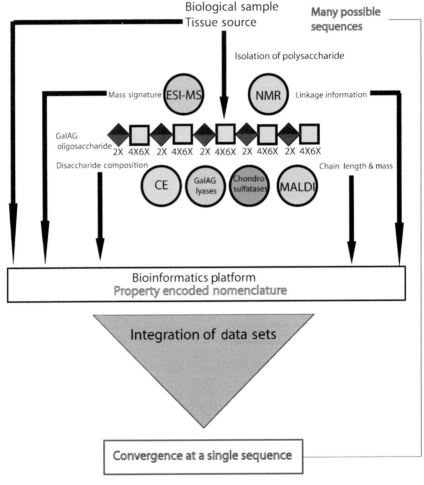

FIGURE 8   Techniques for GalAG sequencing analysis. Three major developments have propelled techniques to characterize the fine structural elements of complex polysaccharides: (1) the development of *enzymatic tools* to specifically degrade functional groups on an oligosaccharide chain, (2) *analytical chemical approaches*, including mass spectrometry, capillary electrophoresis, and nuclear magnetic resonance to establish complementary, orthogonal sets of structural data, and (3) a *bioinformatics platform* to integrate disparate data elements into a numerical strategy for sequencing. These techniques allow for the rapid and bias-free sequencing of complex polysaccharides by considering all possible compositions and converging at a single solution.

TABLE VII   Biotechnological Applications of Chondroitinases

Enzyme	Application	Organization
cABC	Promoting neural plasticity in the central nervous system	Cambridge University; Massachusetts Institute of Technology; Acorda Therapeutics
cB mutants	Rationally-designed polysaccharide lyases for compositional analysis and inhibiting anticoagulant activity and angiogenesis	Massachusetts Institute of Technology
cAC and cB	Attenuation of tumor growth, metastasis, and angiogenesis	IBEX Technologies
cGP	Human chondroitinase glycoprotein	Deliatroph Pharmaceuticals
cABC	Treatment targeting mucus resulting from cystic fibrosis	Beth Israel Deaconess Hospital
cABC	Treatment of chemonucleolysis	Rush Presbyterian/St. Luke's Hospital
cB	Treatment of surface tissue diseases	Seikagaku Corporation
cABC	Clearance of hemorrhagic blood from the vitreous humor of the eye	Advanced Corneal Systems
cB and cAC	Treatment of fibroproliferative diseases	IBEX Technologies
cABC	Treatment for disc herniation	Seikagaku Corporation
cABC	Cleaning and detergent compositions	Procter & Gamble Corporation
cABC I and II	Method for disinserting vitreous body from the neural retina	American Cynamid Company
cAC, cB, cABC I and II, mutants thereof	Compositional analysis of GAG mixtures; treatment of pathologies resultant from the presence of GAGs; the use of defined GAGs and GAG mixtures to treat cancer	Massachusetts Institute of Technology

   The cloning and characterization of heparinase I allowed the first determination of a heparin-binding site (Sasisekharan *et al.*, 1993). Since then, there has been a surge of activity regarding the development of biopolymer-degrading enzymes, including various chondroitinases and exoenzymes. Structural investigations of these enzymes, including crystallographic, spatial modeling, and nuclear magnetic resonance studies, have shed considerable light on enzyme interaction with substrate. Further, the study of GAG biosynthetic and catabolic enzymes *in vivo* has revealed a wealth of insight regarding structural and chemical properties of GAG populations. GAG detection on a variety of platforms has been sensitized by introducing UV chromophores and covalent derivitization with fluorescence or radioactive tags. Mass spectrometric methods have enabled detection of pico- to femtogram quantities of material. Matrix-assisted laser desorption ionization MS of sulfated oligosaccharides is now accurate to within 1 Da. Capillary electrophoresis and liquid chromatography are now being used in tandem with MS to directly identify disaccharides based on mass. These approaches have been coupled with bioinformatics methodologies, including property-encoded nomenclature, to form sequencing strategies (Fig. 8) to elucidate the fine structural elements of complex polysaccharides (Sasisekharan and Venkataraman, 2000; Turnbull *et al.*, 1999; Venkataraman *et al.*, 1999). These tactics rely on the integration of disparate experimentally derived data sets, each of which reinforce each other to provide a solution set of possible polysaccharide sequences. Numerical constraints, including established rules for linkage susceptibility to cleavage, further allow convergence to a single sequence. These attempts at sequence elucidation will be crucial in extending our understanding of the emerging paradigm of sequence-specific binding and modulation of proteins by polysaccharides.

The sweeping involvement of complex polysaccharides like GalAGs within critical biochemical pathways and disease processes heralds a coming age in which glycan biotechnologies will be central elements in diagnostic strategies and therapeutic interventions (Table VII). Such biomedical technologies will include glycan-based approaches for multicellular diseases (Shriver *et al.*, 2004), glycan-based drug improvement strategies, enzyme replacement therapies, and glycome profiling both to screen disease severity in patients and to develop novel medical interventions.

References

Abeijon, C., Mandon, E. C., and Hirschberg, C. B. (1997). Transporters of nucleotide sugars, nucleotide sulfate and ATP in the Golgi apparatus. *Trends Biochem. Sci.* **22**(6), 203–207.

Achur, R. N., Valiyaveettil, M., Alkhalil, A., Ockenhouse, C. F., and Gowda, D. C. (2000). Characterization of proteoglycans of human placenta and identification of unique chondroitin sulfate proteoglycans of the intervillous spaces that mediate the adherence of *Plasmodium falciparum*-infected erythrocytes to the placenta. *J. Biol. Chem.* **275**(51), 40344–40356.

Achur, R. N., Valiyaveettil, M., and Gowda, D. C. (2003). The low sulfated chondroitin sulfate proteoglycans of human placenta have sulfate group-clustered domains that can efficiently bind *Plasmodium falciparum*-infected erythrocytes. *J. Biol. Chem.* **278**(13), 11705–11713.

Alkhalil, A., Achur, R. N., Valiyaveettil, M., Ockenhouse, C. F., and Gowda, D. C. (2000). Structural requirements for the adherence of *Plasmodium falciparum*-infected erythrocytes to chondroitin sulfate proteoglycans of human placenta. *J. Biol. Chem.* **275**(51), 40357–40364.

Bai, X., Zhou, D., Brown, J. R., Crawford, B. E., Hennet, T., and Esko, J. D. (2001). Biosynthesis of the linkage region of glycosaminoglycans: Cloning and activity of galactosyltransferase II, the sixth member of the beta 1,3-galactosyltransferase family (beta 3GalT6). *J. Biol. Chem.* **276**(51), 48189–48195.

Bechard, D., Gentina, T., Delehedde, M., Scherpereel, A., Lyon, M., Aumercier, M., Vazeux, R., Richet, C., Degand, P., Jude, B., Janin, A., Fernig, D. G., *et al.* (2001). Endocan is a novel chondroitin sulfate/dermatan sulfate proteoglycan that promotes hepatocyte growth factor/scatter factor mitogenic activity*J. Biol. Chem.* **276**(51), 48341–48349.

Beggah, A. T., Dours-Zimmermann, M. T., Barras, F. M., Brosius, A., Zimmermann, D. R., and Zurn, A. D. (2005). Lesion-induced differential expression and cell association of neurocan, brevican, versican V1 and V2 in the mouse dorsal root entry zone. *Neuroscience* **133**(3), 749–762.

Bendayan, P., Boccalon, H., Dupouy, D., and Boneu, B. (1994). Dermatan sulfate is a more potent inhibitor of clot-bound thrombin than unfractionated and low molecular weight heparins. *Thromb. Haemost.* **71**(5), 576–580.

Bielicki, J., Hopwood, J. J., Wilson, P. J., and Anson, D. S. (1993). Recombinant human iduronate-2-sulphatase: Correction of mucopolysaccharidosis-type II fibroblasts and characterization of the purified enzyme. *Biochem. J.* **289**(Pt 1), 241–246.

Bishop, P. N. (2000). Structural macromolecules and supramolecular organization of the vitreous gel. *Prog. Retin. Eye Res.* **19**(3), 323–344.

Blakemore, W. F., Chari, D. M., Gilson, J. M., and Crang, A. J. (2002). Modelling large areas of demyelination in the rat reveals the potential and possible limitations of transplanted glial cells for remyelination in the CNS. *Glia* **38**(2), 155–168.

Bradbury, E. J., Moon, L. D., Popat, R. J., King, V. R., Bennett, G. S., Patel, P. N., Fawcett, J. W., and McMahon, S. B. (2002). Chondroitinase ABC promotes functional recovery after spinal cord injury. *Nature* **416**(6881), 636–640.

Brakebusch, C., Seidenbecher, C. I., Asztely, F., Rauch, U., Matthies, H., Meyer, H., Krug, M., Bockers, T. M., Zhou, X., Kreutz, M. R., Montag, D., Gundelfinger, E. D., *et al.* (2002). Brevican-deficient mice display impaired hippocampal CA1 long-term potentiation but show no obvious deficits in learning and memory. *Mol. Cell. Biol.* **22**(21), 7417–7427.

Brooks, B., Briggs, D. M., Eastmond, N. C., Fernig, D. G., and Coleman, J. W. (2000). Presentation of IFN-gamma to nitric oxide-producing cells: A novel function for mast cells. *J. Immunol.* **164**(2), 573–579.

Brooks, D. A. (2002). Alpha-L-iduronidase and enzyme replacement therapy for mucopolysaccharidosis I. *Expert Opin. Biol. Ther.* **2**(8), 967–976.

Buchanan, M. R., and Brister, S. J. (2000). Anticoagulant and antithrombin effects of intimatan, a heparin cofactor II agonist. *Thromb. Res.* **99**(6), 603–612.

Buchanan, M. R., Maclean, G. A., and Brister, S. J. (2001). Selective and sustained inhibition of surface-bound thrombin activity by intimatan/heparin cofactor II and its relevance to assessing systemic anticoagulation *in vivo*, *ex vivo* and *in vitro*. *Thromb. Haemost.* **86**(3), 909–913.

Cardin, A. D., and Weintraub, H. J. (1989). Molecular modeling of protein-glycosaminoglycan interactions. *Arteriosclerosis* **9**(1), 21–32.

Casu, B., Choay, J., Ferro, D. R., Gatti, G., Jacquinet, J. C., Petitou, M., Provasoli, A., Ragazzi, M., Sinay, P., and Torri, G. (1986). Controversial glycosaminoglycan conformations. *Nature* **322** (6076), 215–216.

Casu, B., Guerrini, M., and Torri, G. (2004). Structural and conformational aspects of the anticoagulant and anti-thrombotic activity of heparin and dermatan sulfate. *Curr. Pharm. Des.* **10**(9), 939–949.

Casu, B., Petitou, M., Provasoli, M., and Sinay, P. (1988). Conformational flexibility: A new concept for explaining binding and biological properties of iduronic acid-containing glycosaminoglycans. *Trends Biochem. Sci.* **13**(6), 221–225.

Catlow, K., Deakin, J. A., Delehedde, M., Fernig, D. G., Gallagher, J. T., Pavao, M. S., and Lyon, M. (2003). Hepatocyte growth factor/scatter factor and its interaction with heparan sulphate and dermatan sulphate. *Biochem. Soc. Trans.* **31**(2), 352–353.

Chai, W., Beeson, J. G., and Lawson, A. M. (2002). The structural motif in chondroitin sulfate for adhesion of *Plasmodium falciparum*-infected erythrocytes comprises disaccharide units of 4-O-sulfated and non-sulfated N-acetylgalactosamine linked to glucuronic acid. *J. Biol. Chem.* **277**(25), 22438–22446.

Cheng, F., Yoshida, K., Heinegard, D., and Fransson, L. A. (1992). A new method for sequence analysis of glycosaminoglycans from heavily substituted proteoglycans reveals nonrandom positioning of 4- and 6-*O*-sulphated N-acetylgalactosamine in aggrecan-derived chondroitin sulphate. *Glycobiology* **2**(6), 553–561.

Coccheri, S., Scondotto, G., Agnelli, G., Aloisi, D., Palazzini, E., and Zamboni, V. (2002a). Randomised, double blind, multicentre, placebo controlled study of sulodexide in the treatment of venous leg ulcers. *Thromb. Haemost.* **87**(6), 947–952.

Coccheri, S., Scondotto, G., Agnelli, G., Palazzini, E., and Zamboni, V. (2002b). Sulodexide in the treatment of intermittent claudication: Results of a randomized, double-blind, multicentre, placebo-controlled study. *Eur. Heart J.* **23**(13), 1057–1065.

Cogburn, J. N., and Silbert, J. E. (1986). The effect of penultimate N-acetylgalactosamine 4-sulfate on chondroitin chain elongation. *Carbohydr. Res.* **151**, 207–212.

Daniele, A., Tomanin, R., Villani, G. R., Zacchello, F., Scarpa, M., and Di Natale, P. (2002). Uptake of recombinant iduronate-2-sulfatase into neuronal and glial cells *in vitro*. *Biochim. Biophys. Acta* **1588**(3), 203–209.

DeAngelis, P. L., and Padgett-McCue, A. J. (2000). Identification and molecular cloning of a chondroitin synthase from *Pasteurella multocida* type F. *J. Biol. Chem.* **275**(31), 24124–24129.

Deepa, S. S., Yamada, S., Zako, M., Goldberger, O., and Sugahara, K. (2004). Chondroitin sulfate chains on syndecan-1 and syndecan-4 from normal murine mammary gland epithelial cells are structurally and functionally distinct and cooperate with heparan sulfate chains to bind growth factors: A novel function to control binding of midkine, pleiotrophin, and basic fibroblast growth factor. *J. Biol. Chem.* **279**(36), 37368–37376.

Denholm, E. M., Cauchon, E., Poulin, C., and Silver, P. J. (2000). Inhibition of human dermal fibroblast proliferation by removal of dermatan sulfate. *Eur. J. Pharmacol.* **400**(2–3), 145–153.

Denholm, E. M., Lin, Y. Q., and Silver, P. J. (2001). Anti-tumor activities of chondroitinase AC and chondroitinase B: Inhibition of angiogenesis, proliferation and invasion. *Eur. J. Pharmacol.* **416**(3), 213–221.

Denti, A., Sini, P., Tira, M. E., and Balduini, C. (1995). Structural heterogeneity of dermatan sulfate chains: Correlation with heparin cofactor II activating properties. *Thromb. Res.* **79**(2), 187–198.

Edgell, C. J., BaSalamah, M. A., and Marr, H. S. (2004). Testican-1: A differentially expressed proteoglycan with protease inhibiting activities. *Int. Rev. Cytol.* **236**, 101–122.

Elefteriou, F., Exposito, J. Y., Garrone, R., and Lethias, C. (2001). Binding of tenascin-X to decorin. *FEBS Lett.* **495**(1–2), 44–47.

Enghild, J. J., Salvesen, G., Hefta, S. A., Thogersen, I. B., Rutherfurd, S., and Pizzo, S. V. (1991). Chondroitin 4-sulfate covalently cross-links the chains of the human blood protein pre-alpha-inhibitor. *J. Biol. Chem.* **266**(2), 747–751.

Ernst, S., Langer, R., Cooney, C. L., and Sasisekharan, R. (1995). Enzymatic degradation of glycosaminoglycans. *Crit. Rev. Biochem. Mol. Biol.* **30**(5), 387–444.

Esko, J. D. (1999). Proteoglycans and glycosaminoglycans. *In* "Essentials of Glycobiology" (A. Varki, Ed.), pp. 145–159. Cold Spring Harbor Laboratory Press, Cold Spring Harbor, NY.

Esko, J. D., and Zhang, L. (1996). Influence of core protein sequence on glycosaminoglycan assembly. *Curr. Opin. Struct. Biol.* **6**(5), 663–670.

Evers, M. R., Xia, G., Kang, H. G., Schachner, M., and Baenziger, J. U. (2001). Molecular cloning and characterization of a dermatan-specific N-acetylgalactosamine 4-*O*-sulfotransferase. *J. Biol. Chem.* **276**(39), 36344–36353.

Fawcett, J. W., and Asher, R. A. (1999). The glial scar and central nervous system repair. *Brain Res. Bull.* **49**(6), 377–391.

Fernandez, J. A., Petaja, J., and Griffin, J. H. (1999). Dermatan sulfate and LMW heparin enhance the anticoagulant action of activated protein C. *Thromb. Haemost.* **82**, 1462–1468.

Ferro, D. R., Provasoli, A., Ragazzi, M., Casu, B., Torri, G., Bossennec, V., Perly, B., Sinay, P., Petitou, M., and Choay, J. (1990). Conformer populations of L-iduronic acid residues in glycosaminoglycan sequences. *Carbohydr. Res.* **195**(2), 157–167.

Fethiere, J., Eggimann, B., and Cygler, M. (1999). Crystal structure of chondroitin AC lyase, a representative of a family of glycosaminoglycan degrading enzymes. *J. Mol. Biol.* **288**(4), 635–647.

Fransson, L. A., and Coster, L. (1979). Interaction between dermatan sulphate chains. II. Structural studies on aggregating glycan chains and oligosaccharides with affinity for dermatan sulphate-substituted agarose. *Biochim. Biophys. Acta* **582**(1), 132–144.

Fransson, L. A., Havsmark, B., and Silverberg, I. (1990). A method for the sequence analysis of dermatan sulphate. *Biochem. J.* **269**(2), 381–388.

Freeze, H. H. (1999). Degradation and turnover of glycans. *In* "Essentials of Glycobiology" (A. Varki, Ed.), pp. 267–283. Cold Spring Harbor Laboratory Press, Cold Spring Harbor, NY.

Frevert, C. W., Kinsella, M. G., Vathanaprida, C., Goodman, R. B., Baskin, D. G., Proudfoot, A., Wells, T. N., Wight, T. N., and Martin, T. R. (2003). Binding of interleukin-8 to heparan sulfate and chondroitin sulfate in lung tissue. *Am. J. Respir. Cell Mol. Biol.* **28**(4), 464–472.

Frick, I. M., Schmidtchen, A., and Sjobring, U. (2003). Interactions between M proteins of *Streptococcus pyogenes* and glycosaminoglycans promote bacterial adhesion to host cells. *Eur. J. Biochem.* **270**(10), 2303–2311.

Fukuta, M., Kobayashi, Y., Uchimura, K., Kimata, K., and Habuchi, O. (1998). Molecular cloning and expression of human chondroitin 6-sulfotransferase. *Biochim. Biophys. Acta* **1399**(1), 57–61.

Fukuta, M., Uchimura, K., Nakashima, K., Kato, M., Kimata, K., Shinomura, T., and Habuchi, O. (1995). Molecular cloning and expression of chick chondrocyte chondroitin 6-sulfotransferase. *J. Biol. Chem.* **270**(31), 18575–18580.

Gamain, B., Gratepanche, S., Miller, L. H., and Baruch, D. I. (2002). Molecular basis for the dichotomy in *Plasmodium falciparum* adhesion to CD36 and chondroitin sulfate A. *Proc. Natl. Acad. Sci. USA* **99**(15), 10020–10024.

Garcia-Olivas, R., Hoebeke, J., Castel, S., Reina, M., Fager, G., Lustig, F., and Vilaro, S. (2003). Differential binding of platelet-derived growth factor isoforms to glycosaminoglycans. *Histochem. Cell Biol.* **120**(5), 371–382.

Garwood, J., Rigato, F., Heck, N., and Faissner, A. (2001). Tenascin glycoproteins and the complementary ligand DSD-1-PG/phosphacan: Structuring the neural extracellular matrix during development and repair. *Restor. Neurol. Neurosci.* **19**(1–2), 51–64.

Ghiselli, G., and Iozzo, R. V. (2000). Overexpression of bamacan/SMC3 causes transformation. *J. Biol. Chem.* **275**(27), 20235–20238.

Gotoh, M., Yada, T., Sato, T., Akashima, T., Iwasaki, H., Mochizuki, H., Inaba, N., Togayachi, A., Kudo, T., Watanabe, H., Kimata, K., and Narimatsu, H. (2002). Molecular cloning and characterization of a novel chondroitin sulfate glucuronyltransferase that transfers glucuronic acid to N-acetylgalactosamine. *J. Biol. Chem.* **277**(41), 38179–38188.

Gotting, C., Kuhn, J., Zahn, R., Brinkmann, T., and Kleesiek, K. (2000). Molecular cloning and expression of human UDP-d-xylose: Proteoglycan core protein beta-d-xylosyltransferase and its first isoform XT-II. *J. Mol. Biol.* **304**(4), 517–528.

Grootenhuis, P. D., van Boeckel, C. A., and Haasnoot, C. A. (1994). Carbohydrates and drug discovery: The role of computer simulation. *Trends Biotechnol.* **12**(1), 9–14.

Gu, K., Liu, J., Pervin, A., and Linhardt, R. J. (1993). Comparison of the activity of two chondroitin AC lyases on dermatan sulfate. *Carbohydr. Res.* **244**(2), 369–377.

Guo, S., Sato, T., Shirane, K., and Furukawa, K. (2001). Galactosylation of N-linked oligosaccharides by human beta-1,4-galactosyltransferases I, II, III, IV, V, and VI expressed in Sf-9 cells. *Glycobiology* **11**(10), 813–820.

Guthrie, E. P., Shoemaker, N. B., and Salyers, A. A. (1985). Cloning and expression in *Escherichia coli* of a gene coding for a chondroitin lyase from *Bacteroides thetaiotaomicron*. *J. Bacteriol.* **164**(2), 510–515.

Habuchi, H., Tanaka, M., Habuchi, O., Yoshida, K., Suzuki, H., Ban, K., and Kimata, K. (2000). The occurrence of three isoforms of heparan sulfate 6-O-sulfotransferase having different specificities for hexuronic acid adjacent to the targeted N-sulfoglucosamine. *J. Biol. Chem.* **275**(4), 2859–2868.

Habuchi, O., Matsui, Y., Kotoya, Y., Aoyama, Y., Yasuda, Y., and Noda, M. (1993). Purification of chondroitin 6-sulfotransferase secreted from cultured chick embryo chondrocytes. *J. Biol. Chem.* **268**(29), 21968–21974.

Hamai, A., Hashimoto, N., Mochizuki, H., Kato, F., Makiguchi, Y., Horie, K., and Suzuki, S. (1997). Two distinct chondroitin sulfate ABC lyases: An endoeliminase yielding tetrasaccharides and an exoeliminase preferentially acting on oligosaccharides. *J. Biol. Chem.* **272**(14), 9123–9130.

Hardingham, T. E., and Fosang, A. J. (1992). Proteoglycans: Many forms and many functions. *FASEB J.* **6**(3), 861–870.

Harenberg, J. (1998). Review of pharmacodynamics, pharmacokinetics, and therapeutic properties of sulodexide. *Med. Res. Rev.* **18**(1), 1–20.

Harroch, S., Palmeri, M., Rosenbluth, J., Custer, A., Okigaki, M., Shrager, P., Blum, M., Buxbaum, J. D., and Schlessinger, J. (2000). No obvious abnormality in mice deficient in receptor protein tyrosine phosphatase beta. *Mol. Cell. Biol.* **20**(20), 7706–7715.

Hartmann, U., and Maurer, P. (2001). Proteoglycans in the nervous system: The quest for functional roles *in vivo*. *Matrix Biol.* **20**(1), 23–35.

Hayashi, N., Miyata, S., Yamada, M., Kamei, K., and Oohira, A. (2005). Neuronal expression of the chondroitin sulfate proteoglycans receptor-type protein-tyrosine phosphatase beta and phosphacan. *Neuroscience* **131**(2), 331–348.

Hildebrand, A., Romaris, M., Rasmussen, L. M., Heinegard, D., Twardzik, D. R., Border, W. A., and Ruoslahti, E. (1994). Interaction of the small interstitial proteoglycans biglycan, decorin and fibromodulin with transforming growth factor beta. *Biochem. J.* **302**(Pt 2), 527–534.

Hiraoka, N., Nakagawa, H., Ong, E., Akama, T. O., Fukuda, M. N., and Fukuda, M. (2000). Molecular cloning and expression of two distinct human chondroitin 4-O-sulfotransferases that belong to the HNK-1 sulfotransferase gene family. *J. Biol. Chem.* **275**(26), 20188–20196.

Hiyama, K., and Okada, S. (1976). Action of chondroitinases. I. The mode of action of two chondroitinase-AC preparations of different origin. *J. Biochem. (Tokyo)* **80**(6), 1201–1207.

Hiyama, K., and Okada, S. (1977). Action of chondroitinases. III. Ionic strength effects and kinetics in the action of chondroitinase AC. *J. Biochem. (Tokyo)* **82**(2), 429–436.

Holland, S. J., Peles, E., Pawson, T., and Schlessinger, J. (1998). Cell-contact-dependent signalling in axon growth and guidance: Eph receptor tyrosine kinases and receptor protein tyrosine phosphatase beta. *Curr. Opin. Neurobiol.* **8**(1), 117–127.

Huang, W., Boju, L., Tkalec, L., Su, H., Yang, H. O., Gunay, N. S., Linhardt, R. J., Kim, Y. S., Matte, A., and Cygler, M. (2001). Active site of chondroitin AC lyase revealed by the structure of enzyme-oligosaccharide complexes and mutagenesis. *Biochemistry* **40**(8), 2359–2372.

Huang, W., Lunin, V. V., Li, Y., Suzuki, S., Sugiura, N., Miyazono, H., and Cygler, M. (2003). Crystal structure of *Proteus vulgaris* chondroitin sulfate ABC lyase I at 1.9A resolution. *J. Mol. Biol.* **328**(3), 623–634.

Huang, W., Matte, A., Li, Y., Kim, Y. S., Linhardt, R. J., Su, H., and Cygler, M. (1999). Crystal structure of chondroitinase B from *Flavobacterium heparinum* and its complex with a disaccharide product at 1.7 Å resolution. *J. Mol. Biol.* **294**(5), 1257–1269.

Hwa, V., and Salyers, A. A. (1992a). Analysis of two chondroitin sulfate utilization mutants of *Bacteroides thetaiotaomicron* that differ in their abilities to compete with the wild type in the gastrointestinal tracts of germfree mice. *Appl. Environ. Microbiol.* 58(3), 869–876.

Hwa, V., and Salyers, A. A. (1992b). Evidence for differential regulation of genes in the chondroitin sulfate utilization pathway of *Bacteroides thetaiotaomicron*. *J. Bacteriol.* 174(1), 342–344.

Hwang, H. Y., Olson, S. K., Esko, J. D., and Horvitz, H. R. (2003). *Caenorhabditis elegans* early embryogenesis and vulval morphogenesis require chondroitin biosynthesis. *Nature* 423(6938), 439–443.

Imberti, D., Verso, M., Silvestrini, E., Taliani, M. R., and Agnelli, G. (2003). Successful treatment with dermatan sulfate in six patients with heparin-induced thrombocytopenia and acute venous thromboembolism. *J. Thromb. Haemost.* 1(12), 2696–2697.

Iozzo, R. V. (1997). The family of the small leucine-rich proteoglycans: Key regulators of matrix assembly and cellular growth. *Crit. Rev. Biochem. Mol. Biol.* 32(2), 141–174.

Iozzo, R. V. (1998). Matrix proteoglycans: From molecular design to cellular function. *Annu. Rev. Biochem.* 67, 609–652.

Iwata, M., and Carlson, S. S. (1991). A large chondroitin sulfate basement membrane-associated proteoglycan exists as a disulfide-stabilized complex of several proteins. *J. Biol. Chem.* 266(1), 323–333.

Jackson, R. L., Busch, S. J., and Cardin, A. D. (1991). Glycosaminoglycans: Molecular properties, protein interactions, and role in physiological processes. *Physiol. Rev.* 71(2), 481–539.

Jandik, K. A., Gu, K., and Linhardt, R. J. (1994). Action pattern of polysaccharide lyases on glycosaminoglycans. *Glycobiology* 4(3), 289–296.

Jedrzejas, M. J. (2000). Structural and functional comparison of polysaccharide-degrading enzymes. *Crit. Rev. Biochem. Mol. Biol.* 35(3), 221–251.

Johnson, W. E., Caterson, B., Eisenstein, S. M., and Roberts, S. (2005). Human intervertebral disc aggrecan inhibits endothelial cell adhesion and cell migration *in vitro*. *Spine* 30(10), 1139–1147.

Jourdian, G. W. (1996). Normal and pathological catabolism of glycoproteins. *New Compr. Biochem.* 30, 3–54.

Ju, T., Brewer, K., D'Souza, A., Cummings, R. D., and Canfield, W. M. (2002). Cloning and expression of human core 1 beta1,3-galactosyltransferase. *J. Biol. Chem.* 277(1), 178–186.

Kang, H. G., Evers, M. R., Xia, G., Baenziger, J. U., and Schachner, M. (2002). Molecular cloning and characterization of chondroitin-4-O-sulfotransferase-3. A novel member of the HNK-1 family of sulfotransferases. *J. Biol. Chem.* 277(38), 34766–34772.

Kawachi, H., Fujikawa, A., Maeda, N., and Noda, M. (2001). Identification of GIT1/Cat-1 as a substrate molecule of protein tyrosine phosphatase zeta/beta by the yeast substrate-trapping system. *Proc. Natl. Acad. Sci. USA* 98(12), 6593–6598.

Kawashima, H., Atarashi, K., Hirose, M., Hirose, J., Yamada, S., Sugahara, K., and Miyasaka, M. (2002). Oversulfated chondroitin/dermatan sulfates containing GlcAbeta1/IdoAalpha1-3GalNAc(4,6-O-disulfate) interact with L- and P-selectin and chemokines. *J. Biol. Chem.* 277(15), 12921–12930.

Kearns, A. E., Vertel, B. M., and Schwartz, N. B. (1993). Topography of glycosylation and UDP-xylose production. *J. Biol. Chem.* 268(15), 11097–11104.

Keyhani, N. O., and Roseman, S. (1996). The chitin catabolic cascade in the marine bacterium *Vibrio furnissii*: Molecular cloning, isolation, and characterization of a periplasmic beta-N-acetylglucosaminidase. *J. Biol. Chem.* 271(52), 33425–33432.

Kinsella, M. G., Bressler, S. L., and Wight, T. N. (2004). The regulated synthesis of versican, decorin, and biglycan: Extracellular matrix proteoglycans that influence cellular phenotype. *Crit. Rev. Eukaryot. Gene Expr.* 14(3), 203–234.

Kitagawa, H., Tanaka, Y., Yamada, S., Seno, N., Haslam, S. M., Morris, H. R., Dell, A., and Sugahara, K. (1997). A novel pentasaccharide sequence GlcA(3-sulfate)(beta1-3)GalNAc

(4-sulfate)(beta1–4)(Fuc alpha1–3)GlcA(beta1–3)GalNAc(4-sulfate) in the oligosaccharides isolated from king crab cartilage chondroitin sulfate K and its differential susceptibility to chondroitinases and hyaluronidase. *Biochemistry* **36**(13), 3998–4008.

Kitagawa, H., Fujita, M., Ito, N., and Sugahara, K. (2000). Molecular cloning and expression of a novel chondroitin 6-*O*-sulfotransferase. *J. Biol. Chem.* **275**(28), 21075–21080.

Kitagawa, H., Tone, Y., Tamura, J., Neumann, K. W., Ogawa, T., Oka, S., Kawasaki, T., and Sugahara, K. (1998). Molecular cloning and expression of glucuronyltransferase I involved in the biosynthesis of the glycosaminoglycan-protein linkage region of proteoglycans. *J. Biol. Chem.* **273**(12), 6615–6618.

Kitagawa, H., Uyama, T., and Sugahara, K. (2001). Molecular cloning and expression of a human chondroitin synthase. *J. Biol. Chem.* **276**(42), 38721–38726.

Kitamikado, M., and Lee, Y. Z. (1975). Chondroitinase-producing bacteria in natural habitats. *Appl. Microbiol.* **29**(3), 414–421.

Knudson, C. B., and Knudson, W. (2001). Cartilage proteoglycans. *Semin. Cell Dev. Biol.* **12**(2), 69–78.

Kobayashi, M., Sugumaran, G., Liu, J., Shworak, N. W., Silbert, J. E., and Rosenberg, R. D. (1999). Molecular cloning and characterization of a human uronyl 2-sulfotransferase that sulfates iduronyl and glucuronyl residues in dermatan/chondroitin sulfate. *J. Biol. Chem.* **274**(15), 10474–10480.

Kolbinger, F., Streiff, M. B., and Katopodis, A. G. (1998). Cloning of a human UDP-galactose: 2-acetamido-2-deoxy-D-glucose 3beta-galactosyltransferase catalyzing the formation of type I chains. *J. Biol. Chem.* **273**(1), 433–440.

Kovanen, P. T., and Pentikainen, M. O. (1999). Decorin links low-density lipoproteins (LDL) to collagen: A novel mechanism for retention of LDL in the atherosclerotic plaque. *Trends Cardiovasc. Med.* **9**(3–4), 86–91.

Kusche-Gullberg, M., and Kjellen, L. (2003). Sulfotransferases in glycosaminoglycan biosynthesis. *Curr. Opin. Struct. Biol.* **13**(5), 605–611.

Lander, C., Kind, P., Maleski, M., and Hockfield, S. (1997). A family of activity-dependent neuronal cell-surface chondroitin sulfate proteoglycans in cat visual cortex. *J. Neurosci.* **17**(6), 1928–1939.

Lee, P. H., Trowbridge, J. M., Taylor, K. R., Morhenn, V. B., and Gallo, R. L. (2004). Dermatan sulfate proteoglycan and glycosaminoglycan synthesis is induced in fibroblasts by transfer to a three-dimensional extracellular environment. *J. Biol. Chem.* **279**(47), 48640–48646.

Lesley, J., Hyman, R., English, N., Catterall, J. B., and Turner, G. A. (1997). CD44 in inflammation and metastasis. *Glycoconj. J.* **14**(5), 611–622.

Liaw, P. C., Austin, R. C., Fredenburgh, J. C., Stafford, A. R., and Weitz, J. I. (1999). Comparison of heparin- and dermatan sulfate-mediated catalysis of thrombin inactivation by heparin cofactor II. *J. Biol. Chem.* **274**(39), 27597–27604.

Liaw, P. C., Becker, D. L., Stafford, A. R., Fredenburgh, J. C., and Weitz, J. I. (2001). Molecular basis for the susceptibility of fibrin-bound thrombin to inactivation by heparin cofactor ii in the presence of dermatan sulfate but not heparin. *J. Biol. Chem.* **276**(24), 20959–20965.

Linhardt, R. J., al-Hakim, A., Liu, J. A., Hoppensteadt, D., Mascellani, G., Bianchini, P., and Fareed, J. (1991). Structural features of dermatan sulfates and their relationship to anticoagulant and antithrombotic activities. *Biochem. Pharmacol.* **42**(8), 1609–1619.

Linhardt, R. J., Galliher, P. M., and Cooney, C. L. (1986). Polysaccharide lyases. *Appl. Biochem. Biotechnol.* **12**(2), 135–176.

Linn, S., Chan, T., Lipeski, L., and Salyers, A. A. (1983). Isolation and characterization of two chondroitin lyases from *Bacteroides thetaiotaomicron*. *J. Bacteriol.* **156**(2), 859–866.

Litjens, T., Brooks, D. A., Peters, C., Gibson, G. J., and Hopwood, J. J. (1996). Identification, expression, and biochemical characterization of N-acetylgalactosamine-4-sulfatase mutations and relationship with clinical phenotype in MPS-VI patients. *Am. J. Hum. Genet.* 58(6), 1127–1134.

Liu, D., Shriver, Z., Venkataraman, G., El Shabrawi, Y., and Sasisekharan, R. (2002). Tumor cell surface heparan sulfate as cryptic promoters or inhibitors of tumor growth and metastasis. *Proc. Natl. Acad. Sci. USA* 99(2), 568–573.

Lunin, V. V., Li, Y., Linhardt, R. J., Miyazono, H., Kyogashima, M., Kaneko, T., Bell, A. W., and Cygler, M. (2004). High-resolution crystal structure of *Arthrobacter aurescens* chondroitin AC lyase: An enzyme-substrate complex defines the catalytic mechanism. *J. Mol. Biol.* 337(2), 367–386.

Lyle, S., Stanczak, J., Ng, K., and Schwartz, N. B. (1994). Rat chondrosarcoma ATP sulfurylase and adenosine 5'-phosphosulfate kinase reside on a single bifunctional protein. *Biochemistry* 33(19), 5920–5925.

Lyon, M., Deakin, J. A., and Gallagher, J. T. (2002). The mode of action of heparan and dermatan sulfates in the regulation of hepatocyte growth factor/scatter factor. *J. Biol. Chem.* 277(2), 1040–1046.

Lyon, M., Deakin, J. A., Rahmoune, H., Fernig, D. G., Nakamura, T., and Gallagher, J. T. (1998). Hepatocyte growth factor/scatter factor binds with high affinity to dermatan sulfate. *J. Biol. Chem.* 273(1), 271–278.

Maimone, M. M., and Tollefsen, D. M. (1990). Structure of a dermatan sulfate hexasaccharide that binds to heparin cofactor II with high affinity. *J. Biol. Chem.* 265(30), 18263–18271.

Maimone, M. M., and Tollefsen, D. M. (1991). Structure of a dermatan sulfate hexasaccharide that binds to heparin cofactor II with high affinity. *J. Biol. Chem.* 266(22), 14830.

Mardberg, K., Trybala, E., Tufaro, F., and Bergstrom, T. (2002). Herpes simplex virus type 1 glycoprotein C is necessary for efficient infection of chondroitin sulfate-expressing gro2C cells. *J. Gen. Virol.* 83(Pt 2), 291–300.

Margolis, R. K., and Margolis, R. U. (1993). Nervous tissue proteoglycans. *Experientia* 49(5), 429–446.

Marino, M., Lisi, S., Pinchera, A., Marcocci, C., Menconi, F., Morabito, E., Macchia, M., Sellari-Franceschini, S., McCluskey, R. T., and Chiovato, L. (2003). Glycosaminoglycans provide a binding site for thyroglobulin in orbital tissues of patients with thyroid-associated ophthalmopathy. *Thyroid* 13(9), 851–859.

Mascellani, G., Liverani, L., Bianchini, P., Parma, B., Torri, G., Bisio, A., Guerrini, M., and Casu, B. (1993). Structure and contribution to the heparin cofactor II-mediated inhibition of thrombin of naturally oversulphated sequences of dermatan sulphate. *Biochem. J.* 296(Pt 3), 639–648.

Masuno, M., Tomatsu, S., Nakashima, Y., Hori, T., Fukuda, S., Masue, M., Sukegawa, K., and Orii, T. (1993). Mucopolysaccharidosis IV A: Assignment of the human N-acetylgalacto-samine-6-sulfate sulfatase (GALNS) gene to chromosome 16q24. *Genomics* 16(3), 777–778.

Menozzi, F. D., Pethe, K., Bifani, P., Soncin, F., Brennan, M. J., and Locht, C. (2002). Enhanced bacterial virulence through exploitation of host glycosaminoglycans. *Mol. Microbiol.* 43(6), 1379–1386.

Michalski, J.-C. (1996). Normal and pathological catabolism of glycoproteins. *New Compr. Biochem.* 30, 55–97.

Michel, G., Pojasek, K., Li, Y., Sulea, T., Linhardt, R. J., Raman, R., Prabhakar, V., Sasisekharan, R., and Cygler, M. (2004). The structure of chondroitin B lyase complexed with glycosaminoglycan oligosaccharides unravels a calcium-dependent catalytic machinery. *J. Biol. Chem.* 279(31), 32882–32896.

Michelacci, Y. M., Horton, D. S., and Poblacion, C. A. (1987). Isolation and characterization of an induced chondroitinase ABC from *Flavobacterium heparinum*. *Biochim. Biophys. Acta* 923(2), 291–301.

Mishima, N., and Hoffman, S. (2003). Neurocan in the embryonic avian heart and vasculature. *Anat. Rec. A Discov. Mol. Cell Evol. Biol.* **272**(2), 556–562.

Mitra, A. K., Arnott, S., Atkins, E. D., and Isaac, D. H. (1983). Dermatan sulfate: Molecular conformations and interactions in the condensed state. *J. Mol. Biol.* **169**(4), 873–901.

Mizuguchi, S., Uyama, T., Kitagawa, H., Nomura, K. H., Dejima, K., Gengyo-Ando, K., Mitani, S., Sugahara, K., and Nomura, K. (2003). Chondroitin proteoglycans are involved in cell division of *Caenorhabditis elegans*. *Nature* **423**(6938), 443–448.

Monagle, P., Berry, L., O'Brodovich, H., Andrew, M., and Chan, A. (1998). Covalent heparin cofactor II-heparin and heparin cofactor II-dermatan sulfate complexes: Characterization of novel anticoagulants. *J. Biol. Chem.* **273**(50), 33566–33571.

Monnier, P. P., Sierra, A., Schwab, J. M., Henke-Fahle, S., and Mueller, B. K. (2003). The Rho/ROCK pathway mediates neurite growth-inhibitory activity associated with the chondroitin sulfate proteoglycans of the CNS glial scar. *Mol. Cell. Neurosci.* **22**(3), 319–330.

Moon, L. D., Asher, R. A., Rhodes, K. E., and Fawcett, J. W. (2001). Regeneration of CNS axons back to their target following treatment of adult rat brain with chondroitinase ABC. *Nat. Neurosci.* **4**(5), 465–466.

Morgenstern, D. A., Asher, R. A., and Fawcett, J. W. (2002). Chondroitin sulphate proteoglycans in the CNS injury response. *Prog. Brain Res.* **137**, 313–332.

Morris, C. P., Guo, X. H., Apostolou, S., Hopwood, J. J., and Scott, H. S. (1994). Morquio A syndrome: Cloning, sequence, and structure of the human N-acetylgalactosamine 6-sulfatase (GALNS) gene. *Genomics* **22**(3), 652–654.

Moses, J., Oldberg, A., Eklund, E., and Fransson, L. A. (1997). Biosynthesis of the proteoglycan decorin: Identification of intermediates in galactosaminoglycan assembly. *Eur. J. Biochem.* **248**(3), 767–774.

Moses, J., Oldberg, A., and Fransson, L. A. (1999). Initiation of galactosaminoglycan biosynthesis: Separate galactosylation and dephosphorylation pathways for phosphoxylosylated decorin protein and exogenous xyloside. *Eur. J. Biochem.* **260**(3), 879–884.

Murai, S., Umemiya, T., Seiki, M., and Harigaya, K. (2004). Expression and localization of membrane-type-1 matrix metalloproteinase, CD 44, and laminin-5gamma2 chain during colorectal carcinoma tumor progression. *Virchows Arch.* **445**(3), 271–278.

Nadanaka, S., Fujita, M., and Sugahara, K. (1999). Demonstration of a novel sulfotransferase in fetal bovine serum, which transfers sulfate to the C6 position of the GalNAc residue in the sequence iduronic acid alpha1-3GalNAc beta1-4iduronic acid in dermatan sulfate. *FEBS Lett.* **452**(3), 185–189.

Nadanaka, S., and Sugahara, K. (1997). The unusual tetrasaccharide sequence GlcA beta 1-3GalNAc(4-sulfate)beta 1-4GlcA(2-sulfate)beta 1-3GalNAc(6-sulfate) found in the hexasaccharides prepared by testicular hyaluronidase digestion of shark cartilage chondroitin sulfate D. *Glycobiology* **7**(2), 253–263.

Nakanishi, Y., Shimizu, M., Otsu, K., Kato, S., Tsuji, M., and Suzuki, S. (1981). A terminal 6-sulfotransferase catalyzing a synthesis of N-acetylgalactosamine 4,6-bissulfate residue at the nonreducing terminal position of chondroitin sulfate. *J. Biol. Chem.* **256**(11), 5443–5449.

Natowicz, M. R., Short, M. P., Wang, Y., Dickersin, G. R., Gebhardt, M. C., Rosenthal, D. I., Sims, K. B., and Rosenberg, A. E. (1996). Clinical and biochemical manifestations of hyaluronidase deficiency. *New Engl. J. Med.* **335**(14), 1029–1033.

Nelimarkka, L., Salminen, H., Kuopio, T., Nikkari, S., Ekfors, T., Laine, J., Pelliniemi, L., and Jarvelainen, H. (2001). Decorin is produced by capillary endothelial cells in inflammation-associated angiogenesis. *Am. J. Pathol.* **158**(2), 345–353.

Nenci, G. G. (2002). Dermatan sulphate as an antithrombotic drug. *Pathophysiol. Haemost. Thromb.* **32**(5–6), 303–307.

Nenci, G. G., Gresele, P., Ferrari, G., Santoro, L., and Gianese, F. (2001). Treatment of intermittent claudication with mesoglycan—a placebo-controlled, double-blind study. *Thromb. Haemostasis* **86**(5), 1181–1187.

Neufeld, E. F., and Muenzer, J. (2001). The mucopolysaccharidoses. *In* "The Metabolic and Molecular Bases of Inherited Disease" (C. R. Scriver, A. L. Beaudet, W. S. Sly, and D. Valle, Eds.), Vol. 3, pp. 3421–3452. McGraw-Hill, New York.

Ninomiya, T., Sugiura, N., Tawada, A., Sugimoto, K., Watanabe, H., and Kimata, K. (2002). Molecular cloning and characterization of chondroitin polymerase from *Escherichia coli* strain K4. *J. Biol. Chem.* **277**(24), 21567–21575.

Nyberg, K., Ekblad, M., Bergstrom, T., Freeman, C., Parish, C. R., Ferro, V., and Trybala, E. (2004). The low molecular weight heparan sulfate-mimetic, PI-88, inhibits cell-to-cell spread of herpes simplex virus. *Antivir. Res.* **63**(1), 15–24.

Oegema, T. R., Jr., Kraft, E. L., Jourdian, G. W., and Van Valen, T. R. (1984). Phosphorylation of chondroitin sulfate in proteoglycans from the swarm rat chondrosarcoma. *J. Biol. Chem.* **259**(3), 1720–1726.

Ofosu, F. A. (1998). Pharmacological actions of sulodexide. *Semin. Thromb. Hemost.* **24**(2), 127–138.

Ohtake, S., Ito, Y., Fukuta, M., and Habuchi, O. (2001). Human N-acetylgalactosamine 4-sulfate 6-O-sulfotransferase cDNA is related to human B cell recombination activating gene-associated gene. *J. Biol. Chem.* **276**(47), 43894–43900.

Okajima, T., Yoshida, K., Kondo, T., and Furukawa, K. (1999). Human homolog of *Caenorhabditis elegans* sqv-3 gene is galactosyltransferase I involved in the biosynthesis of the glycosaminoglycan-protein linkage region of proteoglycans. *J. Biol. Chem.* **274** (33), 22915–22918.

Olsson, M., Thyberg, J., and Nilsson, J. (1999). Presence of oxidized low density lipoprotein in nonrheumatic stenotic aortic valves. *Arterioscl. Throm. Vas.* **19**(5), 1218–1222.

Oohira, A., Matsui, F., Tokita, Y., Yamauchi, S., and Aono, S. (2000). Molecular interactions of neural chondroitin sulfate proteoglycans in the brain development. *Arch. Biochem. Biophys.* **374**(1), 24–34.

Oohira, A., Shuo, T., Tokita, Y., Nakanishi, K., and Aono, S. (2004). Neuroglycan C, a brain-specific part-time proteoglycan, with a particular multidomain structure. *Glycoconjugate J.* **21**(1–2), 53–57.

Ornitz, D. M., Herr, A. B., Nilsson, M., Westman, J., Svahn, C. M., and Waksman, G. (1995). FGF binding and FGF receptor activation by synthetic heparan-derived di- and trisaccharides. *Science* **268**(5209), 432–436.

Oshima, A., Kyle, J. W., Miller, R. D., Hoffmann, J. W., Powell, P. P., Grubb, J. H., Sly, W. S., Tropak, M., Guise, K. S., and Gravel, R. A. (1987). Cloning, sequencing, and expression of cDNA for human beta-glucuronidase. *Proc. Natl. Acad. Sci. USA* **84**(3), 685–689.

Otsu, K., Inoue, H., Nakanishi, Y., Kato, S., Tsuji, M., and Suzuki, S. (1984). A sulfotransferase-sulfatase system in avian oviduct which catalyzes a conversion of UDP-N-acetylgalactosamine 4-sulfate to the 6-sulfate isomer. *J. Biol. Chem.* **259**(10), 6403–6410.

Parveen, N., Caimano, M., Radolf, J. D., and Leong, J. M. (2003). Adaptation of the Lyme disease spirochaete to the mammalian host environment results in enhanced glycosaminoglycan and host cell binding. *Mol. Microbiol.* **47**(5), 1433–1444.

Pennybacker, M., Liessem, B., Moczall, H., Tifft, C. J., Sandhoff, K., and Proia, R. L. (1996). Identification of domains in human beta-hexosaminidase that determine substrate specificity. *J. Biol. Chem.* **271**(29), 17377–17382.

Petersen, F., Bock, L., Flad, H. D., and Brandt, E. (1998). A chondroitin sulfate proteoglycan on human neutrophils specifically binds platelet factor 4 and is involved in cell activation. *J. Immunol.* **161**(8), 4347–4355.

Petersen, F., Brandt, E., Lindahl, U., and Spillmann, D. (1999). Characterization of a neutrophil cell surface glycosaminoglycan that mediates binding of platelet factor 4. *J. Biol. Chem.* **274**(18), 12376–12382.

Plaas, A. H., West, L., Midura, R. J., and Hascall, V. C. (2001). Disaccharide composition of hyaluronan and chondroitin/dermatan sulfate: Analysis with fluorophore-assisted carbohydrate electrophoresis. *Methods Mol. Biol.* **171**, 117–128.

Plaas, A. H., West, L. A., Wong-Palms, S., and Nelson, F. R. (1998). Glycosaminoglycan sulfation in human osteoarthritis: Disease-related alterations at the non-reducing termini of chondroitin and dermatan sulfate. *J. Biol. Chem.* **273**(20), 12642–12649.

Pojasek, K., Raman, R., Kiley, P., Venkataraman, G., and Sasisekharan, R. (2002). Biochemical characterization of the chondroitinase B active site. *J. Biol. Chem.* **277**(34), 31179–31186.

Pojasek, K., Shriver, Z., Kiley, P., Venkataraman, G., and Sasisekharan, R. (2001). Recombinant expression, purification, and kinetic characterization of chondroitinase AC and chondroitinase B from *Flavobacterium heparinum*. *Biochem. Biophys. Res. Commun.* **286**(2), 343–351.

Poole, A. R. (1986). Proteoglycans in health and disease: Structures and functions. *Biochem. J.* **236**(1), 1–14.

Popp, S., Andersen, J. S., Maurel, P., and Margolis, R. U. (2003). Localization of aggrecan and versican in the developing rat central nervous system. *Dev. Dynam.* **227**(1), 143–149.

Prabhakar, V., Capila, I., Bosques, C. J., Pojasek, K., and Sasisekharan, R. (2005). Chondroitinase ABC I from *Proteus vulgaris*: Cloning, recombinant expression and active site identification. *Biochem. J.* **386**(Pt 1), 103–112.

Priglinger, U., Geiger, M., Bielek, E., Vanyek, E., and Binder, B. R. (1994). Binding of urinary protein C inhibitor to cultured human epithelial kidney tumor cells (TCL-598): The role of glycosaminoglycans present on the luminal cell surface. *J. Biol. Chem.* **269**(20), 14705–14710.

Properzi, F., Asher, R. A., and Fawcett, J. W. (2003). Chondroitin sulphate proteoglycans in the central nervous system: Changes and synthesis after injury. *Biochem. Soc. Trans.* **31**(2), 335–336.

Proudfoot, A. E., Fritchley, S., Borlat, F., Shaw, J. P., Vilbois, F., Zwahlen, C., Trkola, A., Marchant, D., Clapham, P. R., and Wells, T. N. (2001). The BBXB motif of RANTES is the principal site for heparin binding and controls receptor selectivity. *J. Biol. Chem.* **276**(14), 10620–10626.

Prydz, K., and Dalen, K. T. (2000). Synthesis and sorting of proteoglycans. *J. Cell Sci.* **113**(Pt 2), 193–205.

Ragan, P. M., Chin, V. I., Hung, H. H., Masuda, K., Thonar, E. J., Arner, E. C., Grodzinsky, A. J., and Sandy, J. D. (2000). Chondrocyte extracellular matrix synthesis and turnover are influenced by static compression in a new alginate disk culture system. *Arch. Biochem. Biophys.* **383**(2), 256–264.

Rauch, U., Zhou, X. H., and Roos, G. (2005). Extracellular matrix alterations in brains lacking four of its components. *Biochem. Biophys Res. Commun.* **328**(2), 608–617.

Rautela, G. S., and Abramson, C. (1973). Crystallization and partial characterization of *Staphylococcus aureus* hyaluronate lyase. *Arch. Biochem. Biophys.* **158**(2), 687–694.

Reed, C. C., Waterhouse, A., Kirby, S., Kay, P., Owens, R. T., McQuillan, D. J., and Iozzo, R. V. (2005). Decorin prevents metastatic spreading of breast cancer. *Oncogene* **24**(6), 1104–1110.

Ryan, M. J., Khandke, K. M., Tilley, B. C., and Lotvin, J. A. (1994). Cloning and expression of the chondroitinase I and II genes from *P. vulgaris*. (international application published under the patent cooperation treaty) WO 94/25567.

Rye, C. S., and Withers, S. G. (2002a). Development of an assay and determination of kinetic parameters for chondroitin AC lyase using defined synthetic substrates. *Anal. Biochem.* **308**(1), 77–82.

Rye, C. S., and Withers, S. G. (2002b). Elucidation of the mechanism of polysaccharide cleavage by chondroitin AC lyase from *Flavobacterium heparinum*. *J. Am. Chem. Soc.* **124**(33), 9756–9767.

Rye, C. S., and Withers, S. G. (2002c). Synthesis and evaluation of potential inhibitors of chondroitin AC lyase from *Flavobacterium heparinum*. *J. Org. Chem.* **67**(13), 4505–4512.

Sadler, J. E. (1997). Thrombomodulin structure and function. *Thromb. Haemostasis* **78**(1), 392–395.

Saito, H., Yamagata, T., and Suzuki, S. (1968). Enzymatic methods for the determination of small quantities of isomeric chondroitin sulfates. *J. Biol. Chem.* **243**(7), 1536–1542.

Sanderson, R. D., Yang, Y., Suva, L. J., and Kelly, T. (2004). Heparan sulfate proteoglycans and heparanase—partners in osteolytic tumor growth and metastasis. *Matrix Biol.* **23**(6), 341–352.

Sasisekharan, R., Bulmer, M., Moremen, K. W., Cooney, C. L., and Langer, R. (1993). Cloning and expression of heparinase I gene from *Flavobacterium heparinum*. *Proc. Natl. Acad. Sci. USA* **90**(8), 3660–3664.

Sasisekharan, R., and Venkataraman, G. (2000). Heparin and heparan sulfate: Biosynthesis, structure and function. *Curr. Opin. Chem. Biol.* **4**(6), 626–631.

Sato, N., Shimada, M., Nakajima, H., Oda, H., and Kimura, S. (1994). Cloning and expression in *Escherichia coli* of the gene encoding the *Proteus vulgaris* chondroitin ABC lyase. *Appl. Microbiol. Biotechnol.* **41**(1), 39–46.

Saunders, S., Paine-Saunders, S., and Lander, A. D. (1997). Expression of the cell surface proteoglycan glypican-5 is developmentally regulated in kidney, limb, and brain. *Dev. Biol.* **190**(1), 78–93.

Schmidtchen, A., Frick, I. M., and Bjorck, L. (2001). Dermatan sulphate is released by proteinases of common pathogenic bacteria and inactivates antibacterial alpha-defensin. *Mol. Microbiol.* **39**(3), 708–713.

Schreuder, H. A., de Boer, B., Dijkema, R., Mulders, J., Theunissen, H. J., Grootenhuis, P. D., and Hol, W. G. (1994). The intact and cleaved human antithrombin III complex as a model for serpin-proteinase interactions. *Nat. Struct. Biol.* **1**(1), 48–54.

Schumacher, S., Volkmer, H., Buck, F., Otto, A., Tarnok, A., Roth, S., and Rathjen, F. G. (1997). Chicken acidic leucine-rich EGF-like domain containing brain protein (CALEB), a neural member of the EGF family of differentiation factors, is implicated in neurite formation. *J. Cell. Biol.* **136**(4), 895–906.

Scott, H. S., Anson, D. S., Orsborn, A. M., Nelson, P. V., Clements, P. R., Morris, C. P., and Hopwood, J. J. (1991). Human alpha-L-iduronidase: cDNA isolation and expression. *Proc. Natl. Acad. Sci. USA* **88**(21), 9695–9699.

Scott, J. E., Chen, Y., and Brass, A. (1992). Secondary and tertiary structures involving chondroitin and chondroitin sulphates in solution, investigated by rotary shadowing/ electron microscopy and computer simulation. *Eur. J. Biochem.* **209**(2), 675–680.

Sheng, W., Wang, G., Wang, Y., Liang, J., Wen, J., Zheng, P. S., Wu, Y., Lee, V., Slingerland, J., Dumont, D., and Yang, B. B. (2005). The roles of versican V1 and V2 isoforms in cell proliferation and apoptosis. *Mol. Biol. Cell* **16**(3), 1330–1340.

Shipley, J. M., Grubb, J. H., and Sly, W. S. (1993). The role of glycosylation and phosphorylation in the expression of active human beta-glucuronidase. *J. Biol. Chem.* **268**(16), 12193–12198.

Shriver, Z., Raguram, S., and Sasisekharan, R. (2004). Glycomics: A pathway to a class of new and improved therapeutics. *Nat. Rev. Drug Discov.* **3**(10), 863–873.

Silbert, J. E. (1978). Biosynthesis of chondroitin sulfate: Chain termination. *J. Biol. Chem.* **253** (19), 6888–6892.

Silbert, J. E., and DeLuca, S. (1969). Biosynthesis of chondroitin sulfate. 3. Formation of a sulfated glycosaminoglycan with a microsomal preparation from chick embryo cartilage. *J. Biol. Chem.* **244**(3), 876–881.

Silbert, J. E., and Freilich, L. S. (1980). Biosynthesis of chondroitin sulphate by a Golgi-apparatus-enriched preparation from cultures of mouse mastocytoma cells. *Biochem. J.* **190**(2), 307–313.

Silbert, J. E., and Reppucci, A. C., Jr. (1976). Biosynthesis of chondroitin sulfate: Independent addition of glucuronic acid and N-acetylgalactosamine to oligosaccharides. *J. Biol. Chem.* **251**(13), 3942–3947.

Silbert, J. E., and Sugumaran, G. (2002). Biosynthesis of chondroitin/dermatan sulfate. *IUBMB Life* **54**(4), 177–186.

Stacey, M., Chang, G. W., Davies, J. Q., Kwakkenbos, M. J., Sanderson, R. D., Hamann, J., Gordon, S., and Lin, H. H. (2003). The epidermal growth factor-like domains of the human EMR2 receptor mediate cell attachment through chondroitin sulfate glycosaminoglycans. *Blood* **102**(8), 2916–2924.

Streit, A., Nolte, C., Rasony, T., and Schachner, M. (1993). Interaction of astrochondrin with extracellular matrix components and its involvement in astrocyte process formation and cerebellar granule cell migration. *J. Cell Biol.* **120**(3), 799–814.

Sugahara, K., and Kitagawa, H. (2002). Heparin and heparan sulfate biosynthesis. *IUBMB Life* **54**(4), 163–175.

Sugahara, K., Masuda, M., Harada, T., Yamashina, I., de Waard, P., and Vliegenthart, J. F. (1991). Structural studies on sulfated oligosaccharides derived from the carbohydrate-protein linkage region of chondroitin sulfate proteoglycans of whale cartilage. *Eur. J. Biochem.* **202**(3), 805–811.

Sugahara, K., Mikami, T., Uyama, T., Mizuguchi, S., Nomura, K., and Kitagawa, H. (2003). Recent advances in the structural biology of chondroitin sulfate and dermatan sulfate. *Curr. Opin. Struct. Biol.* **13**(5), 612–620.

Sugahara, K., Mizuno, N., Okumura, Y., and Kawasaki, T. (1992a). The phosphorylated and/or sulfated structure of the carbohydrate-protein-linkage region isolated from chondroitin sulfate in the hybrid proteoglycans of Engelbreth-Holm-Swarm mouse tumor. *Eur. J. Biochem.* **204**(1), 401–406.

Sugahara, K., Ohi, Y., Harada, T., de Waard, P., and Vliegenthart, J. F. (1992b). Structural studies on sulfated oligosaccharides derived from the carbohydrate-protein linkage region of chondroitin 6-sulfate proteoglycans of shark cartilage. I. Six compounds containing 0 or 1 sulfate and/or phosphate residues. *J. Biol. Chem.* **267**(9), 6027–6035.

Sugahara, K., Tanaka, Y., Yamada, S., Seno, N., Kitagawa, H., Haslam, S. M., Morris, H. R., and Dell, A. (1996). Novel sulfated oligosaccharides containing 3-O-sulfated glucuronic acid from king crab cartilage chondroitin sulfate K: Unexpected degradation by chondroitinase ABC. *J. Biol. Chem.* **271**(43), 26745–26754.

Sugahara, K., Yamada, S., Yoshida, K., de Waard, P., and Vliegenthart, J. F. (1992c). A novel sulfated structure in the carbohydrate-protein linkage region isolated from porcine intestinal heparin. *J. Biol. Chem.* **267**(3), 1528–1533.

Sugahara, K., Yamashina, I., De Waard, P., Van Halbeek, H., and Vliegenthart, J. F. (1988). Structural studies on sulfated glycopeptides from the carbohydrate-protein linkage region of chondroitin 4-sulfate proteoglycans of swarm rat chondrosarcoma. Demonstration of the structure Gal(4-O-sulfate)beta 1-3Gal beta 1-4XYL beta 1-O-Ser. *J. Biol. Chem.* **263**(21), 10168–10174.

Sugumaran, G., Katsman, M., and Drake, R. R. (1995). Purification, photoaffinity labeling, and characterization of a single enzyme for 6-sulfation of both chondroitin sulfate and keratan sulfate. *J. Biol. Chem.* **270**(38), 22483–22487.

Sugumaran, G., and Silbert, J. E. (1990). Relationship of sulfation to ongoing chondroitin polymerization during biosynthesis of chondroitin 4-sulfate by microsomal preparations from cultured mouse mastocytoma cells. *J. Biol. Chem.* **265**(30), 18284–18288.

Sukegawa, K., Nakamura, H., Kato, Z., Tomatsu, S., Montano, A. M., Fukao, T., Toietta, G., Tortora, P., Orii, T., and Kondo, N. (2000). Biochemical and structural analysis of missense mutations in N-acetylgalactosamine-6-sulfate sulfatase causing mucopolysaccharidosis IVA phenotypes. *Hum. Mol. Genet.* **9**(9), 1283–1290.

Taliani, M. R., Agnelli, G., Nenci, G. G., and Gianese, F. (1999). Dermatan sulphate in patients with heparin-induced thrombocytopenia. *Brit. J. Haematol.* **104**(1), 87–89.

Tam, Y. C., and Chan, E. C. (1985). Purification and characterization of hyaluronidase from oral *Peptostreptococcus* species. *Infect. Immun.* **47**(2), 508–513.

Tanaka, M., Maeda, N., Noda, M., and Marunouchi, T. (2003). A chondroitin sulfate proteoglycan PTPzeta/RPTPbeta regulates the morphogenesis of Purkinje cell dendrites in the developing cerebellum. *J. Neurosci.* **23**(7), 2804–2814.

Thompson, L. D., Pantoliano, M. W., and Springer, B. A. (1994). Energetic characterization of the basic fibroblast growth factor-heparin interaction: Identification of the heparin binding domain. *Biochemistry* **33**(13), 3831–3840.

Tollefsen, D. M., Maimone, M. M., McGuire, E. A., and Peacock, M. E. (1989). Heparin cofactor II activation by dermatan sulfate. *Ann. N Y Acad. Sci.* **556**, 116–122.

Tovar, A. M., de Mattos, D. A., Stelling, M. P., Sarcinelli-Luz, B. S., Nazareth, R. A., and Mourao, P. A. (2005). Dermatan sulfate is the predominant antithrombotic glycosaminoglycan in vessel walls: Implications for a possible physiological function of heparin cofactor II. *Biochim. Biophys. Acta* **1740**(1), 45–53.

Trowbridge, J. M., and Gallo, R. L. (2002). Dermatan sulfate: New functions from an old glycosaminoglycan. *Glycobiology* **12**(9), 117R–125R.

Trowbridge, J. M., Rudisill, J. A., Ron, D., and Gallo, R. L. (2002). Dermatan sulfate binds and potentiates activity of keratinocyte growth factor (FGF-7). *J. Biol. Chem.* **277**(45), 42815–42820.

Tumova, S., Woods, A., and Couchman, J. R. (2000). Heparan sulfate chains from glypican and syndecans bind the Hep II domain of fibronectin similarly despite minor structural differences. *J. Biol. Chem.* **275**(13), 9410–9417.

Turnbull, J. E., Hopwood, J. J., and Gallagher, J. T. (1999). A strategy for rapid sequencing of heparan sulfate and heparin saccharides. *Proc. Natl. Acad. Sci. USA* **96**(6), 2698–2703.

Uchimura, K., Kadomatsu, K., Nishimura, H., Muramatsu, H., Nakamura, E., Kurosawa, N., Habuchi, O., El-Fasakhany, F. M., Yoshikai, Y., and Muramatsu, T. (2002). Functional analysis of the chondroitin 6-sulfotransferase gene in relation to lymphocyte subpopulations, brain development, and oversulfated chondroitin sulfates. *J. Biol. Chem.* **277**(2), 1443–1450.

Umehara, Y., Yamada, S., Nishimura, S., Shioi, J., Robakis, N. K., and Sugahara, K. (2004). Chondroitin sulfate of appican, the proteoglycan form of amyloid precursor protein, produced by C6 glioma cells interacts with heparin-binding neuroregulatory factors. *FEBS Lett.* **557**(1–3), 233–238.

Unger, E. G., Durrant, J., Anson, D. S., and Hopwood, J. J. (1994). Recombinant alpha-L-iduronidase: Characterization of the purified enzyme and correction of mucopolysaccharidosis type I fibroblasts. *Biochem. J.* **304**(Pt 1), 43–49.

Uyama, T., Kitagawa, H., Tanaka, J., Tamura, J., Ogawa, T., and Sugahara, K. (2003). Molecular cloning and expression of a second chondroitin N-acetylgalactosaminyltransferase involved in the initiation and elongation of chondroitin/dermatan sulfate. *J. Biol. Chem.* **278**(5), 3072–3078.

Valiyaveettil, M., Achur, R. N., Muthusamy, A., and Gowda, D. C. (2004). Chondroitin sulfate proteoglycans of the endothelia of human umbilical vein and arteries and assessment for the adherence of *Plasmodium falciparum*-infected erythrocytes. *Mol. Biochem. Parasitol.* **134**(1), 115–126.

Venkataraman, G., Sasisekharan, V., Cooney, C. L., Langer, R., and Sasisekharan, R. (1994). A stereochemical approach to pyranose ring flexibility: Its implications for the conformation of dermatan sulfate. *Proc. Natl. Acad. Sci. USA* **91**(13), 6171–6175.

Venkataraman, G., Shriver, Z., Raman, R., and Sasisekharan, R. (1999). Sequencing complex polysaccharides. *Science* **286**(5439), 537–542.

Vertel, B. M., Walters, L. M., Flay, N., Kearns, A. E., and Schwartz, N. B. (1993). Xylosylation is an endoplasmic reticulum to Golgi event. *J. Biol. Chem.* **268**(15), 11105–11112.

Vesterberg, O. (1968). Studies on extracellular proteins from *Staphylococcus aureus*. 3. Investigations on the heterogeneity of hyaluronate lyase using the method of isoelectric focusing. *Biochim. Biophys. Acta* **168**(2), 218–227.

Wadhwa, S., Embree, M. C., Bi, Y., and Young, M. F. (2004). Regulation, regulatory activities, and function of biglycan. *Crit. Rev. Eukaryot. Gene Expr.* **14**(4), 301–315.

Watanabe, H., Yamada, Y., and Kimata, K. (1998). Roles of aggrecan, a large chondroitin sulfate proteoglycan, in cartilage structure and function. *J. Biochem. (Tokyo)* **124**(4), 687–693.

Wei, G., Bai, X., Sarkar, A. K., and Esko, J. D. (1999). Formation of HNK-1 determinants and the glycosaminoglycan tetrasaccharide linkage region by UDP-GlcUA:Galactose beta1, 3-glucuronosyltransferases. *J. Biol. Chem.* **274**(12), 7857–7864.

Williams, C., Hinton, D. R., and Miller, C. A. (1994). Somataglycan-S: A neuronal surface proteoglycan defines the spinocerebellar system. *J. Neurochem.* **62**(4), 1615–1630.

Wilson, P. J., Meaney, C. A., Hopwood, J. J., and Morris, C. P. (1993). Sequence of the human iduronate 2-sulfatase (IDS) gene. *Genomics* **17**(3), 773–775.

Winter, W. T., Taylor, M. G., Stevens, E. S., Morris, E. R., and Rees, D. A. (1986). Solid-state 13C NMR and X-ray diffraction of dermatan sulfate. *Biochem. Biophys. Res. Commun.* **137**(1), 87–93.

Wisniewski, H. G., Snitkin, E. S., Mindrescu, C., Sweet, M. H., and Vilcek, J. (2005). TSG-6 protein binding to glycosaminoglycans: Formation of stable complexes with hyaluronan and binding to chondroitin sulfates. *J. Biol. Chem.* **280**(15), 14476–14484.

Yada, T., Gotoh, M., Sato, T., Shionyu, M., Go, M., Kaseyama, H., Iwasaki, H., Kikuchi, N., Kwon, Y. D., Togayachi, A., Kudo, T., Watanabe, H., *et al.* (2003a). Chondroitin sulfate synthase-2: Molecular cloning and characterization of a novel human glycosyltransferase homologous to chondroitin sulfate glucuronyltransferase, which has dual enzymatic activities. *J. Biol. Chem.* **278**(32), 30235–30247.

Yada, T., Sato, T., Kaseyama, H., Gotoh, M., Iwasaki, H., Kikuchi, N., Kwon, Y. D., Togayachi, A., Kudo, T., Watanabe, H., Narimatsu, H., and Kimata, K. (2003b). Chondroitin sulfate synthase-3: Molecular cloning and characterization. *J. Biol. Chem.* **278**(41), 39711–39725.

Yamagata, T., Saito, H., Habuchi, O., and Suzuki, S. (1968). Purification and properties of bacterial chondroitinases and chondrosulfatases. *J. Biol. Chem.* **243**(7), 1523–1535.

Yamauchi, S., Mita, S., Matsubara, T., Fukuta, M., Habuchi, H., Kimata, K., and Habuchi, O. (2000). Molecular cloning and expression of chondroitin 4-sulfotransferase. *J. Biol. Chem.* **275**(12), 8975–8981.

Yang, Y., Macleod, V., Bendre, M., Huang, Y., Theus, A. M., Miao, H. Q., Kussie, P., Yaccoby, S., Epstein, J., Suva, L. J., Kelly, T., and Sanderson, R. D. (2005). Heparanase promotes the spontaneous metastasis of myeloma cells to bone. *Blood* **105**(3), 1303–1309.

Zhang, Y., Rauch, U., and Perez, M. T. (2003). Accumulation of neurocan, a brain chondroitin sulfate proteoglycan, in association with the retinal vasculature in RCS rats. *Invest. Ophth. Vis. Sci.* **44**(3), 1252–1261.

Zhou, X. H., Brakebusch, C., Matthies, H., Oohashi, T., Hirsch, E., Moser, M., Krug, M., Seidenbecher, C. I., Boeckers, T. M., Rauch, U., Buettner, R., Gundelfinger, E. D., *et al.*

(2001). Neurocan is dispensable for brain development. *Mol. Cell Biol.* **21**(17), 5970–5978.

Zuo, J., Neubauer, D., Dyess, K., Ferguson, T. A., and Muir, D. (1998). Degradation of chondroitin sulfate proteoglycan enhances the neurite-promoting potential of spinal cord tissue. *Exp. Neurol.* **154**(2), 654–662.

Zuo, J., Neubauer, D., Graham, J., Krekoski, C. A., Ferguson, T. A., and Muir, D. (2002). Regeneration of axons after nerve transection repair is enhanced by degradation of chondroitin sulfate proteoglycan. *Exp. Neurol.* **176**(1), 221–228.

Mauro S. G. Pavão, Ana Cristina Vilela-Silva, and Paulo A. S. Mourão

Laboratório de Tecido Conjuntivo
Hospital Universitário Clementino Fraga Filho
Instituto de Bioquímica Médica and
Instituto de Ciências Biomédicas
Universidade Federal do Rio de Janeiro
RJ 21941-590, Brazil

Biosynthesis of Chondroitin Sulfate: From the Early, Precursor Discoveries to Nowadays, Genetics Approaches

I. Chapter Overview

Chondroitin sulfate (CS) is a linear heteropolymer of the glycosamino-glycan (GAG) family of polysaccharides formed by alternating residues of N-acetylgalactosamine and glucuronic acid with varying sites and degrees of sulfation. Biosynthesis of this GAG has been investigated since 1960s, initially with classic biochemical assays and more recently using genetic approaches. The synthesis of CS occurs in the Golgi compartment by the action of several glycosyltransferases and sulfotransferases and involves basically three steps, namely the formation of the linkage region, followed by polymerization and modification of the polysaccharide chain. The linkage region, which is common to most of the GAGs, is formed by the addition of one xylose residue to a specific serine on a polypeptide chain followed by two galactoses and one glucuronic acid. These reactions are catalyzed by specific glycosyltransferases, which add individual sugars from

Advances in Pharmacology, Volume 53
1054-3589/06 $35.00
DOI: 10.1016/S1054-3589(05)53006-0

their respective uridine diphosphate nucleotides. Chain polymerization involves the sequential addition of N-acetylgalactosamine and glucuronic acid residues by the action of different N-acetylgalactosyltransferases and glucuronyltransferases (GlcATs), respectively, and occurs concomitantly with modifications of the polymer by the action of several sulfotransferases. The action of an additional glucuronic acid-iduronic acid C-5-epimerase contributes for the generation of dermatan sulfate (DS), an isomer of chondroitin-4-sulfate. *Medial/trans* Golgi-resident sulfotransferases catalyze the transfer of sulfate groups from the sulfate donor 3′-phosphoadenosine-5′-phosphate to hydroxyl groups at specific positions on both N-acetylgalactosamine and glucuronic/iduronic acid residues on the growing polysaccharide chain, generating unique binding sequences within CS and DS with the potential of recognizing specific ligands involved in normal and pathological processes.

II. Introduction

Chondroitin sulfate is a linear heteropolymer of the GAG family of polysaccharides, whose building blocks consist of N-acetyl-D-galactosamine (GalNAc) and D-glucuronic acid (GlcA), varying in size up to a hundred or more disaccharide-repeating units. The GalNAc residues are substituted with sulfate linked to 4- or 6-hydroxyl positions, giving rise to the 4-sulfated (originally denominated as CS-A) and 6-sulfated (CS-C) isomers (Fig. 1A and B). In addition to the typical disaccharide units shown in Fig. 1A and B, several other types of disaccharides have been observed in CS variants, especially in those obtained from nonmammalian sources. Thus, a CS with 4,6-disulfated GalNAc was isolated from squid cartilage (denominated as CS-E) while another chondroitin form, containing $GlcA-2(SO_4)-\beta-1\rightarrow3-GalNAc-6(SO_4)$ disaccharides, was isolated from shark cartilage (CS-D) (Sugahara *et al.*, 2003). The occurrence of 3-sulfated GlcA units was reported on a CS from sea cucumber (Vieira *et al.*, 1991). Furthermore, CSs containing branches of either α-L-fucose (Vieira and Mourão, 1988), D-glucose (Habuchi *et al.*, 1977), or β-fructofuranose (Rodriguez *et al.*, 1988) were found in sea cucumber and squid cartilages and in a uropathogenic bacteria, respectively.

Dermatan sulfate is another form of chondroitin-4-sulfate in which the GlcA has been epimerized to iduronic acid (IdoA) (originally denominated as CS-B) (Fig. 1C). As reported for CS, several DS variants with different sulfation patterns have been described. Thus, tunicates (ascidians) contain oversulfated DSs, all of them 2-sulfated on the IdoA units but differing on the pattern of sulfation of the GalNAc residues (either 4- or 6-sulfated) (Pavão *et al.*, 1995, 1998).

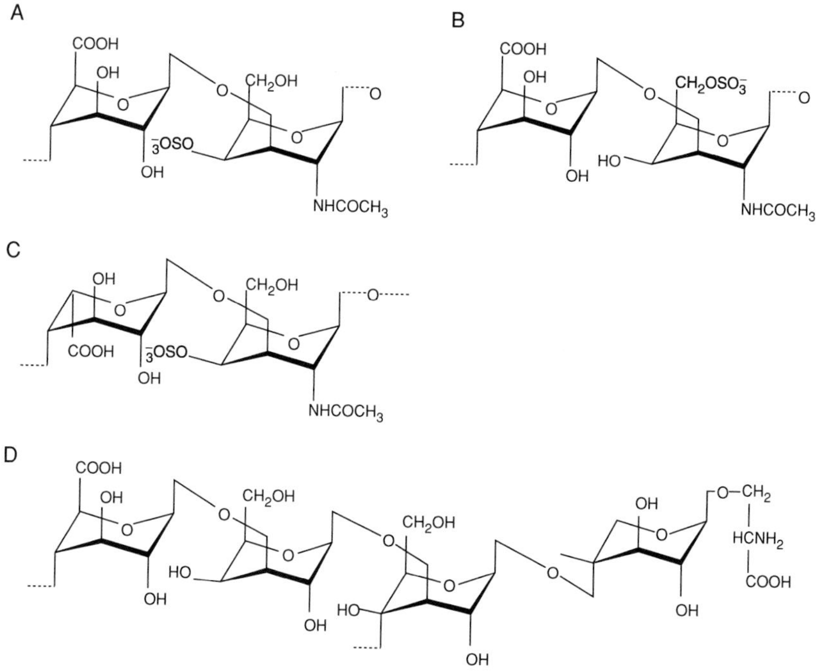

FIGURE I   Structures of the disaccharides found in chondroitin-4-sulfate (A), chondroitin-6-sulfate (B), and DS (C). The GAG chains are attached O-glycosidically to a specific serine residue in core proteins through a β-D-GlcA-1→3-β-D-Gal-1→3-β-D-Gal-1→4-β-D-Xyl tetrasaccharide, denominated as "linkage region" (D).

III. Precursor Discoveries on the Biosynthesis of CS _____

On the basis of the structure of CS (Fig. 1A and B), at least four enzymes could be predicted in its biosynthesis, including two glycosyltransferases for the polymerization of GalNAc and GlcA units, and two sulfotransferases for sulfation at positions 4 and 6 of the GalNAc residues. However, we presently know a larger number of enzymes involved in the biosynthesis of CS, as we will discuss later. But we will initially refer to some precursor studies, in the 1960s and 1970s, concerning the biosynthesis of CS. This was a period of fundamental discoveries on the biosynthesis of glycoconjugates. At that time the basic questions about the biosynthesis of CS were related with the mechanisms of polymerization and sulfation of the polysaccharide.

In 1957, Robbins and Lipmann (1957) isolated 3′-phosphoadenosine 5′-phosphosulfate (PAPS, "active sulfate") from rabbit and lamb livers. They also purified a phenol sulfokinase, which catalyzes the transfer of sulfate from PAPS to nitrophenol. These findings called the attention that PAPS could also be the sulfate donor in the biosynthesis of CS (and also of others GAGs), as in fact, it was demonstrated by the studies of Suzuki and Strominger (1960a) and D'Abramo and Lipmann (1957), using soluble enzyme preparation from chicken oviduct and from embryonic chick cartilage, respectively.

In the case of hen oviduct, the tissue also contained high concentrations of unusual nucleotides, including uridine diphospho-N-acetyl-galactosamine 4-sulfate [UDP-GalNAc-4(SO_4)]. This raised the possibility that sulfate might be transferred from PAPS to the nucleotide and only then incorporated into the GAG chain. Suzuki and Strominger (1960b) investigated this possibility using low-molecular weight oligo-saccharides and clearly demonstrated that sulfate was introduced directly into the acceptor without the simultaneous addition of monosaccharide units.

These initial studies have utilized soluble enzyme preparations with commercial CS or chemically desulfated CS as sulfate acceptor. However, in these studies, the amount of sulfate incorporated into the GAG was too small to affect measurably the anionic characteristic of the acceptor. This aspect was overcome when microsomal preparations from chick embryo epiphyseal cartilage were employed to study incorporation of ^{35}S-sulfate into endogenous acceptor. A highly sulfated CS was indeed formed by the microsomal preparation (DeLuca *et al.*, 1973; Silbert and DeLuca, 1969).

Almost in parallel with the studies concerning the sulfation of CS and subsequent to the discovery that sugar nucleotides were the intermediate in the biosynthesis of several polysaccharides (including hyaluronic acid), it became clear that UDP-GalNAc e UDP-GlcA were the donors of the sugar units of the CS chains.

In a pioneer study, Silbert (1964) described the simultaneous and equimolar incorporation of GalNAc and GlcA into polysaccharides using a microsomal preparation from chick embryo epiphyseal cartilage and incubation mixtures containing labeled and nonlabeled sugar nucleotides (Table I). When the reaction mixture contained a single nucleotide, the incorporation of radioactive precursors into the endogenous acceptor reduced markedly (c and f in Table I). In contrast, when the two nucleotides were added to the mixture, high amount of labeled polysaccharide was observed (a, d, and e, Table I). This clearly indicated that the biosynthesis of CS proceed through alternating transfer of GalNAc and GlcA units from the sugar nucleotides to the polysaccharide. Furthermore, the incorporation of GlcA was approximately one-third when UDP-GalNAc was replaced by uridine diphospho-N-acetyl-glucosamine (UDP-GlcNAc) (b, Table I). Several other studies demonstrated that a single GlcA was transferred from UDP-GlcA to a GalNAc residue at the nonreducing end of an odd numbered oligosaccharide and a single GalNAc can similarly be transferred

TABLE I Incorporation of ^{3}H and ^{14}C from Sugar Nucleotides into Polysaccharide Fraction of a Microsomal Preparation from Chicken Embryo Epiphyseal Cartilage*

	Radioactivity incorporated into polysaccharides (total cpm)	
Nucleotide added	^{3}H	^{14}C
a. ^{3}H-UDP-GalNAc + UDP-GlcA	3000	–
b. ^{3}H-UDP-GlcNAc + UDP-GlcA	1010	–
c. ^{3}H-UDP-GalNAc	290	–
d. ^{3}H-UDP-GalNAc + ^{14}C-UDP-GlcA	3635 (0.091)**	1335 (0.089)**
e. UDP-GalNAc + ^{14}C-UDP-GlcA	–	990
f. ^{14}C-UDP-GlcA	–	110

*Data from Silbert, 1964.
**Values in parenthesis are mμmol of labeled sugar incorporated into the polysaccharide.

from UDP-GalNAc to the GlcA of the nonreducing end of an even number oligosaccharide (Silbert *et al.*, 1976).

It became clear in these initial studies that enzymes involved in the sulfation and polymerization of CS were located together on the microsomal preparation. This suggested that sulfation of the polysaccharide proceeds during polymerization or immediately following polymerization.

IV. The Biosynthesis of the CS Starts with the Formation of the Linkage Region

The CS chain is attached glycosidically to serine in core proteins through a β-D-GlcA-1→3-β-D-Gal-1→3-β-D-Gal-1→4-β-D-Xyl tetrasaccharide, denominated as "linkage region" (Fig. 1D). This observation raises another question concerning the biosynthesis of CS/DS proteoglycans (PGs), related with the incorporation of the four sugar units of the linkage region.

Initial studies revealed that xylose and galactose were transferred from their respective uridine diphosphate derivatives to endogenous acceptors in cell-free systems (Grebner *et al.*, 1966; Telser *et al.*, 1966). A further step was the use of several well-characterized exogenous acceptors, which permitted the development of simple assays for each one of the transfer reactions. Thus, different fragments of the carbohydrate-protein region, such as β-D-Xyl-L-serine, β-D-Gal-1→4-β-Xyl, and β-D-Gal-β-1→4-D-Xyl-L-serine, were used as substrates for the transfer reactions and permitted to distinguish the two galactosyltransferases involved in the biosynthesis of the linkage region (Helting and Roden, 1969a).

Since the first glucuronic acid residue in the CS/DS chains is linked to galactose rather than to GalNAc, two GlcAT could conceivably be involved in the biosynthesis of the polysaccharide. Information regarding this problem was obtained by mixed substrate experiments in which β-Gal-1→3-D-Gal was incubated together with CS trisaccharide or pentasaccharide containing GalNAc-6(SO$_4$) at their reducing terminals (Helting and Roden, 1969b). Glucuronyl transfer to the trisaccharide proceeded equally well in the presence of an excess of β-Gal-1→3-D-Gal (a in Table II). In contrast, the pentasaccharide almost completely abolished glucuronyl transfer to the homologous trisaccharide under similar conditions (b in Table II). These findings indicated that the transfer of GlcA to the galactose residue of the linkage region is mediated by an enzyme distinct from that involved in the formation of the remainder of the CS chain.

Therefore, it is now clear that the biosynthesis of CS starts with xylose addition to specific serine residues in a consensus sequence of a PG core protein (Bourdon *et al.*, 1987), followed by the sequential addition of two galactose residues and a glucuronic acid. Then, chondroitin polymerization takes place, by alternating incorporation of GalNAc and GlcA to constitute the repeating disaccharide region. In these glycosyltransferase reactions the sugar donors are always their respective uridine diphosphate derivatives. Sulfation of the polymer by specific sulfotransferases occurs as the chain is growing. The various steps involved in the biosynthesis of CS are summarized in Fig. 2.

The four glycosyltransferases involved in the synthesis of the linkage region (Fig. 2A), named O-xylosyltransferase-I (XylT-I), galactosyltransferase-I (GalT-I), galactosyltransferase-II (GalT-II), and glucuronyltransferase-I (GlcAT-I), have already been cloned (Almeida *et al.*, 1999; Bai *et al.*, 2001; Gotting *et al.*, 2000; Kitagawa *et al.*, 1998).[1]

Peptide O-xylosyltransferase was one of the first glycosyltransferase to be described (Gregory *et al.*, 1964). Although this enzyme has great ability to transfer xylose to Ser-Gly motifs in the core protein, it has been shown that this is not an absolute requirement. There is evidence, using site-directed mutagenesis, that it may also transfer xylose to threonine (Rodén *et al.*, 1985).

---

[1] Glycosyltransferases are a superfamily of enzymes responsible for the transfer of specific glycosyl residues from activated sugar-nucleotide donors to specific acceptor molecules. Thus, these enzymes are involved in the synthesis of carbohydrate chains of GAGs, glycolipids, and glycoproteins. Members of this superfamily of enzymes are usually named after the sugar moiety that they transfer and are divided into subfamilies based on the linkage established between the donor and acceptor such as β-1→4-, β-1→3-, α-1→4-galactosyltransferase, xylosyltransferase, N-acetylgalactosaminyltransferase, sialyltransferase, and others. For example, β-1→4-GalT forms a family including seven enzymes, from β-1→4-GalT1 through β-1→4-GalT7. All of them transfer galactose from UDP-Gal to the acceptor through β-1→4-linkage, basically differing in the sugar acceptor used.

TABLE II Mixed Substrate Experiments, Which Provided the Initial Evidence that the Transfer of GlcA from UDP-GlcA to the Linkage Region of CS is Mediated by an Enzyme Distinct from that Involved in the Formation of the Remainder of the CS Chain*

Substrates added to the reaction mixtures			Reaction monitored on the assay	
●—●	○—□—○<	○—□—□—○<	○<—□—○< → ○<—□—○—□ (GalNAc/GlcA units)	●—● + □ → ●—□—●
μmol			Total cpm incorporated into the oligosaccharide	
a.				
0	0.1	—	1459	—
0.5	0.1	—	1333	25300
1.0	0.1	—	949	29890
2.0	0.1	—	1580	39400
b.				
—	0.1	—	1040	—
—	0.1	0.07	73	—
—	0.1	0.10	80	—

*Data from Helting and Roden, 1969b.

●—● represents β-D-Gal-1→3-D-Gal disaccharide; ○< the β-D-GalNAc-6(SO4) units of CS; and □ β-D-GlcA residues of either the linkage region or of the major CS structure.

A   Synthesis of the linkage region

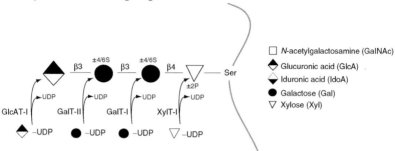

B   Chain polymerization

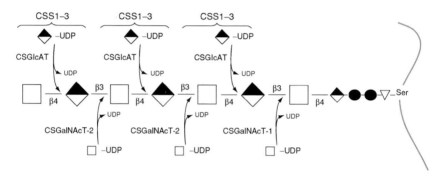

C   Sulfation of chondroitin sulfate

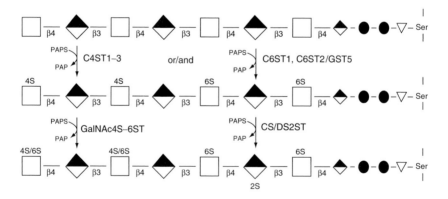

D Polymer modification and sulfation of dermatan sulfate

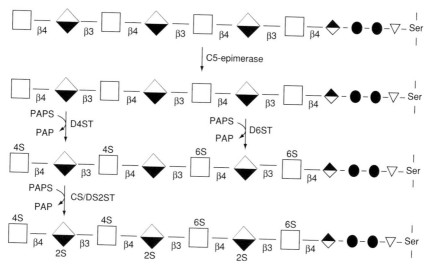

FIGURE 2 Schematic representation of the biosynthesis of CS/DS. (A) Formation of the linkage region: The linkage region is formed by sequential addition of xylose, two galactoses, and glucuronic acid catalyzed by xylosyltransferase I (XylT-I), galactosyltransferase I (GalT-I), galactosyltransferase II (GalT-II), and glucuronyltransferase I (GlcAT-I), respectively. Sulfation (S) and/or phosphorylation (P) of these units are regulatory mechanisms, which select the type of GAG chain that will be synthesized, either a GalAG or a glucosaminoglycan. (B) Chain polymerization: The transfer of the first GalNAc to the linkage region is catalyzed by a chondroitin sulfate N-acetylgalactosaminyltransferase-1 (CSGalNAcT-1). Subsequently, GlcA and GalNAc units are added in an orchestrated and organized manner by the action of chondrotin sulfate glucuronyltransferase (CSGlcAT) and chondroitin sulfate N-acetylgalacto-saminyltransferase-2 (CSGalNAcT-2), respectively. The addition of GlcA and GalNAc can also be carried out by recently cloned enzymes namely chondroitin synthases 1–3 (CSS1–3). These enzymes possess two catalytic domains for the transfer of GlcA and GalNAc units. The sugar donors in all these glycosyltransferase reactions are their respective uridine diphosphate nucleotides. In the panel we refer exclusively to glycosyltransferases that have already been cloned. (C) Sulfation of CS: These reactions involve the transfer of a sulfate group from the activated sulfate donor PAPS into specific position of the CS. Sulfation of position 6 of the CS is catalyzed by C6ST1 or by C6ST2 or GST5. Another enzyme, named chondroitin 6-O-sulfate sulfotransferase (GalNAc4S-6ST), catalyzes transfer of sulfate to position 6 of nonreducing GalNAc-4-sulfate residues and even to internal units in some invertebrate species. Three chondroitin-4-sulfate sulfotransferases (C4ST1-3) are involved in 4-O-sulfation of GalNAc units. Finally, sulfation at position 2 of the GlcA involves a CS/DS 2-O-sulfotransferase (CS/DS2ST). (D) Polymer modification and sulfation of DS: Biosynthesis of DS has an additional step of C5-epimerization of GlcA into IdoA. Thereafter, the polysaccharide is sulfated by a dermatan 4-sulfate sulfotransferase (D4ST) and, at a lower extension, by a dermatan 6-sulfate sulfotransferase (D6ST). Finally, position 2 of the IdoA can be sulfated on a reaction catalyzed by the CS/DS 2-O-sulfotransferase (CS/DS2ST). Interestingly, sulfation prevents back-epimerization of the newly formed IdoA into GlcA. The monosaccharide units are represented in the panels by symbols. These monosaccharides are assumed to be in the D-configuration, except for L-iduronic acid, all in the pyranose form.

V. Post-Translational Modifications of the Linkage Region Regulate the Synthesis of the GAG chain _____

Different types of GAGs are assembled to the protein core through the common linkage tetrasaccharide shown in Fig. 1D. The homogeneity of the linkage region contrasts with the structural diversity of the repeating disaccharides found in each GAG chain. These observations led to speculations concerning the reason why different types of GAG chains are synthesized, starting from the same protein linkage region. What is the molecular signal determinant for the type of glycan chain to be synthesized?

A clarification to this question came when several groups found sulfation at position O-4 and/or O-6 of the galactose residues in the linkage region of CS, which does not occur in heparan sulfate (HS) (de Waard et al., 1992; Sugahara and Kitagawa, 2000; Sugahara et al., 1988), even when these two GAGs are attached to the same PG (Ueno et al., 2001). In contrast, a 2-phosphorylation in xylose residue has been found in all types of GAG chains (Fransson et al., 1985; Moses et al., 1997). Furthermore, chondroitin-4-sulfate and chondroitin-6-sulfate contain galactose residues 4- and 6-sulfated in the linkage region, respectively (Silbert and Sugumaran, 2002). Thus, sulfation and phosphorylation of the sugar residues found in the linkage region may constitute molecular signals to determine the type of GAG chain that will be synthesized.

All these modifications of the linkage region occur as an early posttranslational event (Lohmander et al., 1986) and have been shown to occur in several tissues among different animals (Lauder et al., 2000; Sugahara et al., 1992; Ueno et al., 2001). Sulfation of galactose and phosphorylation of xylose are mutually exclusive events and also are not found in all chains (Ueno et al., 2001). These observations suggest that sulfate and phosphate may be added to specific sugar units of the linkage region as a signaling marker and then removed, as a dynamic process. Certainly, these two major modifications of the linkage region influence the specificity of the glycosyltransferases. Thus, phosphorylation of xylose occurs only after the addition of the first galactose residue since GalT-I is not able to catalyze the incorporation of galactose into phosphorylated xylose (Gulberti et al., 2005). Moses (1997) reported that xylose residue is transiently phosphorylated during decorin biosynthesis, while the linkage region is synthesized. Phosphorylation is essentially complete after the synthesis of the galactose-galactose-xylose, but when the GlcA residue is added dephosphorylation takes place. Therefore, the occurrence of phosphorylated xylose is an important determinant for the GlcAT-I activity. However, phosphorylation of xylose on aggrecan appears to be stable (Oegema et al., 1984).

Overall, these observations suggest that phosphorylation of xylose can arrest the biosynthesis of some GAG chains, representing a regulatory mechanism in their biosynthetic rate. Likewise, sulfation can also be a regulatory mechanism. GlcAT-I is not active toward 4-sulfated galactose residues (Gulberti *et al.*, 2005). Moreover, sulfated galactose is hypothesized to be recognized by an *N*-acetylgalactosaminyltransferase (GalNAcT), named as chondroitin sulfate *N*-acetylgalactosaminyltransferase-1 (CSGalNAcT-1) (Fig. 2B), specific for the linkage region and might be a molecular signal that promotes synthesis of CS rather than HS chain (Sugahara and Kitagawa, 2000). Also, 4-sulfation of GalNAc seems to stimulate CSGalNAcT-2, an enzyme involved in elongation of CS chains (Sato *et al.*, 2003), whereas a terminal 3-sulfated GlcA or penultimate 4,6-disulfated GalNAc residues inhibit the enzyme activity (Kitagawa *et al.*, 1997).

Despite all these data, there is still strong evidence of signals in the structure of core protein that determine the selection of the type of GAG chain that will be synthesized (Esko and Zhang, 1996).

VI. Chain Initiation and Polymerization of CS/DS _____

The transfer of a GalNAc to the linkage region by CSGalNAcT-1 is the initial step for the polymerization of CS/DS chain and will drive the synthesis of a galactosaminoglycan (GalAG) rather than of a glucosaminoglycan. Subsequently, alternating addition of GlcA and GalNAc units goes on in a highly organized mechanism of polymerization in which the enzymes act in an orchestrated manner, adding each individual sugar to the nonreducing end of the acceptor. Different glycosyltransferases are involved in elongation of the CS chain (Rohrmann *et al.*, 1985), as described in Fig. 2B.

Recently, two GalNAcTs involved in the addition of GalNAc to CS chains have been cloned (Uyama *et al.*, 2002, 2003). One is the CSGalNAcT-1, which exhibits a strong activity toward the linkage region, as we referred earlier, and does not use CS chains as acceptor. Another enzyme, named as CSGalNAcT-2, shows high activity toward CS substrate and does not recognize the tetrasaccharide-serine of the linkage region as acceptor. *In vivo* studies have not completely corroborated the *in vitro* studies yet. Possibly, there are some factors regulating the activity of these enzymes such as sulfation in the linkage region or the peptide sequence of the core protein. In addition, the existence of a multimeric complex has been suggested (Uyama *et al.*, 2003).

The transfer of GlcA to elongate CS is achieved by a GlcAT-II, distinct from the GlcAT-I that is involved in the addition of the ultimate residue of the linkage region (Sugumaran *et al.*, 1997). Searching the database for homology to known genes allowed the cloning of a new GlcAT, known as chondroitin sulfate glucuronyltransferase (CSGlcAT), which shows only GlcAT-II activity (Gotoh *et al.*, 2002).

A new enzyme, named CS synthase (CSS1) was cloned and showed both GlcAT-II and GalNAcT-II activities involved in CS polymerization

(Kitagawa *et al.*, 2001). This enzyme possesses two catalytic domains, one containing the β4GT motif that functions by transferring GalNAc to GlcA via β1,4 linkage and other containing a β3GT motif that transfers GlcA to GalNAc via β1,3 linkage. However, a chondroitin polymerization activity has not been observed with the recombinant enzyme *in vitro*. This fact can be explained by the requirement of the coexpression of another protein, the recently cloned chondroitin polymerizing factor (ChPF). Perhaps CSS1 and ChPF exist *in vivo* as a single protein complex. In fact, ChPF is a member of the gene family of CS glycosyltranferases, as it presents homology to the others enzymes previously cloned but shows little GalNAcT-II or GlcAT-II activity (Kitagawa *et al.*, 2003).

Despite all these reports, it is not clear which enzyme really acts on each step of the chain polymerization. Both CSS1 and CSGlcAT possess GlcAT-II activity, however, they have different acceptor specificities. While CSGlcAT prefers short acceptors, CSS1 acts on longer sequences (Gotoh *et al.*, 2002b). This could indicate that both enzymes take part in different stages of CS polymerization. However, the activity and substrate specificity observed *in vitro* might not represent the real situation *in vivo*.

Additional complexities on the mechanism of CS biosynthesis were revealed on studies with the nematode *Caenorhabditis elegans*. In this invertebrate, sqv-5 and PAR2.4, CSS1 and ChPF orthologs, respectively, were cloned (Hwang *et al.*, 2003a; Izumikawa *et al.*, 2004). In addition, two new CSSs were cloned (named as CSS2 and CSS3). These enzymes possess both GalNAcT-II and GlcAT-II activities, as CSS1. However, the specific activity and the rate of expression in tissues of CSS1 are much more significant than their counterparts, although the three enzymes are ubiquitously expressed in animal tissues (Yada *et al.*, 2003a,b).

Overall, the recent purification, cloning, expression, and characterization of many glycosyltransferases have revealed new enzymes involved in the polymerization of the CS chains. However, additional information is required in order to determine the role and specificity of each enzyme under *in vivo* conditions. Furthermore, it is still necessary to clarify the coordination of the event, which probably requires the formation of complex machinery. Finally, the molecular mechanism of gene expression is a critical step to determine the role of each one of these enzymes during CS biosynthesis under normal and pathological conditions.

VII. Sulfation of CS: General Properties of the Sulfotransferases

The sulfation of GAGs occurs in the Golgi compartment and is catalyzed by sulfotransferases, which catalyze the transfer of a sulfate group from the universal activated sulfate donor PAPS to hydroxyl group of a specific position of the sugar residue. PAPS is synthesized in the cytosol and enters the Golgi compartment via a PAPS/PAP (3′-phosphoadenosine-5′-phosphate) translocase shuttle (Ozeran *et al.*, 1996). Some sulfotransferases recognize not only the kind and position of acceptor sugar but also the structure of the neighboring residues. The core protein to which the GAG chains are linked does not determine specificity of sulfation (Uchimura *et al.*, 2002).

Several GAG sulfotransferases have been identified, cloned, and/or purified from vertebrates, such as human (Okuda *et al.*, 2000; Shworak *et al.*, 1999), mouse (Kusche-Gullberg *et al.*, 1998; Yamauchi *et al.*, 2000), chicken (Fukuta *et al.*, 1995), and fish (Bink *et al.*, 2003), in addition to insect (*Drosophila*) (Kamimura *et al.*, 2001) and worms (*C. elegans*) (Turnbull *et al.*, 2003), providing information about their structural organization. Similar to other Golgi-resident enzymes, such as glycosyltransferases, sulfotransferases have a type II transmembrane topology consisting of a short amino-terminal cytoplasmic domain followed by a single transmembrane domain and a carboxy-terminal domain containing the catalytic site faced to the lumen of the Golgi.

X-ray crystallographic studies of sulfotransferases revealed the structural features and the reaction mechanism that can be applied to all sulfotransferases (Kakuta *et al.*, 1997). These enzymes are a single α/β globular protein with a characteristic five-stranded parallel β-sheet flanked by α-helices on both sides of the sheet (Negishi *et al.*, 2001). Studies on the reaction mechanism indicate that sulfotransferases form a ternary complex involving the enzyme, PAPS, and the acceptor substrate. Both the binding of the cosubstrate to the enzyme and the release of the product occur in an ordered manner. PAPS binds first, followed by the acceptor substrate (carbohydrate). After sulfuryl transfer, the sulfated product is released followed by PAP (Negishi *et al.*, 2001).

The sulfation heterogeneity of CS/DS is a result of the action of several sulfotransferases with different isoforms, substrate specificity, and patterns of expression. These enzymes can be grouped into three families, which transfer sulfuryl groups to positions 4 and 6 of GalNAc residues and to position 2 of GlcA or IdoA (in the case of DS). The actions of these enzymes are summarized in Fig. 2C and D.

VIII. 6-*O*-Sulfotransferase

Sulfation at position 6 of the CS is catalyzed by chondroitin-6-sulfate sulfotransferase (C6ST1). The enzyme was first identified in extracts from chick embryo epiphyseal cartilage (Habuchi and Miyashita, 1982) and subsequently purified (Habuchi *et al.*, 1993) and cloned (Fukuta *et al.*, 1995) from cultured chick embryo chondrocytes. The purified enzyme catalyzes the transfer of sulfate group from PAPS to the 6-position of GalNAc residues in GlcA-rich region of CS, in addition to the galactose residues of keratan sulfate (KS) (Fukuta *et al.*, 1995; Uchimura *et al.*, 2002). The cDNA of the chicken C6ST1 predicts a type II transmembrane protein, composed of 458 amino acid residues, containing 6 potential sites for N-glycosylation (Fukuta *et al.*, 1995).

Human and mouse C6ST1 cDNAs were isolated and cloned, based on the avian C6ST1 sequence (Fukuta *et al.*, 1998; Mazany *et al.*, 1998; Tsutsumi *et al.*, 1998; Uchimura *et al.*, 1998). The human C6ST1 displays 74% amino acid sequence identity to the chicken counterpart, and the major difference between the human and chicken enzymes resides in the presence of a unique hydrophilic domain in the human enzyme. Analysis of the reaction products demonstrated that C6ST1 transfers sulfate to position 6 of GalNAc in GlcA-β-1→3-GalNAc sequences. No reaction is observed when GalNAc is 4-sulfated or flanked by IdoA at the nonreducing terminal (Tsutsumi *et al.*, 1998). C6ST1 is ubiquitously expressed in various adult human tissues, indicating that it may be involved in diverse biological processes (Fukuta *et al.*, 1998). Mouse C6ST1 is composed by 472 amino acid residues and exhibits 71% sequence identity to the chicken enzyme. Similarly to the avian enzyme, mouse C6ST1 also displays KS sulfotransferase activity, but in this case it is significantly lower (Uchimura *et al.*, 1998). Analysis of C6ST1 mRNA in mouse tissues indicates that it is strongly expressed in spleen, lung, and eye.

Using the sequence of the human C6ST1, a novel human C6ST was identified and named C6ST2 or GST5. The cDNA sequence of human C6ST2/GST5 reveals a protein of 486 amino acids, which displays 24% sequence identity to human C6ST1 (Kitagawa *et al.*, 2000). A homologous C6ST2/GST5 has also been identified in mouse (Bhakta *et al.*, 2000). Based on functional and structural similarities C6ST2/GST5 has been suggested to belong to the Gal/GalNAc/GlcNAc 6-O-sulfotransferase (GST) family of enzymes, which includes mainly Golgi-resident GlcNAc 6-O-sulfotransferases (Bhakta *et al.*, 2000). The substrate specificities as well as the tissue distribution of the C6ST2/GST5 remain to be clearly determined.

A chondroitin 6-O-sulfate sulfotransferase (GalNAc4S-6ST) that sulfates GalNAc 4-sulfate residues on CS and DS was purified from human serum (Inoue *et al.*, 1986a) and from squid cartilage (Ito and Habuchi, 2000). The human enzyme transfers sulfate from PAPS mainly to position 6 of the nonreducing GalNAc 4-sulfate residues (Inoue *et al.*, 1986b), whereas the squid counterpart transfers sulfate mainly to position 6 of internal GalNAc 4-sulfate residues (Ito and Habuchi, 2000). Human GalNAc4S-6ST was subsequently cloned based on the amino acid sequence of the purified squid enzyme (Ohtake *et al.*, 2001). Its cDNA predicts a type II transmembrane protein, composed of 561 amino acid residues. Nucleotide sequence of the human GalNAc4S-6ST cDNA indicates that it is nearly identical to the sequence of human B cell RAG-associated gene. Based on the analysis of substrate specificities of human GalNAc4S-6ST, it was suggested that the enzyme is involved in the generation of highly sulfated nonreducing terminal sequence in chondroitin-4-sulfate (Ohtake *et al.*, 2003).

A novel DS-specific 6-O-sulfotransferase has been detected in bovine fetal serum. The enzyme transfers sulfate to position 6 of GalNAc residues in the sequence IdoA-α-1$\rightarrow$3-GalNAc-β-1$\rightarrow$4-IdoA of DS. No DS 6-O-sulfotransferase activity is observed toward CS or when the GalNAc residues in the sequence IdoA-α-1$\rightarrow$3-GalNAc-β-1$\rightarrow$4-IdoA are 4-sulfated (Nadanaka *et al.*, 1999). IdoA-α-1$\rightarrow$3-GalNAc-6(SO_4) disaccharide units are common in DS from nonmammalian sources, such as hagfish notocord (Anno *et al.*, 1971), and embryonic and adult sea urchin (Vilela-Silva *et al.*, 2001), implying the occurrence in these animals of 6-O-sulfotransferases with substrate specificities similar to that of bovine fetal serum.

IX. 4-O-Sulfotransferase

4-O-sulfation of GalNAc is the most frequent modification of CS and DS and is carried out by three chondroitin-4-sulfate sulfotransferases (C4ST1–3) and one dermatan 4-sulfate sulfotransferase (D4ST1), which have been cloned and characterized (Evers *et al.*, 2001; Hiraoka *et al.*, 2000; Kang *et al.*, 2002; Yamauchi *et al.*, 2000). These enzymes have different degrees of homologies with HNK-1ST, an enzyme that transfers sulfate from PAPS to position 3 of terminal GlcA residues in the sequence GlcA-β-1$\rightarrow$3-Gal-β-1$\rightarrow$4-GlcNAc found in natural killer cell antigen (HNK-1) (Baenzinger, 2003). C4ST1–3 transfer sulfate from PAPS to position 4 of GalNAc residues in GlcA-rich regions in both desulfated CS and DS.

C4ST1 was first purified to apparent homogeneity from the serum-free cultured medium of rat chondrosarcoma cells (Yamauchi *et al.*, 2000). It is a glycoprotein containing about 35% N-linked oligosaccharides that contribute to the production and stability of the active form of the enzyme (Yusa *et al.*, 2005). Subsequently, C4ST1 cDNAs were isolated from mouse brain and human fetal brain and cloned, based on the amino acid sequences of peptides obtained from the purified rat enzyme (Okuda *et al.*, 2000; Yamauchi *et al.*, 1999). Mouse and human C4ST1 share 96% of amino acid sequence homology and are broadly expressed in adult human (predominant expression in hematopoetic tissues, peripheral blood leucocytes) and mouse (predominant expression in brain and kidney) tissues, as indicated by Northern blot analysis.

Using the conserved RDP motif in HNK-1ST as a probe, which is a part of the binding site for 3'-phosphate group of PAPS, the cDNA of the C4ST2 was cloned. The enzyme shares only 41.8% identity at the amino acid level with C4ST1. Similar to C4ST1, C4ST2 transfers sulfate to position 4 of the

GalNAc, located at GlcA-GalNAc-GlcA sequence in desulfated CS and DS but not to chondrotin-6-sulfate. Northern blot analysis indicates that C4ST2 has a more widely expression than C4ST1 (Hiraoka *et al.*, 2000).

A new C4ST namely C4ST3 has been identified based on its homology to HNK-1ST. Its cDNA encodes a 341-amino acid protein with 45% and 27% sequence identity with C4ST1 and C4ST2, respectively. It has a highly restricted pattern of expression, being expressed predominantly in adult liver and at lower levels in adult kidney (Kang *et al.*, 2002). Although all C4ST share the same substrate specificities they have different patterns of expression. This fact may suggest that these enzymes are involved in different biological events.

D4ST1 has also been cloned based on its homology to HNK-1ST (Evers *et al.*, 2001). Its cDNA encodes a 376-amino acid protein containing two potential N-linked glycosylation sites at the cytoplasmic domain. D4ST1 has 27.3% and 22.8% amino acid identity to C4ST1 and C4ST2, respectively. Enzymatic and structural analysis of the reaction products indicate that the sulfotransferase is able to transfer sulfate group to position 4 of GalNAc in DS, located not only in the sequence IdoA-GalNAc-IdoA but also in GlcA-GalNAc-IdoA and IdoA-GalNAc-GlcA. In addition, it has been suggested that 4-sulfation stimulates subsequent 4-sulfation of GalNAc in the neighboring disaccharide unit. Enzymatic studies using microsomes showed that 4-sulfation follows C5-epimerization of GlcA into IdoA, and the sulfation prevents back epimerization of the newly formed IdoA into GlcA (Mikami *et al.*, 2003; Silbert and Sugumaran, 2002). This epimerization reaction is shown in Fig. 2D.

X. 2-O-Sulfotransferase

Sulfation at position 2 of IdoA is a frequent modification found in DS. It creates unique motifs within the polymer necessary for specific interactions with several molecules. For example, 2-sulfation of IdoA in IdoA-GalNAc-4 (SO_4)-rich region in DS accounts for the presence of a specific sequence required for binding and activation of heparin cofactor II (Maimone and Tollefsen, 1990; Pavão *et al.*, 1998). Sulfation at position 2 of GlcA on CS may also occur, but it is less frequent. The transfer of sulfate groups to IdoA/GlcA is catalyzed CS/DS 2-O-sulfotransferase (CS/DS2ST). 2-sulfation of IdoA during biosynthesis of DS polymers normally occurs next to 4-sulfated GalNAc residues (Silbert *et al.*, 1986). A probable exception to this rule occurs during the biosynthesis of DS in the ascidian *Ascidia nigra*. The DS of this marine invertebrate is composed mainly by IdoA-2(SO_4)-GalNAc-6 (SO_4) disaccharide unities, indicating that 2-sulfation occurs exclusively next to 6-sulfated GalNAc (Pavão *et al.*, 1995, 1998) by a 2-O-sulfotransferase with different substrate specificity, which remains to be identified.

Human CS/DS2ST had been cloned based on the amino acid sequence of the HS iduronyl 2-O-sulfotransferase (Kobayashi *et al.*, 1999). The full-length cDNA encodes a 406-amino acid protein possessing the characteristic type II transmembrane topology of other Golgi-resident sulfotransferases. The fact that 2-sulfation takes place preferentially after sulfation of GalNAc suggests that it is probably the last step in the biosynthesis of CS/DS and would occur in a relatively late Golgi trans network. Northern blot analysis demonstrated that it has a ubiquitous expression in various human tissues and in several human cancer cell lines (Kobayashi *et al.*, 1999).

XI. Genetic Defects Affecting the Biosynthesis of CS _____

Only few heritable disorders involving the biosynthesis of CS have been described. A C6S with low sulfate content was reported in the urine of patients with an unusual form of spondyloepiphyseal dysplasia, having an autosomal recessive inheritance (Mourão *et al.*, 1973). This undersulfated CS possibly results from a low activity of a CS sulfotransferase (Mourão *et al.*, 1981). Another study reported that homozygous brachymorphic mice have a considerable increase in the amounts of nonsulfated disaccharide units in the CS extracted from the abnormal cartilage (Orkin *et al.*, 1976). Additional studies on these mice indicated a defect in the synthesis of PAPS from ATP and sulfate, the availability of PAPS possibly being the rate-limiting factor in the sulfation of the CS. Curiously, no abnormalities were found in skin fibroblasts of the patients with spondyloepiphyseal dysplasia (Mourão *et al.*, 1981) or of the brachymorphic mice (Sugahara *et al.*, 1986). Both genetic defects were restricted to cartilage. These were very early evidences that differences may exist in the distribution of enzymes involved in the biosynthesis of CS.

Now it is clear that a great number of glycosyltransferases and sulfo-transferases genes participate in the biosynthesis of CS, as we already discussed. As various enzymes are involved in CS synthesis, it is complicate to investigate the mechanism of biosynthesis of this GAG by gene knockout and, besides, in some cases, this approach results in animal lethality (Narimatsu, 2004; Sugahara and Kitagawa, 2000). Nevertheless, the genetic approach may constitute an advance in the understanding of CS biosynthesis and also may help to clarify the molecular mechanisms underlying the pathology of various diseases that involve CS or DS.

Mutations in genes that encode glycosyltransferases involved in the formation of the linkage region, which affects both GalAGs and GAGs synthesis, have demonstrated the importance of GAG in some diseases. This is the case of a progeroid variant of Ehlers-Danlos syndrome, caused by two mutations in gene encoding galactosyltransferase I (Furukawa and Okajima, 2002). Also, mutations in *sqv-2* and *sqv-6* genes, which encode xylosyltransferase and galactosyltransferase II, respectively, have shown to influence *C. elegans* development (Hwang *et al.*, 2003a).

It is known that CS plays several roles in cell adhesion, migration, recognition, proliferation, morphogenesis and recently becomes implicated in the formation of neural network during the development of mammalian brain (Sugahara *et al.*, 2003). However, we still have little knowledge about the involvement of specific enzymes of CS biosynthesis in diseases. Cloning of a homolog of human chondroitin synthase in *C. elegans* showed that CS is essential for embryonic cytokinesis and cell division. The depleted expression of the enzyme resulted in cytokinesis defects in early embryogenesis and in an interruption of cell division, which produced an early embryonic death (Hwang *et al.*, 2003b).

XII. Future Perspectives

The recent cloning of various enzymes involved in the biosynthesis of CS may help to understand the molecular basis of several biological events compromised by alterations in the pathways of CS biosynthesis. Another possible avenue to follow is the study of the biosynthesis of CS/DS with unusual structures in invertebrate tissues. These GAGs with unique structure already revealed useful tools to determine structure vs. biological activity or the involvement of rare sulfation pattern on biological events in mammalian tissues. These were the case of studies concerning the anticoagulant activity of DS (Pavão *et al.*, 1995, 1998) and the importance of disulfated disaccharide units found in DS for the formation of neural network during the development of mammalian brain (Hikino *et al.*, 2003). It may be difficult to discover genes and enzymes implicated in the biosynthesis of these rare structures found in mammalian CS/DS. But, as an alternative, the invertebrates may provide a clue.

References

Almeida, R., Levery, S. B., Mandel, U., Kresse, H., Schwientek, T., Bennett, E. P., and Clausen, H. (1999). Cloning and expression of a proteoglycan UDP-galactose:beta-xylose beta1,4-galactosyltransferase I. A seventh member of the human beta4-galactosyltransferase gene family. *J. Biol. Chem.* **274**, 26165–26171.

Anno, K., Seno, N., Mathews, M. B., Yamagata, T., and Suzuki, S. (1971). A new dermatan polysulfate, chondroitin sulfate H, from hagfish notochord. *Biochim. Biophys. Acta* **237**, 173–177.

Baenzinger, J. U. (2003). Glycoprotein hormone GalNAc-4-sulphotransferase. *Biochem. Soc. Trans.* **31**, 326–330.

Bai, X., Zhou, D., Brown, J. R., Crawford, B. E., Hennet, T., and Esko, J. D. (2001). Biosynthesis of the linkage region of glycosaminoglycans: Cloning and activity of galactosyltransferase II, the sixth member of the β1,3-galactosyltransferase family (β3GalT6). *J. Biol. Chem.* **276**, 48189–48195.

Bhakta, S., Bartes, A., Bowman, K. G., Kao, W. M., Polsky, I., Lee, J. K., Cook, B. N., Bruehl, R. E., Rosen, S. D., Bertozzi, C. R., and Hemmerich, S. (2000). Sulfation of N-acetylglucosamine by chondroitin 6-sulfotransferase 2 (GST-5). *J. Biol. Chem.* 275, 40226–40234.

Bink, R. J., Habuchi, H., Lele, Z., Dolk, E., Joore, J., Rauch, G. J., Geisler, R., Wilson, S. W., den Hertog, J., Kimata, K., and Zivkovic, D. (2003). Heparan sulfate 6-O-sulfotransferase is essential for muscle development in zebrafish. *J. Biol. Chem.* 278, 31118–31127.

Bourdon, M. A., Krusius, T., Campbell, S., Schwartz, N. B., and Ruoslahti, E. (1987). Identification and synthesis of a recognition signal for the attachment of glycosaminoglycans to proteins. *Proc. Natl. Acad. Sci.* 84, 3194–3198.

D'Abramo, F., and Lipmann, F. (1957). The formation of adenosine-3'-phosphate-5'-phosphosulfate in extracts of chick embryo cartilage and its conversion into chondroitin sulfate. *Biochim. Biophys. Acta* 25, 211–213.

de Waard, P., Vliegenthart, J. F., Harada, T., and Sugahara, K. (1992). Structural studies on sulfated oligosaccharides derived from the carbohydrate-protein linkage region of chondroitin 6-sulfate proteoglycans of shark cartilage. II. Seven compounds containing 2 or 3 sulfate residues. *J. Biol. Chem.* 267, 6036–6043.

DeLuca, S., Richmond, M. E., and Silbert, J. E. (1973). Biosynthesis of chondroitin sulfate: Sulfation of the polysaccharide chain. *Biochemistry* 12, 3911–3915.

Esko, J. D., and Zhang, L. (1996). Influence of core protein sequence on glycosaminoglycan assembly. *Curr. Opin. Struct. Biol.* 6, 663–670.

Evers, M. R., Xia, G., Kang, H. G., Schachner, M., and Baenziger, J. U. (2001). Molecular cloning and characterization of a dermatan-specific N-acetylgalactosamine 4-O-sulfotransferase. *J. Biol. Chem.* 276, 36344–36353.

Fransson, L. A., Silverberg, I., and Carlstedt, I. (1985). Structure of the heparan sulfate-protein linkage region: Demonstration of the sequence galactosyl-galactosyl-xylose-2-phosphate. *J. Biol. Chem.* 260(27), 14722–14726.

Fukuta, M., Uchimura, K., Nakashima, K., Kato, M., Kimata, K., Shinomura, T., and Habuchi, O. (1995). Molecular cloning and expression of chick chondrocyte chondroitin 6-sulfotransferase. *J. Biol. Chem.* 270, 18575–18580.

Fukuta, M., Kobayashi, Y., Uchimura, K., Kimata, K., and Habuchi, O. (1998). Molecular cloning and expression of human chondroitin 6-sulfotransferase. *Biochim. Biophys. Acta* 1399, 57–61.

Furukawa, K., and Okajima, T. (2002). Galactosyltransferase I is a gene responsible for progeroid variant of Ehlers-Danlos syndrome: Molecular cloning and identification of mutations. *Biochim. Biophys. Acta* 1573, 377–381.

Gotoh, M., Sato, T., Akashima, T., Iwasaki, H., Kameyama, A., Mochizuki, H., Yada, T., Inaba, N., Zhang, Y., Kikuchi, N., Kwon, Y. D., Togayachi, A., *et al.* (2002). Enzymatic synthesis of chondroitin with a novel chondroitin sulfate N-acetylgalactosaminyltransferase that transfers N-acetylgalactosamine to glucuronic acid in initiation and elongation of chondroitin sulfate synthesis. *J. Biol. Chem.* 277, 38189–38196.

Gotting, C., Kuhn, J., Zahn, R., Brinkmann, T., and Kleesiek, K. (2000). Molecular cloning and expression of human UDP-d-Xylose:proteoglycan core protein beta-d-xylosyltransferase and its first isoform XT-II. *J. Mol. Biol.* 304, 517–528.

Grebner, E. E., Hall, C. W., and Neufeld, E. F. (1966). Incorporation of D-xylose-C^{14} into glycoprotein by particles from hen oviduct. *Biochem. Biophys. Res. Commun.* 22, 672–677.

Gregory, J. D., Laurent, T. C., and Rodén, L. (1964). Enzymatic degradation of chondromucoprotein. *J. Biol. Chem.* 239, 3312–3320.

Gulberti, S., Lattard, V., Fondeur, M., Jacquinet, J., Mulliert, G., Netter, P., Magdalou, J., Ouzzine, M., and Fournel-Gigleux, S. (2005). Phosphorylation and sulfation of oligosaccharide substrates critically influence the activity of human beta1,4-galactosyltransferase 7 (GalT-I) and beta1,3-glucuronosyltransferase I (GlcAT-I) involved in the biosynthesis of the glycosaminoglycan-protein linkage region of proteoglycans. *J. Biol. Chem.* **280**, 1417–1425.

Habuchi, O., Sugiura, K., Kawai, N., and Suzuki, S. (1977). Glucose branches in chondroitin sulfates from squid cartilage. *J. Biol. Chem.* **252**, 4570–4576.

Habuchi, O., and Miyashita, N. (1982). Separation and characterization of chondroitin 6-sulfotransferase and chondroitin 4-sulfotransferase from chick embryo cartilage. *Biochim. Biophys. Acta* **717**, 414–421.

Habuchi, O., Matsui, Y., Kotoya, Y., Aoyama, Y., Yasuda, Y., and Noda, M. (1993). Purification of chondroitin 6-sulfotransferase secreted from cultured chick embryo chondrocytes. *J. Biol. Chem.* **268**, 21968–21974.

Helting, T., and Roden, L. (1969a). Biosynthesis of chondroitin sulfate. II. Glucuronosyl transfer in the formation of the carbohydrate-protein linkage region. *J. Biol. Chem.* **244**, 2799–2805.

Helting, T., and Roden, L. (1969b). Biosynthesis of chondroitin sulfate. I. Galactosyl transfer in the formation of the carbohydrate-protein linkage region. *J. Biol. Chem.* **244**, 2790–2798.

Hikino, M., Mikami, T., Faissner, A., Vilela-Silva, A. C. E. S., Pavão, M. S. G., and Sugahara, K. (2003). Oversulfated dermatan sulfate exhibits neurite outgrowth-promoting activity toward embryonic mouse hippocampal neurons. *J. Biol. Chem.* **278**, 43744–43754.

Hiraoka, N., Nakagawa, H., Ong, E., Akama, T. O., Fukuda, M. N., and Fukuda, M. (2000a). Molecular cloning and expression of two distinct human chondroitin4-O-sulfotransferases that belong to the HNK-1 sulfotransferase gene family. *J. Biol. Chem.* **275**, 20188–20196.

Hwang, H. Y., Olson, S. K., Esko, J. D., and Horvitz, H. R. (2003a). *Caenorhabditis elegans* early embryogenesis and vulval morphogenesis require chondroitin biosynthesis. *Nature* **423**, 439–443.

Hwang, H. Y., Olson, S. K., Brown, J. R., Esko, J. D., and Horvitz, H. R. (2003b). The *Caenorhabditis elegans* genes sqv-2 and sqv-6, which are required for vulval morphogenesis, encode glycosaminoglycan galactosyltransferase II and xylosyltransferase. *J. Biol. Chem.* **278**, 11735–11738.

Inoue, H., Otsu, K., Yoneda, M., Kimata, K., Suzuki, S., and Nakanishi, Y. (1986a). Glycosaminoglycan sulfotransferases in human and animal sera. *J. Biol. Chem.* **261**, 4460–4469.

Inoue, H., Otsu, K., Suzuki, S., and Nakanishi, Y. (1986b). Difference between N-acetylgalactosamine 4-sulfate 6-O-sulfotransferases from human serum and squid cartilage in specificity toward the terminal and interior portion of chondroitin sulfate. *J. Biol. Chem.* **261**, 4470–4475.

Ito, Y., and Habuchi, O. (2000). Purification and characterization of N-acetylgalactosamine 4-sulfate 6-O-sulfotransferase from the squid cartilage. *J. Biol. Chem.* **275**, 34728–34736.

Izumikawa, T., Kitagawa, H., Mizuguchi, S., Nomura, K. H., Nomura, K., Tamura, J., Gengyo-Ando, K., Mitani, S., and Sugahara, K. (2004). Nematode chondroitin polymerizing factor showing cell-/organ-specific expression is indispensable for chondroitin synthesis and embryonic cell division. *J. Biol. Chem.* **279**, 53755–53761.

Kamimura, K., Fujise, M., Villa, F., Izumi, S., Habuchi, H., Kimata, K., and Nakato, H. (2001). Drosophila heparan sulfate 6-O-sulfotransferase (dHS6ST) gene. Structure, expression, and function in the formation of the tracheal system. *J. Biol. Chem.* **276**, 17014–17021.

Kakuta, Y., Pedersen, L. G., Carter, C. W., Negishi, M., and Pedersen, L. C. (1997). Crystal structure of estrogen sulphotransferase. *Nat. Struct. Biol.* **4**, 904–908.

Kang, H. G., Evers, M. R., Xia, G., Baenziger, J. U., and Schachner, M. (2002). Molecular cloning and characterization of chondroitin-4-O-sulfotransferase-3: A novel member of the HNK-1 family of sulfotransferases. *J. Biol. Chem.* **277**, 34766–73472.

Kitagawa, H., Tsutsumi, K., Ujikawa, M., Goto, F., Tamura, J., Neumann, K. W., Ogawa, T., and Sugahara, K. (1997). Regulation of chondroitin sulfate biosynthesis by specific sulfation: Acceptor specificity of serum beta-GalNAc transferase revealed by structurally defined oligosaccharides. *Glycobiology* 7, 531–537.

Kitagawa, H., Tone, Y., Tamura, J., Neumann, K. W., Ogawa, T., Oka, S., Kawasaki, T., and Sugahara, K. (1998). Molecular cloning and expression of glucuronyltransferase I involved in the biosynthesis of the glycosaminoglycan-protein linkage region of proteoglycans. *J. Biol. Chem.* 273, 6615–6618.

Kitagawa, H., Fujita, M., Ito, N., and Sugahara, K. (2000). Molecular cloning and expression of a novel chondroitin 6-O-sulfotransferase. *J. Biol. Chem.* 275, 21075–21080.

Kitagawa, H., Uyama, T., and Sugahara, K. (2001). Molecular cloning and expression of a human chondroitin synthase. *J. Biol. Chem.* 276, 38721–38726.

Kitagawa, H., Izumikawa, T., Uyama, T., and Sugahara, K. (2003). Molecular cloning of a chondroitin sulfate polymerizing factor that cooperates with chondroitin synthase for chondroitin polymerization. *J. Biol. Chem.* 278, 23666–23671.

Kobayashi, M., Sugumaran, G., Liu, J., Shworak, N. W., Silbert, J. E., and Rosenberg, R. D. (1999). Molecular cloning and characterization of a human uronyl 2-sulfotransferase that sulfates iduronyl and glucuronyl residues in dermatan/chondroitin sulfate. *J. Biol. Chem.* 274, 10474–10480.

Kusche-Gullberg, M., Eriksson, I., Pikas, D. S., and Kjellen, L. (1998). Identification and expression in mouse of two heparan sulfate glucosaminyl N-deacetylase/N-sulfotransferase genes. *J. Biol. Chem.* 273, 11902–11907.

Lauder, R. M., Huckerby, T. N., and Nieduszynski, I. A. (2000). Increased incidence of unsulphated and 4-sulphated residues in the chondroitin sulphate linkage region observed by high-pH anion-exchange chromatography. *Biochem. J.* 347, 339–348.

Lohmander, L. S., Hascall, V. C., Yanagishita, M., Kuettner, K. E., and Kimura, J. H. (1986). Post-translational events in proteoglycan synthesis: Kinetics of synthesis of chondroitin sulfate and oligosaccharides on the core protein. *Arch. Biochem. Biophys.* 250, 211–227.

Maimone, M. M., and Tollefsen, D. M. (1990). Structure of a dermatan sulfate hexasaccharide that binds to heparin cofactor II with high affinity. *J. Biol. Chem.* 265, 18263–18271.

Mazany, K. D., Peng, T., Watson, C. E., Tabas, I., and Williams, K. J. (1998). Human chondroitin 6-sulfotransferase: cloning, gene structure, and chromosomal localization. *Biochim. Biophys. Acta* 1407, 92–97.

Mikami, T., Mizumoto, S., Kago, N., Kitagawa, H., and Sugahara, K. (2003). Specificities of three distinct human chondroitin/dermatan N-acetylgalactosamine 4-O-sulfotransferases demonstrated using partially desulfated dermatan sulfate as an acceptor: Implication of differential roles in dermatan sulfate biosynthesis. *J. Biol. Chem.* 278, 36115–36127.

Moses, J., Oldberg, A., Cheng, F., and Fransson, L.-A. (1997). Biosynthesis of the proteoglycan decorin: Transient 2-phoshorylation of xylose during formation of the tetrasaccharide linkage region. *Eur. J. Biochem.* 248, 521–526.

Mourão, P. A. S., Toledo, S. P. A., Nader, H. B., and Dietrich, C. P. (1973). Excretion of chondroitin sulfate C with low sulfate content by patients with generalized platyspondyly (brachyolmia). *Biochem. Med.* 7, 415–423.

Mourão, P. A. S., Kato, S., and Donnelly, P. V. (1981). Spondyloepiphyseal dysplasia, chondroitin sulfate type: a possible defect of PAPS: Chondroitin sulfate sulfotransferase in humans. *Biochem. Biophys. Res. Commun.* 98, 388–396.

Nadanaka, S., Fujita, M., and Sugahara, K. (1999). Demonstration of a novel sulfotransferase in fetal bovine serum, which transfers sulfate to the C6 position of the GalNAc residue in the sequence iduronic acid alpha1–3GalNAc beta1–4iduronic acid in dermatan sulfate. *FEBS Lett.* 452, 185–189.

Narimatsu, H. (2004). Construction of a human glycogene library and comprehensive functional analysis. *Glycoconj. J.* **21**, 17–24.

Negishi, M., Pedersen, L. G., Petrotchenko, E., Shevtsov, S., Gorokhov, A., Kakuta, Y., and Pedersen, L. C. (2001). Structure and function of sulfotransferases. *Arch. Biochem. Biophys.* **390**, 149–157.

Oegema, T. R., Kraft, E. L., Jr., Jourdian, G. W., and Van Valen, T. R. (1984). Phosphorylation of chondroitin sulfate in proteoglycans from the swarm rat chondrosarcoma. *J. Biol. Chem.* **259**, 1720–1726.

Ohtake, S., Ito, Y., Fukuta, M., and Habuchi, O. (2001). Human N-acetylgalactosamine 4-sulfate 6-O sulfotransferase cDNA is related to human B cell recombination activating gene-associated gene. *J. Biol. Chem.* **276**, 43894–43900.

Ohtake, S., Kimata, K., and Habuchi, O. (2003). A unique nonreducing terminal modification of chondroitin sulfate by N-acetylgalactosamine 4-sulfate 6-o-sulfotransferase. *J. Biol. Chem.* **278**, 38443–38452.

Okuda, T., Mita, S., Yamauchi, S., Matsubara, T., Yagi, F., Yamamori, D., Fukuta, M., Kuroiwa, A., Matsuda, Y., and Habuchi, O. (2000). Molecular cloning, expression, and chromosomal mapping of human chondroitin 4-sulfotransferase, whose expression pattern in human tissues is different from that of chondroitin 6-sulfotransferase. *J. Biochem. (Tokyo)*, 763–770.

Orkin, R. W., Pratt, R. M., and Martin, G. R. (1976). Undersulfated chondroitin sulfate in the cartilage matrix of brachymorphic mice. *Dev. Biol.* **50**, 82–94.

Ozeran, J. D., Westley, J., and Schwartz, N. B. (1996). Identification and partial purification of PAPS translocase. *Biochemistry* **35**, 3695–3703.

Pavão, M. S., Mourão, P. A., Mulloy, B., and Tollefsen, D. M. (1995). A unique dermatan sulfate-like glycosaminoglycan from ascidian: Its structure and the effect of its unusual sulfation pattern on anticoagulant activity. *J. Biol. Chem.* **270**, 31027–31036.

Pavão, M. S., Aiello, K. R., Werneck, C. C., Silva, L. C., Valente, A. P., Mulloy, B., Colwell, N. S., Tollefsen, D. M., and Mourão, P. A. (1998). Highly sulfated dermatan sulfates from ascidians: Structure versus anticoagulant activity of these glycosaminoglycans. *J. Biol. Chem.* **273**, 27848–27857.

Robbins, P. W., and Lipmann, F. (1957). Isolation and identification of active sulfate. *J. Biol. Chem.* **229**, 837–851.

Rodén, L., Koerner, T., Olson, C., and Schwartz, N. B. (1985). Mechanisms of chain initiation in the biosynthesis of connective tissue polysaccharides. *Fed. Proc.* **44**, 373–380.

Rodriguez, M. L., Jann, B., and Jann, K. (1988). Structure and serological characteristics of the capsular K4 antigen of *Escherichia coli* O5:K4:H4, a fructose-containing polysaccharide with a chondroitin backbone. *Eur. J. Biochem.* **177**, 117–124.

Rohrmann, K., Niemann, R., and Buddecke, E. (1985). Two N-acetylgalactosaminyltransferase are involved in the biosynthesis of chondroitin sulfate. *Eur. J. Biochem.* **148**, 463–469.

Sato, T., Gotoh, M., Kiyohara, K., Akashima, T., Iwasaki, H., Kameyama, A., Mochizuki, H., Yada, T., Inaba, N., Togayachi, A., Kudo, T., Asada, M., et al. (2003). Differential roles of two N-acetylgalactosaminyltransferases, CSGalNAcT-1, and a novel enzyme, CSGalNAcT-2: Initiation and elongation in synthesis of chondroitin sulfate. *J. Biol. Chem.* **278**, 3063–3071.

Shworak, N. W., Liu, J., Petros, L. M., Zhang, L., Kobayashi, M., Copeland, N. G., Jenkins, N. A., and Rosenberg, R. D. (1999). Multiple isoforms of heparan sulfate D-glucosaminyl 3-O-sulfotransferase: Isolation, characterization, and expression of human cDNAs and identification of distinct genomic loci. *J. Biol. Chem.* **274**, 5170–5184.

Silbert, J. E. (1964). Incorporation of ^{14}C and ^{3}H from labeled nucleotide sugars into a polysaccharide in the presence of a cell-free preparation from cartilage. *J. Biol. Chem.* **239**, 1310–1315.

Silbert, J. E., and DeLuca, S. (1969). Biosynthesis of chondroitin sulfate. III. Formation of a sulfated glycosaminoglycan with a microsomal preparation from chick embryo cartilage. *J. Biol. Chem.* **244**, 876–881.

Silbert, J. E., and Reppucci, A. C., Jr. (1976). Biosynthesis of chondroitin sulfate. Independent addition of glucuronic acid N-acetylgalactosamine to oligosaccharides. *J. Biol. Chem.* **251**, 3942–3947.

Silbert, J. E., Palmer, M. E., Humphries, D. E., and Silbert, C. K. (1986). Formation of dermatan sulfate by cultured human skin fibroblasts: Effects of sulfate concentration on proportions of dermatan/chondroitin. *J. Biol. Chem.* **261**, 13397–13400.

Silbert, J. E., and Sugumaran, G. (2002). Biosynthesis of chondroitin/dermatan sulfate. *IUBMB Life* **54**, 177–186.

Sugahara, K., Yamashina, I., De Waard, P., Van Halbeek, H., and Vliegenthart, J. F. (1988). Structural studies on sulfated glycopeptides from the carbohydrate-protein linkage region of chondroitin 4-sulfate proteoglycans of swarm rat chondrosarcoma: Demonstration of the structure Gal(4-O-sulfate)beta 1–3Gal beta 1–4XYL beta 1-O-Ser. *J. Biol. Chem.* **263**, 10168–10174.

Sugahara, K., Ohi, Y., Harada, T., de Waard, P., and Vliegenthart, J. F. (1992). Structural studies on sulfated oligosaccharides derived from the carbohydrate-protein linkage region of chondroitin 6-sulfate proteoglycans of shark cartilage. I. Six compounds containing 0 or 1 sulfate and/or phosphate residues. *J. Biol. Chem.* **267**, 6027–6035.

Sugahara, K., and Kitagawa, H. (2000). Recent advances in the study of the biosynthesis and functions of sulfated glycosaminoglycans. *Curr. Opin. Struct. Biol.* **10**, 518–527.

Sugahara, K., Mikami, T., Uyama, T., Mizuguchi, S., Nomura, K., and Kitagawa, H. (2003). Recent advances in the structural biology of chondroitin sulfate and dermatan sulfate. *Curr. Opin. Struct. Biol.* **13**, 612–620.

Sugumaran, G., Katsman, M., Sunthankar, P., and Drake, R. R. (1997). Biosynthesis of chondroitin sulfate: Purification of glucuronosyl transferase II and use of photoaffinity labeling for characterization of the enzyme as an 80-kDa protein. *J. Biol. Chem.* **272**, 14399–14403.

Suzuki, S., and Strominger, J. L. (1960a). Enzymatic sulfation of mucopolysaccharides in hen oviduct. I. Transfer of sulfate from 3′-phosphoadenosine 5′-phosphosulfate to mucopo-lysaccharides. *J. Biol. Chem.* **235**, 257–266.

Suzuki, S., and Strominger, J. L. (1960b). Enzymatic sulfation of mucopolysaccharides in hen oviduct. II. Mechanism of the reaction studied with oligosaccharides and monosacchar-ides as acceptors. *J. Biol. Chem.* **235**, 267–273.

Telser, A., Robinson, H. C., and Dorfman, A. (1966). The biosynthesis of chondroitin sulfate. *Arch. Biochem. Biophys.* **116**, 458–465.

Tsutsumi, K., Shimakawa, H., Kitagawa, H., and Sugahara, K. (1998). Functional expression and genomic structure of human chondroitin 6-sulfotransferase. *FEBS Lett.* **441**, 235–241.

Turnbull, J., Drummond, K., Huang, Z., Kinnunen, T., Ford-Perriss, M., Murphy, M., and Guimond, S. (2003). Heparan sulphate sulphotransferase expression in mice and *Caenorhabditis elegans. Biochem. Soc. Trans.* **31**, 343–348.

Uchimura, K., Kadomatsu, K., Fan, Q. W., Muramatsu, H., Kurosawa, N., Kaname, T., Yamamura, Y., Fukuta, M., Habuchi, O., and Muramatsu, T. (1998). Mouse chondroitin 6-sulfotransferase: Molecular cloning, characterization and chromosomal mapping. *Glycobiology* **8**, 489–496.

Uchimura, K., Kadomatsu, K., Nishimura, H., Muramatsu, H., Nakamura, E., Kurosawa, N., Habuchi, O., El-Fasakhany, F. M., Yoshikai, Y., and Muramatsu, T. (2002). Functional analysis of the chondroitin 6-sulfotransferase gene in relation to lymphocyte subpopulations, brain development, and oversulfated chondroitin sulfates. *J. Biol. Chem.* **277**, 1443–1450.

Ueno, M., Yamada, S., Zako, M., Bernfield, M., and Sugahara, K. (2001). Structural charac-terization of heparan sulfate and chondroitin sulfate of syndecan-1 purified from normal murine mammary gland epithelial cells: Common phosphorylation of xylose and differential sulfation of galactose in the protein linkage region tetrasaccharide sequence. *J. Biol. Chem.* **276**, 29134–29140.

Uyama, T., Kitagawa, H., Tamura, Ji. J., and Sugahara, K. (2002). Molecular cloning and expression of human chondroitin N-acetylgalactosaminyltransferase: The key enzyme for chain initiation and elongation of chondroitin/dermatan sulfate on the protein linkage region tetrasaccharide shared by heparin/heparan sulfate. *J. Biol. Chem.* **277**, 8841–8846.

Uyama, T., Kitagawa, H., and Sugahara, K. (2003). Proteoglycan core glycosyltransferases. *Tanpakushitsu Kakusan Koso* **48**, 1019–1026.

Vieira, R. P., and Mourão, P. A. S. (1988). Occurrence of a unique fucose-branched chondroitin sulfate in the body wall of a sea cucumber. *J. Biol. Chem.* **263**, 18176–18183.

Vieira, R. P., Mulloy, B., and Mourão, P. A. S. (1991). Structure of a fucose-branched chondroitin sulfate from sea cucumber: Evidence for the presence of 3-O-sulfo-β-D-glucuronosyl residues. *J. Biol. Chem.* **266**, 13530–13536.

Vilela-Silva, A. C., Werneck, C. C., Valente, A. P., Vacquier, V. D., and Mourão, P. A. (2001). Embryos of the sea urchin *Strongylocentrotus purpuratus* synthesize a dermatan sulfate enriched in 4-O- and 6-O-disulfated galactosamine units. *Glycobiology* **11**, 433–440.

Yada, T., Gotoh, M., Sato, T., Shionyu, M., Go, M., Kaseyama, H., Iwasaki, H., Kikuchi, N., Kwon, Y. D., Togayachi, A., Kudo, T., Watanabe, H., *et al.* (2003a). Chondroitin sulfate synthase-2: Molecular cloning and characterization of a novel human glycosyltransferase homologous to chondroitin sulfate glucuronyltransferase, which has dual enzymatic activities. *J. Biol. Chem.* **278**, 30235–30247.

Yada, T., Sato, T., Kaseyama, H., Gotoh, M., Iwasaki, H., Kikuchi, N., Kwon, Y. D., Togayachi, A., Kudo, T., Watanabe, H., Narimatsu, H., and Kimata, K. (2003b). Chondroitin sulfate synthase-3: Molecular cloning and characterization. *J. Biol. Chem.* **278**, 39711–39725.

Yamauchi, S., Hirahara, Y., Usui, H., Takeda, Y., Hoshino, M., Fukuta, M., Kimura, J. H., and Habuchi, O. (1999). Purification and characterization of chondroitin 4-sulfotransferase from the culture medium of a rat chondrosarcoma cell line. *J. Biol. Chem.* **274**, 2456–2463.

Yamauchi, S., Mita, S., Matsubara, T., Fukuta, M., Habuchi, H., Kimata, K., and Habuchi, O. (2000). Molecular cloning and expression of chondroitin 4-sulfotransferase. *J. Biol. Chem.* **275**, 8975–8981.

Yusa, A., Kitajima, K., and Habuchi, O. (2005). N-linked oligosaccharides are required to produce and stabilize the active form of chondroitin 4-sulfotransferase-1. *Biochem. J.* **388**, 115–121.

M. Stylianou, I.-E. Triantaphyllidou, and D. H. Vynios

Laboratory of Biochemistry
Department of Chemistry
University of Patras
26500 Patras, Greece

Advances in the Analysis of Chondroitin/Dermatan Sulfate

I. Chapter Overview

Chondroitin/dermatan sulfate (CS/DS) is a glycosaminoglycan (GAG) found in extracellular matrix (ECM) and cell surface, and participates in various ECM and cell-ECM interactions. It is made from the alternate addition of glucuronic acid (GlcA) and N-acetylgalactosamine (GalNAc). However, during biosynthesis, CS/DS is sulfated on C-4 and/or C-6 of the GalNAc and of C-2 of GlcA and part of GlcA is epimerized on C-5 to obtain iduronic acid (IdoA), all steps depending on the tissue or cell status, making the molecule more complex. Due to the complexity of CS/DS, its analysis is useful to characterize the molecules present in a sample and identify alterations with respect to their amounts and fine structural features in various pathological conditions. In this chapter we present the various techniques developed to analyze and characterize CS/DS.

Advances in Pharmacology, Volume 53
Copyright 2006, Elsevier Inc. All rights reserved.

1054-3589/06 $35.00
DOI: 10.1016/S1054-3589(05)53007-2

II. Introduction

Chondroitin/dermatan sulfate is a member of GAG family, a specific class of biological macromolecules distributed among all organisms that are carbohydrate polymers of a repeating disaccharide unit. Five different types of GAGs are known, namely hyaluronan, CS/DS, keratan sulfate (KS), heparan sulfate (HS), and heparin. CS/DS is composed of variable number of repeating disaccharide units (20–50) consisting of one N-acetyl-D-galac-tosamine (GalNAc) and one uronic acid (D-GlcA or L-IdoA). According to the type of the uronic acid present, the polysaccharide is termed CS (100% GlcA) or DS (variable amounts of IdoA).

CS/DS, as all other GAGs with the exception of hyaluronan, is synthesized under the form of proteoglycans (PGs) in the Golgi apparatus by elaborate biosynthetic machinery. Biosynthesis is initiated by a linkage region composed of four monosaccharides (GlcA1β→3Gal1β→ 3Gal1β→4Xyl1β→) linked via an O-glycosidic bond to certain serine or threonine residues on a specific protein, the core protein. The GAG chain is elongated on this tetrasaccharide by alternative additions to the nonreducing termini of GlcA and GalNAc, both derived from UDP-sugar donors. During chain elongation, a series of enzymatic modifications of the growing poly-saccharide chain determines its final structure.

CS is constructed by the repeating disaccharide unit →4GlcAβ1→ 3GalNAcβ1→, which is then sulfated at the C-4 or C-6 positions of GalNAc (Fig. 1) with 3′-phosphor-adenosine-5′-phosphosulfate as a donor of sulfate group. Few of these positions remain unsulfated. Thus, CS may be sulfated at C-4 (CS-A) and C-6 (CS-C), whereas in tissues of invertebrate origin different or mixed sulfation occurs and the GAG is termed CS-D, CS-E, and CS-K. In these cases, its main disaccharide unit contains two sulfate ester groups at C-2 of GlcA and C-6 of GalNAc, at C-4 and C-6 of GalNAc, and at C-3 of GlcA and C-4 of GalNAc, respectively (Fig. 1).

In the case of DS, further enzymatic modifications complete its final structure such as C-5 epimerization of GlcA to IdoA and O-sulfation at C-2 of IdoA. The characteristic disaccharide unit of DS is →4IdoAα1→ 3GalNAcβ1→ (Fig. 1). Although the principles of the biosynthetic process are not yet fully elucidated, it is well known that this process results in the generation of highly modified oligosaccharide domains within the polymer chain, which are separated by regions of relatively low-degree structural modifications. Thus, DS has a hybrid copolymeric structure consisting of low modified (CS) and highly modified (DS) domains (Karamanos *et al.*, 1994). The IdoA-containing units are often sulfated at C-4 of the GalNAc, while sulfation at C-6 is frequently associated with GlcA-containing disac-charides (Karamanos *et al.*, 1995a).

The detailed structure of CS/DS is modified during development (Carulli *et al.*, 2005; Domowicz *et al.*, 2000, 2003; Masuda and Shiga, 2005; Pinto

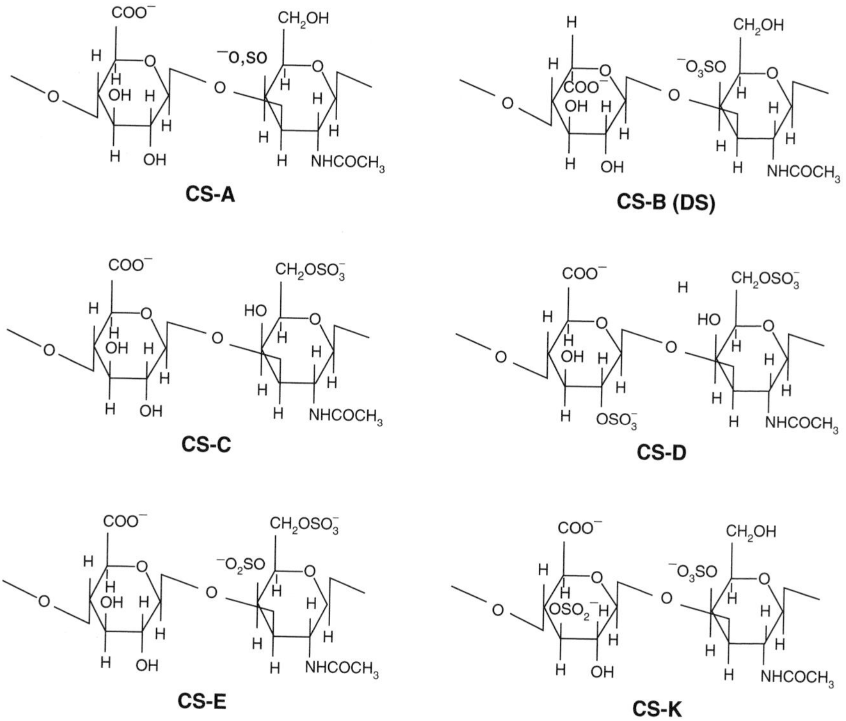

FIGURE I Chemical structure of the main disaccharide repeating unit of the various CSs.

et al., 2004; Rauch, 2004) and in most diseases (Vynios *et al.*, 2002). The well-described structural modifications involve changes in ratios of IdoA to GlcA and of 4-sulfated to 6- and nonsulfated disaccharides. Changes in the size of chains are also described. Many of these alterations can be observed after analysis of CS/DS not only in the tissue or organ affected but also in the urine of patients.

A. Properties of CS/DS

The strong negative charge of CS/DS and its presence under the form of PGs is responsible for water retention within the tissues and space filling ability (Carney and Muir, 1988; Hardingham *et al.*, 1994a). Chemical structure characterization of CS/DS has shown that both these properties are influenced by the presence and position of sulfate ester groups. Non-sulfated or less-sulfated CS/DS, which is not a normal figure for this GAG, possesses decreased ability for water retention and space filling, as compared with normally sulfated or oversulfated CS/DS. Furthermore, the axial position of sulfate at C-4 of GalNAc seems to be responsible for higher space filling ability, as compared with the equatorial position of sulfate at C-6. In addition to the position of sulfate, the epimerization of GlcA to IdoA plays also very critical role, and DS seems to occupy less space and have higher negative charge as compared with CS.

CS possesses the ability to interact with a number of proteins or cells, usually due to its high-negative charge (Caroulli et al., 2005; Kinsella et al., 2004; Kresse et al., 1994; Pan et al., 2002; Schwartz and Domowicz, 2004; Sugahara et al., 2003; Wadstrom and Ljungh, 1999). In some cases adhesion properties were observed (Johnson et al., 2005; Kokenyesi, 2001; Masuda and Shiga, 2005; Sherman et al., 2003). DS, due to the complexity of its structure, can either selfinteract to produce high molecular mass aggregates (Cöster et al., 1981; Fransson et al., 1982) or interact with a variety of extracellular macromolecules, thus regulating their biological functions (Iozzo, 1997; Kresse et al., 1993). DS interactions seem to be regulated by its fine chemical structure, and therefore, analysis may provide information about cell and tissue status.

B. Enzymes Applied in CS/DS Analysis

The first known enzyme degrading GAGs is testicular hyaluronidase that hydrolyzes randomly glycosidic linkages within hyaluronan and CS. It is an endo-N-acetyl-β-D-hexosaminidase (EC 3.2.1.35) with final products mainly tetra- and hexasaccharides. It also cleaves DS but only in GlcA-rich sequences. Hyaluronidase from *Streptomyces hyalurolyticus* (EC 4.2.2.1) is a lyase that specifically cleaves hyaluronan in a similar manner.

The most helpful enzymes in the analysis of CS/DS were isolated from bacteria. They belong to the class of lyases (EC 4.2.2.-), and they specifically degrade CS/DS according to its fine chemical structure. Chondroitinase ABC from *Proteus vulgaris* attacks the same glycosidic bond as hyaluronidase and produces unsaturated disaccharides (Δ-disaccharides). It acts also to hyaluronan; however, quantification is performed after Δ-disaccharides separation, so the enzyme is extensively used for quantitative purposes. Chondroitinase ACI and ACII, from *Flavobacterium heparinum* and *Arthrobacter aurescence*, respectively, act like chondroitinase ABC but without cleaving IdoA-containing glycosidic bonds. Chondroitinase B from *Flavobacterium heparinum* degrades only IdoA-containing glycosidic bonds within CS/DS, similarly as the other chondroitinases. Chondroitinases ACI, ACII, and B are applied to distinguish between CS and DS structures.

Flavobacterium heparinum is a source of two additional classes of GAG-degrading enzymes. The first one is that of heparin lyases I (EC 4.2.2.7), II, and III (EC 4.2.2.8). They possess different activities against specific structures within heparin or HS and are used in a mixture to degrade both in about 90% as Δ-disaccharides. The second one is keratanase (EC

3.2.1.103) that hydrolyzes β-galactosidic linkages in KS in which nonsulfated galactosyl residues participate. Its major products are monosulfated disaccharides.

The analysis of only CS/DS in a biological sample requires its purification or digestion of the preparation with *Streptomyces* hyaluronidase, heparin lyases, and keratanase to obtain intact CS/DS. However, in most of the cases, analysis of CS/DS is performed after its specific degradation with chondroitinases, followed by separation and quantification of the resulting Δ-disaccharides.

III. Chromogenic Quantitative Methods

The detection and quantification of CS/DS in purified preparations is accomplished by colorimetric assays based on either uronic acids or galactosamine. In addition, simplified quantitative assays, based on the reaction of CS/DS with cationic dyes due to its negative charge, are used.

A. Uronic Acids

It was initially proposed that hydrolysis of GAGs with concentrated sulfuric acid for 20 min at 100 °C and subsequent reaction with carbazole for 30 min at room temperature produced a color, from the absorbance of which at 530 nm their uronic acid content can be determined. Since the chromogens formed by both GlcA and IdoA are sensitive to light and that of IdoA is unstable, Bitter and Muir (1962) introduce 0.025 M borax during the hydrolysis step to stabilize them and decrease hydrolysis time to 10 min, followed by reaction with carbazole (0.125% w/v in absolute ethanol) for 15 min at 100 °C. The colored product is detected at 530 nm, and exactly the same sensitivity for GlcA and IdoA is obtained. The detection range is 5–100 μg/ml with detection limit at about 500 ng.

B. Hexosamines

The first assay for the determination of hexosamines was described by Elson and Morgan (1933). It is based on their reaction with acetylacetone, which produces a colored product with maximum absorbance at 525 nm. According to the assay, GAGs are hydrolyzed with 8 M HCl for 3 h at 95 °C, hexosamines are liberated and left to react with acetylacetone for 15 min at room temperature. The color produced from galactosamine and glucosamine is the same, so the assay can be applied only in purified CS/DS. The method is subjected to several modifications, due to its sensitivity to pH, salt content, and presence of interfering substances (Herbert *et al.*, 1971; Immers and Vasseur, 1950; Jang *et al.*, 2005).

Another assay is described by Tsuji *et al.* (1969). The samples are hydrolyzed with 2 M HCl for 2 h at 100°C, followed by deamination of the liberated hexosamines by nitrous acid. The anhydrohexoses produced react with 3-methyl-2-benzo-thiazolone in the presence of $FeCl_3$ to develop a color with maximum absorbance at 650 nm. Its advantages are the great sensitivity (less than 1 μg of hexosamines) and the short time required for the analysis.

In pure CS/DS preparations, whatever of the above assays can be directly applied, whereas in GAG mixtures, separation of hexosamines is required after their liberation (Hayes and Castellino, 1979). Alternatively, various high performance liquid chromatography (HPLC) procedures with pre- or postcolumn derivatization are proposed with highly increased sensitivity (Hjerpe *et al.*, 1980; Honda *et al.*, 1983).

C. Application of Cationic Dyes

The presence of negatively charged macromolecules in biological samples may be examined after reaction with a cationic dye (Fig. 2). Since the reaction is not specific for CS/DS and highly affected by salts and pH, it is used for rapid screening of biological samples for the presence of GAGs. However, under well-defined conditions, it can be applied for quantitative purposes, and by introducing specific enzymatic degradation steps, the quantification of CS/DS is achieved.

I. Alcian Blue

Alcian blue is a tetravalent cation with a hydrophobic core (Fig. 2), through which it is bound to variously negatively charged polymers. Binding of alcian blue is effective at high ionic strength but only with highly charged polyanions, such as CS/DS, in contrast to other cationic dyes. The assay is performed at a pH value low enough to neutralize all other than sulfate groups and at an ionic strength high enough to eliminate ionic interactions other than those between the dye and the sulfated GAGs (Björnsson, 1993; Karlsson and Björnsson, 2001). The absorbance is read at 600–620 nm. Hyaluronan, the nonsulfated GAG, does not interfere in this assay. There is not also interference from proteins or nucleic acids, in contrast to other dye binding assays (Björnsson, 1993). The detection range of the assay is 12.5–400 μg/ml.

2. 1,9-Dimethylmethylene Blue

The basic dye 1,9-dimethylmethylene blue (Fig. 2) is one of the most sensitive thiazine compounds, giving a more marked shift when complexed with GAGs than do other thiazine dyes.

The instability of the dye–GAG complexes has been overcome by Farndale *et al.* (1982) who used formate buffer instead of the tribasic

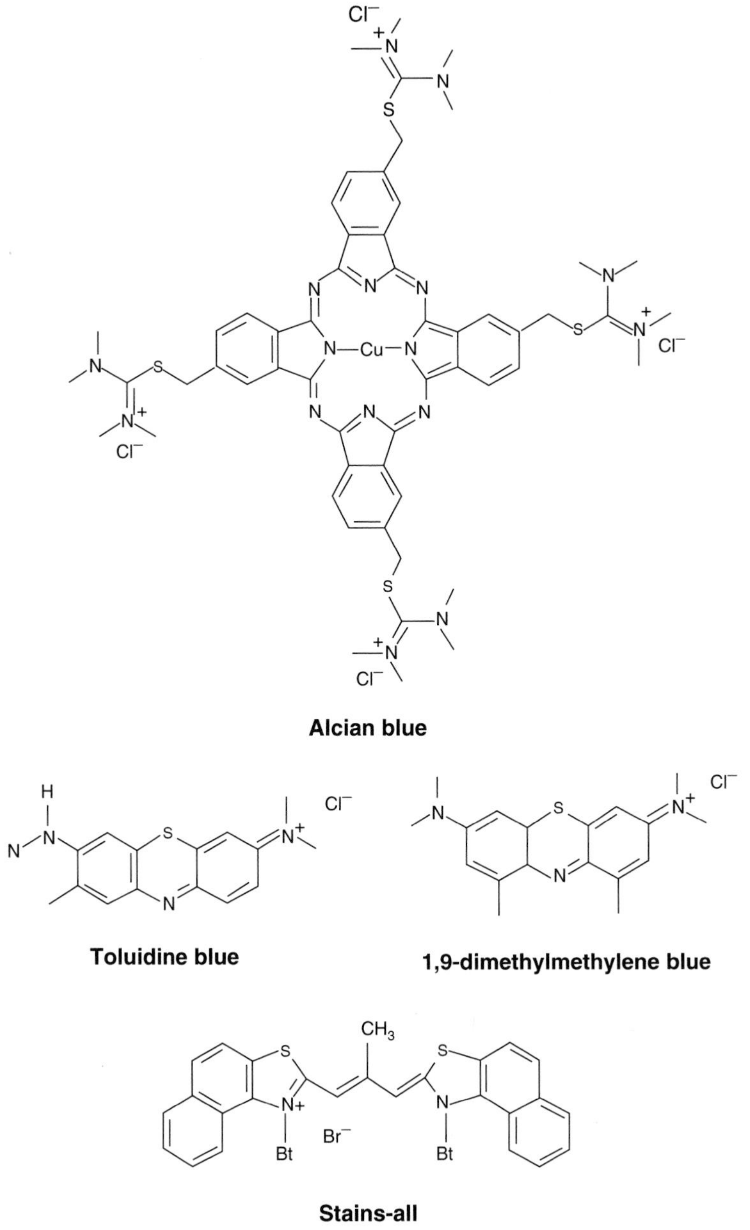

Alcian blue

Toluidine blue

1,9-dimethylmethylene blue

Stains-all

FIGURE 2   Structure of the main cationic dyes used in CS/DS detection and analysis.

citrate/phosphate buffer recommended previously. The pH of the dye solution is set at 3.5 in which the metachromatic color obtained after mixing with sulfated GAGs is stable and linear up to concentrations of about 60 µg/ml, when read at 595 nm. GAG oligosaccharides smaller than decasaccharides do not produce metachromatic color.

However, polyanions other than sulfated GAGs, including hyaluronan, DNA, and RNA, interfere in the assay. Thus, Farndale *et al.* (1986) introduced new modifications of the procedure to eliminate this interference and also showed that the assay can be used after specific "polysaccharidases" treatment to permit quantification of individual sulfated GAGs. The color yields of hyaluronan and DNA are negligible, and this is attributed to suppression of their relatively weak interaction with the dye by the lower pH and higher salt concentration of the modified reagent. The color reagent is prepared in glycine–HCl buffer pH 3, and the absorbance is read at 525 nm. The detection range of the assay is 2–50 µg/ml with detection limit at about 200 ng.

IV. Chromatographic Methods

Chromatographic procedures are widely used for the separation and characterization of CS/DS, which may give information on charge density, polydispersity, and molecular size of the chains.

A. Intact Molecules

1. Ion-Exchange Chromatography

This type of chromatography, by using various types of anion exchangers, is mainly applied for the enrichment in GAGs of a biological sample digested with proteases and/or treated with alkaline borohydride or for the purification of the sulfated GAGs from glycopeptides and hyaluronan and their subsequent characterization and quantification after enzymatic treatment and HPLC or another analytical technique. Nonsulfated carbohydrate structures are removed by washing with 0.1 M NaCl, and sulfated GAGs are recovered following a gradient elution ranging from 0.1 to 1.2 M NaCl. CS/DS elution depends on its charge density and when bears one sulfate ester group per disaccharide unit, it is eluted with 0.5–0.6 M NaCl (Papadas *et al.*, 2002; Vynios *et al.*, 2002).

Ion-exchange chromatography is not usually applied for CS/DS fine characterization due to its natural structural variations. However, under many pathological conditions, charge density changes were observed; therefore, ion-exchange chromatography techniques are helpful, and by combining specific enzymatic treatment, this separational technique becomes a quantitative one. Such alterations are observed in various diseases in which the chains are usually undersulfated (Capon *et al.*, 2003; De Muro *et al.*, 2001; Inazumi *et al.*, 1997; Papadas *et al.*, 2002; Theocharis *et al.*, 2003; Tsara *et al.*, 2002).

2. Gel Permeation Chromatography

Chromatography of purified CS/DS on various gels with different pore sizes provides useful information on the homogeneity of the population according to its size, and its average molecular mass can be determined. In most pathological conditions, especially cancer, there is a decrease of the size of CS/DS, possibly due to the high-biosynthetic rate of PG core protein, which, together with the activity of the various glycosyltransferases, determines the size of CS (Theocharis, 2002; Theocharis *et al.*, 2000, 2003; Tsara *et al.*, 2002). When low amounts are available, traditional gel chromatography should be replaced by gel permeation HPLC.

B. Digested Molecules

Information of the chain composition in absolute quantitative terms can be easily obtained after depolymerization of CS/DS by specific enzymatic degradation, followed by the separation of the obtained products. Digestion is performed by the various chondroitinases, and Δ-disaccharides are obtained, containing a double bond between C-4 and C-5 of the uronic acid that absorbs UV light with a maximum at 232 nm, thus allowing their specific quantification.

I. High-Performance Liquid Chromatography

Over the last 30 years various HPLC methods of normal phase, reverse phase, ion pair, and ion-exchange chromatography have been used for compositional Δ-disaccharide analysis of GAGs. Due to the complexity of CS/DS, its digestion with chondroitinase ABC produces 23 different Δ-disaccharides, 12 of which are derived from DS and 11 from CS structures (Karamanos *et al.*, 1994). By monitoring the absorbance of the effluent at 232 nm the exact chemical composition of CS/DS can be identified.

All differently sulfated Δ-disaccharides can be quantitatively analyzed in nmol range with ion-exchange HPLC using three different elution buffers for non-, mono-, and oversulfated species (Karamanos *et al.*, 1995a). The column is eluted isocratically with 5 mM NaH_2PO_4, pH 2.55, for nonsulfated Δ-disaccharides, 50 mM NaH_2PO_4, pH 2.5, for monosulfated Δ-disaccharides, and 50 mM Na_2SO_4, 10 mM CH_3COONa, pH 5, for di- and trisulfated Δ-disaccharides. This method is very useful for total Δ-disaccharides analysis, since all types of Δ-disaccharides are identified. By using the appropriate enzymatic treatment and well-selected conditions, detailed characterization of CS/DS structure can be performed (Fig. 3).

For the compositional analysis of CS/DS and also its sequence determination after limited digestion with chondroitinases, ion-pair reversed-phase HPLC is proposed (Karamanos *et al.*, 1997), using tetrabutylammonium hydrogen sulfate as ion-pairing agent.

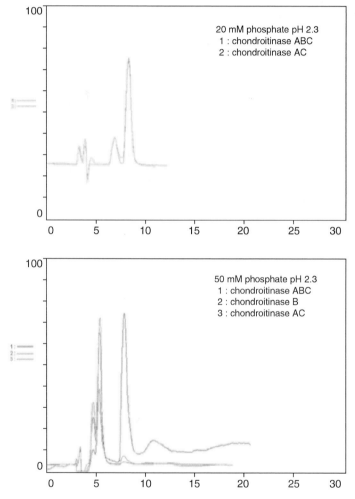

FIGURE 3   HPLC analysis of CS/DS for the identification of low IdoA-containing chains. GAGs were isolated from laryngeal cartilage and then digested with the various chondroitinases and subjected to HPLC eluted with either 20 or 50 mM phosphate buffer to identify IdoA-containing structures, other than disaccharides (D. H. Vynios, unpublished results). (See Color Insert.)

2. Gel Permeation Chromatography

When populations of CS/DS of different fine chemical structure are present in a sample, together or not with other GAGs, degradation with specific enzymes and subsequent gel chromatography does not necessarily result in clear separation of the obtained products, and thus it is difficult or impossible to quantify and characterize the undigested one. This led to the idea of secondary profile determination as extensively described by Theocharis et al. (2001b). The purified CS/DS chains of the sample under study are subjected to chromatography on a well-calibrated gel chromatography column, native and after being treated with chondroitinase B to degrade only DS structures (Fig. 4A). The absolute GAG content in each chromatography fraction before and after the enzymatic treatment is measured, and from the profile shift to the total volume of the column, the determination of the amount of the digested GAG is enabled. In addition, from the difference in GAG content in each fraction from both chromatographies, the elution profile of the digested molecules is derived (Fig. 4B). Thus, by applying this methodology the absolute content and the size distribution of the populations present in a mixture of CS/DS is obtained. This procedure has been successfully applied to determine the net amounts and size distributions of pure CS and DS populations in samples from various cartilages (Theocharis et al., 2001a,b) and from normal and cancerous tissues (Theocharis et al., 2003). The procedure can be applied for similar determination of CS/DS, when it is present in mixtures with KS or HS, by applying suitable treatment of the samples.

V. Electromigration Methods

Electromigration methods are based on the ability of molecules to be separated according to their charge density and/or molecular size on a solid support. This field of research is extensively studied and various methods are developed for the separation of GAGs. Conventional electromigration methods are cellulose acetate electophoresis and gel (agarose or polyacrylamide) electrophoresis. Two additional methods, that is, fluorophore-assisted carbohydrate electrophoresis (FACE) (Fig. 5) and capillary electrophoresis (CE) are developed during the last decade and seem to be very promising for GAG analysis.

A. Cellulose Acetate Electrophoresis

Electrophoresis on cellulose acetate strips is a simple, rapid, and very sensitive method to characterize the GAGs present in biological samples. The method is based on the different mobility of various GAGs when

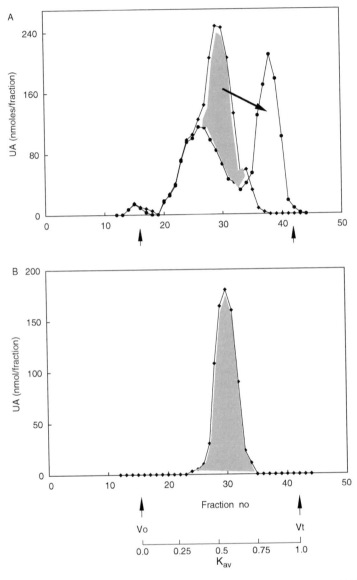

FIGURE 4 Determination and characterization of DS in CS/DS preparations. (A) The CS/DS preparation was chromatographed before (♦) and after (●) digestion with chondroitinase B, and the fractions were analyzed for their uronic acid content. (B) Secondary profile of DS obtained from the positive differences of uronic acid in each fraction of A (from Theocharis *et al.*, 2001b).

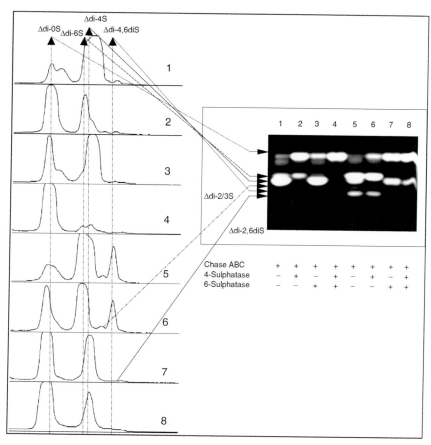

FIGURE 5 Application of FACE in 35% polyacrylamide gels for the analysis and characterization of CS/DS (M. Assouti and D. H. Vynios, unpublished results). Lanes 1–4: CS/DS from pig laryngeal cartilage. Lanes 5–8: CS/DS from shark cartilage. Quantification of the various products is achieved after scanning of the gel (left).

moving on the strip by applying constant current. Electrophoresis can be held in various buffers, as it has been proposed by Hata and Nagai (1972, 1973), the most common being that of 0.2 M $CaCl_2$ pH 7.2, 0.1 M $Ba(CH_3COO)_2$ pH 8.0, and 0.1 M pyridine/0.47M HCOOH pH 3.1 (Table I). The separated GAGs can be stained with various dyes, such as azure A, toluidine blue, or alcian blue (Volpi, 1996), and subjected to densitometric analysis for quantitative purposes. The detection limit is down to 25 pmol. To improve quantification of CS/DS, GAG specimens may be subjected to electrophoresis after specific enzymatic digestion.

In addition, two-dimensional electrophoresis for the improvement of separation is proposed (Hata and Nagai, 1972, 1973; Stevens *et al.*,

TABLE I   Buffer and Staining Conditions for Optimum Separation and Detection of CS/DS upon Cellulose Acetate Electrophoresis

Buffer	Electrophoresis conditions	Staining	Destaining
0.1 M barium acetate pH 5.0 (Volpi, 1996)	(a) 20 mA, 40 min at 10°C	(1) 0.08% azure A in water for 5 min	Water
	(b) 5 V/cm, 180 min at room temperature	(2) 0.2% toluidine blue in ethanol: water:acetic acid (50:49:1) for 5 min	Ethanol:water: acetic acid 50:49:1
		(3) 2.5% alcian blue in water for 5 min	5% acetic acid
0.2 M calcium acetate pH 7.2 (Johansson *et al.*, 2001)	0.6 mA/cm for 5 h at room temperature	0.5% alcian blue in 3% acetic acid for 20 min	1% acetic acid
0.47 M formic acid–0.1 M pyridine pH 3.1 (Papadas *et al.*, 2002)	200 V for 45 min at room temperature	0.2% toluidine blue in 15% ethanol	Water
0.47 M formic acid–0.1 M pyridine pH 3.1 (Papakonstantinou *et al.*, 2003)	7 mA for 70 min at room temperature	0.2% alcian blue in 0.1% acetic acid for 10 min	0.1% acetic acid

1976; Toyoki *et al.*, 1997). The first solvent is 0.1 M pyridine/0.47 M HCOOH, and the electrophoresis is performed at 185 V for 80 min or at 1 mA/cm for 1 h. The second solvent is 0.1 M $Ba(CH_3COO)_2$ pH 8.0, and the electrophoresis is performed at 100 V for 6 h or at 1 mA/cm for 4 h.

B. Gel Electrophoresis

1. Agarose Gel Electrophoresis

The application of gel electrophoretic techniques for GAG analysis is limited due to their high hydrodynamic size and polydispersity, which, in addition with the presence of strong negative charge, results in bands broading. From the various procedures proposed, electrophoresis on agarose gels seems to be very useful tool. The initial protocol uses a separation buffer of 0.1 M Tris/Acetate pH 6.8 in composite gels containing 0.8% agarose and 1.2% polyacrylamide (McDevitt and Muir, 1971). The other protocols proposed are mainly modifications of the above to obtain better separation of the GAGs and decreased broading of the bands (Dietrich *et al.*, 1977; Volpi, 1994). Thus, agarose concentration of 0.5% and running buffers containing Ba(CH₃COO)₂ have been proposed. Staining of the gels is performed with Toluidine blue, however, silver nitrate, Stains-all or sequential staining with Toluidine blue and Stains-all, is also proposed (Volpi and Maccari, 2002; Volpi *et al.*, 2005). Quantification is then achieved by scanning of the gels.

2. Fluorophore-Assisted Carbohydrate Electrophoresis

When the biological sample contains complex mixtures of GAGs, quantification of CS/DS with concomitant structural characterization may be achieved by chondroitinases' degradation of only this GAG, followed by electrophoretic separation of the obtained Δ-disaccharides on polyacrylamide gels of very high concentration of monomer, usually 30% or 35% of acrylamide containing 5% of *N,N'*-methylene-bis-acrylamide. Since the known dyes cannot stain Δ-disaccharides, the degradation products, prior to electrophoresis, are subjected to labeling by reductive amination with specific fluorescent substances, such as 2-aminoacridone (2-AMAC), 2-aminopyridine, 7-aminonaphthalene-1,3-disulfonic acid, and 8-aminonaphthalene-1,3,6-trisulfonic acid (Gao, 2005; Jackson, 1996), the preferred substance being 2-AMAC. The final characterization of the Δ-disaccharides is performed after removal of their sulfate ester groups (Fig. 6), which, in addition, can be used for their quantitative analysis. The detection limit is down to attomol level. The assay can be applied for the characterization of GAGs present in tissues or biological fluids, such as plasma and urine, in various diseases (Calabro *et al.*, 2000, 2001; Karousou *et al.*, 2004, 2005; Mielke *et al.*, 1999; Plaas *et al.*, 2001; Volpi and Maccari, 2005).

C. Capillary Electrophoresis

Capillary electrophoresis is considered to be a unique method since it utilizes the principles of both the electrophoresis technique and the liquid chromatography, combining by this way resolution and sensitivity. CE is commonly used in the analysis and the structural characterization of various GAGs. Various modes of CE have been developed up to now, according to the molecules under study.

I. Conventional Techniques

Capillary zone electrophoresis (CZE) is a widely used mode because it is simple and accurate. It can be applied as long as the molecule is charged. Upon the application of a constant voltage, the negatively charged wall of the uncoated fused-silica capillary causes electroosmotic flow (EOF) of buffer species, which moves all molecules toward the negative electrode.

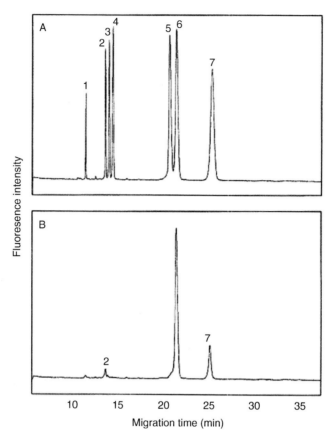

FIGURE 6 Typical electropherograms showing the separation of reference sulfated Δ-disaccharides (A) and of those of CSA obtained after digestion with chondroitinases ABC and AC (B). CE was performed with 15 mM orthophosphate buffer (pH 3.0) as operating buffer at 20 kV and 258 °C using LIF detection with Ar-ion laser source. 1: Δ-tri(2,4,6)S; 2: Δ-di(2,6)S; 3: Δ-di(2,4)S; 4: Δ-di(4,6)S; 5: Δ-mono2S; 6: Δ-mono4S; 7: Δ-mono6S (From Lamari *et al.*, 1999).

The separation of the molecules is accomplished by the vector sum of EOF and their electrophoretic mobility (EM). The EM is depending on the charge to mass ratio of the molecule.

CZE analysis of variously sulfated Δ-disaccharides of the GAGs involves two operating systems, reverse polarity at low pH or normal polarity at high pH. The first provides a rapid resolution of all Δ-disaccharides derived from various GAGs (Karamanos *et al.*, 1995b; Lamari *et al.*, 1999; Mitropoulou *et al.*, 2001). The only problem observed in this system is the lack of reproducibility of the migration time of nonsulfated disaccharide, which may be attributed to the stability of the capillary used. The second involves triethylamine as additive in alkaline borate buffer (pH 8.8–10.4), which suppresses EOF and EM and provides efficient separation of eight CS Δ-disaccharides (Scapol et al., 1996). The same separation conditions can be applied for the separation of 2-AMAC-derivatives of Δ-disaccharides.

Micellar electrokinetic capillary chromatography (MECC) mimics reversed-phase HPLC conditions, since the analyzed molecules interact with micelles of surfactants in the operating buffer. The elution of the analyzed molecules therefore depends on their hydrophobicity. MECC is applied to analyze both charged and neutral molecules bearing either hydrophobic or hydrophilic characteristics. GAGs Δ-disaccharides analysis can be performed by the addition of various detergents and additives such as sodium dodecyl sulfate (SDS) and cetyltrimethylammonium bromide in the alkaline borate buffers commonly used (Michaelsen et al., 1993).

Microemulsion electrokinetic capillary chromatography (MEEKC) is another mode of CE in which neutral and charged molecules can be analyzed. Separation is based on their partitioning into oil droplets moving in the operating buffer. The microemulsion droplets are generally formed by mixing immiscible solvents, such as heptane or octane, with high pH aqueous buffers such as borate and phosphate. SDS at relatively high concentrations stabilizes the emulsion by coating the outside part of the droplet. A solvent miscible with water, such as butan-1-ol, further stabilizes the microemulsion. The electrophoretic migration of the droplet, due to the SDS-derived negative charge, attempts to oppose the EOF, which is directed to positive electrode. Hydrophobic solutes prefer their partitioning into the oil droplet and therefore are more retarded than hydrophilic ones. MEEKC is applied to determine Δ-disaccharide composition of GAGs after treatment with chondroitinases and derivatization with 2-AMAC (Mastrogianni et al., 2001).

All CE modes, predominantly CZE, are applied for the characterization of GAGs in biological samples revealing differences between normal and pathological conditions and also during the development of the disease (Mitropoulou and Stagiannis, 2004; Mitropoulou et al., 2001; Theocharis and Theocharis, 2002). They can also be applied for simple quantification of CS/DS after its digestion with chondroitinases and chondrosulfatases, especially in small-sized samples.

2. Hyphenated Techniques

Conventional CE methodology by measuring either the absorbance at 232 nm of Δ-disaccharides or the fluorescence obtained by the specific derivatization of the Δ-disaccharides permits CS/DS quantitative analysis and structural characterization with high accuracy and sensitivity. However, the establishment of the fine structure of CS/DS can be facilitated by using a variety of spectroscopic techniques such as NMR spectroscopy and mass spectroscopy (MS). NMR and MS are widely used in the characterization and analysis of various natural products and drugs, but their use is limited in CS/DS analysis.

In hyphenated CE, the first step in the analysis is the isolation and/or subfractionation of the specific CS/DS products, followed by CE and characterization of the separated products by NMR or MS. Hyphenated techniques have been used in studies concerning the presence of specific structures within CS/DS chains (Kinoshita *et al.*, 2001; Nadanaka and Sugahara, 1997). Zamfir *et al.* (2004) developed an on-line sheathless CE/ nanoelectrospray ionization-tandem MS for the analysis of GAG oligosaccharides of large size. By this method, in data-dependent acquisition mode, the oversulfated oligosaccharides species can be sequenced and the localization of the additional sulfate group along the chain can be determined.

VI. Solid Phase Assays, ELISA and ELISA-Based Procedures ───────────────

After the pioneering work of Kohler and Milstein (1976), scientists working with glycoconjugates have directed their efforts to prepare MAbs against GAGs. The first report describing the isolation of such MAbs was that from Bruce Caterson's group (Caterson *et al.*, 1985; Couchman *et al.*, 1984). They used chondroitinase ABC degraded aggrecan as antigen, and a lot of MAbs has been obtained, the most famous being 3-B-3, 2-B-6, and 1-B-5, which recognize the Δ-di-mono6S, Δ-di-mono4S, and Δ-di-nonS, respectively, and are commercially available. Thereafter, the analysis of CS/DS can be performed by using the various immunochemical techniques already established. The main advantage of the application of immunochemical techniques is that they do not normally require purified samples in contrast to chromatography and electromigration procedures.

A. Immunohistochemistry

Immunohistochemistry is a very helpful tool for CS/DS analysis, since it can be applied in several kinds of tissues and is able to determine the sulfation pattern. It is very simple and of high sensitivity. The analyzed specimens are usually treated with specific enzymes, and after blocking for avoiding non-specific reactions, they are incubated with the suitable antibody. The obtained antigen–antibody complex is left to react with the secondary antibody conjugated with peroxidase, and staining is developed with diaminobenzidine. The technique is widely used for structural analysis of CS/DS in various pathological conditions (Detamore *et al.*, 2005; Skandalis *et al.*, 2004; Worrall *et al.*, 1994). As an alternative, labeling of the antibodies can be performed with colloidal gold (Chan *et al.*, 1997; Iozzo and Clark, 1987). Both types of the technique are qualitative, however, by using the suitable scanning system they may give quantitative results.

B. Immunoblotting

Immunoblotting is a technique for the detection of macromolecules immobilized on solid supports, which follows their electrophoretic separation. Various types of solid supports are used, the most familiar being nitrocellulose (NC), nylon, or polyvilylidene fluoride membranes. NC membranes are treated with cetylpyridinium chloride prior to GAG electrotransfer to ensure their efficient immobilization (Maccari and Volpi, 2003; Rosen et al., 2002). The visualization of GAGs is achieved immunochemically as described earlier or by the use of enhanced chemiluminescense reaction. The assay is usually applied for qualitative purposes; however, quantification can also be done.

C. ELISA and ELISA-Like Techniques

ELISA and ELISA-like techniques are widely used in the analysis of various macromolecule components of either inter- or extracellular origin. They are very important tools in the analysis, since they combine increased sensitivity together with the ability to analyze numerous of samples in 2–3 h. The isolation of MAbs against GAGs substructures has facilitated CS/DS quantitative analysis, together or not with its fine chemical structure determination (Hardingham et al., 1994b). The techniques usually applied are of competitive nature, and alterations observed under pathological conditions can be expressed in quantitative terms.

Quantitative analysis of intact CS/DS can also be performed by an ELISA-like methodology. In this case, the available MAbs cannot be used, thus labeling of the chains should be followed, the most preferable being biotinylation (Vynios et al., 1999). In addition, and since CS/DS cannot be immobilized directly on to the hydrophobic polysterene, due to its hydrophilic character, an activation step is required to incorporate positive charged groups on the plate wells (Grigoreas et al., 2003; Vynios, 1999; Vynios et al., 1998). Application of this methodology gives information on the total amount of CS/DS in a biological sample, especially when it is combined with the analysis of the same sample after specific enzymatic degradation (Vynios et al., 2001). The assay is very simple and of high sensitivity, since its detection limit is down to 10 ng of GAG and it can be automated, thus it is applicable in clinical diagnosis.

VII. General Conclusions

Analysis of CS/DS is used for either quantitative purposes or its characterization. Very simple assays of high efficiency are developed for analytical determinations, with or without prior separation or degradation of the other

GAGs such as chromogenic, electrophoretic, and solid phase assays. In addition, more sophisticated techniques are proposed for CS/DS structural characterization in highly purified samples, such as HPLC and CE, and very recently hyphenated CE.

The analytical methodology depends on the type and the size of the sample, the type of analysis required and the type and the amount of other GAGs present. In samples with high-GAG content, a purification step is introduced to separate CS/DS from other GAGs. On the contrary, in samples with low-GAG content, additional steps prior to analysis resulted in decreased recovery of CS/DS and therefore should be avoided. However, direct chondroitinases' and/or chondrosulfatases' treatment of samples with very low CS/DS content in order to be subjected in quantitative analysis results in significant variations, thus an enrichment of the samples in CS/DS is a prerequisite. A very smart procedure for such enrichment is proposed (Volpi and Maccari, 2005).

Analysis of CS/DS is required to elucidate the state of a biological sample. GAGs, generally, may be implicated in a disease for a variety of reasons. There may be an inbuilt structural defect in the GAGs, or alternatively, defects may be present, for example, in matrix proteins with which GAG chains are involved or deficiencies may be present in GAGs metabolism. Among the latter, characteristic examples are many types of cancer in which impairment in the biosynthesis of GAGs is observed and all mucopolysaccharidoses in which an inherited deficiency of at least in one enzyme involved in GAG catabolism is found. All these result in the alteration of the content of GAG in the tissue and the plasma, and its excretion with the urine. Quantitative analysis of CS/DS alone may be sufficient only for a small number of cases and especially when extreme differences appeared. However, in most of the cases when healthy and pathological samples have to be analyzed, their quantitative differences in CS/DS amounts are not substantial and additional information regarding CS/DS fine chemical structure is required. In those cases, separational techniques should be applied in partially or totally digested CS/DS for its fingerprinting (Lauder et al., 2000; Volpi, 2004). From the various separational techniques proposed, each one provides different information and the selection of the appropriate depends on the type of CS/DS alterations observed in a disease and the amount of the sample required.

The use of MAbs for quantification and/or structural characterization of CS/DS is an alternate methodology, which is applicable in most of the cases and especially in samples with very low-CS/DS content. All the known types of immunochemical techniques may be applied, depending on the answer required. Analysis through MAbs may also give information on the distribution of different types of CS/DS in a tissue without any requirement of GAGs purification, by applying immunochemical staining. This type of analysis can also be applied in biopsy specimens for diagnostic purposes.

Acknowledgments

The financial support of the Research Committee of the University of Patras (Program K. Karatheodori) to I.-E. Triantaphyllidou is acknowledged.

References

Bitter, T., and Muir, H. M. (1962). A modified uronic acid-carbazole reaction. *Anal. Biochem.* 4, 330–334.

Björnsson, S. (1993). Size dependent separation of proteoglycans by electrophoresis in gels of pure agarose. *Anal. Biochem.* 210, 282–291.

Calabro, A., Hascall, V. C., and Midura, R. J. (2000). Adaptation of FACE methodology for microanalysis of total hyaluronan and chondroitin sulfate composition from cartilage. *Glycobiology* 10, 283–293.

Calabro, A., Midura, R., Wang, A., West, L., Plaas, A., and Hascall, V. C. (2001). Fluorophore-assisted carbohydrate electrophoresis (FACE) of glycosaminoglycans. *Osteoarthritis Cartilage* 9(Suppl A), S16–S22.

Capon, C., Mizon, C., Lemoine, J., Rodie-Talbere, P., and Mizon, J. (2003). In acute inflammation, the chondroitin-4 sulphate carried by bikunin is not only longer, it is also undersulphated. *Biochimie* 85, 101–107.

Carney, S. L., and Muir, H. (1988). The structure and function of cartilage proteoglycans. *Physiol. Rev.* 68, 858–910.

Carulli, D., Laabs, T., Geller, H. M., and Fawcett, J. W. (2005). Chondroitin sulfate proteoglycans in neural development and regeneration. *Curr. Opin. Neurobiol.* 15, 116–120.

Caterson, B., Christner, J. E., Baker, J. R., and Couchman, J. R. (1985). Production and characterization of monoclonal antibodies directed against connective tissue proteoglycans. *Fed. Proc.* 44, 386–393.

Chan, F. L., Choi, H. L., and Underhill, C. B. (1997). Hyaluronan and chondroitin sulfate proteoglycans are colocalized to the ciliary zonule of the rat eye: A histochemical and immunocytochemical study. *Histochem. Cell Biol.* 107, 289–301.

Cöster, L., Fransson, L. A., Sheehan, J., Nieduszynski, I. A., and Phelps, C. F. (1981). Self-association of dermatan sulphate proteoglycans from bovine sclera. *Biochem. J.* 197, 483–490.

Couchman, J. R., Caterson, B., Christner, J. E., and Baker, J. R. (1984). Mapping by monoclonal antibody detection of glycosaminoglycans in connective tissues. *Nature* 307, 650–652.

De Muro, P., Faedda, R., Formato, M., Re, F., Satta, A., Cherchi, G. M., and Carcassi, A. (2001). Urinary glycosaminoglycans in patients with systemic lupus erythematosus. *Clin. Exp. Rheumatol.* 19, 125–130.

Detamore, M. S., Orfanos, J. G., Almarza, A. J., French, M. M., Wong, M. E., and Athanasiou, K. A. (2005). Quantitative analysis and comparative regional investigation of the extracellular matrix of the porcine temporomandibular joint disc. *Matrix Biol.* 24, 45–57.

Dietrich, C. P., McDuffie, N., and Sampaio, L. O. (1977). Identification of acidic mucopolysaccharides by agarose gel electrophoresis. *J. Chromatogr.* 130, 299–304.

Domowicz, M., Mangoura, D., and Schwartz, N. B. (2000). Cell specific-chondroitin sulfate proteoglycan expression during CNS morphogenesis in the chick embryo. *Int. J. Dev. Neurosci.* 18, 629–641.

Domowicz, M. S., Mueller, M. M., Novak, T. E., Schwartz, L. E., and Schwartz, N. B. (2003). Developmental expression of the HNK-1 carbohydrate epitope on aggrecan during chondrogenesis. *Dev. Dyn.* 226, 42–50.

Elson, L. A., and Morgan, W. T. J. (1933). A colorimetric method for the determination of glucosamine and chondrosamine. *Biochem. J.* 27, 1824–1933.

Farndale, R. W., Sayers, C. A., and Barrett, A. J. (1982). A direct spectophotometric microassay for sulphated glycosaminoglycans in cartilage cultures. *Connect. Tissue Res.* 9, 274–278.

Farndale, R. W., Buttle, D. J., and Barrett, A. J. (1986). Improved quantitation and discrimination of sulphated glycosaminoglycans by use of dimethylmethylene blue. *Biochim. Biophys. Acta* 883, 173–177.

Fransson, L. A., Cöster, L., Malmström, A., and Sheehan, J. K. (1982). Self-association of scleral proteodermatan sulfate: Evidence for interaction via the dermatan sulfate side chains. *J. Biol. Chem.* 257, 6333–6338.

Gao, N. (2005). Fluorophore-assisted carbohydrate electrophoresis a: A sensitive and accurate method for the direct analysis of dolichol pyrophosphate-linked oligosaccharides in cell cultures and tissues. *Methods* 35, 323–327.

Grigoreas, G. H., Anagnostides, S. T., and Vynios, D. H. (2003). A solid-phase assay for the quantitative analysis of hyaluronic acid at the nanogram level. *Anal. Biochem.* 320, 179–184.

Hardingham, T. E., Fosang, A. J., and Dudhia, J. (1994a). The structure, function and turnover of aggrecan, the large aggregating proteoglycan from cartilage. *Eur. J. Clin. Chem. Clin.* 32, 249–257.

Hardingham, T. E., Fosang, A. J., Hey, N. J., Hazell, P. K., Kee, W. J., and Ewins, R. J. (1994b). The sulphation pattern in chondroitin sulphate chains investigated by chondroitinase ABC and ACII digestion and reactivity with monoclonal antibodies. *Carbohydr. Res.* 255, 241–254.

Hata, R., and Nagai, Y. (1972). A rapid and micro method for the separation of acidic glycosaminoglycans by two-dimensional electrophoresis. *Anal. Biochem.* 45, 462–468.

Hata, R., and Nagai, Y. (1973). A micro colorimetric determination of acidic glycosaminoglycans by two-dimensional electrophoresis on a cellulose acetate strip. *Anal. Biochem.* 52, 652–656.

Hayes, M. L., and Castellino, F. J. (1979). Carbohydrate of the human plasminogen variants. III. Structure of the O-glycosidically linked oligosaccharide unit. *J. Biol. Chem.* 254, 8777–8780.

Herbert, D., Phipps, P. J., and Strange, R. E. (1971). Clinical analysis of microbial cells. *Methods Enzymol.* 5B, 209–344.

Hjerpe, A., Antonopoulos, C. A., Classon, B., and Engfeldt, B. (1980). Separation and quantitative determination of galactosamine and glucosamine at the nanogram level by sulphonyl chloride reaction and high-performance liquid chromatography. *J. Chromatogr.* A 202, 453–459.

Honda, S., Konishi, T., Suzuki, S., Takahashi, M., Kakehi, K., and Ganno, S. (1983). Automated analysis of hexosamines by high-performance liquid chromatography with photometric and fluorimetric postcolumn labeling using 2-cyanoacetamide. *Anal. Biochem.* 134, 483–488.

Immers, J., and Vasseur, E. (1950). Influence of sugars and amines on the colorimetric hexosamine method of Elson and Morgan and its possible climination. *Nature* 165, 898–899.

Inazumi, T., Tajima, S., and Nishikawa, T. (1997). Overexcretion of low-sulphated chondroitin sulphate in the urine of the patient resembling progeroid. *Dermatology* 195, 296–300.

Iozzo, R. V. (1997). The family of the small leucine-rich proteoglycans: Key regulators of matrix assembly and cellular growth. *Crit. Rev. Biochem. Mol. Biol.* 32, 141–174.

Iozzo, R. V., and Clark, C. C. (1987). Chondroitin sulfate proteoglycan is a constituent of the basement membrane in the rat embryo parietal yolk sac. *Histochemistry* 88, 23–29.

Jackson, P. (1996). The analysis of fluorophore-labeled carbohydrates by polyacrylamide gel electrophoresis. *Mol. Biotechnol.* 2, 101–123.

Jang, J. H., Hia, H. C., Ike, M., Inoue, C., Fujita, M., and Yoshida, T. (2005). Acid hydrolysis and quantitative determination of total hexosamines of an exopolysaccharide produced by *Citrobacter sp. Biotechnol. Lett.* **27**, 13–18.

Johansson, B., Smedberg, J.-I., Langley, M., and Embery, G. (2001). Glycosaminoglycans in peri-implant sulcus fluid from implants placed in *Martin* sinus-inlay bone grafts. *Clin. Oral Implants Res.* **12**, 202–206.

Johnson, W. E., Caterson, B., Eisenstein, S. M., and Roberts, S. (2005). Human intervertebral disc aggrecan inhibits endothelial cell adhesion and cell migration *in vitro. Spine* **30**, 1139–1147.

Karamanos, N. K., Syrokou, A., Vanky, P., Nurminen, M., and Hjerpe, A. (1994). Determination of 24 variously sulfated galactosaminoglycan- and hyaluronan-derived disaccharides by high-performance liquid chromatography. *Anal. Biochem.* **221**, 189–199.

Karamanos, N. K., Vanky, P., Syrokou, A., and Hjerpe, A. (1995a). Identity of dermatan and chondroitin sequences in dermatan sulfate chains determined by using fragmentation with chondroitinases and ion-pair high-performance liquid chromatography. *Anal. Biochem.* **225**, 220–230.

Karamanos, N. K., Axelsson, S., Vanky, P., Tzanakakis, G. N., and Hjerpe, A. (1995b). Determination of hyaluronan and galactosaminoglycan disaccharides by high-performance capillary electrophoresis at the attomole level: Applications to analyses of tissue and cell culture proteoglycans. *J. Chromatogr. A* **696**, 295–305.

Karamanos, N. K., Vanky, P., Tzanakakis, G. N., Tsegenidis, T., and Hjerpe, A. (1997). Ion-pair high performance liquid chromatography for determining disaccharide composition of heparin and heparan sulfate. *J. Chromatogr. A* **756**, 169–179.

Karlsson, M., and Björnsson, S. (2001). Quantitation of proteoglycans in biological fluids using Alcian blue. *Methods Mol. Biol.* **171**, 159–173.

Karousou, E. G., Militsopoulou, M., Porta, G., DeLuca, G., Hascall, V. C., and Passi, A. (2004). Polyacrylamide gel electrophoresis of fluorophore-labeled hyaluronan and chondroitin sulfate disaccharides: Application to the analysis in cells and tissues. *Electrophoresis* **25**, 2919–2925.

Karousou, E. G., Viola, M., Genasetti, A., Vigetti, D., DeLuca, G., Karamanos, N. K., and Passi, A. (2005). Application of polyacrylamide gel electrophoresis of fluorophore-labeled saccharides for analysis of hyaluronan and chondroitin sulfate in human and animal tissues and cell cultures. *Biomed. Chromatogr.* **19**, 761–765.

Kinoshita, A., Yamada, S., Haslam, S. M., Morris, H. R., Dell, A., and Sugahara, K. (2001). Isolation and structural determination of novel sulfated hexasaccharides from squid cartilage chondroitin sulfate E that exhibits neuroregulatory activities. *Biochemistry* **40**, 12654–12665.

Kinsella, M. G., Bressler, S. L., and Wight, T. N. (2004). The regulated synthesis of versican, decorin, and biglycan: Extracellular matrix proteoglycans that influence cellular phenotype. *Crit. Rev. Eukaryot. Gene Expr.* **14**, 203–234.

Kohler, G., and Milstein, C. (1976). Derivation of specific antibody-producing tissue culture and tumor lines by cell fusion. *Eur. J. Immunol.* **6**, 511–519.

Kokenyesi, R. (2001). Ovarian carcinoma cells synthesize both chondroitin sulfate and heparan sulfate cell surface proteoglycans that mediate cell adhesion to interstitial matrix. *J. Cell Biochem.* **83**, 259–270.

Kresse, H., Hauser, H., and Schönherr, E. (1993). Small proteoglycans. *Experientia* **49**, 403–416.

Kresse, H., Hausser, H., Schonherr, E., and Bittner, K. (1994). Biosynthesis and interactions of small chondroitin/dermatan sulphate proteoglycans. *Eur. J. Clin. Chem. Clin.* **32**, 259–264.

Lamari, F., Theocharis, A., Hjerpe, A., and Karamanos, N. K. (1999). Ultrasensitive capillary electrophoresis of sulfated disaccharides in chondroitin/dermatan sulfates by laser-induced fluorescence after derivatization with 2-aminoacridone. *J. Chromatogr. B Biomed Sci. Appl.* **730**, 129–133.

Lauder, R. M., Huckerby, T. N., and Nieduszynski, I. A. (2000). A fingerprinting method for chondroitin/dermatan sulphate and hyaluronanoligosaccharides. *Glycobiology* **10**, 393–401.

Maccari, F., and Volpi, N. (2003). Direct and specific recognition of glycosaminoglycans by antibodies after their separation by agarose gel electrophoresis and blotting on cetylpyridinium chloride-treated nitrocellulose membranes. *Electrophoresis* **24**, 1347–1352.

Mastrogianni, O., Lamari, F., Syrokou, A., Militsopoulou, M., Hjerpe, A., and Karamanos, N. K. (2001). Microemulsion electrokinetic capillary chromatography of sulfated disaccharides derived from glycosaminoglycans. *Electrophoresis* **22**, 2743–2745.

Masuda, T., and Shiga, T. (2005). Chemorepulsion and cell adhesion molecules in patterning initial trajectories of sensory axons. *Neurosci. Res.* **51**, 337–347.

McDevitt, C. A., and Muir, H. (1971). Gel electrophoresis of proteoglycans and glycosaminoglycans on large-pore composite polyacrylamide-agarose gels. *Anal. Biochem.* **44**, 612–622.

Michaelsen, S., Schroder, M. B., and Sorensen, H. (1993). Separation and determination of glycosaminoglycan disaccharides by micellar electrokinetic capillary chromatography for studies of pelt glycosaminoglycans. *J. Chromatogr. A* **652**, 503–515.

Mielke, C. H., Jr., Starr, C. M., Klock, J. C., Devereaux, D., Mielke, M. R., Baker, D. E., Broemeling, L., Wacksman, M., White, J. R., Jr., Oliver, S. A., Ens, G., Gavin, P., *et al.* (1999). Direct measurement of unfractionated heparin using a biochemical assay. *Clin. Appl. Thromb. Hemost.* **5**, 267–276.

Mitropoulou, T. N., Lamari, F., Syrokou, A., Hjerpe, A., and Karamanos, N. K. (2001). Identification of oligomeric domains within dermatan sulfate chains using differential enzymic treatments, derivatization with 2-aminoacridone and capillary electrophoresis. *Electrophoresis* **22**, 2458–2463.

Mitropoulou, T. N., and Stagiannis, K. D. (2004). Variation in sulfation pattern of galactosaminoglycan containing proteoglycans is associated with the development of uterine leiomyoma. *Biomed. Chromatogr.* **18**, 411–413.

Mitropoulou, T. N., Theocharis, A. D., Stagiannis, K. D., and Karamanos, N. K. (2001). Identification, quantification and fine structural characterization of glycosaminoglycans from uterine leiomyoma and normal myometrium. *Biochimie* **83**, 529–536.

Nadanaka, S., and Sugahara, K. (1997). The unusual tetrasaccharide sequence GlcA beta 1-3GalNAc(4-sulfate)beta 1-4GlcA(2-sulfate)beta 1-3GalNAc(6-sulfate) found in the hexasaccharides prepared by testicular hyaluronidase digestion of shark cartilage chondroitin sulfate D. *Glycobiology* **7**, 253–263.

Pan, T., Wong, B. S., Liu, T., Li, R., Petersen, R. B., and Sy, M. S. (2002). Cell-surface prion protein interacts with glycosaminoglycans. *Biochem. J.* **368**, 81–90.

Papadas, Th. A., Stylianou, M., Mastronikolis, N. S., Papageorgakopoulou, N., Skandalis, S., Goumas, P., Theocharis, D. A., and Vynios, D. H. (2002). Alterations in the content and composition of glycosaminoglycans in human laryngeal carcinoma. *Acta Otolaryngol.* **122**, 330–337.

Papakonstantinou, E., Dionyssopoulos, A., Pesintzaki, C., Minas, A., and Karakiulakis, G. (2003). Expression of proteoglycans and glycosaminoglycans in angiofibroma and fibrous plaque skin lesions from patients with tuberous sclerosis. *Arch. Dermatol. Res.* **295**, 138–145.

Pinto, D. O., Ferreira, P. L., Andrade, L. R., Petrs-Silva, H., Linden, R., Abdelhay, E., Araújo, H. M. M., Alonso, C.-E. V., and Pavão, M. S. G. (2004). Biosynthesis and metabolism of sulfated glycosaminoglycans during *Drosophila melanogaster* development. *Glycobiology* **14**, 529–536.

Plaas, A. H., West, L. A., Thonar, E. J., Karcioglu, Z. A., Smith, C. J., Klintworth, G. K., and Hascall, V. C. (2001). Altered fine structures of corneal and skeletal keratan sulfate and chondroitin/dermatan sulfate in macular corneal dystrophy. *J. Biol. Chem.* **276**, 39788–39796.

Rauch, U. (2004). Extracellular matrix components associated with remodeling processes in brain. *Cell. Mol. Life Sci.* **61**, 2031–2045.

Rosen, M., Edfors-Lilja, I., and Bjornsson, S. (2002). Quantitation of repetitive epitopes in glycosaminoglycans immobilized on hydrophobic membranes treated with cationic detergents. *Anal. Biochem.* **308**, 210–222.

Scapol, L., Marchi, E., and Viscomi, G. C. (1996). Capillary electrophoresis of heparin and dermatan sulfate unsaturated disaccharides with triethylamine and acetonitrile as electrolyte additives. *J. Chromatogr. A* **735**, 367–374.

Schwartz, N. B., and Domowicz, M. (2004). Proteoglycans in brain development. *Glycoconj. J.* **21**, 329–341.

Sherman, I. W., Eda, S., and Winograd, E. (2003). Cytoadherence and sequestration in *Plasmodium falciparum*: Defining the ties that bind. *Microbes Infect.* **5**, 897–909.

Skandalis, S. S., Theocharis, A. D., Theocharis, D. A., Papadas, Th. A., Vynios, D. H., and Papageorgakopoulou, N. (2004). Matrix proteoglycans are markedly affected in advanced laryngeal squamous cell carcinoma. *Biochim. Biophys. Acta Mol. Basis Dis.* **1689**, 152–161.

Stevens, R. L., Colombo, M., Gonzales, J. J., Hollander, W., and Schmid, K. (1976). The glycosaminoglycans of the human artery and their changes in atherosclerosis. *J. Clin. Invest.* **58**, 470–481.

Sugahara, K., Mikami, T., Uyama, T., Mizuguchi, S., Nomura, K., and Kitagawa, H. (2003). Recent advances in the structural biology of chondroitin sulfate and dermatan sulfate. *Curr. Opin. Struct. Biol.* **13**, 612–620.

Theocharis, A. D. (2002). Human colon adenocarcinoma is associated with specific post-translational modifications of versican and decorin. *Biochim. Biophys. Acta* **1588**, 165–172.

Theocharis, A. D., and Theocharis, D. A. (2002). High-performance capillary electrophoretic analysis of hyaluronan and galactosaminoglycan-disaccharides in gastrointestinal carcinomas. Differential disaccharide composition as a possible tool-indicator for malignancies. *Biomed. Chromatogr.* **16**, 157–161.

Theocharis, A. D., Tsara, M. E., Papageorgacopoulou, N., Karavias, D. D., and Theocharis, D. A. (2000). Pancreatic carcinoma is characterized by elevated content of hyaluronan and chondroitin sulfate with altered disaccharide composition. *Biochim. Biophys. Acta* **1502**, 201–206.

Theocharis, A. D., Tsara, M. E., Papageorgakopoulou, N., Vynios, D. H., and Theocharis, D. A. (2001a). Characterization of glycosaminoglycans from human normal and scoliotic nasal cartilage with particular reference to dermatan sulphate. *Biochim. Biophys. Acta* **1528**, 81–88.

Theocharis, A. D., Vynios, D. H., Papageorgakopoulou, N., Skandalis, S. S., and Theocharis, D. A. (2003). Altered content composition and structure of glycosaminoglycans and proteoglycans in gastric carcinoma. *Int. J. Biochem. Cell Biol.* **35**, 376–390.

Theocharis, D. A., Papageorgakopoulou, N., Vynios, D. H., Anagnostides, S., Th., and Tsiganos, C. P. (2001b). Determination and structural characterization of dermatan sulfate in the presence of other galactosaminoglycans. *J. Chromatogr. B* **754**, 297–309.

Tsara, M. E., Theocharis, A. D., and Theocharis, D. A. (2002). Compositional and structural alterations of proteoglycans in human rectum carcinoma with special reference to versican and decorin. *Anticancer Res.* **22**, 2893–2898.

Toyoki, Y., Yoshihara, S., Sasaki, M., and Konn, M. (1997). Characterization of glycosaminoglycans in regenerating canine liver. *J. Hepatol.* **26**, 1135–1140.

Tsuji, A., Kinoshita, T., and Hoshino, M. (1969). Microdetermination of hexosamines. *Chem. Pharm. Bull.* **17**, 1505–1510.

Volpi, N. (1994). Fractiontion of heparin, dermatan sulphate and chondroitin sulphate by sequential precipitation: A method to purify a single glycosaminoglycan species from a mixture. *Anal. Biochem.* **218**, 382–391.

Volpi, N. (1996). Electrophoresis separation of glycosaminoglycans on notrocellulose membranes. *Anal. Biochem.* **240**, 114–118.

Volpi, N. (2004). Disaccharide mapping of chondroitin sulphate of different origins by high performance capillary electrophoresis and high performance liquid chromatography. *Carbohydr. Polymers* **55**, 273–281.

Volpi, N., and Maccari, F. (2002). Detection of submicrogram quantities of glycoosaminoglycans on agarose gels by sequential staining with toluidine blue and stains-all. *Electrophoresis* **24**, 4060–4066.

Volpi, N., and Maccari, F. (2005). Microdetermination of chondroitin sulfate in normal human plasma by fluorophore-assisted carbohydrate electrophoresis (FACE). *Clin. Chim. Acta* **356**, 125–133.

Volpi, N., Maccari, F., and Titze, J. (2005). Simultaneous detection of submicrogram quantities of hyaluronic acid and dermatan sulphate on agarose-gel by sequential staining with toluidine blue and stains-all. *J. Chromatogr. B* **820**, 131–135.

Vynios, D. H. (1999). Microscale determinations using solid phase assays: Applications to biochemical, clinical and biotechnological sectors: A review. *J. Liq. Chromatogr. RT* **22**, 2555–2574.

Vynios, D. H., Vamvacas, S. S., Kalpaxis, D. L., and Tsiganos, C. P. (1998). Aggrecan immobilization onto polystyrene plates through electrostatic interactions with spermine. *Anal. Biochem.* **260**, 64–70.

Vynios, D. H., Faraos, A., Spyracopoulou, G., Aletras, A. J., and Tsiganos, C. P. (1999). A solid-phase assay for quantitative analysis of sulfated glycosaminoglycans at the nanogram level: Application to tissue samples. *J. Pharm. Biomed. Anal.* **21**, 859–865.

Vynios, D. H., Papadas, Th. A., Faraos, A., Mastronikolis, N. S., Goumas, P., and Tsiganos, C. P. (2001). A solid phase assay for the determination of heparan sulfate and its application to normal and cancerous human cartilage samples. *J. Immunoass. Immunochem.* **22**, 337–351.

Vynios, D. H., Karamanos, N. K., and Tsiganos, C. P. (2002). Advances in analysis of glycosaminoglygans: Its application for the assessment of physiological and pathological states of connective tissues. *J. Chromatogr. B.* **781**, 21–38.

Wadstrom, T., and Ljungh, A. (1999). Glycosaminoglycan-binding microbial proteins in tissue adhesion and invasion: Key events in microbial pathogenicity. *J. Med. Microbiol.* **48**, 223–233.

Worrall, J. G., Wilkinson, L. S., Bayliss, M. T., and Edwards, J. C. (1994). Zonal distribution of chondroitin-4-sulphate/dermatan sulphate and chondroitin-6-sulphate in normal and diseased human synovium. *Ann. Rheum. Dis.* **53**, 35–38.

Zamfir, A., Seidler, D. G., Schonherr, E., Kresse, H., and Peter-Katalinic, J. (2004). On-line sheathless capillary electrophoresis/nanoelectrospray ionization-tandem mass spectrometry for the analysis of glycosaminoglycan oligosaccharides. *Electrophoresis* **25**, 2010–2016.

Emmanuel Petit*, Cedric Delattre†, Dulce Papy-Garcia‡, and Philippe Michaud§

*Société OTR³ SAS, 75001 Paris, France

†Laboratoire Des Glucides-EPMV CNRS FRE 2779, IUT/GB, UPJV
Avenue Des Facultés, Le Bailly, 80025 Amiens Cedex, France

‡Laboratoire de Recherche sur la Croissance
la Réparation et la Régénération Tissulaires (CRRET), CNRS FRE-2412
Université Paris 12-Val de Marne, 94010 Créteil cedex, France

§Laboratoire de Génie Chimique et Biochimique
Université Blaise Pascal CUST, 63174 Aubière, France

Chondroitin Sulfate Lyases: Applications in Analysis and Glycobiology

I. Chapter Overview

Chondroitin sulfate (CS) and dermatan sulfate (DS) are largely distributed as glycosaminoglycan (GAG) side chains of proteoglycans (PG) found on cellular membranes and in the extracellular matrix (ECM) of mammalian tissues. They are known to participate in various physiological functions as, for example, interactions with matrix proteins, activation of growth factors, regulation of angiogenesis, and melanoma cell invasion and proliferation. So, preparation of CS oligosaccharides is now becoming an important task, first, to investigate their structure–function relationship and second, as an approach to develop new therapeutic agents. For this, CS lyases constitute a powerful tool for generation of CS oligosaccharides. Cleavage of CS glycosidic linkage is conduced by specific sulfatation pattern, thus different CS lyases activities have been reported. This review catalogs the potentialities of these polysaccharide cleavage enzymes in the

Advances in Pharmacology, Volume 53
Copyright 2006, Elsevier Inc. All rights reserved.

structural investigations of sulfated galactosaminoglycans (GalAGs) and in the preparation of novel highly charged oligosaccharides as potential drug.

II. Introduction

There is a large number of polysaccharide degrading enzymes generally classified in two groups: polysaccharide hydrolases (EC 3.2.1.-) and polysaccharide lyases (PL, EC 4.2.2.-). First group catalyzes the hydrolysis of glycosidic bonds in neutral and acidic polysaccharides (Fig. 1A), while the second group cleaves in large majority ($1{\rightarrow}4$) glycosidic bonds on anionic polysaccharides by a β-elimination three stages reaction mechanism. First, the carboxyl group of the substrate is neutralized, probably by formation of a salt bridge with a positively charged amino acyl side chain in the active site of the enzyme (lysine is the most described); second, a base-catalyzed abstraction of the proton at C-5 of the uronic acid occurs, with formation of a resonance-stabilized enolate intermediate. One residue may be required as the proton acceptor and another as the proton donor. Finally, a transfer of electrons from the carboxyl group to form a double bond between C-4 and C-5 results in the elimination of the 4-*O*-glycosidic bond and in the formation of 4-deoxy-L-erythro-hex-4-enopyranosyluronate (Fig. 1B).

The PL classification by EC number considers the PL specificity relative to the substrates but not to the structurally related catalysis. In this context, another classification, based on amino acid sequences similarities, was proposed (Coutinho and Henrissat, 1999; see Carbohydrate-Active enZYmes server at URL: http://afmb.cnrs-mrs.fr/~cazy/CAZY/index. html). In this classification, PL belong to one of the five classes of carbohydrate-acting enzymes with glycosidases and transglycosidases (or glycoside hydrolases), glycosyltransferases, carbohydrate esterases, and carbohydrate-binding modules. In each class, divisions are operated into families. Actually 14 PL families are identified for 491 sequences.

PL are found in many organisms, and in general, they act as endoenzymes even if some exoenzymes are described in literature. Their products are in majority unsaturated oligosaccharides with degree of polymerization (DP) between 2 and 5, and they are significantly inhibited by polysaccharide substitutions as *O*-acetates and sulfates (Michaud *et al.*, 2003). Degradation of GAGs in mammalian systems occurs by the action of hydrolases, whereas bacteria express GAGs lyases. Among them, those acting specifically on chondroitins have been biochemically classified as chondroitinases ABC, AC, B, and C depending to their substrate specificities. This review is focused on these chondroitinases.

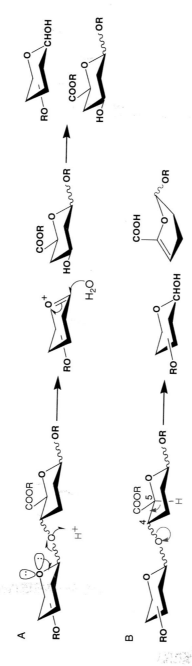

FIGURE I Schematic representations of the polysaccharide depolymerization by the action of polysaccharide hydrolases (A) and polysaccharide lyases (B).

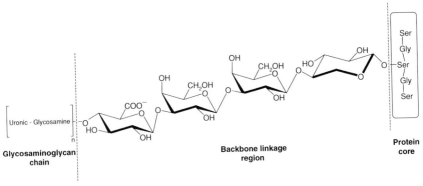

FIGURE 2   Generalized structure of the major forms of PGs.

III. Structures of Chondroitin Sulfates

CS and DS, as HS, are synthesized as GAGs side chains of PGs (Fig. 2). CS are linear polymers constructed from 40 to more than 100 repeating disaccharide units containing a hexosamine, N-acetyl galactosamine (GalNAc), and a glucuronic acid (GlcA) jointed by $\beta(1\rightarrow3)$ and $\beta(1\rightarrow4)$ linkages, respectively. DS contain varying proportions of iduronic acid (IdoA) in place of GlcA. Various types of CS are distinguished in function of their constitutive disaccharides structures. Six typical disaccharide units found in CS and DS backbone are represented in Fig. 3 (Sugahara *et al.*, 2003). Chondroitin-4-sulfate (CS-A) and chondroitin-6-sulfate (CS-C) are respectively characterized by their GalNAc(4S) and GalNAc(6S) units. Some hybrid chains contain units including GalNAc(4S) and GalNAc(6S) in the same GAG and occasionally GalNAc(4S,6S). Some GlcA(2S) or (3S) have also been identified. DS (or CS-B) contains usually GalNAc(4S) and IdoA(2S) with some nonsulfated IdoA and sometimes GalNAc(6S). Hybrid CS/DS structures have been characterized. In addition, in all chondroitins there are variable amounts of unsulfated GalNAc.

The identification of these various sulfated residues in CS/DS depends in some extent on the utilization of the different CS lyases, and this subject has been reviewed here in detail.

IV. Degradation of Chondroitin Backbone by CS Lyases

CS and DS lyases are bacterial enzymes acting on 3)-βGalNAc(4x,6x)/ GluNAc-(1$\rightarrow$4)-βGlcA(2x,3x)/-αIdoA(2x)-(1, in where x is either a sulfated or an unsubstituted site. The chondroitinases AC (EC 4.2.2.5) cleave CS-A and CS-C but not DS. They display a varied degree of activity toward

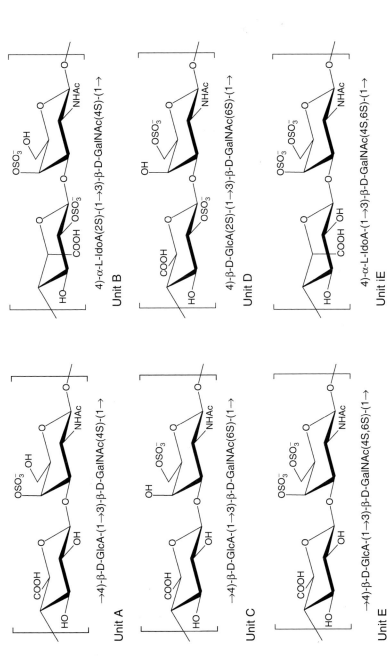

FIGURE 3 Six typical disaccharide units found in CS/DS chains.

hyaluronic acid (HA) (Hiyama and Okada, 1976). The chondroitinases B (no EC number) degrade DS whereas chondroitinases C (EC 4.2.2.-) depolymerise CS-C and HA. Finally, chondroitinases ABC (EC 4.2.2.4) are active on DS and CS (Table I). The majority of data concerning purification of chondroitinases are relative to soil bacterial species that may depend on animal tissues as a nutrient source, notably *Flavobacterium heparinum* (*Pedobacter heparinus*). The enzymes are currently inducible by CS or DS and optimal expressions are reached when CS are used as the sole carbon source (Ernst *et al.*, 1995). Nevertheless, some anaerobic bacteria from the human colonic microflora as *Bacteroides* species are able to metabolise CS.

The lyases cleave CS by a β-elimination endolytic or exolytic mechanisms. Their action is usually optimal at pH values in the range 7.0–8.0, and their products are commonly oligosaccharides ranging in size from a DP of 2 to 4–6. Nonetheless, oligosaccharides with higher DP are sometimes described and may be the result of resistant sequences of the substrate (Gu *et al.*, 1993). We noted the lack of any observed transglycosylation. None of the chondroitinases have any activity toward exclusively (1→4) linked GAGs as heparin. So, even if it is the (1→4) glycosidic bond of CS that is cleaved by chondroitinases, the (1→3) linkage is essential for enzymatic activity. Even if all CS lyases are bacterial proteins, those expressed by *Flavobacterium* are glycosylated (Lechner, 1989). Effectively, this strain unlike most bacteria, is capable of posttranslational glycosylations.

A. Chondroitin Sulfate AC Lyases

CS-AC lyases cleave the glycosidic bond on the nonreducing end of an uronic acid and use as substrate [3)-βGalNAc(4S)-(1→4)-βGlcA(2x,3x)-(1] in CS-A, or [3)-βGalNAc(6S)-(1→4)-βGlcA(2x,3x)-(1] in CS-C and [3)-βGluNAc-(1→4)-β-D-GlcA-(1,] in HA. These enzymes have in majority a random endolytic mode of action (Jandik *et al.*, 1994) affording mixtures of disaccharides and longer products. However, ArthroAC, expressed by *Arthrobacter aurescens*, displays higher activity toward HA than to CS-A and CS-C acting as an exolyase releasing disaccharides (Jandik *et al.*, 1994). By comparison, *F. heparinum* periplasmic chondroitinase AC (FlavoAC) acts as an endolyase and do not produce disaccharides until late in the reaction (Gu *et al.*, 1995). Regarding the relative activity with unsulfated, results are not homogenous. Globally, excepted for ArthroAC, chondroitinases AC are active toward unsulfated substrates with lower relative activity than those detecte with sulfated substrates (Ernst *et al.*, 1995). This observation could indicate that ionic or hydrophobic interactions between enzymes and sulfate substituants contribute to the binding step, as correlated by lower K_M with CS and chondroitin O-methyl ester, than with unsulfated chondroitin (Avci *et al.*, 2003). DS has an inhibitory effect on chondroitinases AC indicating that these enzymes act only on linkage with

TABLE I Biochemical Properties of Chondroitinases from Various Sources

Species and enzyme type	Enzyme	Mol mass (kDa)	pH_{opt}	T_{opt} (°C)	pI	Cleavage mode	Reference
Chondroitinase AC							
Arthrobacter aurescens	ArthroAC	79	6.0	50	5.5	Exo	Hiyama and Okada, 1977; Lunin et al., 2004
Aurebacterium		81	7.5	37		Endo	Takegawa et al., 1991
Aeromonas liquefaciens			6.6	<46			Kitamikado and Lee, 1975
Bacteroides stercoris		170	5.7–6.0	45–50	8.3	Endo	Hong et al., 2002
Flavobacterium heparinum	ChnAC/FlavoAC	74	6.6	40	8.85	Endo	Gu et al., 1995; Hiyama et al., 1976
Flavobacterium columnare							Stringer-Roth et al., 2002
Chondroitinase ABC							
B. stercoris		83	7.0	40	7.9	Exo	Hong et al., 2002
Bacillus sp.		53	5.5–6.0	75–80			Bellamy et al., 1990
P. vulgaris	cABC I	100	8.0	37	8.25/8.50	Endo	Hamai et al., 1997
P. vulgaris	cABC II	105	8.0	40	8.45	Exo	Hamai et al., 1997
Chondroitinase B							
F. heparinum	ChnB	55			9.05	Endo	Gu et al., 1995
Chondroitinase C							
F. heparinum							Ototani and Yosizawa, 1979

GlcA (Gu *et al.*, 1993). However, when the negatively charged carboxyl group of GlcA is replaced with a neutral carboxyl methyl ester, FlavoAC cleaved chondroitin O-methyl ester (Avci *et al.*, 2003).

As shown in Table I, three genes coding for chondroitinase AC have been isolated from *F. heparinum*, *F. columnare*, and *A. aurescens*. Based on deduced amino acid sequence similarities, the proteins have been classified in the family 8 of PL with HA lyase (EC 4.2.2.1), CS-ABC lyase (EC 4.2.2.4), and xanthan lyase (EC 4.2.2.12). Crystal structures of ArthroAC and FlavoAC have been determined (Féthiere *et al.*, 1999; Lunin *et al.*, 2004) (Table II). ArthroAC has an overall $\alpha + \beta$ architecture. This structure supports the lytic mechanism where Tyr242 acts as a base that abstracts the proton from the C-5 position of GlcA, while Asn183 and His233 neutralize the charge on the carboxylate group. The N-terminal α-helical domain includes 13 α-helices, 10 of which form an incomplete double-layered $(\alpha/\alpha)_5$ toroid. The active and substrate-binding sites have been located on a long, deep groove on one side of the toroid. By comparison, FlavoAC is also composed of two domains (Féthière *et al.*, 1999). The N-terminal domain includes 12 α-helices, and 10 of them are arranged into an open toroid. As for ArthroAC, α-helices that do not participate to the double layered toroid closes off the central cleft on one side. The C-terminal domain is built from antiparallel β-strands arranged into four β-sheets as described for ArthroAC. Huang *et al.* (2001) have investigated the crystal structure of FlavoAC bound to various oligosaccharides. His225, Tyr234, Arg288, and Arg292 were the most likely candidates for the active site residues. Authors pointed out that Arg292 was primarily involved in recognition of the N-acetyl and sulfate moieties of GalNAc. So, despite a low homology (24%) of their amino acid sequences, ArthroAC and FlavoAC present a common fold, similar to the other GAG lyases with a $(\alpha/\alpha)_5$ fold. The closest similarity of ArthroAC is with *S. pneumonia* HA lyase (SpHL; Jedrzejas *et al.*, 2002). However, the two CS-AC lyases act differently toward their polysaccharidic substrate (Capila *et al.*, 2002). Comparison of the two enzyme structures showed that ArthroAC has two insertions in the N-terminal domain relative to FlavoAC. The limited space in the cavity can accommodate only two or three sugars and is responsible of the exolytic activity. In opposite, the cleft of FlavoAC allows binding to the middle of a long carbohydrate. However, the Arg to Ala292 mutation on FlavoAC leads to a subsequent processive stepwise exolytic mechanism due to a loss of high-affinity contact (Capila *et al.*, 2002). As a residue corresponding to this amino acid involved in N-acetyl or O-sulfate moieties of galactosamin residues, is maintained in sequences of HA lyases (Huang *et al.*, 2001) and has been shown to interact with the N-acetyl moiety of HA GlcNAc (Ponnuraj and Jedrzejas, 2000), authors concluded that this amino acid have a similar function in the HA lyases.

TABLE II Genes Encoding Chondroitinases and their Assignment to the PL Families

Species	Activity	Gene	Glycosidase family	Database accession no.	PDB/3D	Reference
Flavobacterium heparinum	Chondroitinase AC	cslA	8	U27583	1CB8A	Fethiere et al., 1999
Arthrobacter aurescens	Chondroitinase AC		8		1RW9A	Lunin et al., 2004
Flavobacterium heparinum	Chondroitinase B	cslB	6	U27584	1DBGA	Tkalec et al., 2000
Flavobacterium columnare	Chondroitinase AC		8	AY912281		Unpublished
Proteus vulgaris	Chondroitinase ABC		8	P59807	1HN0A	Huang et al., 2003
Proteus vulgaris	Chondroitinase ABC		8	AAB43333		Unpublished

B. Chondroitin Sulfate B Lyases

Chondroitinase B from *F. heparinum*, the only example of chondroitin lyase active toward DS, is a periplasmic O-glycosylated protein that cleaves the following glycosidic bond [3]-βGalNAc(4x6x)-(1→4)-αIdoA(2x)-(1] in a random endolytic manner to produce unsaturated disaccharides (Gu *et al.*, 1995). Its gene was cloned and the deduced amino acid sequence was classified in PL family 6 that includes only three proteins and notably an alginate lyase. The structure of this enzyme has been resolved with and without a disaccharidic product (Huang *et al.*, 1999) (Table II). The protein assumes a right-handed parallel β-helix fold as described in pectate lyase. Authors suggested that the substrate specificity of chondroitinase B acting only on DS is due to Arg318 and Arg363 that make polar interactions with the carboxyl group of the unsaturated IdoA. Moreover, DS is sulfated in majority on the C4 of the GalNAc (Ernst *et al.*, 1995) and Arg 364 interacts directly with this C-4 sulfate group to reinforce the specificity. Pojasek *et al.* (2002) have identified Lys250, His-272, and Arg364 as residues potentially involved in substrate binding and catalysis. The cocrystal structure of the enzyme complexed with DS and CS oligosaccharides has been undertaken (Michel *et al.*, 2004) and revealed a Ca^{2+} ion coordinated with amino acids in the protein site. As for other enzymes that degrade polysaccharides (Herron *et al.*, 2003; Liu *et al.*, 1999), the Ca^{2+} ion participate in substrate binding and is directly involved in enzymatic activity.

C. Chondroitin Sulfate ABC Lyases

CS-ABC lyases (EC 4.2.2.4) are mainly expressed by *Proteus vulgaris*, and the conventional preparations from this bacteria contained two distinct enzymes, an endo and an exolyase (Hamai *et al.*, 1997). The first (cABC I) catalyzes the endolytic cleavage of CS and the other (cABC II) split off disaccharide residues from the nonreducing ends of both polymeric CSs and their oligosaccharides. These two CS-ABC lyases show activity with CS-A, CS-B, and DS (Hamai *et al.*, 1997). Their genes have been cloned (Sato *et al.*, 1994 and unpublished data) and deduced amino acid sequences were classified in the family 8 of the PL. The two sequences comparisons with other proteins show a clear homology with the C-terminal domains of CS-AC lyase (Fethière *et al.*, 1999) and bacterial HA lyase (Li and Jedrzejas, 2001; Li *et al.*, 2000). It is notable that despite little sequence homologies between CS-B lyase and cABC I, this last depolymerizes DS. The crystal structure of the cABC I (Table II) reveals three domains arranged in a linear fashion with a catalytic domain in a wide-open cleft (Huang *et al.*, 2003). Authors propose that substrate binding provokes a closure of the binding site, within which a flexible side chain of an Arg residue can interact with the carboxylic group of GlcA or IdoA explaining the enzyme ability to cleave the two substrates. The N-terminal domain has a jellyroll fold and consists of a two-layered bent β-sheet sandwich with one short α-helix. The central catalytic domain is a helical domain formed by α-helices arranged into an incomplete toroid. The fold of this domain is similar to that of the catalytic domain in other GAG lyases despite the lack of detectable sequence homology. The C-terminal domain, composed of a stack of four antiparallel β-sheets, exhibits structural similarity with CS-AC lyase from *F. heparinum* sequence homology. Recombinant expression in *Escherichia coli* of the cABC I as expected from *P. vulgaris*, and mutagenesis revealed that a tetrad residue (His501, Tyr508, Arg560, and Glu653) is crucial for enzyme activity. As observed previously with other GAG lyases, it seems that this group of residue is potentially capable of performing the stabilization of the proton shuffling responsibilities required for GAGs degradation (Prabhakar *et al.*, 2005).

V. Applications of Chondroitin Sulfates Lyases

A. CS Lyases for Production of Oligosaccharide Libraries

Several studies have been directed to gain insights into the chemical structure of CS/DS through the preparation and structural characterization of pure oligosaccharides. Enzymatic digestion of CS/DS with CS lyases is one of the more rapid and reliable strategies developed to access to the construction of oligosaccharides libraries. Other approaches to production of CS oligosaccharides libraries, including chemical, chemoenzymatic, or enzymatic synthesis, are still expensive and long time consuming (Hanson *et al.*, 2004; Karst and Linhardt, 2003; Perugino *et al.*, 2004). CS lyases are commercially available and optimal digestion conditions have clearly been reported (Hernaiz and Linhardt, 2001). Several authors have described the application of CS lyases to prepare CS oligosaccharides from diverse biological sources including porcine intestinal mucosal and skin CS-B (Karamanos *et al.*, 1995; Yang *et al.*, 2000), shark cartilage CS-D (Sugahara *et al.*, 1996), hagfish notochord CS-H (Ueoka *et al.*, 1999), human articular cartilage (Lauder *et al.*, 2001), and so on. Squid cartilage CS-E chains have been extensively digested with chondroitinase AC-II to yield highly sulfated tetrasaccharides containing an internal GlcA(3S) residue (Kinoshita-Toyoda *et al.*, 2004), supposed to be decomposed by digestion with chondroitin ABC lyase (Kinoshita *et al.*, 1997). Homogeneous, structurally characterized CS/DS-oligosaccharides standards are useful to facilitate the development of new GAG sequencing technologies. They help to better understand the structure and size specificities of the binding sites within CS with biologically important proteins and with chondroitin lyases and hydrolases (Huang *et al.*, 1999).

B. Structural Analyses

Structural analysis of CS/DS chains are often realized by determination of the disaccharide composition after treatment with CS lyases. By enzymatic digestion, numerous disaccharides, containing an unsaturation at the nonreducing end, which is detected by UV absorbance at 232 nm, have been isolated from diverse sources. Imanari *et al.* (1996) reported a review on the separation and detection of unsaturated disaccharides by high-performance liquid chromatography (HPLC) techniques. Unsaturated disaccharides are also easily separated by capillary electrophoresis (CE) (Al-Hakim and Linhardt, 1991).

Disaccharide derivatization with UV-absorbing or fluorescent molecules significantly enhances detection sensitivity of HPLC, CE, and gel electrophoresis. Review by Lamari *et al.* (2003) details various kinds of labeling reagents and methods for carbohydrates analysis.

Nuclear magnetic resonance (NMR) and mass spectroscopies have been highly valuable to fully determine the disaccharides and oligosaccharide structures (Huckerby *et al.*, 2001). Fast atom bombardment was used to identify oligosaccharides resistant to chondroitinase ABC digestion (Sugahara *et al.*, 1994) or GlcA(3S) residues on CS from various sources (Kitagawa *et al.*, 1997). Electrospray mass spectrometry (ESI) has also been used along (Yang *et al.*, 2000) or coupled with HPLC (Zaia and Costello, 2001) or CE techniques (Zamfir *et al.*, 2002). Matrix-assisted laser desorption ionization and time of flight mass spectrometry (MALDI-TOF) has proved to be highly useful for the analysis of heparin oligosaccharides by using their ionic complex with synthetic arginine–glycine peptide (Juhasz and Biemann, 1995) or other matrix (Dai *et al.*, 1997). By using this technique, no previous derivatization is required for analyzing oligosaccharide obtained from the action of CS-ABC lyase on cartilage (Schiller *et al.*, 1999).

The progress in the analytical technologies have brought an important gain in sensitivity, the biological effects of some CS/DS structures could be highlighted by analyzing their particular residue composition. The CS lyases play a key role in this determination.

C. CS Oligosaccharides of Biological Interest

One of the first examples of specific CS oligosaccharides of biological interest concerned the sequences required for the binding and activation of heparin cofactor II (Tollefsen *et al.*, 1986). The finding that DS from wound fluid is an activator for fibroblast growth factor (FGF-2) signaling indicated the importance of discrete domain structures on CS/DS in efficient signaling (Penc *et al.*, 1998). CS-B lyase digestion of CS/DS from human skin fibroblasts allowed the detection and partial identification of a pentasulfated hexasaccharide, containing either the αIdoA(yS)-(1→3)-βGalNAc(yS)-(1→4)-βGlcA(yS)-(1→3)-βGalNAc(yS) or the αIdoA(yS)-(1→3)-βGalNAc(yS)-(1→4)-βGlcA-(1→3)-βGalNAc(yS) moiety (in where y is position of sulfate group) that showed to interact with FGF-2. This hexasaccharide and larger oligosaccharides bind to FGF-2, albeit with lower capacity than the intact GAG chains, showing their potential relevance for *in vivo* protein interactions (Zamfir *et al.*, 2003).

Other authors have established that for binding to type V collagen, CS-E oligosaccharides must have, at least, an octasaccharide size with a continuous sequence of three 4)-βGlcA-(1→3)-βGalNAc(4S,6S)-(1 units together with either a 4)-βGlcA-(1→3)-βGalNAc(4S,6S)-(1, or 4)-βGlcA-(1→3)-βGalNAc(4S)-(1 or 4)-βGlcA-(1→3)-βGalNAc(6S)-(1 unit at the reducing terminal. It is likely that these oversulfated oligosaccharide sequences play key roles in cell adhesion and ECM assembly (Takagaki *et al.*, 2002).

Oversulfated CS/DS chains containing 4)-βGlcA/αIdoA-(1→3)-βGalNAc(4S,6S)-(1 have been found in mast cells (Katz *et al.*, 1986), neutrophils (Ohhashi *et al.*, 1984), monocytes (Uhlin-Hansen *et al.*, 1989), glomeruli (Kobayashi *et al.*, 1985), and mesangial cells (Yaoita *et al.*, 1990) and have been supposed to interact with various biologically active molecules and regulate their functions *in vitro*.

Analogously, the oversulfated tetrasaccharide 4)-βGlcA/αIdoA-(1→3)-βGalNAc(4S,6S)-(1→4)-βGlcA/αIdoA-(1→3)-βGalNAc(4S,6S)-(1 was found to bind preferentially to L- and P- selectins and to chemokines and to regulate their activities (Kawashima *et al.*, 2002). This tetrasaccharide has also been detected in CS-H from hagfish notochord (Ueoka *et al.*, 1999) and in CS-E from shark cartilage, which exhibits axonic and dendritic neuritogenic activities for mouse hippocampal neurons (Nadanaka *et al.*, 1998) and binding activities for a number of growth factors and a few major neurotrophic factors expressed in brain (including FGF-2, FGF-10, FGF-18, midkine (MK), and pleiotrophin (PTN) and heparin-binding epidermal growth factor (Nandini *et al.*, 2004). A different CS-E structure containing 4)-βGlcA-(1→3)-βGalNAc(4S)-(1 or 4)-βGlcA-(1→3)-βGalNAc(6S)-(1 appears to interact with CD44 (Kawashima *et al.*, 2002). It has been demonstrated that mono- and disaccharides including a GalNAc residue with (4S), (6S), or (4S,6S) substitution bind the Aβ peptide implicated in the major pathological features of Alzheimer's disease with a potent effect on the formation and structure of Aβ fibrils. GAG-derived disaccharides were suggested as a template for designing GAG mimetics for potential amyloid therapeutics (Fraser *et al.*, 2001).

CS-A derived oligosaccharides with antihyaluronidase activity reduce polyspermy during *in vitro* fertilization of porcine oocytes. These oligosaccharides constitutes an efficient probe for promoting normal fertilization process in terms of an effective decrease in the incidence of polysperm during IVB of porcine oocytes (Tatemoto *et al.*, 2005).

The new carbohydrate microarray technologies are now developed for glycoconjugates and glycans including CS (Feizi and Chai, 2004; Park et al., 2004). The approach opens the way for discovering new carbohydrate-recognizing proteins and for mapping the repertoire of carbohydrate recognition structures. New leads to biological pathways and new therapeutic targets are among biomedically important outcomes anticipated from applications of these technologies. Werz and Seeberger (2005) have reviewed applications concerning the therapeutic potential of synthetic oligosaccharides.

D. CS Lyases as Therapeutic Use

It has been well established that the variation in the sulfation profile of CS/DS chains regulates central nervous system (CNS) development in vertebrates (Hwang et al., 2003; Zou et al., 2003).

One of the major advances in CNS regeneration has been assessed with the use of CS-ABC lyases to treat injury of CNS in vivo models (Rhodes and Fawcett, 2004). For many neurons, the migration and axon elongation occurs through the ECM, which is filled with a network of glycoproteins, HA, and PGs including CSPGs. CS-ABC lyases has proven to be highly beneficial toward regenerating axons, by degrading the axon-inhibitory HA and CS chains in the ECM in astroglial scar (Bradbury et al., 2002; Moon et al., 2001; Zuo et al., 2002). This enzyme has shown to restore synaptic plasticity in visual cortex of adult rats (Pizzorusso et al., 2002). The combined treatment with brain-derived neurotrophic factor and chondroitinase ABC shows synergistic regenerative effects on axon growth in damaged retinal fibers (Tropea et al., 2003).

Degrading the GAG components of perineuronal nets restore the ability of cortical neurons to interact with one another more freely, and neuronal processes, such as axon and dendrite, should be able to grow in the extracellular space. These findings suggest that treatment with chondroitinase ABC can be relevant in therapies for the repair of the damaged adult CNS, however, interference with protective roles of CS have to be clarified. For instance, it has been suggested that CS functions in memory and learning (Brakebusch et al., 2002; Zhou et al., 2001) and that chondroitinase ABC treatment of normal mice hippocampal slices reduces 50% of long-term potentialization (Bukalo et al., 2001). Moreover, CS chains with particular oversulfated structures containing the E and/or D disaccharide units known to be involved in neuronal migration, adhesion, and neuritogenesis. These CS chains are present in the signal transducing receptor-type protein tyrosine phosphatase PTPζ (also known as RPTPβ) and in its variant phosphocan (also known as DSD-1-PG), both of them mainly expressed in glial cells and neurons. The typical ligands of these CSPG are the heparin-binding growth factors MK and PTN. CS-ABC lyase removal of the CS chains leads to aberrant morphogenesis of neurons in a cerebellar organotypic slice culture (Tanaka *et al.*, 2003). Moreover, CS-ABC or CS-B lyases treatment abolished the neuritogenic activity of phosphocan on embryonic mesencephalic and hippocampal mice neurons (Clement *et al.*, 1998).

VI. Conclusions

In summary, this review covers advances on structure characterization and active site chemistry of chondroitinases and their implication for advancing knowledge on the CS/DS degradation mechanism. Chondroitinases constitute until now a valuable tool for the generation of disaccharides indispensable for fine CS analyses assisted by analytical techniques. Similarly, generation of biological active oligosaccharides affords tools for the study of carbohydrate–protein interactions and to the development of new therapeutic solutions. The use of chondroitinase ABC to treat CNS injury has proven to be highly beneficial toward regeneration of axons and restoring synaptic plasticity in the visual cortex. This suggests exiting prospects in the use of these enzymes in therapeutics for CNS.

References

Al-Hakim, A., and Linhardt, R. J. (1991). Capillary electrophoresis for the analysis of chondroitin sulfate and dermatan sulfate derived disaccharides. *Anal. Biochem.* **195**, 68–73.

Avci, F. Y., Toida, T., and Linhardt, R. J. (2003). Chondroitin O-methyl ester: An unusual substrate for chondroitin AC lyase. *Carbohyd. Polym.* **338**, 2101–2104.

Bellamy, W. R. (1990). A novel *Bacillus* sp. capable of degrading sulfated glycosaminoglycans. *In* "Superbugs, Microorganisms in Extreme Environments" (K. Horikoshi, and W. D. Grant, Eds.), pp. 143–157. Japan Scientific Societies Press, Tokyo.

Bradbury, E. J., Moon, L. D. F., Popat, R. J., King, V. R., Bennett, G. S., Patel, P. N., Fawcett, J. W., and McMahon, S. B. (2002). Chondroitinase ABC promotes functional recovery after spinal cord injury. *Nature* **416**, 636–640.

Brakebusch, C., Seidenbecher, C. I., Asztely, F., Rauch, U., Matthies, H., Meyer, H., Krug, M., Bockers, T. M., Zhou, X., Kreutz, M. R., Montag, D., Gundelfinger, E. D., *et al.* (2002). Brevican-deficient mice display impaired hippocampal CA1 long-term potentiation but show no obvious deficits in learning and memory. *Mol. Cell. Biol.* **22**, 7417–7427.

Bukalo, O., Schachner, M., and Dityatev, A. (2001). Modification of extracellular matrix by enzymatic removal of chondroitin sulfate and by lack of tenascin-R differentially affects several forms of synaptic plasticity in the hippocampus. *Neuroscience* **104**, 359–369.

Capila, I., Wu, Y., Rethwisch, D. W., Matte, A., Cygler, M., and Linhardt, R. J. (2002). Role of arginine 292 in the catalytic activity of chondroitin AC lyase from *Flavobacterium heparinum. Biochim. Biophys. Acta* **1597**, 260–270.

Clement, A. M., Nadanaka, S., Masayama, K., Mandl, C., Sugahara, K., and Faissner, A. (1998). The DSD-1 carbohydrate epitope depends on sulfation, correlates with chondroitin sulfate D motifs, and is sufficient to promote neurite outgrowth. *J. Biol. Chem.* **273**, 28444–28453.

Coutinho, P. M., and Henrissat, B. (1999). Carbohydrate-active enzymes: An integrated database approach. *In* "Recent Advances in Carbohydrate Bioengineering" (H. J. Gilbert, G. Davies, B. Henrissat, and B. Svensson, Eds.), pp. 3–12. The Royal Society of Chemistry, Cambridge.

Dai, Y., Whittal, R. M., Bridges, C. A., Isogai, Y., Hindsgaul, O., and Li, L. (1997). Matrix-assisted laser desorption ionization mass spectrometry for the analysis of monosulfated oligosaccharides. *Carbohyd. Res.* **304**, 1–9.

Ernst, S., Langer, R., Cooney, C. L., and Sasisekharan, R. (1995). Enzymic degradation of glycosaminoglycans. *Crit. Rev. Biochem. Mol.* **30**, 387–444.

Feizi, T., and Chai, W. (2004). Oligosaccharide microarrays to decipher the glyco code. *Nat. Rev. Mol. Cell. Biol.* **5**, 582–588.

Féthière, J., Eggimann, B., and Cygler, M. (1999). Crystal structure of chondroitin AC lyase, a representative of a family of glycosaminoglycan degrading enzymes. *J. Mol. Biol.* **288**, 635–647.

Fraser, P. E., Darabie, A. A., and McLaurin, J. A. (2001). Amyloid-beta interactions with chondroitin sulfate-derived monosaccharides and disaccharides: Implications for drug development. *J. Biol. Chem.* **276**, 6412–6419.

Gu, K., Linhardt, R. J., Laliberte, M., Gu, K., and Zimmermann, J. (1995). Purification, characterization and specificity of chondroitin lyases and glycuronidase from *Flavobacterium heparinum. Biochem. J.* **312**, 569–577.

Gu, K., Liu, J., Pervin, A., and Linhardt, R. J. (1993). Comparison of the activity of two chondroitin AC lyases on dermatan sulfate. *Carbohyd. Res.* **244**, 369–377.

Hamai, A., Hashimoto, N., Mochizuki, H., Kato, F., Makiguchi, Y., Horie, K., and Suzuki, S. (1997). Two distinct chondroitin sulfate ABC lyases: An endoeliminase yielding tetrasaccharides and an exoeliminase preferentially acting on oligosaccharides. *J. Biol. Chem.* **272**(14), 9123–9130.

Hanson, S., Best, M., Bryan, M. C., and Wong, C. H. (2004). Chemoenzymatic synthesis of oligosaccharides and glycoproteins. *Trends Biochem. Sci.* **29**, 656–663.

Hernaiz, M. J., and Linhardt, R. J. (2001). Degradation of chondroitin sulfate and dermatan sulfate with chondroitin lyases. *Methods Mol. Biol.* **171**, 363–371.

Herron, S. R., Scavetta, R. D., Garrett, M., Legner, M., and Jurnak, F. (2003). Characterization and Implications of Ca^{2+} Binding to Pectate Lyase C. *J. Biol. Chem.* **278**, 12271–12277.

Hiyama, K., and Okada, S. (1976). Action of chondroitinases I. *J. Biochem.* **80**, 1201–1207.

Hiyama, K., and Okada, S. (1977). Action of chondroitinases III. *J. Biochem.* **82**, 429–436.

Hong, S. W., Kim, B. T., Shin, H. Y., Kim, W. S., Lee, K. S., Kim, Y. S., and Kim, D. H. (2002). Purification and characterization of novel chondroitin ABC and AC lyases from *Bacteroides stercoris* HJ-15, a human intestinal anaerobic bacterium. *Eur. J. Biochem.* **269**, 2934–2940.

Huang, W., Boju, L., Tkalec, L., Su, H., Yang, H. O., Gunay, N. S., Linhardt, R. J., Kim, Y. S., Matte, A., and Cygler, M. (2001). Active site of chondroitin AC lyase revealed by the structure of enzyme-oligosaccharide complexes and mutagenesis. *Biochemistry* **40**, 2359–2372.

Huang, W., Lunin, V. V., Li, Y., Suzuki, S., Sugiura, N., Miyazono, H., and Cygler., M. (2003). Crystal structure of *Proteus vulgaris* chondroitin sulfate ABC lyase I at 1.9 A resolution. *J. Mol. Biol.* **328**, 623–634.

Huang, W., Matte, A., Li, Y., Kim, Y. S., Linhardt, R. J., Su, H., and Cygler, M. (1999). Crystal structure of chondroitinase B from *Flavobacterium heparinum* and its complex with a disaccharide product at 1.7 Å resolution. *J. Mol. Biol.* **294**, 1257–1269.

Huckerby, T. N., Lauder, R. M., Brown, G. M., Nieduszynski, I. A., Anderson, K., Boocock, J., Sandall, P. L., and Weeks, S. D. (2001). Characterization of oligosaccharides from the chondroitin sulfates. ^{1}H-NMR and ^{13}C-NMR studies of reduced disaccharides and tetrasaccharides. *Eur. J. Biochem.* **268**, 1181–1189.

Hwang, H. Y., Olsen, S. K., Esko, J. D., and Horvitz, H. R. (2003). *Caenorhabditis elegans* early embryogenesis and vulval morphogenesis depend on chondroitin biosynthesis. *Nature* **423**, 439–443.

Imanari, T., Toida, T., Koshiishi, I., and Toyoda, H. (1996). High performance liquid chromatographic analysis of glycosaminoglycans derived oligosaccharides. *J. Chromatogr. A* **720**, 275–293.

Jandik, K. A., Gu, K., and Linhardt, R. J. (1994). Action patterns of polysaccharide lyases on glycosaminoglycans. *Glycobiology* **4**, 286–296.

Jedrzejas, M. J., Mello, L. V., De Groot, B. L., and Li, S. (2002). Mechanism of hyaluronan degradation by *Streptococcus pneumoniae* hyaluronate lyase: Structures of complexes with the substrate. *J. Biol. Chem.* **277**, 28287–28297.

Juhasz, P., and Biemann, K. (1995). Utility of non-covalent complexes in the matrix-assisted laser desorption ionization mass spectrometry of heparin-derived oligosaccharides. *Carbohydr. Res.* **270**, 131–147.

Karamanos, N. K., Vanky, P., Syrokou, A., and Hjerpe, A. (1995). Identity of dermatan and chondroitin sequences in dermatan sulfate chains by using fragmentation with chondroitinases and ion pair high performance liquid chromatography. *Anal. Biochem.* **225**, 220–230.

Karst, N. A., and Linhardt, R. J. (2003). Recent chemical and enzymatic approaches to the synthesis of glycosaminoglycan oligosaccharides. *Curr. Med. Chem.* **10**, 1993–2031.

Katz, H. R., Austen, K. F., Caterson, B., and Stevens, R. L. (1986). Secretory granules of heparin-containing rat serosal mast cells also possess highly sulfated chondroitin sulfate proteoglycans. *J. Biol. Chem.* **261**, 13393–13396.

Kawashima, H., Atarashi, K., Hirose, M., Hirose, J., Yamada, S., Sugahara, K., and Miyasaka, M. (2002). Oversulfated chondroitin/dermatan sulfates containing GlcAbeta1/IdoAalpha1-3GalNAc(4,6-O-disulfate) interact with L- and P-selectin and chemokines. *J. Biol. Chem.* **277**, 12921–12930.

Kinoshita, A., Yamada, S., Haslam, S. M., Morris, H. R., Dell, A., and Sugahara, K. (1997). Novel tetrasaccharides isolated from squid cartilage chondroitin sulfate E contain unusual sulfated disaccharide units GlcA(3-O-sulfate)β1-3GalNAc(6-O-sulfate) or GlcA (3-O-sulfate)β1-3GalNAc(4,6-O-disulfate). *J. Biol. Chem.* **272**, 19656–19665.

Kinoshita-Toyoda, A., Yamada, S., Haslam, S. M., Khoo, K. H., Sugiura, M., Morris, H. R., Dell, A., and Sugahara, K. (2004). Structural determination of five novel tetrasaccharides containing 3-O-sulfated D-glucuronic acid and two rare oligosaccharides containing a beta-D-glucose branch isolated from squid cartilage chondroitin sulfate E. *Biochemistry* **43**, 11063–11074.

Kitagawa, H., Tanaka, Y., Yamada, S., Seno, N., Haslam, S. M., Morris, H. R., Dell, A., and Sugahara, K. (1997). A novel pentasaccharide sequence GlcA(3-sulfate)(β1-4)GalNAc(4-sulfate)(β1-4)(Fucα1-3)GlcA(β1-3)GalNAc(4-sulfate) in the oligosaccharides isolated from king crab cartilage chondroitin sulfate K and its differential susceptibility to chondroitinases and hyaluronidase. *Biochemistry* **36**, 3998–4008.

Kitamikado, M., and Lee, Y.-Z. (1975). Chondroitinase-producing bacteria in natural habitats. *Appl. Microbiol.* **29**, 414–421.

Kobayashi, S., Oguri, K., Yaoita, E., Kobayashi, K., and Okayama, M. (1985). Highly sulfated proteochondroitin sulfates synthesized *in vitro* by rat glomeruli. *Biochim. Biophys. Acta* **841**, 71–80.

Lamari, F. N., Kuhn, R., and Karamanos, N. K. (2003). Derivatization of carbohydrates for chromatographic, electrophoretic and mass spectrometric structure analysis. *J. Chromatogr. B* **793**, 15–36.

Lauder, R. M., Huckerby, T. N., Brown, G. M., Bayliss, M. T., and Nieduszynski, I. A. (2001). Age-related changes in the sulphation of the chondroitin sulphate linkage region from human articular cartilage aggrecan. *Biochem. J.* **358**, 523–528.

Lechner, J. (1989). Structure and biosynthesis of prokaryotic glycoproteins. *Annu. Rev. Biochem.* **60**, 443–475.

Li, S., and Jedrzejas, M. J. (2001). Hyaluronan binding and degradation by *Streptococcus agalactiae* hyaluronate lyase. *J. Biol. Chem.* **276**, 41407–41416.

Li, S., Kelly, S. J., Lamani, E., Ferraroni, M., and Jedrzejas, M. J. (2000). Structural basis of hyaluronan degradation by *Streptococcus pneumoniae* hyaluronate lyase. *EMBO J.* **19**, 1228–1240.

Liu, D., Shriver, Z., Godavarti, R., Venkataraman, G., and Sasisekharan, R. (1999). The calcium-binding sites of heparinase I from *Flavobacterium heparinum* are essential for enzymatic activity. *J. Biol. Chem.* **274**, 4089–4095.

Lunin, V. V., Li, Y., Linhardt, R. J., Miyazono, H., Kyogashima, M., Kaneko, T., Bell, A. W., and Cygler, M. (2004). High-resolution crystal structure of *Arthrobacter aurescens* chondroitin AC lyase: An enzyme-substrate complex defines the catalytic mechanism. *J. Mol. Biol.* **337**, 367–386.

Michaud, P., Da Costa, A., Courtois, B., and Courtois, J. (2003). Polysaccharides Lyases: Recent developments as biotechnological tools. *Crit. Rev. Biotechnol.* **23**, 233–266.

Michel, G., Pojasek, K., Li, Y., Sulea, T., Linhardt, R. J., Raman, R., Prabhakar, V., Sasisekharan, R., and Cygler, M. (2004). The structure of chondroitin B lyase complexed with glycosaminoglycan oligosaccharides unravels a calcium-dependent catalytic machinery. *J. Biol. Chem.* **279**, 32882–32896.

Moon, L. D. F., Asher, R. A., Rhodes, K. E., and Fawcett, J. W. (2001). Regeneration of CNS axons back to their original target following treatment of adult rat brain with chondroitinase ABC. *Nat. Neurosci.* **4**, 465–466.

Nadanaka, S., Clement, A., Masayama, K., Faissner, A., and Sugahara, K. (1998). Characteristic hexasaccharide sequences in octasaccharides derived from shark cartilage chondroitin sulfate D with a neurite outgrowth promoting activity. *J. Biol. Chem.* **273**, 3296–3307.

Nandini, C. D., Mikami, T., Ohta, M., Itoh, N., Akiyama-Nambu, F., and Sugahara, K. (2004). Structural and functional characterization of oversulfated chondroitin sulfate/dermatan sulfate hybrid chains from the notochord of hagfish: Neuritogenic and binding activities for growth factors and neurotrophic factors. *J. Biol. Chem.* **279**, 50799–50809.

Ohhashi, Y., Hasumi, F., and Mori, Y. (1984). Comparative study on glycosaminoglycans synthesized in peripheral and peritoneal polymorphonuclear leucocytes from guinea pigs. *Biochem. J.* **217**, 199–207.

Ototani, N., and Yosizawa, Z. (1979). Purification of chondroitinase B and chondroitinase C using glycosaminoglycan-bound AH-Sepharose 4B. *Carbohydr. Res.* **70**, 295–306.

Park, S., Lee, M. R., Pyo, S. J., and Shin, I. (2004). Carbohydrate chips for studying high-throughput carbohydrate-protein interactions. *J. Am. Chem. Soc.* **126**, 4812–4819.

Penc, S. F., Pomahac, B., Winkler, T., Dorschner, R. A., Eriksson, E., Herndon, M., and Gallo, R. L. (1998). Dermatan sulfate released after injury is a potent promoter of fibroblast growth factor-2 function. *J. Biol. Chem.* **273**, 28116–28121.

Perugino, G., Trincone, A., Rossi, M., and Moracci, M. (2004). Oligosaccharide synthesis by glycosynthases. *Trends Biotechnol.* **22**, 31–37.

Pizzorusso, T., Medini, P., Berardi, N., Chierzi, S., Fawcett, J. W., and Maffei, L. (2002). Reactivation of ocular dominance plasticity in the adult visual cortex. *Science* **298**, 1248–1251. See commentary, Fox, K., and Caterson, B. (2002). Freeing the brain from the perineuronal net. *Science* **298**, 1187–1189.

Pojasek, K., Raman, R., Kiley, P., and Venkataraman, G. (2002). Biochemical characterization of the chondroitinase B active site. *J. Biol. Chem.* **277**(34), 31179–31186.

Ponnuraj, K., and Jedrzejas, M. J. (2000). Mechanism of hyaluronan binding and degradation: Structure of *Streptococcus pneumoniae* hyaluronate lyase in complex with hyaluronic acid disaccharide at 1.7 A resolution. *J. Mol. Biol.* **299**, 885–895.

Prabhakar, V., Capila, I., Bosques, C. J., Pojasek, K., and Sasisekharan, R. (2005). Chondroitinase ABC I from *Proteus vulgaris:* Cloning, recombinant expression and active site identification. *Biochem. J.* **386**(1), 103–112.

Rhodes, K. E., and Fawcett, J. W. (2004). Chondroitin sulphate proteoglycans: Preventing plasticity or protecting the CNS? *J. Anat.* **204**, 33–48.

Sato, N., Shimada, M., Nakajima, H., Oda, H., and Kimura, S. (1994). Cloning and expression in *Escherichia coli* of the gene encoding the *Proteus vulgaris* chondroitin ABC lyase. *Appl. Microbiol. Biotechnol.* **41**, 39–46.

Schiller, J., Arnhold, J., Benard, S., Reichl, S., and Arnold, K. (1999). Cartilage degradation by hyaluronate lyase and chondroitin ABC lyase: A MALDI-TOF mass spectrometric study. *Carbohydr. Res.* **318**, 116–122.

Stringer-Roth, K. M., Yunghans, W., and Caslake, L. F. (2002). Differences in chondroitin AC lyase activity of *Flavobacterium columnare* isolates. *J. Fish Dis.* **25**, 687–691.

Sugahara, K., Mikami, T., Uyama, T., Mizuguchi, S., Nomura, K., and Kitagawa, H. (2003). Recent advances in the structural biology of chondroitin sulfate and dermatan sulfate. *Curr. Opin. Struct. Biol.* **13**, 612–620.

Sugahara, K., Nadanaka, S., Takeda, K., and Kojima, T. (1996). Structural analysis of unsaturated hexasaccharides isolated from shark cartilage chondroitin sulfate D that are substrates for the exolytic action of chondroitin ABC lyase. *Eur. J. Biochem.* **239**, 871–880.

Sugahara, K., Takemura, Y., Sugiura, M., Kohno, Y., Yoshida, K., Takeda, K., Khoo, K. H., Morris, H. R., and Dell, A. (1994). Chondroitinase ABC-resistant sulfated trisaccharides isolated from digests of chondroitin/dermatan sulfate chains. *Carbohydr. Res.* **255**, 165–182.

Takagaki, K., Munakata, H., Kakizaki, I., Iwafune, M., Itabashi, T., and Endo, M. (2002). Domain structure of chondroitin sulfate E octasaccharides binding to type V collagen. *J. Biol. Chem.* **277**, 8882–8889.

Takegawa, K., Iwahara, K., and Iwahara, S. (1991). Purification and properties of chondroitinase produced by a bacterium isolated from soil. *J. Ferment. Bioeng.* **72**, 128–131.

Tanaka, M., Maeda, N., Noda, M., and Marunouchi, T. (2003). A chondroitin sulfate proteoglycan PTPζ/RPTPβ regulates the morphogenesis of Purkinje cell dendrites in the developing cerebellum. *J. Neurosci.* **23**, 2804–2814.

Tatemoto, H., Muto, N., Yim, S. D., and Nakada, T. (2005). Anti-hyaluronidase oligosaccharide derived from chondroitin sulfate a effectively reduces polyspermy during *in vitro* fertilization of porcine oocytes. *Biol. Reprod.* **72**, 127–134.

Tkalec, A. L., Fink, D., Blain, F., Zhang-Sun, G., Laliberte, M., Bennett, D. C., Gu, K., Zimmermann, J. J., and Su, H. (2000). Isolation and expression in *Escherichia coli* of cslA and cslB, genes coding for the chondroitin sulfate-degrading enzymes chondroitinase AC and chondroitinase B, respectively, from *Flavobacterium heparinum. Appl. Envron. Microbiol.* **66**, 29–35.

Tollefsen, D. M., Peacock, M. E., and Monafo, W. J. (1986). Molecular size of dermatan sulfate oligosaccharides required to bind and activate heparin cofactor II. *J. Biol. Chem.* **261**, 8854–8858.

Tropea, D., Caleo, M., and Maffei, L. (2003). Synergistic effects of brain-derived neurotrophic factor and chondroitinase ABC on retinal fiber sprouting after denervation of the superior colliculus in adult rats. *J. Neurosci.* **23**, 7034–7044.

Ueoka, C., Nadanaka, S., Seno, N., Khoo, K. H., and Sugahara, K. (1999). Structural determination of novel tetra- and hexasaccharide sequences isolated from chondroitin sulfate H (oversulfated dermatan sulfate) of hagfish notochord. *Glycoconj. J.* **16**, 291–305.

Uhlin-Hansen, L., Eskeland, T., and Kolset, S. O. (1989). Modulation of the expression of chondroitin sulfate proteoglycan in stimulated human monocytes. *J. Biol. Chem.* **264**, 14916–14922.

Werz, D. B., and Seeberger, P. H. (2005). Carbohydrates as the next frontier in pharmaceutical research. *Chemistry* **11**, 3194–3206.

Yang, H. O., Gunay, N. S., Toida, T., Kuberan, B., Yu, G., Kim, Y. S., and Linhardt, R. J. (2000). Preparation and structural determination of dermatan sulfate-derived oligosaccharides. *Glycobiology* **10**, 1033–1039.

Yaoita, E., Oguri, K., Okayama, E., Kawasaki, K., Kobayashi, S., Kihara, I., and Okayama, M. (1990). Isolation and characterization of proteoglycans synthesized by cultured mesangial cells. *J. Biol. Chem.* **265**, 522–531.

Zaia, J., and Costello, C. E. (2001). Compositional analysis of glycosaminoglycans by electrospray mass spectrometry. *Anal. Chem.* **73**, 233–239.

Zamfir, A., Seidler, D. G., Kresse, H., and Peter-Katalinic, J. (2003). Structural investigation of chondroitin/dermatan sulfate oligosaccharides from human skin fibroblast decorin. *Glycobiology* **11**, 733–742.

Zamfir, A., Seidler, D. G., Kresse, H., and Peter-Katalinic, J. (2002). Structural characterization of chondroitin/dermatan sulfate oligosaccharides from bovine aorta by capillary electrophoresis and electrospray ionization quadrupole time-of-flight tandem mass spectrometry. *Rapid Commun. Mass Spectrom.* **16**, 2015–2024.

Zhou, X. H., Brakebusch, C., Matthies, H., Oohashi, T., Hirsch, E., Moser, M., Krug, M., Seidenbecher, C. I., Boeckers, T. M., Rauch, U., Buettner, R., Gundelfinger, E. D., *et al.* (2001). Neurocan is dispensable for brain development. *Mol. Cell. Biol.* **21**, 5970–5978.

Zou, P., Zou, K., Muramatsu, H., Ichihara-Tanaka, K., Habuchi, O., Ohtake, S., Ikematsu, S., Sakuma, S., and Muramatsu, T. (2003). Glycosaminoglycan structures required for strong binding to midkine, a heparin-binding growth factor. *Glycobiology* **13**, 35–42.

Zuo, J., Neubauer, D., Graham, J., Krekoski, C. A., Ferguson, T. A., and Muir, D. (2002). Regeneration of axons after nerve transection repair is enhanced by degradation of chondroitin sulfate proteoglycan. *Exp. Neurol.* **176**, 221–228.

Robert J. Linhardt*, Fikri Y. Avci*, Toshihiko Toida[†], Yeong Shik Kim[‡], and Miroslaw Cygler[§]

*Department of Chemistry and Chemical Biology
Biology and Chemical and Biological Engineering
Rensselaer Polytechnic Institute, Troy, New York 12180

[†]Graduate School of Pharmaceutical Sciences
Chiba University, Chiba 263-8522, Japan

[‡]Natural Products Research Institute, College of Pharmacy
Seoul National University, Seoul 110-460, Korea

[§]Biotechnology Research Institute, NRC, Montreal
Quebec H4P2R2, Canada

CS Lyases: Structure, Activity, and Applications in Analysis and the Treatment of Diseases

I. Chondroitin Sulfate Glycosaminoglycans

Glycosaminoglycans (GAGs) are a family of highly sulfated, complex mixture of linear polysaccharides that display a wide array of biological activities (Boneu, 1996; Jackson et al., 1991). GAGs can be classified into four basic types—hyaluronan, chondroitin/dermatan sulfates (CS/DS), heparin/heparan sulfate, and keratan sulfate (Capila and Linhardt, 2002; Esko and Selleck, 2002; Iozzo, 1998; Linhardt and Toida, 2004). Chondroitin/dermatan sulfates are the focus of this chapter. Chondroitin/dermatan sulfates are linear, polydisperse GAGs with a repeating core of disaccharide structure composed of a D-glucopyranosyl uronic (GlcAp) acid or L-idopyranosyl uronic (IdoAp) acid glycosidically linked to 2-deoxy, 2-acetamido-D-galactopyranose (GalpNAc) residue (Fig. 1). The major classes of the chondroitin family of GAGs are: chondroitin; chondroitin-4-sulfate (CS-A); dermatan sulfate (CS-B or DS), and chondroitin-6-sulfate (CS-C).

Advances in Pharmacology, Volume 53
Copyright 2006, Elsevier Inc. All rights reserved.

1054-3589/06 $35.00
DOI: 10.1016/S1054-3589(05)53009-6

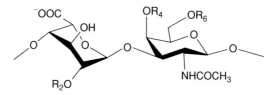

Chondroitin sulfate

CS-A: $R_4=SO_3^-$ R_2, $R_6=H$
CS-C: $R_6=SO_3^-$ R_2, $R_4=H$
Chondroitin: R_2, R_4, $R_6=H$
Oversulfated CS: 2 or 3 sulfo groups at R_2, R_4, R_6

Dermatan sulfate

DS (CS-B): $R_4=SO_3^-$ R_2, $R_6=H$
Oversulfated DS: 2 or 3 sulfo groups at R_2, R_4, R_6

FIGURE 1   CS, oversulfated CS and chondroitin: the molecular weight ranges from 5000–50,000 (average 25 kDa). DS and oversulfated DS: the molecular weight ranges from 5000–50,000 (average 25 kDa).

GAGs are the sulfated polysaccharide side chains of proteoglycans (PGs). These PGs are ubiquitous in animals and found localized on the external cell membrane and extracellular matrix (ECM) in all tissues (Iozzo, 1998). Despite intensive studies on this class of biopolymers, their precise chemical structures and biological functions are still not well understood. The major families of GAGs differ based on their disaccharide repeating unit, their linkage chemistry, and their sulfation pattern. Our current understanding of GAG structure and the biosynthetic pathway of GAG synthesis suggest the presence of defined sequences that specifically interact with an array of GAG-binding proteins (Esko and Selleck, 2002). Among these proteins are several families of growth factors, chemokines, enzymes, and adhesion proteins (Capila and Linhardt, 2002). The GAG chains of PGs act as receptors in signal transduction, controlling cell growth, differentiation, migration, adhesion, and other important physiological and pathophysiological events (Linhardt and Toida, 2004). CS is the predominant GAG present in aggrecan, the major PG of cartilage (Kresse and Schonherr,

2001). Due to the sulfo and carboxyl moieties of their GAG components, PGs concentrate large amounts of negative charge in the ECM. This has direct osmotic effects on these tissues in which the GAGs are under hydrated due to constraints imposed by the collagen fiber network, giving cartilage its shock-absorbing function (Kempson, 1980). GalNpAc O-sulfonation of chondroitin can occur at the 4- and/or 6-positions (CS-A and CS-C, respectively), and it is not known how the sulfated units are distributed throughout the PG molecules or whether particular regions have different biological functions. CS-A, CS-C, and DS are found within the ECM or on cell membranes attached to a variety of proteins, including decorin, biglycan, and aggrecan (Kresse and Schonherr, 2001).

II. Enzymes Mediating GAG Synthesis _____

GAG presence is associated with all animals, ranging from *C. elegans* to man (Esko and Selleck, 2002). These polysaccharide chains are synthesized by a set of specialized enzymes that assemble an initiation tetrasaccharide on specific serine residues of the core protein, followed by successive addition of repeating disaccharide units to the nonreducing end by synthases (Spicer and McDonald, 1998; Yada *et al.*, 2003). GAGs, however, are not unique to eukaryotes. Several specialized microorganisms also produce simpler forms of these polymers. The enzymes mediating GAG synthesis have been characterized, and the ability to express them in large quantities would greatly facilitate the production of defined GAG components (Spicer and McDonald, 1998; Yada *et al.*, 2003).

Glycosaminoglycans are synthesized by the serial addition of UDP-sugars through the action of dedicated membrane anchored glycosyl transferases followed by several sulfotransferases, deacetylases, and epimerases (Esko and Selleck, 2002; Hannesson *et al.*, 1996; Silbert and Sugumaran, 2002; Sugahara and Kitagawa, 2002). Sugar transfer occurs in the Golgi, and the type of GAG added is believed to be dependent on as yet unclear signals present on the core proteins (Iozzo, 1998; Rosenberg *et al.*, 1997). In general, GAGs are added to a specific region of the core protein. In most cases a common tetrasaccharide linkage region is assembled by xylosylation of specific serine residues, followed by addition of two galactose units and glucuronic acid. The next step, addition of *N*-acetyl hexosamine determines whether the resulting chain will be CS/DS or heparan sulfate (HS). The three-dimensional structures of two of these biosynthetic enzymes have been determined (Negishi *et al.*, 2003). The final glycosyl transferases that add repeating disaccharides to extend the growing GAG chain are of greatest interest. These are bifunctional enzymes that alternatively add GlcUAp and GalNpAc or GlcNpAc. Families of these enzymes have been identified for human CS (Kitagawa *et al.*, 2001, 2003; Uyama *et al.*, 2003; Yada *et al.*, 2003) and HS (Esko and Selleck, 2002) synthesis. A gene coding for chondroitin synthase was identified in the K4 strain of *E. coli* (Ninomiya *et al.*, 2002). While the mammalian enzymes can only be expressed in tiny amounts, bacterial chondroitin synthase has been produced as a soluble recombinant protein (Yada *et al.*, 2003).

Since no protein core is associated with hyaluronic acid, a different biosynthetic mechanism is in place for this macromolecule. Two classes of hyaluronan synthases (HAS) have been characterized (DeAngelis, 1999). The class I enzymes are integral membrane proteins whereas the class II members are membrane associated through a C-terminal membrane spanning segment. Mammalian HAS belong to class I and appear to be bifunctional enzymes that add alternating UDP sugars to the growing hyaluronan chain, which is extruded onto the cell surface and into the ECM. Three mammalian genes coding for HAS have been identified, and their gene structures are evolutionarily well conserved (Monslow *et al.*, 2003). These isoforms show high-amino acid sequence identity between themselves and to some bacterial enzymes, for example, *Streptococcus pyogenes* HA synthase. They contain seven putative membrane-spanning regions with a long cytoplasmic loop containing the putative UDP binding and glycosyltransferase catalytic sites (Itano and Kimata, 2002). A soluble and active fragment of human HAS2 was expressed in *E. coli* (Hoshi *et al.*, 2004), opening the door to functional and structural studies of this enzyme.

Assembly of heparan and chondroitin chains involves two additional modifications—sulfation of specific positions of the *N*-acetyl hexosamine and the uronic acid units and epimerization of glucuronic acid residues. C5-epimerases responsible for this step in heparan biosynthesis have been characterized (Li *et al.*, 1997), but those responsible for chondroitin to dermatan conversion remain unclear (Seidler *et al.*, 2002). Finally, a series of sulfotransferases acts to modify the CS/DS and HS/heparin families of PGs. The three-dimensional structures of two of these biosynthetic enzymes have been determined (Moon *et al.*, 2004; Thorp *et al.*, 2004).

III. CS Degrading Enzymes

Two chemically distinct enzymatic mechanisms have evolved for the degradation of GAGs, and the enzymes are accordingly classified as either hydrolases or lyases. Henrissat has divided these enzymes into families based on sequence similarity (http://afmb.cnrs-mrs.fr/CAZY/). Cleavage of the hexuronic acid→hexosamine bond always involves a standard glycosidase mechanism of either inverting or retaining type in which the glycosidic bond is hydrolyzed by addition of a water molecule (Fig. 2) (Zechel and Withers, 2000). In contrast, cleavage of the hexosamine→hexuronic acid bond can occur through either a hydrolytic, catalyzed by hydrolases, or an eliminative mechanism, catalyzed by lyases (Fig. 2) (Ernst *et al.*, 1995; Linhardt *et al.*,

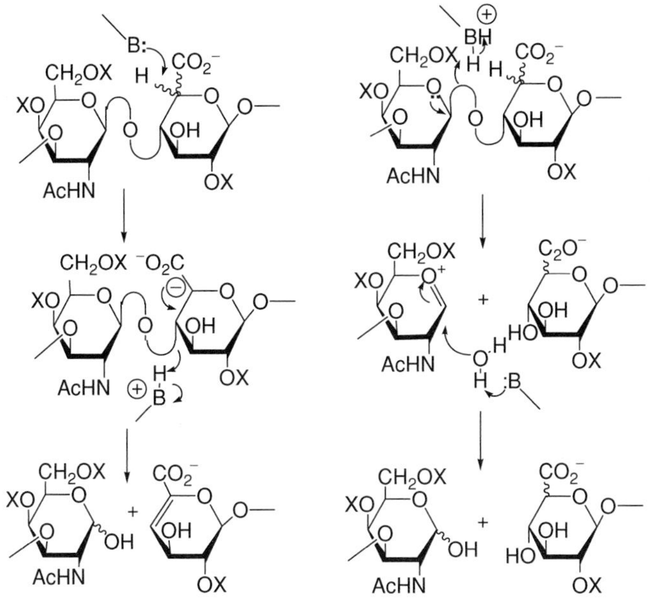

FIGURE 2 Mechanism for the enzymatic breakdown of GAGs. Lyases catalyze eliminative cleavage and hydrolases catalyze hydrolytic cleavage leading to different oligosaccharide products.

1986; Michaud *et al.*, 2003). While polysaccharide hydrolases are found in virtually all organisms, polysaccharide lyases are not found in vertebrates.

In many tissues GAGs undergo rapid turnover. Hyaluronan degradation plays a major part in the release of PGs from cartilage that occurs in normal development and in arthritis (Sztrolovics *et al.*, 2002). It has been estimated that in the dermis, which contains more than half of the HA in the body, 50–75% of this GAG is turned over every 24 h (Frost *et al.*, 1996; McCourt, 1999). Similarly, cell surface HSPGs have a half-life of 3–8 h (Stringer and Gallagher, 1997), indicating the efficiency with which these molecules can be broken down. Following endocytosis of the substrates into the cell, complete GAG disassembly proceeds by an ordered desulfation/exolytic cleavage to yield monosaccharide products. The consequences of defects in enzymes mediating intracellular GAG degradation are evidenced by the different pathologies of the mucopolysaccharidoses (Leroy and Wiesmann, 1993). Extracellular GAG degradation, although of equal importance, is an incompletely understood process. Extracellular endolytic GAG-degrading enzymes, the hyaluronidases (Frost *et al.*, 1996), and heparanase (Vlodavsky *et al.*, 1999) have been characterized, and they play major roles in normal and pathological turnover of the ECM, and specific inhibitors of these enzymes would have important therapeutic benefits.

Testicular hyaluronidase has been known for many years (Kreil, 1995). This membrane-bound hydrolase cleaves hyaluronate but can also degrade CS and plays an important role in fertilization. It has been shown that this GAG hydrolase is the prototype of a six-member human gene family. Five functional hyaluronidases and an expressed pseudogene have been characterized. *Hyal-1*, *-2*, and *-3* occur as a cluster on chromosome 3 at position 3p21, while the well-characterized testicular hyaluronidase (also termed *PH20*) as well as *hyal-4* and the pseudogene (*hyalP1*) are found on chromosome 7q31 (Csóka *et al.*, 1999). While "hyaluronidase" has been generally considered to be a lysosomal enzyme, there is strong evidence for extracellular hyaluronidase activity. Various reports have associated elevated hyaluronidase levels with increased tumorogenicity (Madan *et al.*, 1999a,b; Novak *et al.*, 1999), and it has been demonstrated that hyal-2 is a cell surface receptor for a retrovirus in sheep (Miller, 2003).

A. Microbial CS-Degrading Enzymes (Polysaccharide Lyases)

In contrast to the vertebrates, microorganisms utilize an eliminative mechanism to breakdown GAGs, which involves abstraction of the proton at C-5 of the hexuronic acid by a general base and β-elimination of the 4-O-glycosidic bond with concomitant formation of an unsaturated C4–C5 bond within the hexuronic acid located at the nonreducing end (Fig. 2). The leaving group must be protonated, either by a side chain acting as a general acid or by proton abstraction from a water molecule. Proton abstraction and β-elimination are expected to proceed in a stepwise as opposed to concerted manner (Godavarti and Sasisekharan, 1998; Guthrie and Kluger, 1993). There is an extensive variation in specificity among lyases for different GAG types. Thus, chondroitinase B is specific for cleavage of DS, accepting only an iduronic acid, whereas chondroitinase ABC will accept either glucuronic acid or iduronic acid. Extensive biochemical and mutagenesis studies have been carried out on enzymes obtained from *Flavobacterium heparinum* (*Pedobacter heparinus*) that produces two chondroitinases (FlavoAC and FlavoB) (Gu *et al.*, 1995) and on two general specificity chondroitinases from *Proteus vulgaris* (PvulABCI and PvulABCII) (Hamai *et al.*, 1997). In addition, several hyaluronate lyases contributing to virulence have been characterized from different bacteria and bacteriophage (Hynes and Walton, 2000; Li *et al.*, 2000; Rigden and Jedrzejas, 2003). Of particular interest is the genomic sequence of the commensal bacterium, *Bacteroides thetaiotaomicron* (Xu *et al.*, 2003). *B. thetaiotaomicron* and *B. stercoris* (Ahn *et al.*, 1998; Kim *et al.*, 2000) are dominant members of the intestinal microbiota of humans and other mammals. Most notably the genome of

B. thetaiotaomicron shows a markedly expanded repertoire of genes involved in polysaccharide uptake and degradation, specifically for utilizing a large variety of complex polysaccharides as a source of carbon and energy (Xu *et al.*, 2003). Among these are several chondroitinases (BthetABC and BsterABC) and heparinases, which contribute to the nutrition of the host (Ahn *et al.*, 1998; Kim *et al.*, 2000; Xu *et al.*, 2003).

While glycoside hydrolases display an extraordinary variety of folds (Bourne and Henrissat, 2001), only three folds have been identified for GAG lyases, the $(\alpha/\alpha)_5$-toroid, the right-handed β-helix, and a β-sandwich. The intriguing observation of both eliminative and hydrolytic enzymes within the first two-fold families and similarity of the β-sandwich to the N-terminal domain of PvulABCI suggest that binding of linear uronic acid-containing polysaccharide substrates demands special structural features. Of the 15 classified lyase families and over 25 unclassified sequences, the fold has been established for 9 families encompassing several pectate/pectin lyase families, alginate, chondroitin, and rhamnogalacturonan lyases.

B. Purification and Characterization of Chondroitinases

Chondroitin AC and B lyases from *Flavobacterium heparinum* (FlavoAC and FlavoB) were first purified to homogeneity, and their physical and kinetic constants were determined in the Linhardt laboratory in 1995 (Gu *et al.*, 1995). From the N-terminal sequences that we determined, these enzymes were subsequently cloned and expressed in *E. coli* (Pojasek *et al.*, 2001). Chondroitinase ABC (BsterABC) was first isolated from *B. stercoris* by the Kim laboratory in 1998 (Ahn *et al.*, 1998), and the *B. thetaiotaomicron* chondroitinase ABC (BthetABC) has been cloned and expressed in the Kim laboratory (in preparation). The BsterABC and BthetABC enzymes appear to be structurally and catalytically similar to one another. The *P. vulgaris* chondroitinase ABC (a mixture of PvulABCI and -II) is the only commercially available chondroitinase ABC preparation (Seikagaku, Tokyo, Japan). The endolytic chondroitinase ABC (PvulABCI) was cloned and expressed in *E. coli* (Prabhakar *et al.*, 2005). Some of the well-characterized polysaccharide lyases acting on chondroitins are listed in Table I.

C. Chondroitin Lyase Structures and Mechanism

The Cygler laboratory has determined the three-dimensional structures of representatives of chondroitinases B, AC, and ABC (Fig. 3).

I. Chondroitin AC Lyase

The three-dimensional structures and the enzymatic mechanisms of two chondroitin AC lyases from *F. heparinum* (FlavoAC) and *Arthrobacter aurescens* (ArthroAC) were investigated. Both FlavoAC and ArthroAC act

TABLE I Properties of Polysaccharide Lyases Acting on Chondroitins

Name[a]	Substrates	Linkage specificity[b]	Action pattern	Mr (Da)	$K_M^{c,d}$	$V_{max}^{c,e}$
Chondroitinase AC (Fh) (Gu et al., 1995)	CS-A (4S) CS-C (6S) HA	→3)GalNAc(or GlcNAc) 4X,6X(1→4)GlcA(1→	Endo	74,000	9.3	121
Chondroitinase AC (Aa) (Linhardt, 1994; Lunin et al., 2004)	CS-A (4S) CS-C (6S) HA	→3)GalNAc(or GlcNAc) 4X,6X(1→4)GlcA(1→	Exo	79,840	0.01	
Chondroitinase B (Fh) (Gu et al., 1995)	DS	→3)GalNAc 4X,6X(1→4)IdoA2X(1→	Endo	55,200	7.4	209
Chondroitinase ABC (Bs) (Hong et al., 2002)	CS-A (4S) CS-C (6S) DS	→3)GalNAc 4X,6X(1→4)UA2X(1→	Endo	116,000		45.7
Chondroitinase ABC I (Pv) (Hamai et al., 1997)	CS-A (4S) CS-C (6S) DS	→3)GalNAc 4X,6X(1→4)UA2X(1→	Endo	100,000	66	310
Chondroitinase ABC II (Pv) (Hamai et al., 1997)	CS-A (4S) CS-C (6S) DS	→3)GalNAc 4X,6X(1→4)UA2X(1→	Exo	105,000	80	34
Hyaluronate lyase (Pa) (Ingham et al., 1979)	HA CS-A (4S) CS-C (6S)	→3)GalNAc(or GlcNAc) 4X,6X(1→4)GlcA(1→		85,110		7.75

[a]Fh: *Flavobacterium heparinum*; Aa: *Arthrobacter aurescens*; Pv: *Proteus vulgaris*; Bs: *Bacteroides stercoris*.

[b]The primary sites of action are shown. X = SO_3^- or H, UA = glucuronic or iduronic acid.

[c]Kinetic parameters are given for the primary substrates.

[d]Apparent K_M in μM.

[e]V_{max} in μmol min^{-1} mg^{-1}.

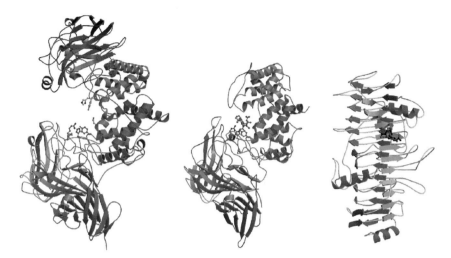

FIGURE 3 Comparison of crystal structures of chondroitinases PvulABCI (left), FlavoAC (center), and FlavoB (right). (See Color Insert.)

on CS-A and CS-C as well as on hyaluronan (Linhardt, 1994). Neither enzyme acts on pure DS, containing only repeating units of →3)GalNpAc4S (1→4)IdoAp(1→, and both AC lyases are inhibited by this GAG (Gu *et al.*, 1993). Studies in the Linhardt laboratory confirmed that both FlavoAC and ArthroAC act on the →3)GalNpAc(4S or 6S)(1→4)GlcAp(1→4) sequences found within CS and in many DS (Gu *et al.*, 1993). FlavoAC is an endolytic, and ArthroAC is an exolytic chondroitin lyase (Jandik *et al.*, 1994). The substrate specificities of both AC lyases have been extensively investigated on natural (Hernáiz and Linhardt, 2001; Linhardt, 1994; Yang *et al.*, 2000) as well as unnatural (Avci *et al.*, 2003) substrates. The structure of FlavoAC was determined at 1.9 Å resolution and revealed a two-domain molecule with the N-terminal α-helical domain and the C-terminal β-sheet domain (Fig. 3) (Féthière *et al.*, 1999). The N-terminal domain is folded into an incomplete double-layered $(\alpha/\alpha)_5$ toroid. This domain contains the catalytic machinery and provides a major part of the substrate-binding site. The C-terminal domain is composed of four antiparallel β-sheets. Since chondroitin AC lyase is inhibited by DS, we investigated complexes of FlavoAC with DS oligosaccharides. The tetrasaccharide binding site [subsites −2, −1, +1, +2 with the cleavage site between −1 and +1 using nomenclature according to Davies and coworkers (Davies *et al.*, 1997)] and four putative catalytic residues—His225, Tyr234, Arg288, and Glu371—have also been identified (Huang *et al.*, 2001). Expression of His225Ala, Tyr234Phe, and Arg288Ala mutants in *F. heparinum*, by integration of the DNA containing the mutated gene into the genomic DNA of the bacterium, rendered the enzyme inactive

(Blain *et al.*, 2002). Candidates for the general base, abstracting the glucuronic acid C-5 proton, were Tyr234 (transiently deprotonated during catalysis) or His225. The Tyr234 was deemed to be the best candidate to protonate the leaving group. Arg288 likely contributes to charge neutralization and stabilization of the enolate anion intermediate during catalysis.

Subsequently, the crystal structure of Tyr234Phe mutant with a CS-A tetrasaccharide was determined, confirming the general features of substrate binding, but this structure was inconclusive in the assignment of the role of general acid to either His225 or Tyr234 due to an enzymatically noncompetent conformation of the substrate (Fig. 4) (Huang *et al.*, 2001).

A breakthrough that allowed the assignment of the catalytic general base came from the investigation of chondroitin AC lyase from *A. aurescens* (ArthroAC). Although the amino acid sequence of this protein was not known at the onset of our investigations, it was likely that it shared homology with FlavoAC. We were fortunate in obtaining crystals diffracting to near atomic (1.25 Å) resolution (Lunin *et al.*, 2004). The resulting electron density maps allowed us to determine the amino acid sequence (Fig. 5), which was confirmed subsequently by mass spectrometry (MS) of tryptic peptides. This sequence showed 24% identity to FlavoAC. Using a series of short soaks of the crystals with CS-A tetrasaccharide, their immediate

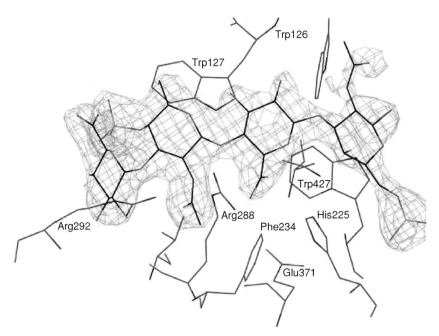

FIGURE 4   Chondroitin-4,6-sulfate tetrasaccharide in the active site of FlavoAC Tyr234Phe mutant. (See Color Insert.)

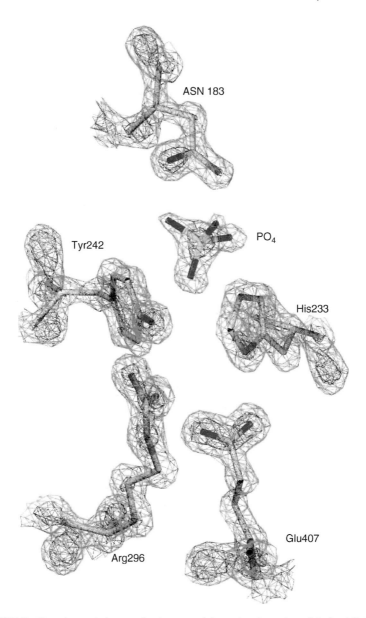

FIGURE 5   Experimental electron density map of the active site region of ArthroAC. Green contours are drawn at 3σ level, red contours at 5σ level. In the native structure, there is a phosphate ion in the active site. Nitrogen atoms are blue, oxygens are red, carbons are gray, and phosphorus is yellow. (See Color Insert.)

freezing in liquid nitrogen, and data collection at the synchrotron, we showed that the enzyme acted slowly in the crystal, allowing us to capture the enzymatically active conformation. This data resolved that Tyr242 acts as the general base that abstracts the proton and His233 helps in deprotonation of Tyr242 and in the proper orientation of the glucuronate acidic group. The glucuronate assumes a distorted boat conformation, much like that observed in lysozyme (Fig. 6).

Chondroitin O-methyl ester (C-OMe) is also depolymerized by chondroitin AC lyase from *F. heparinum* (Avci *et al.*, 2003). The major product isolated from the depolymerization reaction was found to be chondroitin Δdi-O-methyl ester (Fig. 7). Although, in chemical terms, abstraction of an acidic proton at the a-position of methyl ester group is expected, the

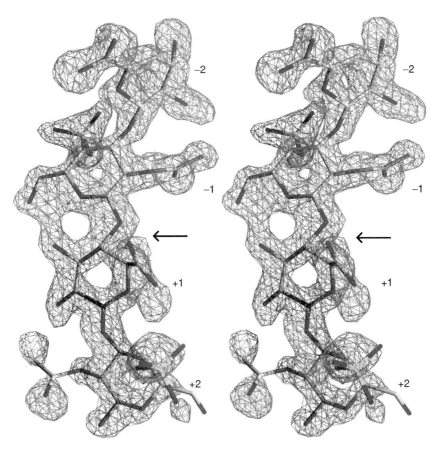

FIGURE 6   Conformation of the chondroitin-4-sulfate tetrasaccharide substrate bound in the active site of ArthroAC. Omit electron density map is drawn at the 3σ level. (See Color Insert.)

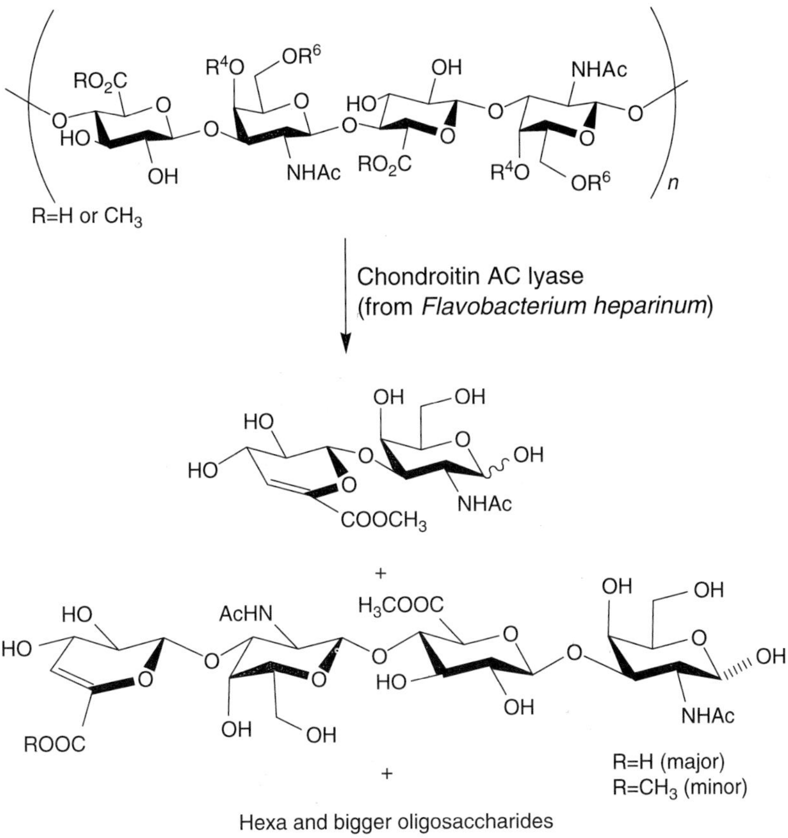

FIGURE 7 Enzymatic depolymerization of chondroitin O-methyl ester.

esterification of the carboxylate group might alter the interaction of anion-stabilizing elements in an enzymatic reaction, adversely impacting catalysis (Fig. 2). Kinetic studies show that the K_M on C-OMe (12.0 µM) is comparable to CS-A (7.0 µM) and lower than that observed on chondroitin (63.0 µM). In contrast, the V_{max} on C-OMe (0.3 µmol min^{-1} mg^{-1}) is significantly lower than on CS-A (2.0 µmol min^{-1} mg^{-1}) or chondroitin (3.3 µmol min^{-1} mg^{-1}) suggesting that the binding step is less adversely impacted than catalytic step by methylation of the carboxyl group. The low K_M observed for C-OMe (comparable to CS-A) might be ascribed to the contribution of hydrophobic interactions between the methyl ester and the enzyme, replacing ionic interactions lost through the desulfonation and methyl esterification of the substrate. Both chondroitinase AC I from *F. heparinum* and chondroitinase AC II from *A. aurescens* were demonstrated by the Toida laboratory to be capable of depolymerizing hyaluronan O-methyl ester (Hirano *et al.*, 2005).

2. Chondroitin B Lyase

The Cygler laboratory has determined the structure of native *F. heparinum* chondroitin B lyase (FlavoB) and its complex with the reaction disaccharide product (Huang *et al.*, 1999). The fold of this lyase is completely different to that of FlavoAC and belongs to the β-helix family with 13 coils. The soaking of chondroitin B lyase crystals with a DS tetrasaccharide resulted in a complex with two DS disaccharide reaction products occupying $(-2, -1)$ and $(+1, +2)$ subsites in the substrate-binding site. Unexpectedly, this structure showed the presence of a Ca^{2+} ion coordinated by conserved acidic residues and by the carboxyl group of the L-iduronic acid at the $+1$ subsite (Fig. 8).

Chondroitin B lyase was subsequently shown to absolutely require calcium for its activity, indicating that the protein-Ca^{2+}-oligosaccharide complex is functionally relevant. We proposed that the Ca^{2+} ion neutralizes the carboxyl moiety of the L-iduronic acid at the cleavage site, while the

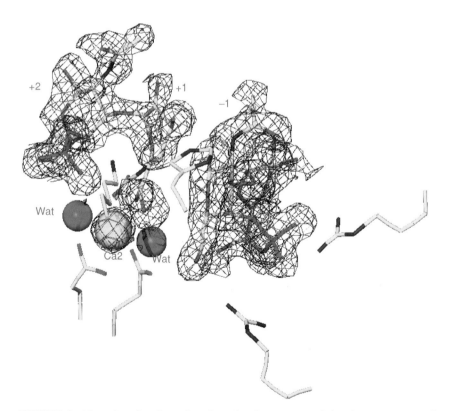

FIGURE 8   Three disaccharide products bound in the active site of chondroitinase B. Bound calcium atom is shown as a yellow sphere, two water molecules as red spheres. (See Color Insert.)

conserved Lys250 and Arg271 act as general base and acid, respectively. Model building showed that a DS substrate would bind in a bent conformation and that this sugar ring adopts a distorted conformation. The requirement of Ca^{2+} for catalysis was further investigated in collaboration with Dr Sasisekharan by measuring K_{cat} and K_M as a function of calcium concentration (Michel *et al.*, 2004).

3. Chondroitin ABC I (endo) Lyase

The Cygler laboratory crystallized (Huang *et al.*, 2000) and determined the structure (Huang *et al.*, 2003) of chondroitin ABC I (endo) lyase from *P. vulgaris* (PvulABCI). This 110 kD protein consists of three domains. The amino acid sequence comparison indicated only that the C-terminal domain is homologous to the C-terminal, noncatalytic domain of FlavoAC, and this was confirmed by the structure. The N-terminal domain has a similar fold to carbohydrate-binding domains of xylanases and some lectins while the middle domain showed, unexpectedly, structural similarity to the catalytic domain of FlavoAC and to hyaluronan lyases. The superposition of these two domains showed the conservation of residues forming the active site tetrad (Fig. 9).

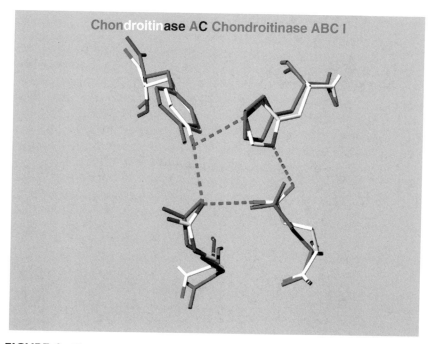

FIGURE 9 The superposition of the active-site tetrad of FlavoAC and PvulABCI. The Asn175 of FlavoAC and Arg500 of PvulABCI are also shown. (See Color Insert.)

The Asn175 of FlavoAC, which plays an essential role in binding the acidic group of glucuronic acid, is not conserved in PvulABCI. Instead, the side chain of Arg500 may perform this function. We speculated that the charged guanidinium group at the end of a long arm provides the flexibility essential for adapting the enzyme's catalytic machinery to two possible configurations of the acidic group at the C-5 position of the uronic acid ring. The substrate binding area in this structure is wide open, and we have not yet been able to obtain complexes with oligosaccharides (Fig. 10). It has not yet been possible to unequivocally deduce from this structure residues that contribute to substrate binding and the key protein–substrate interactions.

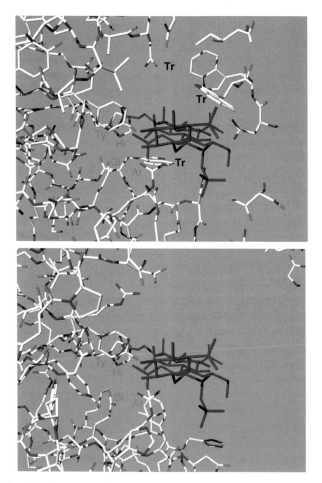

FIGURE 10   The disposition of the substrate in FlavoAC (left) was transferred to PvulABCI (right) based on the superposition of the active site tetrad. In this open form of PvulABCI are very few contacts between the enzyme and its substrate. (See Color Insert.)

Further efforts toward obtaining PvulABCI complexes with substrate or inhibitors are essential for the understanding of the mechanistic properties of these enzymes and their ability to break down CS and DS.

While the PvulABCI is an endolytic lyase, this bacterium also produces a closely homologous enzyme chondroitin ABC II (exo) lyase (PvulABCII) with similar spectrum of substrate specificities while being an exolytic lyase. We have obtained crystals of this protein and would like to determine its structure to understand the mechanism underlying exolytic vs. endolytic selectivity and to detail the catalytic mechanism.

IV. Analytical Applications

Determination of CS/DS oligosaccharide structure is a formidable analytical problem that has limited structure–activity relationship studies, and the development of improved methods is necessary for further progress. Current approaches involve the preparation of CS/DS oligosaccharides using chondroitin lyases followed by separation techniques including gel permeation chromatography (GPC) (Yang *et al.*, 2000), strong anion exhange-high performance liquid chromatography (SAX-HPLC) (Linhardt *et al.*, 1994; Yang *et al.*, 2000), polyacrylamide gel electrophoresis (PAGE) (Linhardt *et al.*, 1991, 1994), and capillary electrophoresis (CE) (Al-Hakim and Linhardt, 1991; Pervin *et al.*, 1993, 1994). These provide important data on composition and domain structure but generally yield indirect and incomplete sequence information. MS has also been applied to the analysis of CS/DS oligosaccharides (Kitagawa *et al.*, 1997; Lamb *et al.*, 1992; Yang *et al.*, 2000). Fast-atom bombardment (FAB-MS), electrospray ionization (ESI-MS), and matrix-assisted laser desorption ionization (MALDI-MS) are capable of determining the molecular weight of oligosaccharides. Nuclear magnetic resonance (NMR) spectroscopy provides for the accurate determination of the chemical fine structure of small CS/DS oligosaccharides (containing 2–14 saccharide units) (Linhardt *et al.*, 1992; Yang *et al.*, 2000).

A. Oligosaccharide Structure Analysis

GAG lyases are used for the structural analysis of GAGs. In a general oligosaccharide structure analysis procedure first, a small quantity of the polysaccharide is exhaustively depolymerized in the reaction using the proper lyase enzyme (Table II) (Linhardt, 1994). Next, a controlled, partial depolymerization is performed to obtain the UV absorbance value at 232 nm (the nonreducing end uronic acid residue absorbs at 232 nm) corresponding to the maximum number of oligosaccharides that can be detected. The partial depolymerization reaction is next scaled up, and the resulting oligosaccharide mixture is next size fractionated by GPC. This

TABLE II Reaction Conditions for Polysaccharide Lyases Acting on Chondroitins with Optimum Buffers and Reaction Conditions

Lyase	Buffer	Optimum temperature (°C)
Chondroitinase ABC	Tris.Cl/sodium acetate, pH 8	37
Chondroitinase AC	Tris.Cl/sodium acetate, pH 8	37
Chondroitinase B	Ethylenediamine/acetic acid/NaCl, pH 8	25
Hyaluronate lyase	Sodium acetate/NaCl, pH 5.2	30

separation affords size-uniform oligosaccharide mixtures corresponding to oligosaccharides ranging in size from disaccharide to octadecasaccharide. PAGE analysis of these size-fractionated oligosaccharides demonstrates the degree of size separation. The size fractions are next purified by semipreparative SAX-HPLC, desalted and lyophilized. Analytical SAX-HPLC is used to assess whether a second semipreparative SAX-HPLC separation step is necessary. Finally, mass spectral analysis and 1D/2D NMR analysis are acquired for their structural elucidation.

Using chondroitin ABC lyase, we prepared eight oligosaccharides from DS and elucidated their structures (Fig. 11) (Yang *et al.*, 2000). Treatment of tetrasaccharide and hexasaccharide fragments with mercuric acetate afforded trisaccharide and pentasaccharide products, respectively. The purity of the oligosaccharides obtained was confirmed by analytical SAX-HPLC and CE. The molecular mass and degree of sulfation of the eight purified oligosaccharides were elucidated using ESI-MS, and their structures were established with NMR. These DS oligosaccharides are being used to study interaction of the DS with biologically important proteins.

B. Oligosaccharide Mapping

Quantitative saccharide compositional analysis of GAGs can be conveniently performed using high resolution, high sensitivity CE. CS and DS can be depolymerized using chondroitin lyases (or hyaluronate lyases) into eight to nine different disaccharides that can be easily resolved by CE (Al-Hakim and Linhardt, 1991). Sensitive (picomole range) UV detection is possible due to the presence of an unsaturated residue formed in each disaccharide through the eliminase action of the polysaccharide lyases. Oligosaccharide mapping of GAGs is comparable in principle to the peptide mapping of protein and has been widely used for the comparison of GAGs from different tissues or species (Linhardt *et al.*, 1991, 1992; Loganathan *et al.*, 1990). A GAG is first treated, either partially or completely, with various depolymerizing chemicals or enzymes, and PAGE maps are prepared using PAGE and SAX-HPLC (Linhardt *et al.*, 1988). Using this approach we have

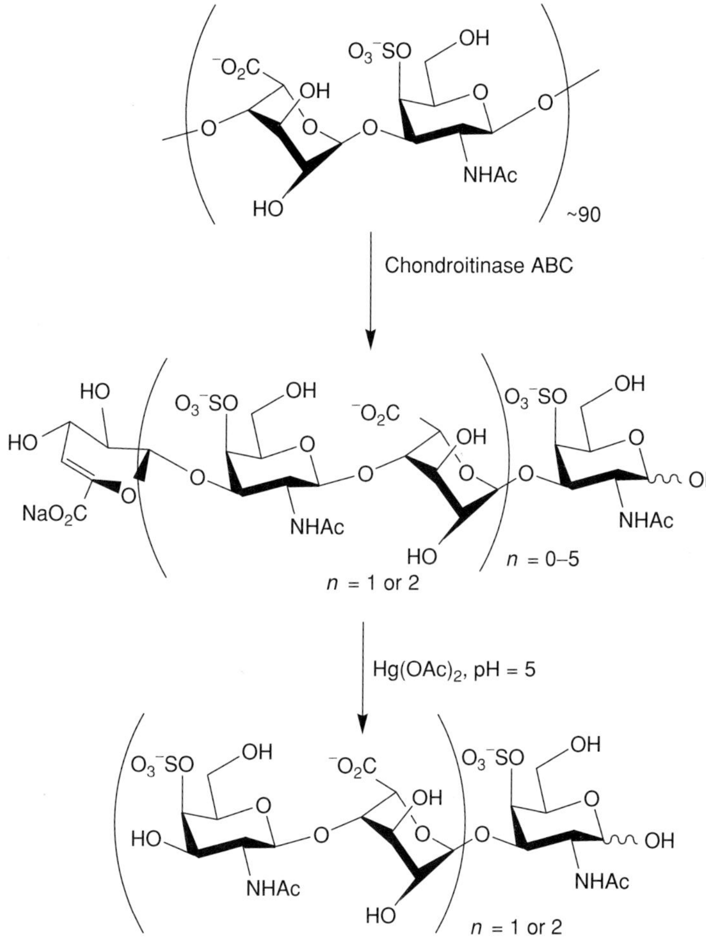

FIGURE 11 Controlled enzymatic depolymerization of DS by chondroitinase ABC and mercuric acetate treatment to remove the unsaturated nonreducing end residue.

studied chondroitinase ABC depolymerized mixtures of DS sample obtained from different species and tissue origins. High molecular weight and low-molecular weight DS as well as charge-fractionated DS, having substantially different heparin cofactor-II (HC-II) mediated antithrombin activities were examined. Gradient PAGE was used to study the DS oligosaccharide mixtures prepared by chondroitinase ABC treatment. Commercially available disaccharide standards have been examined by SAX-HPLC, and their retention times compared with the oligosaccharide mixture obtained from chondroitinase ABC treated DS. On the basis of these studies, certain structural features associated with DS have been established (Linhardt *et al.*, 1988).

C. Disaccharide Analysis

CS is widely used as a neutraceutical and pharmaceutical raw materials. As the number of products containing CS increases, stricter and more accurate evaluation should be required for the manufacture of high-quality products. Disaccharide analysis using HPLC should be useful for evaluation of the quality of CS as a pharmaceutical and nutraceutical ingredient. The pretreatment method followed by enzymatic digestion makes it possible to quantify CS content in soft capsules and liquid preparations and should be applicable for the quality control of CS. The present methods can be applied to confirm the purity and label claim of CS in raw materials, pharmaceuticals, and neutraceuticals.

The Kim laboratory performed the quantitative analysis of CS obtained from raw materials and various pharmaceutical preparations (Sim *et al.*, 2005). To quantify CS content in raw materials and in an ophthalmic solution, each test sample and the authentic CS were first digested by chondroitinase ABC. The CS disaccharides produced were analyzed by HPLC, and CS content was quantified by calculating the total peak areas of the disaccharides derived from a CS calibration curve. In the case of soft capsules, CS was first extracted with hexane followed by phenol-chloroform to remove oil and protein ingredients. The extracted CS samples were depolymerized by chondroitinase ABC, and CS content was determined. Quantitative analysis of the disaccharides derived from raw materials and an ophthalmic solution showed the CS contents (%) were 39.5–105.6 and 103.3, respectively. In case of CS analysis in soft capsules and liquid preparations, the overall recovery (%) of the spiked CS was 96.79–103.54 and 97.10–103.17, respectively (Table III). In conclusion, the quantitative analysis of the disaccharides produced by enzymatic digestion can be used in the direct quantitation of CS containing pharmaceutical formulations.

TABLE III   Quantitation of CS from Pharmaceuticals[a]

Sample	Labeled amount (mg)	Determined amount (mg)	Label claim (%)
Ophthalmic solution	2	2.07	103.33
Liquid preparation	30	29.25	97.48
Soft capsule	120	114.06	95.05

[a] The CS content was quantified by calculating the total peak areas of the disaccharides derived from a CS calibration curve.

V. Synthetic Applications

A. Oligosaccharide Preparation

Polysaccharide lyases have been used to produce Δ^4-uronate disaccharides and higher oligosaccharides from heparin, HS, CS, DS, hyaluronan, and chemically modified GAGs (Linhardt and Al-Hakim, 1991; Pervin *et al.*, 1995; Weiler *et al.*, 1992). Because both the polysaccharide substrates and enzymes are relatively inexpensive, these oligosaccharides can be prepared in large quantities at a low cost. The discovery of new GAGs, such as acharan sulfate (Kim *et al.*, 1996) as well as the mild acid hydrolyzate *E. coli* polysaccharide K5 (Razi *et al.*, 1995), can afford novel structures in large quantities and at low cost.

B. Chemoenzymatic Synthesis

We proposed that the lyase-derived oligosaccharides could be chemically linked together to form larger oligosaccharides with the requisite structure for a wide variety of biological activities. The first objective would be to differentially protect enzymatically prepared desulfated disaccharides and to use these neutral disaccharides to prepare larger target oligosaccharides (Fig. 12) (Islam *et al.*, 2003). The advantages of this approach are (1) disaccharides can be assembled into oligosaccharides with a reduced number of glycosylation reactions and (2) a high level of structural complexity (i.e., stereochemistry, sulfation pattern) is already built into these disaccharides. In addition, we investigated the use of 2,2,2-trifluorodiazoethane as a reagent for sulfo group protection in enzymatically prepared CS disaccharides (Fig. 12) (Avci *et al.*, 2004). This approach was first used for sulfate ester protection in carbohydrates by Flitsch and coworkers (Proud *et al.*, 1997). Once the sulfo groups have been protected, the free hydroxyl and carboxyl groups could be protected in organic solvents used in standard carbohydrate synthesis. This chemistry has been successfully used to selectively protect primary and secondary *O*- and *N*- sulfo groups in unprotected sulfated mono- and disaccharides in high yields (Karst *et al.*, 2003, 2004).

VI. Therapeutic Applications

Bacterial GAG-degrading enzymes also have direct medical applications. Heparinase is an important reagent that can be used to remove anticoagulant heparin from blood in the prevention of excessive bleeding following coronary artery bypass surgery (Langer *et al.*, 1982). *In vitro* experiments have revealed that chondroitinases inhibit melanoma invasion, proliferation, and angiogenesis (Denholm *et al.*, 2001). Subretinal injection of chondroitinase ABC (PvulABCI and PvulABCII) promotes retinal reattachment in rabbits (Yao *et al.*, 1992). Chondroitinase ABC (PvulABCI

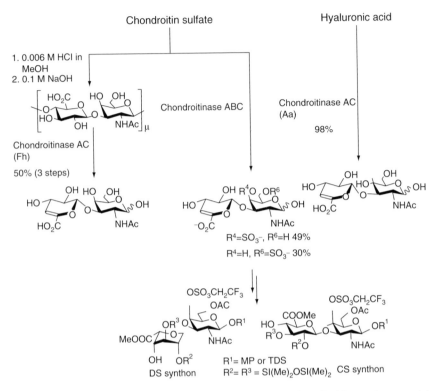

FIGURE 12 Preparation of desulfated and sulfoprotected disaccharide starting materials for the synthesis of CS/DS/HA oligosaccharides.

and -II) has also been applied therapeutically to treat invertebral disc protrusion (Kato *et al.*, 1990).

It has been shown that chondroitinase ABC (PvulABCI and -II) promotes the regeneration of central nervous system axons (Bradbury *et al.*, 2002; Pizzorusso *et al.*, 2002). Permanent paralysis can result in adult mammals following spinal cord injuries due to the inability of axons to regenerate (Fawcett and Asher, 1999). A glial scar develops at the site of the central nervous system injury (Fitch and Silver, 1999). This scar is composed of ECM molecules and is particularly rich in CSPGs (Fawcett and Asher, 1999; Fitch and Silver, 1999). *In vitro* CSPGs inhibit axonal growth (McKeon *et al.*, 1991; Niederost *et al.*, 1999; Smith-Thomas *et al.*, 1994), and *in vivo* regions rich in CSPGs stop regenerating axons (Davies *et al.*, 1999). Chondroitinase ABC catalyzed removal of CS chains *in vitro* can reverse this inhibitory activity (Fidler *et al.*, 1999; McKeon *et al.*, 1995; Moon *et al.*, 2001; Zuo *et al.*, 1998). In a recent *in vivo* study in an adult rat spinal cord injury model, the delivery of chondroitinase ABC directly to the injury site promoted functional recovery (Bradbury *et al.*, 2002). In this study, chondroitinase ABC was delivered intrathecally to lessoned dorsal columns of adult rats. This treatment upregulated regeneration-associated protein in injured neurons, promoting regeneration of both ascended sensory projections and descending corticospinal tract axons. This treatment restored postsynaptic activity below the lesion after electrical stimulation of corticospinal neurons. Chondroitinase ABC also promoted functional recovery of locomotor and proprioceptive behaviors.

VII. Conclusions

Modern analytical methods, including NMR and MS, are widely used for the determination of CS structure. While modern spectroscopic techniques provide limited information on the structure of the intact CS polysaccharide, it is often useful to utilize chondroitin lyases to prepare oligosaccharides for more detailed structural determination. The structure, activity, and specificity of these enzymes were the focus of this chapter. These lyases can be combined with separation methods, such as chromatography and electrophoresis, for the preparation of CS oligosaccharides for biological evaluations as well as for disaccharide analysis, oligosaccharide mapping, and polysaccharide sequencing. These enzymes have also been shown to have direct therapeutic value. This chapter examined the various applications for this important class of enzymes.

References

Ahn, M., Shin, K., Kim, D.-H., Jang, E.-A., Toida, T., Linhardt, R., and Kim, Y. (1998). Characterization of a bacteroides species from human intestine that degrades glycosaminoglycans. *Can. J. Microbiol.* **44**, 423–429.

Al-Hakim, A., and Linhardt, R. J. (1991). Capilary electrophoresis for the analysis of chondroitin sulfate and dermatan sufate derived disaccharides. *Anal. Biochem.* **195**, 68–73.

Avci, F. Y., Toida, T., and Linhardt, R. J. (2003). Chondroitin O-methyl ester: An unusual substrate for chondroitin AC lyase. *Carbohydr. Res.* **338**, 2101–2104.

Avci, F. Y., Karst, N., Islam, T., and Linhardt, R. J. (2004). Trifluoroethylsulfonate protected monosaccharides in glycosylation reactions. 228th ACS National Meeting, Philadelphia.

Blain, F., Tkalec, A. L., Shao, Z., Poulin, C., Pedneault, M., Gu, K., Eggimann, B., Zimmermann, J., and Su, H. (2002). Expression system for high levels of GAG lyase gene expression and study of the hepA upstream region in *Flavobacterium heparinum*. *J. Bacteriol.* **184**, 3242–3252.

Boneu, B. (1996). Glycosaminoglycans: Clinical use. *Sem. Thromb. Hemost.* **22**, 209–212.

Bourne, Y., and Henrissat, B. (2001). Glycoside hydrolases and glycosyltransferases: Families and functional modules. *Curr. Opin. Struct. Biol.* **11**, 593–600.

Bradbury, E. J., Moon, L. D., Popat, R. J., King, V. R., Bennet, G. S., Patel, P. N., Fawcett, J. W., and McMahon, S. B. (2002). Chondroitinase ABC promotes functional recovery after spinal cord injury. *Nature* **416**, 636–640.

Capila, I., and Linhardt, R. J. (2002). Heparin protein interactions. *Angew. Chemie Int. Ed.* **41**, 390–412.

Csóka, A. B., Scherer, S. W., and Stern, R. (1999). Expression analysis of six paralogous human hyaluronidase genes clustered on chromosomes 3p21 and 7q31. *Genomics* **60**, 356–361.

Davies, G. J., Wilson, K. S., and Henrissat, B. (1997). Nomenclature for sugar-binding subsites in glycosyl hydrolases. *Biochem. J.* **321**, 557–559.

Davies, S. J., Gaucher, D. R., Doller, C., and Silver, J. (1999). Robust regeneration of adult sensory axons in degenerating white matter of the adult rat spinal cord. *J. Neurosis.* **19**, 5810–5822.

DeAngelis, P. L. (1999). Hyaluronan synthases: Fascinating glycosyltransferases from vertabrates, bactrerial pathogens and algal viruses. *Cell Mol. Life Sci.* **56**, 670–682.

Denholm, E. M., Lin, Y. Q., and Silver, P. J. (2001). Anti-tumor activities of chondroitinase AC and chondroitinase B: Inhibition of angiogenesis, proliferation and invasion. *Eur. J. Pharmacol.* **416**, 213–221.

Ernst, S., Langer, R., Cooney, C. L., and Sasisekharan, R. (1995). Enzymatic degradation of glycosaminoglycans. *Crit. Rev. Biochem. Mol. Biol.* **30**, 44–45.

Esko, J. D., and Selleck, S. B. (2002). Order out of chaos: Assembly of ligand binding sites in heparan sulfate. *Annu. Rev. Biochem.* **71**, 435–471.

Fawcett, J. W., and Asher, R. A. (1999). The glial scar and central nervous system repair. *Brain Res. Bull.* **49**, 377–391.

Féthière, J., Eggimann, B., and Cygler, M. (1999). Crystal structure of chondroitin AC lyase, a representative of a family of glycosaminoglycan degrading enzymes. *J. Mol. Biol.* **288**, 635–647.

Fidler, P. S., Schuette, K., Asher, R. A., Dobbertin, A., Thornton, S. R., Calle-Patino, Y., Muir, E., Levin, J. M., Geller, H. M., Rogers, J., Faissner, A., and Fawcett, J. W. (1999). Comparing astrocytic cell lines that are inhibitory or permissive for axon growth: The major axon-inhibitory proteoglycans is NG2. *J. Neurosis.* **19**, 8778–8788.

Fitch, M. T., and Silver, J. (1999). CNS regeneration. In "Basic Science and Clinical Advances" (M. H. Tusynski and J. H. Kordower, Eds.), pp. 55–58. Academic Press, San Diego.

Frost, G. I., Csoka, T., and Stern, R. (1996). The hyaluronidases: A chemical, biological and clinical overview. *Trends Glycosci. Glycotechnol.* **44**, 419–434.

Godavarti, R., and Sasisekharan, R. (1998). Heparinase I from *Flavobacterium heparinum*: Role of positive charge in enzymatic activity. *J. Biol. Chem.* **273**, 248–255.

Gu, K., Liu, J., Pervin, A., and Linhardt, R. J. (1993). Comparison of the activity of two chondroitin AC lyases on dermatan sulfate. *Carbohydr. Res.* **244**, 369–377.

Gu, K., Linhardt, R. J., Laliberte, M., Gu, K., and Zimmermann, J. (1995). Purification, characterization and specificity of chondroitin lyases and glycuronidase from *Flavobacterium heparinum*. *Biochem. J.* **312**, 569–577.

Guthrie, J. P., and Kluger, R. (1993). Electrostatic stabilization can explain the unexpected acidity of carbon acids in enzyme-catalyzed reactions. *J. Am. Chem. Soc.* **115**, 11569–11572.

Hamai, A., Hashimoto, N., Mochizuki, H., Kato, F., Makiguchi, Y., Horie, K., and Suzuki, S. (1997). Two distinct chondroitin sulfate ABC lyases: An endoeliminase yielding tetrasaccharides and an exoeliminase preferentially acting on oligosaccharides. *J. Biol. Chem.* **272**, 9123–9130.

Hannesson, H. H., Hagner-McWhirter, A., Tiedemann, K., Lindahl, U., and Malmstrom, A. (1996). Biosynthesis of dermatan sulfate: Defructosylated *Escherichia coli* K4 capsular polysaccharide as a substrate for the D-glucuronyl C-5 epimerase, and an indication of a two-base reaction mechanism. *Biochem. J.* **313**, 589–596.

Hernáiz, M. J., and Linhardt, R. J. (2001). Degradation of chondroitin and dermatan sulfate with chondroitin lyases. In "Methods in Molecular Biology" (R. V. Iozzo, Ed.). Humane Press, New York.

Hirano, K., Sakai, S., Ishikawa, T., Avci, F. Y., Linhardt, R. J., and Toida, T. (2005). Preparation of hyaluronan Omethylester and its enzymatic degradation. *Carbohydr. Res.* **338**, 2101–2104.

Hong, S.-W., Kim, B.-T., Shin, H.-Y., Kim, W.-S., Lee, K.-S., Kim, Y.-S., and Kim, D.-H. (2002). Purification and characterization of novel chondroitin ABC and AC lyases from *Bacteroides stercoris* HJ-15, a human intestinal anaerobic bacterium. *Eur. J. Biochem.* **269**, 2934–2940.

Hoshi, H., Nakagawa, H., Nishiguchi, S., Iwata, K., Niikura, K., Monde, K., and Nishimura, S. (2004). An engineered hyaluronan synthase 2 expressed in *Escherichia coli. J. Biol. Chem.* **279**, 2341–2349.

Huang, W., Matte, A., Li, Y., Kim, Y. S., Linhardt, R. J., Su, H., and Cygler, M. (1999). Crystal structure of chondroitinase B from *Flavobacterium heparinum* and its complex with a disaccharide product at 1.7 Å resolution. *J. Mol. Biol.* **294**, 1257–1269.

Huang, W., Matte, A., Suzuki, S., Sugiura, N., Miyazono, H., and Cygler, M. (2000). Crystallization and preliminary x-ray analysis of chondroitin sulfate ABC lyases I and II from *Proteus vulgaris. Acta Crystallogr.* **D56**, 904–906.

Huang, W., Boju, L., Tkalec, L., Su, H., Yang, H. O., Gunay, N. S., Linhardt, R. J., Kim, Y. S., Matte, A., and Cygler, M. (2001). Active site of chondroitin AC lyase revealed by the structure of enzyme-oligosaccharide complexes and mutagenesis. *Biochemistry* **40**, 2359–2372.

Huang, W., Lunin, V. V., Li, Y., Suzuki, S., Sugiura, N., Miyazono, H., and Cygler, M. (2003). Crystal structure of *Proteus vulgaris* chondroitin sulfate ABC lyase I at 1.9 Å resolution. *J. Mol. Biol.* **328**, 623–634.

Hynes, W. L., and Walton, S. L. (2000). Hyaluronidases of Gram-positive bacteria. *FEMS Microbial. Lett.* **183**, 201–207.

Ingham, E., Holland, K. T., Gowland, G., and Cunliffe, W. J. (1979). Purification and partial characterization of hyaluronate lyase (EC 4.2.2.1) from *Propionibacterium acnes. J. Gen. Microbiol.* **115**, 411–418.

Iozzo, R. V. (1998). Matrix proteoglycans: From molecular design to cellular function. *Annu. Rev. Biochem.* **67**, 609–652.

Islam, T., Avci, F. Y., Karst, N., Zhang, J., and Linhardt, R. J. (2003). Disaccharide approach for the synthesis of glycosaminoglycan oligosaccharides. 226th ACS National Meeting, New York.

Itano, N., and Kimata, K. (2002). Mammalian hyaluronan synthases. *IUMB Life* **54**, 195–199.

Jackson, R. L., Busch, S. J., and Cardin, A. D. (1991). Glycosaminoglycans: Molecular properties, protein interactions, and role in physiological processes. *Physiol. Rev.* **71**, 481–539.

Jandik, K. A., Gu, K., and Linhardt, R. J. (1994). Action pattern of polysaccharide lyases on glycosaminoglycans. *Glycobiology* **4**, 289–296.

Karst, N. A., Islam, T. F., and Linhardt, R. J. (2003). Sulfo-protected hexosamine monosaccharides: Potentially versatile building blocks for glycosaminoglycan synthesis. *Org. Lett.* **5**, 4839–4842.

Karst, N. A., Islam, T. F., Avci, F. Y., and Linhardt, R. J. (2004). Trifluoroethylsulfonate protected monosaccharides in glycosylation reactions. *Tetrahedron Lett.* **45**, 6433–6437.

Kato, F., Iwata, H., Hiatus, K., and Miura, T. (1990). Experimental chemonucleolysis with chondroitinase ABC. *Clin. Ortho.* **253**, 301–308.

Kempson, G. E. (1980). The mechanical properties of articular cartilage. *In* "The Joints and Synovial Fluid" (L. Sokoloff, Ed.), Vol. 2, pp. 177–238. Academic Press, New York.

Kim, B.-T., Kim, W.-S., Kim, Y. S., Linhardt, R. J., and Kim, D.-H. (2000). Purification and characterization of a novel heparinase from *Bacteroides stercoris* HJ-15. *J. Biochem. Tokyo* **128**, 323–328.

Kim, Y. S., Jo, Y. T., Chang, I. M., Toida, T., Park, Y., and Linhardt, R. J. (1996). A new glycosaminoglycan from the giant african snail, *Achatina fulica*. *J. Biol. Chem.* **271**, 11750–11755.

Kim, B.-T., Kim, W.-S., Kim, Y. S., Linhardt, R. J., and Kim, D.-H. (2000). Purification and characterization of a novel heparinase from *Bacteroides stercoris* HJ-15. *J. Biochem. Tokyo* **128**, 323–328.

Kitagawa, H., Tanaka, Y., Yamada, S., Seno, N., Haslam, S. M., Morris, H. R., Dell, A., and Sugahara, K. (1997). A novel pentasaccharide sequence GlcA(3-sulfate)(beta1-3)GalNAc (4-sulfate)(beta1-4)(Fuc alpha1-3)GlcA(beta1-3)GalNAc(4-sulfate) in the oligosaccharides isolated from king crab cartilage chondroitin sulfate K and its differential susceptibility to chondroitinases and hyaluronidase. *Biochemistry* **36**, 3998–4008.

Kitagawa, H., Uyama, T., and Sugahara, K. (2001). Molecular cloning and expression of a human chondroitin synthase. *J. Biol. Chem.* **276**, 38721–38726.

Kitagawa, H., Izumikawa, T., Uyama, T., and Sugahara, K. (2003). Molecular cloning of a chondroitin polymerizing factor that cooperates with chondroitin synthase for chondroitin polymerization. *J. Biol. Chem.* **278**, 23666–23671.

Kreil, G. (1995). Hyaluronidases: A group of neglected enzymes. *Protein Sci.* **4**, 1666–1669.

Kresse, H., and Schonherr, E. (2001). Proteoglycans of the extracellular matrix and growth control. *J. Cell Physiol.* **189**, 266–274.

Lamb, D. J., Wang, H. M., Mallis, L. M., and Linhardt, R. J. (1992). Negative-ion fast atom bombardment tandem mass spectrometry to determine sulfate and linkage position in glycosaminoglycan-derived disaccharides. *J. Am. Soc. Mass Spectrom* **3**, 797–803.

Langer, R., Linhardt, R. J., Hoffberg, S., Larsen, A. K., Cooney, C. L., Topper, D., and Klein, M. (1982). An enzymatic system for removing heparin in extracorporeal therapy. *Science* **217**, 261–263.

Leroy, J. G., and Wiesmann, U. (1993). Disorders of lysosomal enzymes. *In* "Connective Tissue and its Heritable Disorders: Molecular, Genetic, and Medical Aspects" (P. Royce and B. Steinmann, Eds.), pp. 613–639. Wiley, New York.

Li, J. P., Hagner-McWhirter, A., Kjellen, L., Palgi, J., Jalkanen, M., and Lindahl, U. (1997). Biosynthesis of heparin/heparan sulfate: cDNA cloning and expression of D-glucuronyl C5-epimerase from bovine lung. *J. Biol. Chem.* **272**, 28158–28163.

Li, S., Kelly, S. J., Lamani, E., Ferraroni, M., and Jedrzejas, M. J. (2000). Structural basis of hyaluronan degradation by *Streptococcus pneumoniae* hyaluronate lyase. *EMBO J.* **19**, 1228–1240.

Linhardt, R. J., Galliher, P., and Cooney, C. (1986). Plysaccharide lyases. *Appl. Biochem. Biotechnol.* **12**, 135–176.

Linhardt, R. J., Rice, K. G., Kim, Y. S., Lohse, D. L., Wang, H. M., and Loganathan, D. (1988). Mapping and quantification of the major oligosaccharide components of heparin. *Biochem. J.* **254**, 781–787.

Linhardt, R. J., Al-Hakim, A., Liu, J., Hoppensteadt, D., Mascelanni, P., and Fareed, J. (1991). Structural features of dermatan sulfates and their relationship to anticoagulant and antithrombotic activities. *Biochem. Pharm.* **42**, 1609–1619.

Linhardt, R. J., and Al-Hakim, A. (1991). Biocatalysis for the synthesis and modification of biopolymers. *In* "Biocatalysis for Industry: Topics in Applied Chemistry" (J. S. Dordick, Ed.), Vol. 5, pp. 83–112. Plenum Publishing Company, New York.

Linhardt, R. J., Ampofo, S., Fareed, J., Hoppensteadt, D., Mulliken, J., and Folkman, J. (1992). Isolation and characterization of a human heparin. *Biochemistry* **31**, 12441–12445.

Linhardt, R. J. (1994). Analysis of glycosaminoglycans with polysaccharide lyases. *In* "Current Protocols in Molecular Biology, Analysis of Glycoconjugates" (A. Varki, Ed.), Vol. 2, pp. 17.13.17–17.13.32. Wiley Interscience, Boston.

Linhardt, R. J., Desai, U., Liu, J., Pervin, A., Hoppensteadt, D., and Fareed, J. (1994). Low molecular weight dermatan sulfate as an antithrombotic agent. *Biochem. Pharmacol.* **47**, 1241–1252.

Linhardt, R. J., and Toida, T. (2004). Role of glycosaminoglycans in cellular communication. *Acc. Chem. Res.* **37**, 431–438.

Loganathan, D., Wang, H. M., Mallis, L. M., and Linhardt, R. J. (1990). Structural variation of the antithrombin III binding site and its occurrence in heparin from different sources. *Biochemistry* **29**, 4362–4368.

Lunin, V. V., Li, Y., Linhardt, R. J., Miyazano, H., Kyogashima, M., Kaneko, T., Bell, A. W., and Cygler, M. (2004). High-resolution crystal structure of *Arthrobacter aurescens* chondroitin AC lyase: An enzyme-substrate complex defines the catalytic mechanism. *J. Mol. Biol.* **337**, 367–386.

Madan, A. K., Yu, K., Dhurandhar, N., Cullinane, C., Pang, Y., and Beech, D. J. (1999a). Association of hyaluronidase and breast adenocarcinoma invasiveness. *Oncol. Rep.* **6**, 607–609.

Madan, A. K., Pang, Y., Wilkiemeyer, M. B., Yu, D., and Beech, D. J. (1999b). Increased hyaluronidase expression in more aggressive prostate adenocarcinoma. *Oncol. Rep.* **6**, 1431–1433.

McCourt, P. A. G. (1999). How does the hyaluronan scrap-yard operate. *Matrix Biol.* **18**, 427–432.

McKeon, R. J., Schreiber, R. C., Rudge, J. S., and Silver, J. (1991). Reduction of neurite outgrowth in a model of glial scarring following CNS injury is correlated with the expression of inhibitory molecules on reactive astrocytes. *J. Neurosis.* **11**, 3398–3411.

McKeon, R. J., Hoke, A., and Silver, J. (1995). Injury-induced proteoglycans inhibit the potential for laminmediated axon growth on astrocytin scars. *Exp. Neural.* **136**, 32–43.

Michaud, P., Da Costa, A., Courtois, B., and Courtois, J. (2003). Polysaccharide lyases: Recent developments as biotechnological tools. *Crit. Rev. Biotechnol.* **23**, 233–266.

Michel, G., Pojasek, K., Li, Y., Sulfa, T., Linhardt, R. J., Raman, R., Probhakar, V., Sasisekharan, R., and Cygler, M. (2004). The structure of chondroitin B lyase complexed with glycosaminoglycan oligosaccharides unravels a calcium-dependent catalytic machinery. *J. Biol. Chem.* **279**, 32882–32896.

Miller, A. D. (2003). Identification of Hyal2 as the cell-surface receptor for jaagsiekte sheep retrovirus and ovine nasal adenocarcinoma virus. *Curr. Top Microbiol. Immunol.* **275**, 179–199.

Monslow, J., Williams, J. D., Nurton, N., Guy, C. A., Price, I. K., Coleman, S. L., Williams, N. M., Buckland, P. R., Spicer, A. P., and Topley, N. (2003). The human hyaluronan synthase genes: Genomic structures, proximal promoters and polymorphic microsatellite markers. *Int. J. Biochem. Cell Biol.* **35**, 1272–1283.

Moon, A. F., Edavettal, S. C., Krahn, J. M., Munoz, E. M., Negishi, M., Linhardt, R. J., Liu, J., and Pedersen, L. C. (2004). Structural analysis of the sulfotransferase (3-OST-3) involved in the biosynthesis of an entry receptor for herpes simplex virus 1. *J. Biol. Chem.* **279**, 45185–45193.

Moon, L. D., Asher, R. A., Rhodes, K. E., and Fawcett, J. W. (2001). Regeneration of CNS axons back to their target following treatment of adult rat brain with chondroitinases ABC. *Nat. Neurosci.* **4**, 465–466.

Negishi, M., Dong, J., Darden, T. A., Pedersen, L. G., and Pedersen, L. C. (2003). Glycosaminoglycan biosynthesis: What we can learn from the X-ray crystal structures of glycosyl transferases GlcAT1 and EXTL2. *Biochem. Biohys. Res. Commun.* **303**, 393–398.

Niederost, B. P., Zimmermann, D. R., Schwab, M. E., and Bandtlow, C. E. (1999). Bovine CNS myelin contains neurite growth-inhibitory activity associated with chondroitin sulfate proteoglycans. *J. Neurosis.* **19**, 8979–8989.

Ninomiya, T., Sugiura, N., Tawada, A., Sugimoto, K., Watanabe, H., and Kimata, K. (2002). Molecular cloning and characterization of chondroitin polymerase from *Escherichia coli* strain K4. *J. Biol. Chem.* **277**, 21567–21575.

Novak, U., Stylli, S. S., Kaye, A. H., and Lepperdinger, G. (1999). Hyaluronidase-2 overexpression accelerates intracerebral but not subcutaneous tumor formation of murine astrocytoma cells. *Cancer Res.* **59**, 6246–6250.

Pervin, A., Gu, K., and Linhardt, R. J. (1993). Capilary electrophoresis to measure sulfoesterase activity on chondroitin sulfate and heparin derived disaccharides. *Appl. Theor. Electroph.* **3**, 297–303.

Pervin, A., Al-Hakim, A., and Linhardt, R. J. (1994). Separation of glycosamionoglycan derived oligosaccharides by capilary electrophoresis using reverse polarity. *Anal. Biochem.* **221**, 182–188.

Pervin, A., Gallo, C., Jandik, K. A., Han, X. J., and Linhardt, R. J. (1995). Preparation and structural characterization of large heparin-derived oligosaccharides. *Glycobiology* **5**, 83–95.

Pizzorusso, T., Medini, P., Berardi, N., Chierzi, S., Fawcett, J. W., and Maffei, L. (2002). Reactivation of ocular dominance plasticity in the adult visual cortex. *Science* **298**, 1248–1251.

Pojasek, K., Shriver, Z., Kiley, P., Venkataraman, G., and Sasisekharan, R. (2001). Recombinant expression, purification, and kinetic characterization of chondroitinase AC and chondroitinase B from *Flavobacterium heparinum*. *Biochem. Biophys. Res. Commun.* **286**, 343–351.

Prabhakar, V., Capila, I., Bosques, C. J., Pojasek, K., and Sasisekharan, R. (2005). Chondroitinase ABC I from *Proteus vulgaris*: Cloning, recombinant expression and active site identification. *Biochem. J.* **386**, 103–112.

Proud, A. D., Prodger, J. C., and Flitsch, S. L. (1997). Development of a protecting group for sulfate esters. *Tetrahedron Lett.* **38**, 7243–7246.

Razi, N., Feyzi, E., Bjork, I., Naggi, A., Casu, B., and Lindahl, U. (1995). Structural and functional properties of heparin analogs obtained by chemical sulphation of *Escherichia coli* K5 capsular polysaccharide. *Biochem. J.* **309**, 465–472.

Rigden, D. J., and Jedrzejas, M. J. (2003). Structures of *Streptococcus pnemoniae* hyaluronate lyase in complex with chondroitin and chondroitin sulfate disaccharides. *J. Biol. Chem.* **278**, 50596–50606.

Rosenberg, R. D., Shworak, N. W., Liu, J., Schwartz, J. J., and Zhang, L. (1997). Heparan sulfate proteoglycans of the cardiovascular system. Specific structures emerge but how is synthesis regulated? *J. Clin. Invest.* **99**, 2062–2070.

Seidler, D. G., Breuer, E., Grande-Allen, K. J., Hascall, V. C., and Kresse, H. (2002). Core protein dependence of epimerization of glucuronosyl residues in galactosaminoglycans. *J. Biol. Chem.* **279**, 25789–25797.

Silbert, J. E., and Sugumaran, G. (2002). Biosynthesis of chondroitin/dermatan sulfate. *IUMB Life* **54**, 177–186.

Sim, J. S., Jun, G., Toida, T., Cho, S. Y., Choi, D. W., Chang, S. Y., Linhardt, R. J., and Kim, Y. S. (2005). Quantitative analysis of chondroitin sulfate in raw materials, ophthalmic solutions, soft capsules and liquid preparations. *J. Chromatogr. B* **818**, 133–139.

Smith-Thomas, L. C., Fok-seang, J., Stevene, J., Du, J., Muir, E., Faissner, A., Geller, H. M., Rogers, J. H., and Fawcett, J. W. (1994). An inhibitor of neurite outgrowth produced by astrocytes. *J. Cell Sci.* **107**, 1687–1695.

Spicer, A. P., and McDonald, J. A. (1998). Characterization and molecular evolution of a vertabrate hyaluronan synthase gene family. *J. Biol. Chem.* **273**, 1923–1932.

Stringer, S. E., and Callagher, J. T. (1997). Heparan sulphate. *Int. J. Biochem. Cell Biol.* **29**, 709–714.

Sugahara, K., and Kitagawa, H. (2002). Heparin and heparan sulfate biosynthesis. *IUMB Life* **54**, 163–175.

Sztrolovics, R., Recklies, A. D., Roughley, P. J., and Mort, J. (2002). Hyaluronate degradation as an alternate mechanism for proteoglycan release from cartilage during interleukin-1ß-stimulated catabolism. *Biochem. J.* **362**, 473–479.

Thorp, S., Lee, K. A., Negishi, M., Linhardt, R. J., Liu, J., and Pedersen, L. C. (2004). Crystal structure and mutational analysis of heparan sulfate 3-O-sulfotransferase isoform 1. *J. Biol. Chem.* **279**, 25789–25797.

Uyama, T., Kitagawa, H., Tanaka, J., Tamura, J., Ogawa, T., and Sugahara, K. (2003). Molecular cloning and expression of a second chondroitin N-acetylgalactosaminyltrans-ferase involved in the initiation and elongation of chondroitin/dermatan sulfate. *J. Biol. Chem.* **278**, 3072–3078.

Vlodavsky, I., Friedmann, Y., Elkin, M., Aingorn, H., Atzmon, R., Ishai-Michaeli, R., Bitan, M., Pappo, O., Peretz, T., Michal, I., Spector, L., and Pecker, I. (1999). Mammalian heparanse: Gene cloning, expression and function in tumor progression and metastasis. *Nat. Med.* **5**, 793–802.

Weiler, J. M., Edens, R. E., Linhardt, R. J., and Kapelanski, D. P. (1992). Heparin and modified heparin inhibit complement activation *in vivo. J. Immunol.* **148**, 3210–3215.

Xu, J., Bjursell, M. K., Himrod, J., Deng, S., Carmichael, L. K., Chiang, H. C., Hooper, L. V., and Gordon, J. I. (2003). A genomic view of the human-*Bacteroides thetaiotaomicron* symbiosis. *Science* **299**, 2074–2076.

Yada, T., Sato, T., Kaseyama, H., Gotoh, M., Iwasaki, H., Kikuchi, N., Kwon, Y. D., Togayachi, A., Kudo, T., Watanabe, H., Narimatsu, H., and Kimata, K. (2003). Chondroitin sulfate synthase-3: Molecular cloning and characterization. *J. Biol. Chem.* **278**, 39711–39725.

Yang, H. O., Gunay, N. S., Toida, T., Kuberan, B., Yu, G., Kim, Y. S., and Linhardt, R. J. (2000). Preparation and structural determination of dermatan sulfate-derived oligosac-charides. *Glycobiology* **10**, 1033–1040.

Yao, X. Y., Hageman, G. S., and Marmor, M. F. (1992). Recovery of retinal adhesion after enzymatic perturbation of the interphotoreceptor matrix. *Invest. Ophthalmol. Vis. Sci.* **33**, 498–503.

Zechel, D. L., and Withers, S. G. (2000). Glycosidase mechanism: Anatomy of a finely tuned catalyst. *Acc. Chem. Res.* **33**, 11–18.

Zuo, J., Neubauer, D., Dyes, K., Ferguson, T. A., and Muir, D. (1998). Degradation of chondroitin sulfate proteoglycans enhances the neurite-promoting potential of spinal cord tissue. *Exp. Neurol.* **154**, 654–662.

PART II

Biological Role of Chondroitin Sulfate

Christopher J. Handley, Tom Samiric, and Mirna Z. Ilic

School of Human Biosciences
La Trobe University, Melbourne
Victoria 3086, Australia

Structure, Metabolism, and Tissue Roles of Chondroitin Sulfate Proteoglycans

I. Chapter Overview

Proteoglycans (PGs) are a complex group of glycoproteins that are characterized by the presence of one or more sulfated glycosaminoglycan (GAG) chains and various oligosaccharides that are covalently attached to a core protein. The majority of chondroitin sulfate proteoglycans (CSPGs) belongs to the group of large aggregating PGs (hyalectins) and small leucine-rich PGs. The sulfated GAG chains, oligosaccharides, and domains within the core proteins of these macromolecules allow PGs to interact with a large number of macromolecules. As a result PGs have wide-ranging roles in tissues where they are involved in the organization and function of extracellular matrices, matrix cell interactions, and the regulation of cellular processes. The cellular and tissue location of PGs is largely dependent on the interactions of specific domains in the core proteins and the GAG chains with other molecules present in the cell membrane or extracellular structures.

Advances in Pharmacology, Volume 53
Copyright 2006, Elsevier Inc. All rights reserved.

1054-3589/06 $35.00
DOI: 10.1016/S1054-3589(05)53010-2

II. Introduction

Proteoglycans are ubiquitous macromolecules that are expressed to a varying degree by most mammalian cells and are characterized by the presence of sulfated GAG chains that are covalently attached to a core protein (Hascall and Hascall, 1981). Proteoglycans were initially defined as proteins that contain one or more sulfated GAG chains, but it is now clear that different species of PGs have genetically distinct core proteins and can be classified into families on the basis of common structural features of their core proteins (Iozzo, 1998). The core proteins of PGs are also substituted with oligosaccharide groups. This gives rise to a group of macromolecules that have a high degree of complexity and heterogeneity. The GAGs as well as domains present within the core proteins allow PGs to specifically interact with a wide range of molecules (Iozzo, 1998). It was initially thought that the principal role of PGs was in the formation and organization of the extracellular matrix (ECM) of tissues or basement membranes where they contribute directly to the mechanical properties of tissues. However, it is now clear that PGs have far more diverse roles since they are present on or interact with the plasma membranes of cells, where they are involved in cell-matrix interactions and regulation of cellular processes that include differentiation, cell division, and migration (Iozzo, 1998).

III. Major Structural Features of Proteoglycans

The core proteins of all PGs are coded for by the genome of the cell, and the expression of a particular core protein gene will determine the specific type of PG synthesized by a cell. The core proteins contain a number of distinct domains that are made up of protein motifs that are involved in specific interactions with other molecules and therefore contribute to the function of a PG. In addition, the messenger RNA can undergo alternate splicing that is likely to modify the function and distribution of the PGs. Also present in the core proteins of PGs are attachment sites for GAG and oligosaccharide chains, both of which have the potential to interact with a range of molecules. The degradation of PGs in the ECM involves proteolytic processing of the core protein (Campbell *et al.*, 1989; Ilic *et al.*, 1992). There is growing evidence that proteolytic processing of PGs depends on the action of specific proteinases at specific sites within the core proteins (Ilic *et al.*, 1998). Such proteolytic processing of PGs is not only critical for the catabolism of these macromolecules but may also play a role in the functional properties of PGs.

Glycosaminoglycan chains are made up of repeating disaccharides usually composed of hexuronic acid and N-acetylhexosamine sugars that can be sulfated on either monosaccharide unit. In the case of chondroitin sulfate

Glycosaminoglycan	Repeating disaccharide unit	Sulfation
Chondroitin sulfate	[β1–4]-D-Glucuronic acid [β1–3]N-acetyl-D-galactosamine	Carbon 4 or 6 of the hexosamine and occasionally carbon 2 of the hexuronic acid
Dermatan sulfate	[β1–4]-L-Iduronic acid [α1–3]N-acetyl-D-galactosamine	Carbon 4 or 6 of the hexosamine and occasionally carbon 2 of the hexuronic acid
Keratan sulfate	[β1–3]-D-Galactose [β1–4]N-acetyl-D-galactosamine	Carbon 6 of the hexosamine and occasionally carbon 6 of the galactose
Heparan sulfate and heparin	[α1–4]-D-Glucuronic acid [β1–4]N-acetyl-D-glucosamine or [α1–4]-L-Iduronic acid [α1–4]N-acetyl-D-glucosamine	Carbon 2, 3, or 6 of the hexosamine and carbon 2 of the hexuronic acid
Hyaluronan	[β1–4]-D-Glucuronic acid [β1–3]N-acetyl-D-glucosamine	None

FIGURE I   The structure of GAGs.

(CS), the repeating disaccharide unit is made up of glucuronic acid and N-acetylgalactosamine sugars that contain sulfate groups attached to either carbon 4 or 6 of the hexosamine residues or occasionally carbon 2 of the hexuronic acid residue (Fig. 1). In some PGs the hexuronic acid in the disaccharide unit is epimerized to iduronic acid that gives rise to dermatan sulfate (DS). Dermatan sulfate GAGs can contain CS disaccharides. Chondroitin sulfate chains are attached to the core protein through a linkage region made up of glucuronic acid-galactose-galactose-xylose monosaccharides, and the xylose is attached to a serine residue by an O-glycosyl bond (Muir, 1958). Keratan sulfate (KS) is another GAG that is found in some CS-containing PGs, and this GAG is made up of disaccharides consisting of galactose and N-acetylglucosamine sugars.

The synthesis of GAG chains is a complex process and unlike protein synthesis is not based on a template directed by the genetic code but instead relies on the activity of a group of specific glycosyltransferase and sulfotransferase enzymes that are present in the Golgi apparatus of cells (Prydz and Dalen, 2000). The synthesis of PGs containing CSGAGs involves the addition of xylose to selective serine residues in the core protein followed by the addition of two galactose and a glucuronic acid monosaccharides; each step is catalyzed by a specific glycosyltranserase from nucleotide precursors (Robinson *et al.*, 1966). After synthesis of the linkage region, the GAG chains are elongated by the sequential addition of N-acetylgalactosamine and glucuronic acid monosaccharides from nucleotide precursors. The N-acetylgalactosamine residues can be substituted by 4- and/or 6-sulfate groups or the hexuronic acid groups on carbon 2 by the action of specific sulfotransferases. Some or all of the glucuronic acid residues present in the nascent chondroitin chain can undergo isomerization to iduronic acid by the action of an epimerase followed by the addition of sulfate groups to give DS. This synthetic pathway gives rise to GAGs that have complex and variable structures that can also vary in response to changes in physiological conditions including disease. The biological significance of these structures is becoming evident. Good examples of the relationship between the fine structure of the GAGs and their function can be seen from the pioneering work investigating the relationship between the structure of heparin and heparan GAGs and their growth factor binding properties and anticoagulant activity (Gallagher and Lyon, 2000).

Little is known about the regulation of enzymes involved in GAG synthesis. The amino acid sequence around a GAG attachment site in the core protein of a PG determines whether a particular serine residue will be substituted with a GAG chain (Zhang *et al.*, 1995). The availability of nucleotide sugars and precursors of sulfation have been implicated in the regulation of the nature, size, and sulfation patterns of GAG chains (Toma *et al.*, 1996). It has also been suggested that the enzymes involved in GAG chain synthesis are organized into complexes that will synthesize specific GAGs and may be separated from each other within the Golgi apparatus and require the core proteins to be targeted to the respective enzyme complex (Sugumaran *et al.*, 1998). Although a number of potential regulatory mechanisms in GAG synthesis have been identified, it still remains to be established how these are modulated to generate both gross and subtle changes in the structure of GAGs.

IV. Major Species of Chondroitin Sulfate Proteoglycans _____

A. Hyalectins

Hyalectins are a group of large PGs that can form aggregates with hyaluronan (hyaluronic acid), a large nonsulfated linear GAG made up of repeating glucuronic acid and N-acetylglucosamine disaccharide units.

These PGs have a large core protein made up of a number of distinctive domains that are substituted with many CS and KSGAG chains (Fig. 2). Examples of these PGs are aggrecan, versican, neurocan, and brevican.

1. Aggrecan

Aggrecan is the major PG of cartilage but is also present in a number of other connective tissues that include tendon, ligament, joint capsule, and neural tissue. Aggrecan specifically interacts with hyaluronan and link protein to form large complexes comprising of up to 100 aggrecan PGs associated with one molecule of hyaluronan (Buckwalter and Rosenberg, 1982).

The aggrecan core protein is approximately 220 kDa in size and has a number of distinctive globular domains termed the G1, G2, and G3 (Fig. 2). The G1 domain is at the amino-terminal end of the core protein and is involved in the interaction of aggrecan with hyaluronan and link protein to form aggregates. Between the G1 and G2 domains is the interglobular domain that is important in the catabolism of aggrecan since it contains an amino acid sequence that is specifically cleaved by aggrecanase proteinases (Ilic et al., 1992). The G2 domain is unique to aggrecan, but its role is obscure. The G3 domain is at the carboxyl-terminal end of the core protein and has the potential to interact with other matrix components. Between the G2 and G3 domains of aggrecan there are three regions that are substituted with GAG chains. The KS attachment region is directly next to the G2 domain to which are attached KS chains and oligosaccharide chains (Antonsson et al., 1989). Adjacent to the KS attachment region and extending to the G3 domain are the CS attachment regions 1 and 2 that are substituted with approximately 150 CS chains (Doege et al., 1991).

The number, size, and composition of the KS and CS chains associated with aggrecan show variation. In aggrecan from newborn human articular cartilage, CS makes up about 90% of the total GAG content of the PG. The amount of KS increases to about 30% of the total GAGs in aggrecan from mature human cartilage, and this can be explained in part by an increase in the size of the KS chains (Brown et al., 1991). There are age-related changes in the size and fine structure of CS chains associated with aggrecan. Chondroitin sulfate chains present in aggrecan from mature cartilage are approximately 18 kDa in size, which is half the size as that observed for GAGs from newborn individuals. In tissue from young individuals, there are equal levels of both chondroitin 6- and 4-sulfate GAGs present in aggrecan, but in the adult more than 90% of CS chains present are in the form of chondroitin 6-sulfate (Calabro et al., 2000). These age-related changes in the structure of both GAGs associated with aggrecan occur around adolescence and reflect changes in the regulation of the synthesis of these GAG chains.

The role of aggrecan in cartilage is to maintain the hydration of the tissue by attracting and binding water and in doing so gives cartilage its

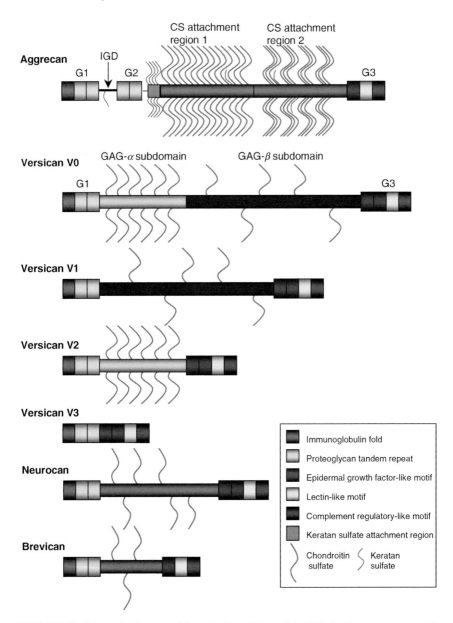

FIGURE 2   Schematic diagrams of the major large CS containing PGs that form aggregates with hyaluronan (hyalectins). CS, chondroitin sulfate; IGD, interglobular domain. (See Color Insert.)

ability to resist compression. This property of attracting water comes from the high density of negative charges that are associated with the GAG chains (Maroudas *et al.*, 1969). Aggrecan appears to be trapped within the collagen network of cartilage as the result of the formation of aggrecan complexes with hyaluronan and link protein (Bolis *et al.*, 1989). There is little evidence of interactions of aggrecan with other molecules in the ECM of cartilage that result in the retention of this PG in the tissue, since after the cleavage of the core protein the carboxyl-terminal fragments rapidly exit the tissue (Campbell *et al.*, 1984). This work also suggests that aggrecan monomers within cartilage may be in a compressed state, thus occupying their own molecular domain that precludes interactions between adjacent aggrecan PGs. In other tissues, such as tendon, aggrecan most likely has a similar role of maintaining tissue hydration and contributing to the mechanical properties of the tissue. However, the G3 domain of aggrecan may be involved in the retention of this PG within tendon (Samiric *et al.*, 2004). The CS chains may also be involved in interactions with other components of the matrix.

2. Versican

Versican is the most common PG in the hyalectin family of PGs and is present in the ECM of most connective tissues as well as smooth muscle, the nervous system and the kidney. This PG can have the largest core protein in this family of PGs (M_r ∼400 kDa), and in mammalian tissues four splice variants of versican have been identified and are termed V0, V1, V2, and V3 (Fig. 2) (Dours-Zimmermann and Zimmermann, 1994). The domain structure of the core proteins of versican shows some similarity to that of aggrecan in that they contain G1 and G3 domains but no G2 domain. A striking feature of versican is that it is less substituted with CS chains than aggrecan and contains no KS chains. The splice variants contain different numbers of CS chains. The size of the CSGAGs of versican varies between 25 and 80 kDa in different tissues. The GAG chains are substituted with both chondroitin 4- and 6-sulfate GAGs, and it appears that chondroitin 6-sulfate is the predominant GAG (Schonherr *et al.*, 1991). However, the ratio of the two isomers of CS can differ between tissues. Versican can also contain DS chains. There is little information about age-related changes in the structure of GAG chains associated with versican.

Versican is likely to have a similar role to that of aggrecan and is important for the maintenance of the hydration of ECM of tissues due to the formation of large complexes with hyaluronan and the water binding properties of CS chains (LeBaron *et al.*, 1992). Versican interacts with a number of extracellular macromolecules and cell surface receptors and therefore is likely to be involved in the organization of the ECM (Aspberg *et al.*, 1999). The V0 and V1 splice variants of versican inhibit the attachment of cells to extracellular proteins such as Type I collagen, fibronectin, and laminin, and this property appears to be due to the CS chains associated with these PGs (Yamagata *et al.*, 1993). Versican can also be involved in the regulation of cell proliferation and migration since there is an increase in the expression of versican by rapidly growing cells (Zimmermann *et al.*,

1994). Versican also appears to be essential in development since versican-knockout mice do not survive *in utero* (Mjaatvedt *et al.*, 1998).

3. Other Hyalectins

Neurocan and brevican are two CSPGs of the hyalectin family of PGs that are expressed specifically by the nervous system (Fig. 2). Their expression by neural tissue is dependent on the developmental stage of the tissue as well as its anatomical location (Bandtlow and Zimmermann, 2000). Neurocan is synthesized by neural cells and has a core protein that contains G1 and G3 domains similar in structure to those found in other hyalectins (Margolis and Margolis, 1994). This PG is involved with neural cell adhesion and outgrowth since it specifically interacts with a number of neural adhesion cell molecules (Ng-CAM and N-CAM) as well as tenascin-C, and there is evidence to suggest that the presence of CS chains is critical for these interactions (Margolis and Margolis, 1997). Neurocan-deficient mice do not appear to have changes in brain structure, development, or physiology compared with wild type animals. This suggests that neurocan may have a limited role or is replaced by other extracellular macromolecules in neurocan-knockout mice (Zhou *et al.*, 2001).

Brevican is expressed by astrocytes of the central nervous system and is the smallest PG in the hyalectin family of PGs. The core protein of this PG has both G1 and G3 domains and a very short CS attachment region that has three CS attachment sites (Yamada *et al.*, 1994). Brevican can be found in tissue either with or without GAG chains. The secreted form of brevican has an intact G3 domain and can undergo proteolytic processing between the G1 and G3 domains (Yamada *et al.*, 1995). Another form of brevican exists and is a product of alternate splicing, where the G3 domain is replaced by a glycosylphosphotidyl-inositol (GPI) anchor and is incorporated into plasma membranes (Seidenbecher *et al.*, 1995). Brevican-deficient mice show some changes in the development of the brain and a decrease in memory, but otherwise the animals have a normal physiology. In brevican-knockout mice, there are changes in the expression of neurocan that may reflect a compensatory process (Brakebusch *et al.*, 2002).

B. Small Leucine-Rich Proteoglycans

A prominent family of CSPGs present in the ECM is small leucine-rich PGs characterized by a core protein that contains repeating leucine-rich motifs (Hocking *et al.*, 1998), and compared with the hyalectin family of PGs the core proteins of these PGs are smaller of approximately 40 kDa in size (Fig. 3). Decorin and biglycan are members of the small leucine-rich family of PGs that are substituted with one or two CS/DSGAG chains, respectively (Fisher *et al.*, 1989).

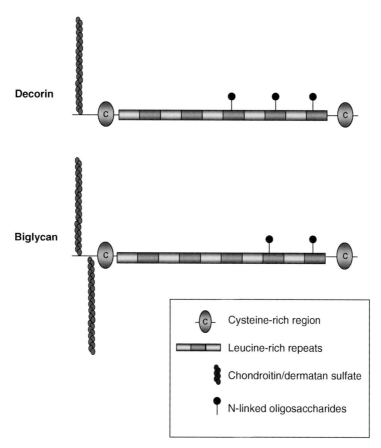

FIGURE 3 Schematic diagrams of decorin and biglycan, two DS/CS containing small leucine-rich PGs.

I. Decorin

Decorin is present in the ECM of most connective tissues and is the predominant PG in dense connective tissues such as tendon and ligament (Vogel and Heinegard, 1985). The central part of the core protein of human decorin is made up of 10 leucine-rich repeat motifs. Between the amino- and carboxyl-terminal ends of the core protein, there are clusters of cysteine residues that are organized into loops stabilized by disulfide bonds (Fig. 3). Decorin contains one GAG chain attached to a serine that is the fourth amino acid residue from the amino-terminus of the core protein (Chopra *et al.*, 1985).

Decorin interacts with Type I and II collagens to inhibit collagen fiber formation that results in thinner collagen fibrils (Vogel *et al.*, 1984). The leucine-rich repeat sequences give decorin a horseshoe shape that allows it to bind to a single molecule of collagen (Weber *et al.*, 1996). The fourth and fifth leucine-rich repeat sequences appear to be important for the binding of decorin to collagen (Kresse *et al.*, 1997). Removal of the GAG chain or the amino-terminal sequence does not alter the ability of decorin to influence collagen fibrillogenesis suggesting that the interaction with collagen depends on the protein core (Vogel *et al.*, 1987). However, the size and the ratio of CS to DS of the glycosaminoglycan chain associated with decorin appear to influence collagen fiber diameter (Kuc and Scott, 1997). Decorin has been reported to interact with other collagens that include Type VI collagen that is associated with Type I collagen, and this interaction may indirectly influence the organization of Type I collagen (Bidanset *et al.*, 1992). Decorin also binds to the nonfibrillar collagens Type XII and XIV collagen, and this interaction appears to require the presence of the GAG chain (Font *et al.*, 1996). The importance of decorin in the organization of the ECM has been demonstrated in work using decorin-knockout mice. In the skin of these animals, the diameter of the collagen fibers shows a greater variation compared with controls, and their arrangement is also different. These changes are also reflected in reduced tensile strength of the skin of these animals (Danielson *et al.*, 1997).

As well as being a component of the ECM, decorin plays a role in the regulation of cell proliferation by interacting directly with cells or with growth factors. The core protein of decorin depresses the rate of cell division, and this occurs as the result of decorin binding to specific cell membrane receptors. The core protein of decorin also binds to transforming growth factor-β and controls the levels of this growth factor that are available to cell signaling. This can influence a number of cellular functions that include cell division, differentiation, adhesion, and synthesis of components of the ECM (Yamaguchi *et al.*, 1990). Decorin also binds to epidermal growth factor receptors and modulates cellular functions associated with this growth factor (Moscatello *et al.*, 1998). These observations are supported by work using decorin-knockout mice where it has been observed that the periodontal ligaments of these animals are more cellular than those observed in wild type animals (Hakkinen *et al.*, 2000).

2. Biglycan

Biglycan is another member of the small leucine-rich family of PGs and is found in a number of tissues that include capillary endothelium, skeletal muscle, cartilage, bone, and tendon (Fisher *et al.*, 1989). In contrast to decorin, biglycan is substituted by two CS/DSGAG chains on serine residues at positions 5 and 10 of the core protein (Fig. 3) (Kresse *et al.*, 2001).

Unlike decorin, biglycan does not inhibit cell division, but there are reports that this PG may activate cell division of bone marrow stromal cells. In biglycan-knockout mice, there is a slower rate of bone growth and the animals show signs of early osteoporosis, which supports the observations that biglycan is involved in bone development and regeneration. Furthermore, in these animals there were changes in the organization of the collagen network of a number of connective tissues, which support the suggestion that biglycan is involved in the organization of collagen fibers (Xu *et al.*, 1998).

V. Concluding Remarks

Proteoglycans are multifunctional macromolecules that have wide ranging functions within the body. Not only are they involved in the organization of extracellular functions, they also have cell regulatory functions. These attributes of PGs arise from structural domains that are present on both the core proteins and the GAG chains of this group of macromolecules. The use of knockout mouse models to understand the tissue and cellular roles of PGs has revealed information that has supported the previous work, which has utilized physical methods to study the interactions of PGs and associated GAG chains with matrix and cell components. Knockout technology has also raised a number of questions especially the ability of animals to develop normally in the absence of a particular PG. Furthermore, protein modeling has given an insight into the potential of the core protein domains and subdomains to interact with other extracellular proteins. It is also evident that the fine structure of GAGs is important for the interactions with other molecules and therefore has an impact on the overall functional properties of a PG. However, the details of such structures within GAG chains have yet to be discovered. The understanding of such structures will give insights into the significance of the changes in CSPGs that occur in ageing and disease. All these changes must involve the modulation of the synthesis of GAG chains, and although the enzymes involved in the synthesis of GAGs have been well described, little is known about their regulation. Gene expression can be routinely measured in the laboratory, but elucidating the mechanisms of regulation of posttranslational modifications of PGs that have been described in this chapter pose an exciting challenge.

References

Antonsson, P., Heinegard, D., and Oldberg, A. (1989). The keratan sulfate-enriched region of bovine cartilage proteoglycan consists of a consecutively repeated hexapeptide motif. *J. Biol. Chem.* **264**, 16170–16173.

Aspberg, A., Adam, S., Kostka, G., Timpl, R., and Heinegard, D. (1999). Fibulin-1 is a ligand for the C-type lectin domains of aggrecan and versican. *J. Biol. Chem.* **274**, 20444–20449.

Bandtlow, C. E., and Zimmermann, D. R. (2000). Proteoglycans in the developing brain: New conceptual insights for old proteins. *Physiol. Rev.* **80**, 1267–1290.

Bidanset, D. J., Guidry, C., Rosenberg, L. C., Choi, H. U., Timpl, R., and Hook, M. (1992). Binding of the proteoglycan decorin to collagen type VI. *J. Biol. Chem.* **267**, 5250–5256.

Bolis, S., Handley, C. J., and Comper, W. D. (1989). Passive loss of proteoglycan from articular cartilage explants. *Biochim. Biophys. Acta* **993**, 157–167.

Brakebusch, C., Seidenbecher, C. I., Asztely, F., Rauch, U., Matties, H., Meyer, H., Krug, M., Bockers, T. M., Zhou, X., Kreutz, M. R., Montag, D., Gundelfinger, E. D., *et al.* (2002). Brevican-deficient mice display impaired hippocampal CA1 long-term potentiation but show no obvious deficits in learning and memory. *Mol. Cell. Biol.* **21**, 7417–7427.

Brown, T. A., Bouchard, T., St John, T., Wayner, E., and Carter, W. G. (1991). Human keratinocytes express a new CD44 core protein (CD44E) as a heparan-sulfate intrinsic membrane proteoglycan with additional exons. *J. Cell Biol.* **113**, 207–221.

Buckwalter, J. A., and Rosenberg, L. C. (1982). Electron microscopic studies of cartilage proteoglycans: Direct evidence for the variable length of the chondroitin sulfate-rich region of proteoglycan subunit core protein. *J. Biol. Chem.* **257**, 9830–9839.

Calabro, A., Midura, R. J., Hascall, V. C., Plaas, A. H., Goodstone, N. J., and Roden, R. (2000). Structure and biosynthesis of chondroitin sulfate and hyaluronan. *In* "Proteoglycans Structure, Biology and Molecular Interactions" (R. V. Iozzo, Ed.), pp. 5–26. Marcel Dekker, New York.

Campbell, M. A., Handley, C. J., Hascall, V. C., Campbell, R. A., and Lowther, D. A. (1984). Turnover of proteoglycans in cultures of bovine articular cartilage. *Arch. Biochem. Biophys.* **234**, 275–289.

Campbell, M. A., Handley, C. J., and D'Souza, S. E. (1989). Turnover of proteoglycans in articular cartilage cultures: Characterisation of proteoglycans released into the medium. *Biochem. J.* **259**, 21–25.

Chopra, R. K., Pearson, C. H., Pringle, G. A., Fackre, D. S., and Scott, P. G. (1985). Dermatan sulphate is located on serine-4 of bovine skin proteodermatan sulphate. *Biochem. J.* **232**, 277–279.

Danielson, K. G., Baribault, H., Holmes, D. F., Graham, H., Kadler, K. E., and Iozzo, R. V. (1997). Targeted disruption of decorin leads to abnormal collagen fibril morphology and skin fragility. *J. Cell Biol.* **136**, 729–743.

Doege, K., Sasaki, M., Kimura, T., and Yamada, Y. (1991). Complete coding sequence and deduced primary structure of the human cartilage large aggregating proteoglycan, aggrecan. *J. Biol. Chem.* **266**, 894–902.

Dours-Zimmermann, M. T., and Zimmermann, D. R. (1994). A novel glycosaminoglycan attachment domain identified in two alternative splice variants of human versican. *J. Biol. Chem.* **269**, 32992–32998.

Fisher, L. W., Termine, J. D., and Young, M. F. (1989). Deduced protein sequence of bone small proteoglycan I (biglycan) shows homology with proteoglycan II (decorin) and several non-connective tissue proteins in a variety of species. *J. Biol. Chem.* **264**, 4571–4576.

Font, B., Eichenberger, D., Rosenberg, L. M., and van der Rest, M. (1996). Characterization of the interactions of type XII collagen with two small proteoglycans from fetal bovine tendon, decorin and fibromodulin. *Matrix Biol.* **15**, 341–348.

Gallagher, J. T., and Lyon, M. (2000). Heparan sulfate: Molecular structure and interactions with growth factors and morphogens. *In* "Proteoglycans Structure, Biology and Molecular Interactions" (R. V. Iozzo, Ed.), pp. 27–60. Marcel Dekker, New York.

Hakkinen, L., Strassburger, S., Kahari, V. M., Scott, P. G., Eichstetter, I., Iozzo, R. V., and Larjava, H. (2000). A role for decorin in the structural organization of periodontal ligament. *Lab. Invest.* **80**, 1869–1880.

Hascall, V. C., and Hascall, G. K. (1981). Proteoglycans. *In* "Cell Biology of Extracellular Matrix" (E. D. Hay, Ed.), pp. 39–63. Plenum Press, New York.

Hocking, A. M., Shinomura, T., and McQuillan, D. J. (1998). Leucine-rich repeat glycoproteins of the extracellular matrix. *Matrix Biology* **17**, 1–19.

Ilic, M. Z., Handley, C. J., Robinson, H. C., and Mok, M. T. (1992). Mechanism of catabolism of aggrecan by articular cartilage. *Arch. Biochem. Biophys.* **294**, 115–122.

Ilic, M. Z., Robinson, H. C., and Handley, C. J. (1998). Characterisation of aggrecan retained and lost from the extracellular matrix of articular cartilage: Involvement of carboxyl-terminal processing in the catabolism of aggrecan. *J. Biol. Chem.* **273**, 17451–17458.

Iozzo, R. V. (1998). Matrix proteoglycans: From molecular design to cellular function. *Annu. Rev. Biochem.* **67**, 609–652.

Kresse, H., Liszio, C., Schonherr, E., and Fisher, L. W. (1997). Critical role of glutamate in a central leucine-rich repeat of decorin for interaction with type I collagen. *J. Biol. Chem.* **272**, 18404–18410.

Kresse, H., Seidler, D. G., Muller, M., Breuer, E., Hausser, H., Roughley, P. J., and Schonherr, E. (2001). Different usage of the glycosaminoglycan-attachment sites of biglycan. *J. Biol. Chem.* **276**, 13411–13416.

Kuc, I. M., and Scott, P. G. (1997). Increased diameters of collagen fibres precipitated *in vitro* in the presence of decorin from various connective tissues. *Connect. Tissue Res.* **36**, 287–296.

LeBaron, R. G., Zimmermann, D. R., and Ruoslahti, E. (1992). Hyaluronate binding properties of versican. *J. Biol. Chem.* **267**, 10003–10010.

Margolis, R. U., and Margolis, R. K. (1994). Aggrecan-versican-neurocan family of proteoglycans. *Method Enzymol.* **245**, 105–126.

Margolis, R. U., and Margolis, R. K. (1997). Chondroitin sulfate proteoglycans as mediators of axon growth and pathfinding. *Cell Tissue Res.* **290**, 343–348.

Maroudas, A., Muir, H., and Wingham, J. (1969). The correlation of fixed negative charge with glycosaminoglycan content of human articular cartilage. *Biochim. Biophys. Acta* **117**, 492–500.

Mjaatvedt, C. H., Yamamura, H., Capehart, A. A., Turner, D., and Markwald, R. R. (1998). The Cspg2 gene, disrupted in the hdf mutant, is required for right cardiac chamber and endocardial cushion formation. *Dev. Biol.* **202**, 56–66.

Moscatello, D. K., Santra, M., Mann, D. M., McQuillan, D. J., Wong, A. J., and Iozzo, R. V. (1998). Decorin suppresses tumor cell growth by activating the epidermal growth factor receptor. *J. Clin. Invest.* **101**, 406–412.

Muir, H. (1958). The nature of the link between proteins and carbohydrates of a chondroitin sulphate complex from articular cartilage. *Biochem. J.* **69**, 195–202.

Prydz, K., and Dalen, K. T. (2000). Synthesis and sorting of proteoglycans. *J. Cell Sci.* **113**, 193–205.

Robinson, H. C., Telser, A., and Dorfman, A. (1966). Studies on the biosynthesis of the linkage region of chondroitin sulfate protein complex. *Proc. Natl. Acad. Sci. USA* **56**, 1859–1864.

Samiric, T., Ilic, M. Z., and Handley, C. J. (2004). Characterization of proteoglycans and their catabolic products in tendon and explant cultures of tendon. *Matrix Biol.* **23**, 127–140.

Schonherr, E., Jarvelainen, H. T., Sandell, L. J., and Wight, T. N. (1991). Effects of platelet-derived growth factor and transforming growth factor-beta 1 on the synthesis of a large versican-like chondroitin sulphate proteoglycan by arterial smooth muscle cells. *J. Biol. Chem.* **266**, 17640–17647.

Seidenbecher, C. I., Richter, K., Rauch, U., Fassler, R., Garner, C. C., and Gundelfinger, E. D. (1995). Brevican, a chondroitin sulphate proteoglycan of rat brain, occurs as secreted and cell surface glycosylphosphatidylinositol-anchored isoforms. *J. Biol. Chem.* **270**, 27206–27212.

Sugumaran, G., Katsman, M., and Silbert, J. E. (1998). Subcellular co-localization and potential interaction of glucuronosyltransferases with nascent proteochondroitin sulfate at Golgi sites of chondroitin synthesis. *Biochem. J.* **329**, 203–208.

Toma, L., Pinhal, M. A., Dietrich, C. P., Nader, H. B., and Hirschberg, C. B. (1996). Transport of UDP-galactose into the Golgi lumen regulates the biosynthesis of proteoglycans. *J. Biol. Chem.* **271**, 13147–13154.

Vogel, K. G., and Heinegard, D. (1985). Characterisation of proteoglycans from adult bovine tendon. *J. Biol. Chem.* **260**, 9298–9306.

Vogel, K. G., Paulsson, M., and Heinegard, D. (1984). Specific inhibition of type I and II collagen fibrillogenesis by the small proteoglycan of tendon. *Biochem. J.* **223**, 587–597.

Vogel, K. G., Koob, T. J., and Fisher, L. W. (1987). Characterisation and interactions of a fragment of the core protein of the small proteoglycan (PGII) from bovine tendon. *Biochem. Biophys. Res. Commun.* **148**, 658–663.

Weber, I. T., Harrison, R. W., and Iozzo, R. V. (1996). Model structure of decorin and implications for collagen fibrillogenesis. *J. Biol. Chem.* **271**, 31767–31770.

Xu, T., Bianco, P., Fisher, L. W., Longenecker, G., Smith, E., Goldstein, S., Bonadio, J., Boskey, A., Heegaard, A. M., Sommer, B., Satomura, K., Dominguez, P., *et al.* (1998). Targeted disruption of the biglycan gene leads to an osteoporosis-like phenotype in mice. *Nat. Genet.* **20**, 78–82.

Yamada, H., Watanabe, K., Shimonaka, M., and Yamaguchi, Y. (1994). Molecular cloning of brevican, a novel brain proteoglycan of the aggrecan/versican family. *J. Biol. Chem.* **269**, 10119–10126.

Yamada, H., Watanabe, H., Shimonaka, M., Yamasaki, M., and Yamaguchi, Y. (1995). cDNA cloning and the identification of an aggrecanase-like cleavage site in rat brevican. *Biochem. Biophys. Res. Commun.* **216**, 957–963.

Yamagata, M., Saga, S., Kato, M., Bernfield, M., and Kimata, K. (1993). Selective distributions of proteoglycans and their ligands in pericellular matrix of cultured fibroblasts: Implications for their roles in cell-substratum adhesion. *J. Cell Sci.* **106**, 55–65.

Yamaguchi, Y., Mann, D. M., and Ruoslahti, E. (1990). Negative regulation of transforming growth factor-β by the proteoglycan decorin. *Nature* **346**, 281–284.

Zhang, L., David, G., and Esko, J. D. (1995). Repetitive Ser-Gly sequences enhance heparan sulfate assembly in proteoglycans. *J. Biol. Chem.* **270**, 27127–27135.

Zhou, X. H., Brakebusch, C., Matties, H., Oohashi, T., Hirsch, E., Moser, M., Krug, M., Seidenbecher, C. I., Boeckers, T. M., Rauch, U., Buettner, R., Gundelfinger, E. D., *et al.* (2001). Neurocan is dispensable for brain development. *Mol. Cell. Biol.* **17**, 5970–5978.

Zimmermann, D. R., Dours-Zimmermann, M. T., Schubert, M., and Bruckner-Tuderman, L. (1994). Versican is expressed in the proliferating zone in the epidermis and in association with the elastic network of the dermis. *J. Cell Biol.* **124**, 817–825.

Lucia O. Sampaio and Helena B. Nader

Disciplina de Biologia Molecular
Departamento de Bioquímica
Universidade Federal de São Paulo
Rua Três de Maio, 100
04044-020 São Paulo
São Paulo, Brazil

Emergence and Structural Characteristics of Chondroitin Sulfates in the Animal Kingdom

I. Chapter Overview

The data reviewed here provides a framework for the selective appearance and special structural characteristics of galactosaminoglycans (GalAGs) and raises questions of how those characteristics evolved during evolution. Analysis of species of the domain eukarya showed the absence of sulfated glycosaminoglycans (GAGs) in protista, plantae, and fungi. In the animal kingdom, the appearance of chondroitin sulfate (CS) coincides with the emergence of eumetazoa, which are animals that display true tissues. This compound is ubiquitously found in all tissues and species analyzed. The occurrence of dermatan sulfate (DS) is a late event in the evolutionary GAG tree, being restricted to the appearance of deuterostomes. The sulfation pattern of the different disaccharides as well as the copolymeric nature of these compounds are discussed related to phylogenetic aspects. Examples of structural branches for the GalAGs in bacteria and animal tissues are also

Advances in Pharmacology, Volume 53
1054-3589/06 $35.00
DOI: 10.1016/S1054-3589(05)53011-4

presented. The divergence in the appearance of DS and heparan sulfate (HS) suggests that the epimerases involved in the biosynthesis of these families of GAGs appeared in the phylogenetic tree at distinct moments. Temporal expression pattern and localization of GAGs during embryonic development of vertebrates and invertebrates are briefly commented.

II. Introduction

Glycosaminoglycans are linear polysaccharides composed of repeating disaccharides units, containing a hexosamine (D-glucosamine or D-galactosamine) linked by a glycosidic linkage to an uronic acid residue (D-glucuronic acid or L-iduronic acid) or a neutral sugar (D-galactose). These polymers are negatively charged due to the presence of sulfate groups in their structure and/or carboxyl groups from the uronic acids, which contribute to the highly polyanionic nature of the GAGs. According to the type of hexosamine, the GAGs can be divided into glucosaminoglycans [hyaluronic acid or hyaluronan, HS, heparin, and keratan sulfate (KS)] and GalAGs (CS and DS). Thus, the GAGs can be differentiated regarding the type of hexosamine and nonnitrogen sugar moieties, degree and position of sulfation, as well as the type of the inter- and intradisaccharide glycosydic linkages. The main structural characteristics of these compounds are summarized in Table I. The hexosamine is always N-acetylated in CS, DS, hyaluronic acid, and KS. On the other hand, in heparin the glucosamine is mostly N-sulfated, whereas in HS both substitutions are found.

Except for hyaluronic acid, all GAG chains occur in the tissues as proteoglycans (PGs), covalently linked to a core protein. Proteoglycans are widely distributed in animal tissues and can be found at the cell surface, in the extracellular matrix (ECM) and in the intracellular compartment, usually as secretory granules. The major classes of PGs are divided according to the core proteins. The ones located at the cell surface comprise the syndecan and glypican families, whereas serglycin corresponds to the PGs usually found in granules. The extracellular matrices comprehend three major classes—the large aggregating PGs that interact with hyaluronan (e.g., aggrecan, versican), the small leucine-rich PGs also named fibrilar PGs (e.g., decorin, biglycan), and the ones specifically found in basement membranes (e.g., perlecan, aggrin) (Bernfield *et al.*, 1999; Iozzo, 1998; Silbert and Sugumaran, 2002a). The diversity in structure and specific cellular and tissue distribution indicate that these glycoconjugates could perform different biological roles. Pivotal functions have been postulated for PGs and their GAG moieties, such as organization and modulation of the ECM, tissue morphogenesis and differentiation, and cellular adhesion and recognition, among others.

TABLE I   Main Structural Features of Glycosaminoglycans

Nomenclature		Monosaccharides[a]	Position of sulfate	Glycosydic linkage
Meyer (1938)	Jeanloz (1960)			
Chondroitin	Chondroitin	N-acetylgalactosamine	–	$\beta(1–4)$
		glucuronic acid		$\beta(1–3)$
Chondroitin sulfate A	Chondroitin 4-sulfate	N-acetylgalactosamine	4	$\beta(1–4)$
		glucuronic acid	–	$\beta(1–3)$
Chondroitin sulfate C	Chondroitin 6-sulfate	N-acetylgalactosamine	6	$\beta(1–4)$
		glucuronic acid	–	$\beta(1–3)$
Chondroitin sulfate B	Dermatan sulfate	N-acetylgalactosamine	4	$\beta(1–4)$
		glucuronic acid	–	$\beta(1–3)$
		Iduronic acid	–	$\alpha(1–3)$
Hyaluronic acid	Hyaluronic acid[b]	N-acetylglucosamine	–	$\beta(1–4)$
		glucuronic acid		$\beta(1–3)$
Kerato sulfate	Keratan sulfate	N-acetylglucosamine	6	$\beta(1–3)$
		galactose	–/6	$\beta(1–4)$
Heparitin sulfate	Heparan sulfate	Glucosamine	2/6	$\alpha(1–4)$
		N-acetylglucosamine	–/6	$\alpha(1–4)$
		Glucuronic acid	–	$\beta(1–4)$
		Iduronic acid	–	$\alpha(1–4)$
Heparin	Heparin	Glucosamine	2/6	$\alpha(1–4)$
		Glucuronic acid	–	$\beta(1–4)$
		Iduronic acid	–/2	$\alpha(1–4)$

[a] All monosaccharides are in the D-configuration, except for iduronic acid, which is in the L-configuration.
[b] Also known as hyaluronan.

Except for KS, the GAG chains are covalently O-linked to specific serine residues in the respective core proteins through a common tetrasaccharide region composed of [GlcUA-Gal-Gal-Xyl-] (Fig. 1). In this chapter, we are not considering the PG nature of the GAGs but rather focusing on the diversity of the GalAG chains (Silbert and Sugumaran, 2002a).

The isolation and characterization of the specificity of several lyases, sulfatases, and glycuronidases from bacteria enabled to perform structural analysis of the GAGs. Figure 2 shows a hypothetic structure for CS/DS indicating the glycosydic bonds that are recognized by some of these enzymes (Linhardt et al., 1986; Michelacci and Dietrich, 1975, 1976).

Degradation with specific enzymes, chemical analysis of the products formed, and NMR spectroscopy of the polymer and fragments had shown the types of disaccharides that can be found in CSs and DSs (Fig. 3). The GalAGs are hybrid compounds, regarding the types of disaccharide units, which alternate in the polymeric chains. In this respect, the nomenclature

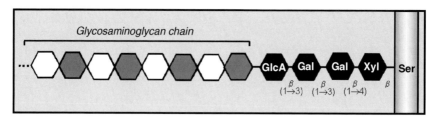

FIGURE 1   Structure of the linkage region of GAGs to the core protein. Ser, serine; Xyl, xylose; Gal, galactose; GlcA, glucuronic acid; open hexagon, uronic acid; gray hexagon, hexosamine.

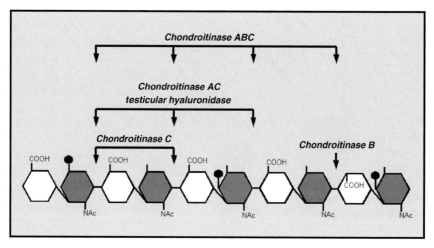

FIGURE 2   Hypothetical structure of a GalAG and site of action of different enzymes. •, Sulfate ester groups; open hexagon, uronic acid; gray hexagon, galactosamine.

used to designate CSs does not take into consideration the hybrid structure of the compounds.

The complexity of the structure of the GalAGs depends on the specificity of different glycosyltrasferases, sulfotransferases, as well as epimerase. The glycosyltransferases catalyze the transfer of sugar residues from nucleotide sugars (donors) to the nonreducing end of the growing polymer through the stepwise addition of each monosaccharide. Thus, the biosynthetic assembly of GalAGPGs is characterized by the following sequential processes: (1) synthesis of the core protein; (2) xylosylation of specific serine moieties of the core protein (xylosyltransferase); (3) addition of two galactose residues to the xylose (galactosyltransferases I and II); (4) completion of common tetrasaccharide linkage region by the addition of a glucuronic acid (GlcUA) residue

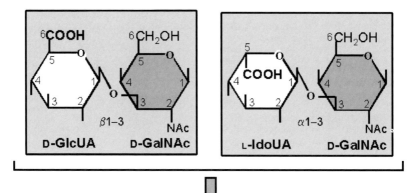

	D-Glucuronic acid		L-Iduronic acid	
Nonsulfated	[GlcUA-GalNAc]		[IdoUA-GalNAc]	
Monosulfated	[GlcUA-GalNAc (4S)]	A	[IdoUA-GalNAc (4S)]	B
	[GlcUA-GalNAc (6S)]	C	[IdoUA-GalNAc (6S)]	
Disulfated	[GlcUA-GalNAc (4S,6S)]	E	[IdoUA-GalNAc (4S,6S)]	iE
	[GlcUA (2S)-GalNAc (6S)]	D	[IdoUA (2S)-GalNAc (6S)]	iD
	[GlcUA (2S)-GalNAc (4S)]		[IdoUA (2S)-GalNAc (4S)]	
	[GlcUA (3S)-GalNAc (6S)]		[IdoUA (3S)-GalNAc (6S)]	
	[GlcUA (3S)-GalNAc (4S)]	K	[IdoUA (3S)-GalNAc (4S)]	iK
Trisulfated	[GlcUA (2S)-GalNAc (4S,6S)]		[IdoUA (2S)-GalNAc (4S,6S)]	
	[GlcUA (3S)-GalNAc (4S,6S)]		[IdoUA (3S)-GalNAc (4S,6S)]	

FIGURE 3   Types of disaccharide units in GalAGs.

(glucuronyltransferase I); (5) addition of an N-acetylgalactosamine (GalNAc) residue to initiate the GalAG chain (N-acetylgalactosaminyltransferase I); (6) repeated addition of GlcUA residues alternating with GalNAc residues to grow the large heteropolymer GAG chains (glucuronyltransferase II and N-acetylgalactosaminyltransferase II); and (7) modification of these growing GAG chains by variable O-sulfation and epimerization of GlcUA to iduronic acid (IdoUA). It has been demonstrated that a single polypeptide had the dual glycosyltransferase activities of glucuronyltransferase II and

N-acetylgalactosaminyltransferase II that are responsible for synthesizing the repeated disaccharide units of CS. Thus, the enzyme that contributes to the synthesis of repeated disaccharide units was designated chondroitin synthase. Different sulfotransferases transfer sulfate to defined position of the sugar residues in the growing polymer from active sulfate donor (3'-phosphoadenosine 5'-phosphosulfate) and, for DS, an epimerase (D-glucuronyl C-5 epimerase) that acts at the polymeric level (Prydz and Dalen, 2000; Silbert and Sugumaran, 2002b; Sugahara et al., 2003).

III. Galactosaminoglycans in an Evolutionary Context _____

In the early 1970s, the data regarding the presence of GAGs in different animal phyla was scattered, and the procedures used for extraction, identification, and structural characterization of the compounds were not comparable among the different reports (Hunt, 1970; Katzman and Jeanloz, 1969). At that time, it was well documented the presence of CSs in cartilaginous tissues of different species of vertebrate (Muir, 1977) and DS in the skin of mammals (Malmström and Fransson, 1971).

The first systematic approach for the search of this class of complex carbohydrates using the same methodology that combined electrophoretical behavior in agarose gels, degradation with specific enzymes and analysis of the products formed showed that the distribution of sulfated GAGs in vertebrate is tissue and species specific. It was shown that each tissue has a characteristic composition differing from each other regarding the relative amount, type, and molecular size of CSs, DS, and HS. Heparan sulfate is a ubiquitous compound present at the cell surface of all species (Gomes and Dietrich, 1982; Toledo and Dietrich, 1977). On the other hand, heparin is present only inside the granules of mast cells (Nader and Dietrich, 1989). Also, the GalAGs are found in all species, but the relative proportion between CS and Ds varies among the different tissues analyzed. For instance, CS is the main GAG in cartilage and brain of all species, whereas DS is predominant in muscle and skin.

The same protocol was then used to address the distribution of sulfated GAG in other living organisms in order to trace the evolutionary pathways back (Cassaro and Dietrich, 1977; Dietrich, 1984; Dietrich et al., 1983; Medeiros et al., 2000). Analysis of species of the domain eukarya, showed the absence of sulfated GAGs in protista, plantae, and fungi. Again, the profile of sulfated GAG is tissue and species specific. The distribution of the GalAGs is depicted in Fig. 4. In the animal kingdom, the appearance of CS coincides with the emergence of eumetazoa, which are animals that display true tissues. This compound is ubiquitously found in all species analyzed. On the other hand, in parazoa (Porifera), which are animals that lack any coherent epithelium, no GAGs were characterized. In fact, sponges contain

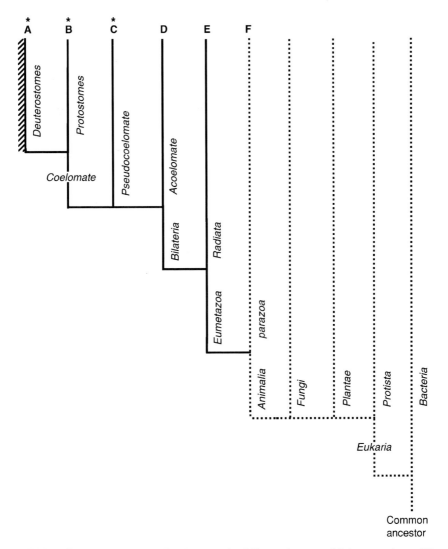

FIGURE 4   The distribution of GalAGs in the different domains of living organisms. (A) Chordata (Vertebrata, Urochordata, Cephalochordata), Echinodermata, Phoronida, Brachiopoda, Bryozoa; (B) Arthropoda, Annelida, Molluska; (C) Rotifera, Nematoda, Nemertea; (D) Platyelminthes; (E) Ctenophora, Cnidaria; (F) Porifera. The symbol (*) indicates the presence of chondroitin synthases; dotted line, absence of GalAGs; solid line, presence of CS; dashed line, presence of dermatan sulfate.

large amounts of other types of sulfated polysaccharides composed among other sugars of galactose, uronic acid, and fucose (Misevic and Burger, 1990; Spillmann *et al.*, 1995; Zierer and Mourão, 2000). The occurrence of DS is a late event in the evolutionary GAG tree, being restricted to the appearance of deuterostomes (Anno *et al.*, 1971; Bao *et al.*, 2005; Cassaro and Dietrich, 1977; Dietrich, 1984; Dietrich *et al.*, 1983; Gomes and Dietrich, 1982; Inestrosa *et al.*, 1987; Kobayashi *et al.*, 1985; Malmström and Fransson, 1971; Medeiros *et al.*, 2000; Nandini *et al.*, 2004; Pavão *et al.*, 1995, 1998; Poblacion and Michelacci, 1986; Sakai *et al.*, 2003; Toledo and Dietrich, 1977; Ueoka *et al.*, 1999; Vicente *et al.*, 2001; Yaoita *et al.*, 1990). Considering that the difference between the GalAGs resides in the types of uronic acid residues (β-D-glucuronic acid and α-L-iduronic acid), one can postulate that the appearance of D-glucuronyl C-5 epimerase involved in DS biosynthesis will be restricted to the emergence of deuterostomes.

It should be pointed out that HS expression also starts in eumetazoa, being a conspicuous compound of all species. On the other hand, heparin is only found in some species of some phyla of eumetazoa and always confined to granules of "mast-like" cells (Dietrich *et al.*, 1985; Nader *et al.*, 1999; Santos *et al.*, 2002). Like DS, heparin and HS also present in their structure α-L-iduronic acid besides β-D-glucuronic acid. Nevertheless, considering the emergence of these compounds we can postulate that the epimerases involved in the biosynthesis of these families of GAGs show divergence time of appearance in the phylogenetic tree, suggesting that the genes have arisen separately. The need for epimerization in the CS chains seems to be restricted to late evolutionary events, suggesting that DS fulfills specific biological functions.

Sulfated GAGs are not present in the kingdom bacteria (Fig. 4). Nevertheless, in capsules of pathogenic bacteria (genera *Streptococcus*, *Escherichia*, *Pasteurella*, and *Moraxella*) are found linear polysaccharides with a repeating disaccharide backbone containing an *N*-acetylated amino sugar and β-D-glucuronic acid, such as hyaluronic acid (hyaluronan), nonsulfated chondroitin (chondrosan) and nonsulfated heparan (heparosan), apparently not covalently linked to a core protein (Roberts, 1996; Rodriguez *et al.*, 1988; Vann *et al.*, 1981; Wilson *et al.*, 2005). The presence of these GAGs in the capsules appears to serve as camouflage, protective shielding, and an adhesive device, as well as a mean of manipulating animal host cell behavior (DeAngelis, 2002; DeAngelis and Padgett-McCue, 2000).

Regarding CS and HS biosynthetic pathways, it has been shown that the polymerization of the repeating disaccharide units involves specific GAG synthases that bear dual glycosyltransferase activities. Genes related to chondroitin synthase and heparan synthase have been cloned and activity of the proteins proved (DeAngelis, 2002; Duncan *et al.*, 2001; Kitagawa *et al.*, 2001; Lind *et al.*, 1998; Silbert and Sugumaran, 2002b). The data of GAG distribution and their absence in parazoa, fungi, plantae, and protista indicate that the synthases emerged in eumetazoa (Fig. 4). So, it seems possible that pathogenic microbial start to express the synthases activities later in their time line evolution in order to deal with infecting the host and survival.

IV. Structural Characteristics of the Galactosaminoglycans ___

As already mentioned, CSs consist of alternating units of D-glucuronic acid (GlcUA) and D-N-acetylgalactosamine (GalNAc) saccharides that are β1-3 and β1-4-linked respectively, with variable amounts and location of the sulfate esters. The disaccharides are usually monosulfated, either at position C-4 (chondroitin 4-sulfate or CS-A) or C-6 (chondroitin 6-sulfate or CS-C) of the GalNAc, or nonsulfated to a minor extent. The relative proportion of these disaccharides in the same chain varies depending on the tissue and animal species. For instance, CSs from platelets and brain tissues of various species contain more than 90% of 4-sulfated disaccharide units (Dietrich et al., 1978; Nader, 1991; Sampaio et al., 1977), whereas nonsulfated disaccharide represents around 50% of the repeating disaccharide unit in GalAGs present in different tissues of some species of mollusks (Gastropoda: Pomacea, Viviparus, and mud snail) (Dietrich et al., 1983; Lee et al., 1998; Nader et al., 1984; Volpi and Mucci, 1988) as well as the major disaccharide in the nematode (C. elegans) and the GalAG chain of plasmatic bikunin (Yamada et al., 1999; Zhuo et al., 2003). On the other hand, some examples of mostly 6-sulfated disaccharides (~85%) are described for adult normal human articular cartilage (Bayliss et al., 1999; Michelacci et al., 1979; Mourão, 1988), shark cartilages (Michelacci and Horton, 1989), and fetal tissues (Sampaio and Dietrich, 1981). It should also be pointed out that for the same tissue the ratio of the different disaccharides may vary with aging (Bayliss et al., 1999).

Disaccharides containing extrasulfate groups in the N-acetylgalactosamine and/or glucuronic acid are also present in some types of CSs (Fig. 3).

(1) *GlcUAβ 1-3GalNAc(4,6S) (unit E)*: in invertebrates, the occurrence of CS E was originally described in squid cartilage (Suzuki et al., 1968). It has also been reported in squid cornea (Karamanos et al., 1991) and the body wall of different species of sea cucumber (Kariya et al., 1990; Vieira et al., 1991). Subclasses of mast cells, natural killer cells, and basophilic leukocytes from different mammals possess a distinct CSPG rich in this type of disaccharide unit (Razin et al., 1982; Rothenberg et al., 1987; Stevens, 1986; Thompson et al., 1988). This epitope has also been described in PGs from brain tissues, such as the amyloid precursor protein (appican) (Tsuchida et al., 2001).

(2) *GlcUA(2S)β 1-3GalNAc(4S) or GlcUA(2S)β 1-3GalNAc(6S) (unit D)*: the presence of type D unit in CS was originally observed in shark cartilage (Mathews, 1962; Suzuki, 1960). The location of this unit in the shark cartilage CS chain has been investigated (Nadanaka and Sugahara, 1997). Synthesis of CS D in murine lymph node-derived mast cells has been described (Davidson et al., 1990). Also, using different monoclonal antibodies, a variation was shown in the sulfation profile of the CS

chains of brain PGs (phosphacan) related to the disulfated disaccharide D unit, which apparently is involved in the central nervous system development in vertebrates (Ito *et al.*, 2005; Maeda *et al.*, 2003).

(3) *GlcUA(3S)β 1-3GalNAc(4S)* or *GlcUA(3S)β 1-3GalNAc(6S) (unit K)*: sulfation of CS at the C-3 position of the glucuronic acid was first considered in shark cartilage (Suzuki, 1960). In king crab cartilage, disulfated disaccharide K-unit was fully characterized (Kitagawa *et al.*, 1997; Seno and Sekizuka, 1978; Sugahara *et al.*, 1996). This type of unit has also been characterized in CSs from the body wall of sea cucumber (Vieira *et al.*, 1991) and squid cartilage (Kinoshita *et al.*, 1997; Kinoshita-Toyoda *et al.*, 2004).

(4) *GlcUA(2S)β 1-3GalNAc(4,6S)* or *GlcUA(3S)β 1-3GalNAc(4,6S)*: trisulfated disaccharides are also described in CSs of squid cartilage (Kinoshita *et al.*, 1997, 2001; Kinoshita-Toyoda *et al.*, 2004).

Dermatan sulfates contain variable amounts of L-iduronic acid disaccharide units besides the typical CSs disaccharides arranged in a copolymeric chain. The typical disaccharide in DS known as unit B corresponds to IdoUA α 1-3 GalNAc(4S). Nevertheless, differences in the sulfation of the iduronic acid containing units can also be observed, as shown in Fig. 3. The relative proportion of the glucuronic and iduronic acid containing disaccharides in the same chain varies depending on the tissue and animal species (Chatziioannidis *et al.*, 1999; Poblacion and Michelacci, 1986; Sampaio *et al.*, 1988; Toledo and Dietrich, 1977). Some examples of iduronic acid containing disaccharide units with different degree and location of sulfation are described further.

(1) *IdoUAα 1-3 GalNAc(4,6S) (unit iE)*: GalAGs containing IdoA-Gal-NAc(4,6-SO$_4$) units have been reported in the hagfish notochord (Anno *et al.*, 1971; Nandini *et al.*, 2004; Ueoka *et al.*, 1999), rat glomeruli and mesangial cells (Hadad *et al.*, 1996; Kobayashi *et al.*, 1985; Yaoita *et al.*, 1990), porcine intestine (Yamada *et al.*, 1998), and sea urchin species (Vilela-Silva *et al.*, 2001). Dermatan sulfate consisting mainly of this type of disaccharide unit is also known as CS H.

(2) *IdoUA(2S)α 1-3GalNAc(4S)* or *IdoUA(2S)α 1-3GalNAc(6S) (unit iD)*: sulfation in the C-4 of the GalNAc has been described in DSs from mammalian tissues as well as from eel skin (Sakai *et al.*, 2003) and ascidia (*Styela plicata* and *Halocynthia pyriformis*) (Pavão *et al.*, 1998). This type of unit is also present in hagfish notochord (Nandini *et al.*, 2004; Ueoka *et al.*, 1999). Sulfation in the C-6 of the GalNAc is present in the body of *Ascidia nigra*. This same epitope is found in mouse brain (Bao *et al.*, 2005; Pavão *et al.*, 1995).

(3) *IdoUA(3S)α 1-3GalNAc(4S)* or *IdoUA(3S) α 1-3GalNAc(6S) (unit iK)*: these type of units have been suggested in skin of the eel *Anguilla japonica*. The NMR spectra also suggests the presence of IdoUA 2S,3S (Sakai *et al.*, 2003).

(4) *IdoUA(2S)α 1-3GalNAc(4,6S)* or *IdoUA(3S)α 1-3GalNAc(4,6S)*: trisulfated disaccharides are present in significant amounts in DS from hagfish notochord (Nandini *et al.*, 2004; Ueoka *et al.*, 1999).

Oversulfated DSs have also been described in granules of mast cells and basophilic cells, but the position of sulfate esters has not been investigated further (Enerback *et al.*, 1985; Nader *et al.*, 1980; Seldin *et al.*, 1985).

Galactosaminoglycans from specific tissues of some animal species and some bacteria can occasionally exhibit ramifications. The main types of branched-GalAG are delineated in Fig. 5. For some species of invertebrates, glucose branches are present in CS from squid cartilage (Habuchi *et al.*, 1977; Kinoshita-Toyoda *et al.*, 2004) and skin (Karamanos *et al.*, 1992), whereas fucose branches, for king crab (Kitagawa *et al.*, 1997) and sea cucumber (Kariya *et al.*, 1997; Vieira and Mourão, 1988). On the other hand, fructose ramifications are also found in nonsulfated CS from pathogenic bacteria (Rodriguez *et al.*, 1988). Bikunin is a small low-sulfated CSPG that occurs in blood of several mammals as the light chain of inter-a-trypsin inhibitor (ITI) family members. The distal portion of the CS chain of bikunin is linked to the heavy chain via a unique ester bond between the C-6 of an internal *N*-acetylgalactosamine and the α-carboxyl group of the C-terminal of an aspartic acid residue (Zhuo *et al.*, 2003).

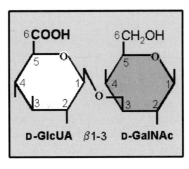

FIGURE 5 Types of branches found in some galactosaminoglycans.

The detailed structural data on GalAGs can give important clues for the understanding of the evolutionary aspects of enzymes involved in the biosynthesis of these compounds. D-Glucuronyl C-5 epimerase involved in GalAG biosynthesis seems to be a late acquisition in evolution, being found only in deuterostomes, whereas different sulfotransferases should be found throughout the eumetazoa. In this respect, it should be pointed out that the fine structure of CSs from the phylum Mollusca varies between the bivalves (*Tagelus* and *Anomalocardia*) and the Gastropoda (*Pomacea*). For instance, no 6-sulfated or disulfated disaccharide could be found in the CS of *Pomacea*. In all tissues of this species, CS is a copolymer of nonsulfated and 4-sulfated disaccharide units (Dietrich *et al.*, 1983). Since the class Gastropoda is less evolved than the class bivalve, the sulfotransferase responsible for the 6-sulfation of chondroitin might be a later acquisition in evolution (Nader *et al.*, 1984). Results of another species of Gastropoda (*Viviparus*) (Volpi and Mucci, 1988) reinforce this hypothesis.

Regarding GAG concentration, it was shown that the degree of salinity of the habitat influences the total content of the compounds. Studies with 15 species of 3 different classes of invertebrates show a direct correlation between the concentration of the sulfated GAGs and the degree of salinity of the natural habitat. This is particularly evident with the vicarious species (Nader *et al.*, 1983).

The differences in concentration, sulfation profile, and epimerization have been correlated with biological properties of the CSs, such as cell migration/adhesion/differentiation, growth control, neuroregulatory functions, anticoagulant activity, among others, through molecular interactions with specific proteins (growth factors, serpins, selectins, chemokines, cell adhesion proteins, and so on). The findings also imply that temporal and spatial expression besides the structural diversity of the GalAGs should be involved in tissue homeostasis, modulating several biological processes.

An example involving specific localization and different temporal expression pattern of GAGs is the embryonic development, especially during the progressive steps of morphogenesis and tissue differentiation. A few examples are commented below.

A sequential order of appearance of each of the acidic polysaccharides is observed coinciding with the major processes of the ontogeny. In mammals, hyaluronic acid is the first GAG synthesized during morphogenesis (Toole, 2001). This GAG is then replaced by chondroitin 6-sulfate prior to tissue differentiation. Heparan sulfate, DS, and chondroitin 4-sulfate appear during cell differentiation (Cutler *et al.*, 1991; Galbraith *et al.*, 1992; Mark *et al.*, 1990a,b; Sampaio and Dietrich, 1981). The same general pattern is also observed in molluscs except that hyaluronic acid is replaced by an acidic galactan in the morphogenetic process (Nader *et al.*, 1985, 1996). Significant amount of 6-sulfated units in CS has been described during embryonic and larval tissues of the fly *Drosophila melanogaster* (Pinto *et al.*, 2004). In sea urchin embryos (echinoderms) an acidic glycan, containing sulfate and uronic acid, performs the role of hyaluronic acid during early blastula to the end of gastrula (Papakonstantinou and Misevic, 1993; Papakonstantinou *et al.*, 1994). Regarding the sulfated GAGs, it was observed that sea urchin embryos synthesize high amounts of GalAGs bearing disulfated units as well as iduronic acid containing disaccharides. It should be noted that the 4-*O*-sulfate in the galactosamine unit decreases in the polymer found in adult as compared to larvae (Lane and Solursh, 1991; Vilela-Silva *et al.*, 2001). Data shows that expression of chondroitin synthase is required for embryonic cytokinesis and cell division (Izumikawa *et al.*, 2004; Mizuguchi *et al.*, 2003).

Even though it is not the scope of this review, it should be mentioned that structural modifications, variation in the topography, and fluctuations in content, among other aspects occur for GalAGs in different physiopathological conditions, such as cell cycle, aging, tumor formation, inflammation, and so on.

V. Concluding Remarks

The new results that are coming out in the literature regarding cloning of enzymes involved in the biosynthesis and degradation of the GAGs, as well as the families of core proteins add to the distribution and characterization of the compounds that were discussed.

The data reviewed here provides a framework for the selective appearance and special structural characteristics of GalAGs and raises questions of how those characteristics evolved during evolution. This broad scenario of information can bring new insights in the investigation of the biology of these compounds. The information stored in these molecules and its dynamics guided by the diversity of the GAGs coupled with the new tools of genomics and proteomics will certainly bring out new aspects to the knowledge of the field.

In honor of Professor Carl P. Dietrich.

References

Anno, K., Seno, N., Mathews, M. B., Yamagata, T., and Suzuki, S. (1971). A new dermatan polysulfate, chondroitin sulfate H, from hagfish notochord. *Biochim. Biophys. Acta* **237**, 173–177.

Bao, X., Pavão, M. S., Dos Santos, J. C., and Sugahara, K. (2005). A functional dermatan sulfate epitope containing iduronate(2-*O*-sulfate)alpha1–3GalNAc(6-*O*-sulfate) disaccharide in the mouse brain: Demonstration using a novel monoclonal antibody raised against dermatan sulfate of ascidian. *Ascidia nigra. Biol. Chem.* **280**, 23184–23193.

Bayliss, M. T., Osborne, D., Woodhouse, S., and Davidson, C. (1999). Sulfation of chondroitin sulfate in human articular cartilage. *J. Biol. Chem.* **274**, 15892–15900.

Bernfield, M., Gotte, M., Park, P. W., Reizes, O., Fitzgerald, M. L., Lincecum, J., and Zako, M. (1999). Functions of cell surface heparan sulfate proteoglycans. *Annu. Rev. Biochem.* **68**, 729–777.

Cassaro, C. M., and Dietrich, C. P. (1977). Distribution of sulfated mucopolysaccharides in invertebrates. *J. Biol. Chem.* **252**, 2254–2261.

Chatziioannidis, C. C., Karamanos, N. K., Anagnostides, S. T., and Tsegenidis, T. (1999). Purification and characterisation of a minor low-sulphated dermatan sulphate-proteoglycan from ray skin. *Biochimie* **81**, 187–196.

Cutler, L. S., Christian, C. P., and Rendell, J. K. (1991). Sulphated glycosaminoglycan synthesis by developing rat submandibular gland secretory units. *Arch. Oral. Biol.* **36**, 389–395.

Davidson, S., Gilead, L., Amira, M., Ginsburg, H., and Razin, E. (1990). Synthesis of chondroitin sulfate D and heparin proteoglycans in murine lymph node-derived mast cells: The dependence on fibroblasts. *J. Biol. Chem.* **265**, 12324–12330.

DeAngelis, P. L. (2002). Evolution of glycosaminoglycans and their glycosyltransferases: Implications for the extracellular matrices of animals and the capsules of pathogenic bacteria. *Anat. Rec.* **268**, 317–326.

DeAngelis, P. L., and Padgett-McCue, A. J. (2000). Identification and molecular cloning of a chondroitin synthase from *Pasteurella multocida* type F. *J. Biol. Chem.* **275**, 24124–24129.

Dietrich, C. P. (1984). A model for cell-cell recognition and control of cell growth mediated by sulfated glycosaminoglycans. *Braz. J. Med. Biol. Res.* **17**, 5–15.

Dietrich, C. P., Schibuola, C. T., Sampaio, L. O., and Ibara, I. (1978). Changes in the composition of sulfated mucopolysaccharides during neoplastic transformation of cerebral tissue. *Cancer Res.* **38**, 3969–3971.

Dietrich, C. P., Paiva, V. M. P., Jerônimo, S. M. B., Ferreira, T. M. P. C., Medeiros, M. G. L., Paiva, J. F., and Nader, H. B. (1983). Characteristic distribution of heparan sulfates and chondroitin sulfates in tissues and organs of the Ampularidae *Pomacea sp. Comp. Biochem. Physiol.* **76B**, 695–698.

Dietrich, C. P., de Paiva, J. F., Moraes, C. T., Takahashi, H. K., Porcionatto, M. A., and Nader, H. B. (1985). Isolation and characterization of a heparin with high anticoagulant activity from *Anomalocardia brasiliana. Biochim. Biophys. Acta* **843**, 1–7.

Duncan, G., McCormick, C., and Tufaro, F. (2001). The link between heparan sulfate and hereditary bone disease: Finding a function for the EXT family of putative tumor suppressor proteins. *J. Clin. Invest.* **108**, 511–516.

Enerback, L., Kolset, S. O., Kusche, M., Hjerpe, A., and Lindahl, U. (1985). Glycosaminoglycans in rat mucosal mast cells. *Biochem. J.* **227**, 661–668.

Galbraith, D. B., Cutler, L. S., and Kollar, E. J. (1992). The correlation of temporal regulation of glycosaminoglycan synthesis with morphogenetic events in mouse tooth development. *Arch. Oral. Biol.* **37**, 623–628.

Gomes, P. B., and Dietrich, C. P. (1982). Distribution of heparin and other sulfated glycosaminoglycans in vertebrates. *Comp. Biochem. Physiol.* **73B**, 857–863.

Habuchi, O., Sugiura, K., and Kawai, N. (1977). Glucose branches in chondroitin sulfates from squid cartilage. *J. Biol. Chem.* **252**, 4570–4576.

Hadad, S. J., Michelacci, Y. M., and Schor, N. (1996). Proteoglycans and glycosaminoglycans synthesized *in vitro* by mesangial cells from normal and diabetic rats. *Biochim. Biophys. Acta* **1290**, 18–28.

Hunt, S. (1970). Evolution of mucopolysaccharides and related molecules. *In* "Polysaccharide-Protein Complexes in Invertebrates," pp. 287–305. Academic Press, New York.

Inestrosa, N. C., Nader, H. B., Garrido, J., Sampaio, L. O., Brandan, E., and Dietrich, C. P. (1987). Glycosaminoglycan composition of electric organ basement membranes. *J. Neurosci. Res.* **17**, 256–264.

Iozzo, R. V. (1998). Matrix proteoglycans: From molecular design to cellular function. *Annu. Rev. Biochem.* **67**, 609–652.

Ito, Y., Hikino, M., Yajima, Y., Mikami, T., Sirko, S., von Holst, A., Faissner, A., Fukui, S., and Sugahara, K. (2005). Structural characterization of the epitopes of the monoclonal antibodies 473HD, CS-56, and MO-225 specific for chondroitin sulfate D-type using the oligosaccharide library. *Glycobiology* **15**, 593–603.

Izumikawa, T., Kitagawa, H., Mizuguchi, S., Nomura, K. H., Nomura, K., Tamura, J., Gengyo-Ando, K., Mitani, S., and Sugahara, K. (2004). Nematode chondroitin polymerizing factor showing cell-/organ-specific expression is indispensable for chondroitin synthesis and embryonic cell division. *J. Biol. Chem.* **279**, 53755–53761.

Jeanloz, R. W. (1960). The nomenclature of mucopolysaccharides. *Arthritis Rheum.* **3**, 233–237.

Karamanos, N. K., Manouras, A., Tsegenidis, T., and Antonopoulos, C. A. (1991). Isolation and chemical study of the glycosaminoglycans from squid cornea. *Int. J. Biochem.* **23**, 67–72.

Karamanos, N. K., Aletras, A. J., Tsegenidis, T., Tsiganos, C. P., and Antonopoulos, C. A. (1992). Isolation, characterization and properties of the oversulphated chondroitin sulphate proteoglycan from squid skin with peculiar glycosaminoglycan sulphation pattern. *Eur. J. Biochem.* **204**, 553–560.

Kariya, Y., Watabe, S., Hashimoto, K., and Yoshida, K. (1990). Occurrence of chondroitin sulfate E in glycosaminoglycan isolated from the body wall of sea cucumber *Stichopus japonicus*. *J. Biol. Chem.* **265**, 5081–5085.

Kariya, Y., Watabe, S., Kyogashima, M., Ishihara, M., and Ishii, T. (1997). Structure of fucose branches in the glycosaminoglycan from the body wall of the sea cucumber *Stichopus japonicus*. *Carbohydr. Res.* **297**, 273–279.

Katzman, R. L., and Jeanloz, R. W. (1969). Acid polysaccharides from invertebrate connective tissue: Phylogenetic aspects. *Science* **166**, 758–759.

Kinoshita, A., Yamada, S., Haslam, S. M., Morris, H. R., Dell, A., and Sugahara, K. (1997). Novel tetrasaccharides isolated from squid cartilage chondroitin sulfate E contain unusual sulfated disaccharide units GlcA(3-O-sulfate)beta1–3GalNAc(6-O-sulfate) or GlcA(3-O-sulfate)beta1-3GalNAc. *J. Biol. Chem.* **272**, 19656–19665.

Kinoshita, A., Yamada, S., Haslam, S. M., Morris, H. R., Dell, A., and Sugahara, K. (2001). Isolation and structural determination of novel sulfated hexasaccharides from squid cartilage chondroitin sulfate E that exhibits neuroregulatory activities. *Biochemistry* **40**, 12654–12665.

Kinoshita-Toyoda, A., Yamada, S., Haslam, S. M., Khoo, K. H., Sugiura, M., Morris, H. R., Dell, A., and Sugahara, K. (2004). Structural determination of five novel tetrasaccharides containing 3-O-sulfated D-glucuronic acid and two rare oligosaccharides containing a beta-D-glucose branch isolated from squid cartilage chondroitin sulfate E. *Biochemistry* **43**, 11063–11074.

Kitagawa, H., Tanaka, Y., Yamada, S., Seno, N., Haslam, S. M., Morris, H. R., Dell, A., and Sugahara, K. (1997). A novel pentasaccharide sequence GlcA(3-sulfate)(beta1–3)GalNAc (4-sulfate)(beta1–4)(Fuc alpha1 3)GlcA(beta1–3)GalNAc(4-sulfate) in the oligosaccharides isolated from king crab cartilage chondroitin sulfate K and its differential susceptibility to chondroitinases and hyaluronidase. *Biochemistry* **36**, 3998–4008.

Kitagawa, H., Uyama, T., and Sugahara, K. (2001). Molecular cloning and expression of a human chondroitin synthase. *J. Biol. Chem.* **276**, 38721–38726.

Kobayashi, S., Oguri, K., Yaoita, E., Kobayashi, K., and Okayama, M. (1985). Highly sulfated proteochondroitin sulfates synthesized *in vitro* by rat glomeruli. *Biochim. Biophys. Acta* **841**, 71–80.

Lane, M. C., and Solursh, M. (1991). Primary mesenchyme cell migration requires a chondroitin sulfate/dermatan sulfate proteoglycan. *Dev. Biol.* **143**, 389–397.

Lee, K. B., Kim, J. S., Kwak, S. T., Sim, W., Kwak, J. H., and Kim, Y. S. (1998). Isolation and identification of chondroitin sulfates from the mud snail. *Arch. Pharm. Res.* **21**, 555–558.

Lind, T., Tufaro, F., McCormick, C., Lindahl, U., and Lidholt, K. (1998). The putative tumor suppressors EXT1 and EXT2 are glycosyltransferases required for the biosynthesis of heparan sulfate. *J. Biol. Chem.* **273**, 26265–26268.

Linhardt, R. J., Galliher, P. M., and Cooney, C. L. (1986). Polysaccharide lyases. *Appl. Biochem. Biotechnol.* **12**, 135–176.

Maeda, N., He, J., Yajima, Y., Mikami, T., Sugahara, K., and Yabe, T. (2003). Heterogeneity of the chondroitin sulfate portion of phosphacan/6B4 proteoglycan regulates its binding affinity for pleiotrophin/heparin binding growth-associated molecule. *J. Biol. Chem.* **278**, 35805–35811.

Malmström, A., and Fransson, L. A. (1971). Structure of pig skin dermatan sulfate. 2. Demonstration of sulfated iduronic acid residues. *Eur. J. Biochem.* **18**, 431–435.

Mark, M. P., Baker, J. R., Morrison, K., and Ruch, J. V. (1990a). Chondroitin sulfates in developing mouse tooth germs. An immunohistochemical study with monoclonal antibodies against chondroitin-4 and chondroitin-6 sulfates. *Differentiation* **43**, 37–50.

Mark, M. P., Baker, J. R., Kimata, K., and Ruch, J. V. (1990b). Regulated changes in chondroitin sulfation during embryogenesis: An immunohistochemical approach. *Int. J. Dev. Biol.* **34**, 191–204.

Mathews, M. B. (1962). Sodium chondroitin sulfate-protein complexes of cartilage. III. Preparation from shark. *Biochim. Biophys. Acta* **58**, 92–101.

Medeiros, G. F., Mendes, A., Castro, R. A., Bau, E. C., Nader, H. B., and Dietrich, C. P. (2000). Distribution of sulfated glycosaminoglycans in the animal kingdom: Widespread occurrence of heparin-like compounds in invertebrates. *Biochim. Biophys. Acta* **1475**, 287–294.

Meyer, K. (1938). The chemistry and biology of mucopolysaccharides and glycoproteins. *Cold Spring Harbor Symp. Quant. Biol.* **6**, 91–102.

Michelacci, Y. M., and Dietrich, C. P. (1975). A comparative study between a chondroitinase B and a chondroitinase AC from *Flavobacterium heparinum*: Isolation of a chondroitinase AC-susceptible dodecasaccharide from chondroitin sulphate B. *Biochem. J.* **151**, 121–129.

Michelacci, Y. M., and Dietrich, C. P. (1976). Chondroitinase C from *Flavobacterium heparinum*. *J. Biol. Chem.* **251**, 1154–1158.

Michelacci, Y. M., and Horton, D. S. P. Q. (1989). Proteoglycans from the cartilage of young hammerhead shark *Sphyrna-lewini*. *Comp. Biochem. Physiol.* **92B**, 651–658.

Michelacci, Y. M., Mourão, P. A., Laredo, J., and Dietrich, C. P. (1979). Chondroitin sulfates and proteoglycans from normal and arthrosic human cartilage. *Connect. Tissue Res.* **7**, 29–36.

Misevic, G. N., and Burger, M. M. (1990). The species-specific cell-binding site of the aggregation factor from the sponge *Microciona prolifera* is a highly repetitive novel glycan containing glucuronic acid, fucose, and mannose. *J. Biol. Chem.* **265**, 20577–20584.

Mizuguchi, S., Uyama, T., Kitagawa, H., Nomura, K. H., Dejima, K., Gengyo-Ando, K., Mitani, S., Sugahara, K., and Nomura, K. (2003). Chondroitin proteoglycans are involved in cell division of *Caenorhabditis elegans*. *Nature* **423**, 443–448.

Mourão, P. A. (1988). Distribution of chondroitin 4-sulfate and chondroitin 6-sulfate in human articular and growth cartilage. *Arthritis Rheum.* **31**, 1028–1033.

Muir, H. (1977). Structure and function of proteoglycans of cartilage and cell-matrix interactions. *Soc. Gen. Physiol. Ser.* **32**, 87–99.

Nadanaka, S., and Sugahara, K. (1997). The unusual tetrasaccharide sequence GlcA beta 1-3GalNAc(4-sulfate)beta 1-4GlcA(2-sulfate)beta 1-3GalNAc(6-sulfate) found in the hexasaccharides prepared by testicular hyaluronidase digestion of shark cartilage chondroitin sulfate D. *Glycobiology* **7**, 253–263.

Nader, H. B. (1991). Characterization of a heparan sulfate and a peculiar chondroitin 4-sulfate proteoglycan from platelets: Inhibition of the aggregation process by platelet chondroitin sulfate proteoglycan. *J. Biol. Chem.* **266**, 10518–10523.

Nader, H. B., and Dietrich, C. P. (1989). Natural occurrence, and possible biological role of heparin. *In* "Heparin. Chemical and Biological Properties. Clinical Applications" (D. A. Lane and U. Lindahl, Eds.), pp. 81–96. Edward Arnold, London.

Nader, H. B., Marx, W., and Spolter, L. (1980). Glycosaminoglycans of some mouse mastocytomas. *Biochim. Biophys. Acta* **631**, 463–478.

Nader, H. B., Medeiros, M. G. L., Paiva, J. F., Paiva, V. M. P., Jerônimo, S. M. B., Ferreira, T. M. P. C., and Dietrich, C. P. (1983). A correlation between the sulfated glycosaminoglycan concentration and degree of salinity of the habitat in fifteen species of the classes Crustacea, Pelecypoda and Gastropoda. *Comp. Biochem. Physiol.* **76B**, 433–436.

Nader, H. B., Ferreira, T. M., Paiva, J. F., Medeiros, M. G., Jeronimo, S. M., Paiva, V. M., and Dietrich, C. P. (1984). Isolation and structural studies of heparan sulfates and chondroitin sulfates from three species of molluscs. *J. Biol. Chem.* **259**, 1431–1435.

Nader, H. B., Jeronimo, S. M. B., Porcionatto, M. A., and Dietrich, C. P. (1985). Biosynthesis of acidic galactan and sulfated glycosaminoglycans during embryonic development of the mollusk *Pomacea sp. Biochim. Biophys. Acta* **840**, 187–192.

Nader, H. B., Oliveira, F. W., Jeronimo, S. M., Chavante, S. F., Sampaio, L. O., and Dietrich, C. P. (1996). Synchronized order of appearance of hyaluronic acid (or acidic galactan) –> chondroitin C-6 sulfate –> chondroitin C-4/C-6 sulfate, heparan sulfate, dermatan sulfate –> heparin during morphogenesis, differentiation and development. *Braz. J. Med. Biol. Res.* **29**, 1221–1226.

Nader, H. B., Chavante, S. F., dos-Santos, E. A., Oliveira, T. W., Paiva, J. F., Jerônimo, S. M., Medeiros, G. F., de-Abreu, L. R., Leite, E. L., de-Sousa-Filho, J. F., Castro, R. A.Toma, L., *et al.* (1999). Heparan sulfates and heparins: Similar compounds performing the same functions in vertebrates and invertebrates? *Braz. J. Med. Biol. Res.* **32**, 529–538.

Nandini, C. D., Mikami, T., Ohta, M., Itoh, N., Akiyama-Nambu, F., and Sugahara, K. (2004). Structural and functional characterization of oversulfated chondroitin sulfate/dermatan sulfate hybrid chains from the notochord of hagfish. Neuritogenic and binding activities for growth factors and neurotrophic factors. *J. Biol. Chem.* **279**, 50799–50809.

Papakonstantinou, E., and Misevic, G. N. (1993). Isolation and characterization of a new class of acidic glycans implicated in sea urchin embryonal cell adhesion. *J. Cell Biochem.* **53**, 98–113.

Papakonstantinou, E., Karakiulakis, G., Aletras, A. J., and Misevic, G. N. (1994). A novel class of adhesion acidic glycans in sea urchin embryos. Isolation, characterization and immunological studies during early embryonal development. *Eur. J. Biochem.* **224**, 1067–1077.

Pavão, M. S., Mourão, P. A., Mulloy, B., and Tollefsen, D. M. (1995). A unique dermatan sulfate-like glycosaminoglycan from ascidian. Its structure and the effect of its unusual sulfation pattern on anticoagulant activity. *J. Biol. Chem.* **270**, 31027–31036.

Pavão, M. S., Aiello, K. R., Werneck, C. C., Silva, L. C., Valente, A. P., Mulloy, B., Colwell, N. S., Tollefsen, D. M., and Mourão, P. A. (1998). Highly sulfated dermatan sulfates from Ascidians. Structure versus anticoagulant activity of these glycosaminoglycans. *J. Biol. Chem.* **273**, 27848–27857.

Pinto, D. O., Ferreira, P. L., Andrade, L. R., Petrs-Silva, H., Linden, R., Abdelhay, E., Araújo, H. M., Alonso, C. E., and Pavão, M. S. (2004). Biosynthesis and metabolism of sulfated glycosaminoglycans during *Drosophila melanogaster* development. *Glycobiology* **14**, 529–536.

Poblacion, C. A., and Michelacci, Y. M. (1986). Structural differences of dermatan sulfates from different origins. *Carbohydr. Res.* **147**, 87–100.

Prydz, K., and Dalen, K. T. (2000). Synthesis and sorting of proteoglycans. *J. Cell Sci.* **113**, 193–205.

Razin, E., Stevens, R. L., Akiyama, F., Schmid, K., and Austen, K. F. (1982). Culture from mouse bone marrow of a subclass of mast cells possessing a distinct chondroitin sulfate proteoglycan with glycosaminoglycans rich in N-acetylgalactosamine-4,6-disulfate. *J. Biol. Chem.* **257**, 7229–7236.

Roberts, I. S. (1996). The biochemistry and genetics of capsular polysaccharide production in bacteria. *Annu. Rev. Microbiol.* **50**, 285–315.

Rodriguez, M. L., Jann, B., and Jann, K. (1988). Structure and serological characteristics of the capsular K4 antigen of *Escherichia coli* O5:K4:H4, a fructose-containing polysaccharide with a chondroitin backbone. *Eur. J. Biochem.* **177**, 117–124.

Rothenberg, M. E., Caulfield, J. P., Austen, K. F., Hein, A., Edmiston, K., Newburger, P. E., and Stevens, R. L. (1987). Biochemical and morphological characterization of basophilic leukocytes from two patients with myelogenous leukemia. *J. Immunol.* **138**, 2616–2625.

Sakai, S., Kim, W. S., Lee, I. S., Kim, Y. S., Nakamura, A., Toida, T., and Imanari, T. (2003). Purification and characterization of dermatan sulfate from the skin of the eel. *Anguilla japonica. Carbohydr. Res.* **338**, 263–269.

Sampaio, L. O., and Dietrich, C. P. (1981). Changes of sulfated mucopolysaccharides and mucopolysaccharidases during fetal development. *J. Biol. Chem.* **256**, 9205–9210.

Sampaio, L. O., Dietrich, C. P., and Gianotti-Filho, O. G. (1977). Changes in sulfated mucopolysaccharide composition of mammalian tissues during growth and in cancer tissues. *Biochim. Biophys. Acta* **498**, 123–131.

Sampaio, L. O., Bayliss, M. T., Hardingham, T. E., and Muir, H. (1988). Dermatan sulphate proteoglycan from human articular cartilage: Variation in its content with age and its structural comparison with a small chondroitin sulphate proteoglycan from pig laryngeal cartilage. *Biochem. J.* **254**, 757–764.

Santos, E. A., Rocha, L. R., Pereira, N. M., Andrade, G. P., Nader, H. B., and Dietrich, C. P. (2002). Mast cells are present in epithelial layers of different tissues of the mollusc *Anomalocardia brasiliana. In situ* characterization of heparin and a correlation of heparin and histamine concentration. *Histochem. J.* **34**, 553–558.

Seldin, D. C., Austen, K. F., and Stevens, R. L. (1985). Purification and characterization of protease-resistant secretory granule proteoglycans containing chondroitin sulfate di-B and heparin-like glycosaminoglycans from rat basophilic leukemia cells. *J. Biol. Chem.* **260**, 11131–11139.

Seno, N., and Sekizuka, E. (1978). Structure of linkage region between chondroitin polysulfates and peptides. *J. Biochem.* **83**, 953–956.

Silbert, J. E., and Sugumaran, G. (2002a). A starting place for the road to function. *Glycoconj. J.* **19**, 227–237.

Silbert, J. E., and Sugumaran, G. (2002b). Biosynthesis of chondroitin/dermatan sulfate. *IUBMB Life* **54**, 177–186.

Spillmann, D., Thomas-Oates, J. E., van Kuik, J. A., Vliegenthart, J. F., Misevic, G., Burger, M. M., and Finne, J. (1995). Characterization of a novel sulfated carbohydrate unit implicated in the carbohydrate-carbohydrate-mediated cell aggregation of the marine sponge *Microciona prolifera. J. Biol. Chem.* **270**, 5089–5097.

Stevens, R. L. (1986). Secretory granule proteoglycans of mast cells and natural killer cells. *Ciba Found. Symp.* **124**, 272–285.

Sugahara, K., Tanaka, Y., Yamada, S., Seno, N., Kitagawa, H., Haslam, S. M., Morris, H. R., and Dell, A. (1996). Novel sulfated oligosaccharides containing 3-O-sulfated glucuronic acid from king crab cartilage chondroitin sulfate K. Unexpected degradation by chondroitinase ABC. *J. Biol. Chem.* **271**, 26745–26754.

Sugahara, K., Mikami, T., Uyama, T., Mizuguchi, S., Nomura, K., and Kitagawa, H. (2003). Recent advances in the structural biology of chondroitin sulfate and dermatan sulfate. *Curr. Opin. Struct. Biol.* **13**, 612–620.

Suzuki, S. (1960). Isolation of novel disaccharides from chondroitin sulfates. *J. Biol. Chem.* **235**, 3580–3588.

Suzuki, S., Saito, H., Yamagata, T., Anno, K., Seno, N., Kawai, Y., and Furuhashi, T. (1968). Formation of three types of disulfated disaccharides from chondroitin sulfates by chondroitinase digestion. *J. Biol. Chem.* **243**, 1543–1550.

Thompson, H. L., Schulman, E. S., and Metcalfe, D. D. (1988). Identification of chondroitin sulfate E in human lung mast cells. *J. Immunol.* **140**, 2708–2713.

Toledo, O. M., and Dietrich, C. P. (1977). Tissue specific distribution of sulfated mucopoly-saccharides in mammals. *Biochim. Biophys. Acta* **498**, 114–122.

Toole, B. P. (2001). Hyaluronan in morphogenesis. *Sem. Cell Develop. Biol.* **12**, 79–87.

Tsuchida, K., Shioi, J., Yamada, S., Boghosian, G., Wu, A., Cai, H., Sugahara, K., and Robakis, N. K. (2001). Appican, the proteoglycan form of the amyloid precursor protein, contains chondroitin sulfate E in the repeating disaccharide region and 4-O-sulfated galactose in the linkage region. *J. Biol. Chem.* **276**, 37155–37160.

Ueoka, C., Nadanaka, S., Seno, N., Khoo, K.-H., and Sugahara, K. (1999). Structural determination of novel tetra- and hexasaccharide sequences isolated from chondroitin sulfate H (oversulfated dermatan sulfate) of hagfish notochord. *Glycoconj. J.* **16**, 291–305.

Vann, W. F., Schmidt, M. A., Jann, B., and Jann, K. (1981). The structure of the capsular polysaccharide (K5 antigen) of urinary-tract-infective *Escherichia coli* 010:K5:H4. A polymer similar to desulfo-heparin. *Eur. J. Biochem.* **116**, 359–364.

Vicente, C. P., Zancan, P., Peixoto, L. L., Alves-Sa, R., Araujo, F. S., Mourão, P. A., and Pavão, M. S. (2001). Unbalanced effects of dermatan sulfates with different sulfation patterns on coagulation, thrombosis and bleeding. *Thromb. Haemost.* **86**, 1215–1220.

Vieira, R. P., and Mourão, P. A. (1988). Occurrence of a unique fucose-branched chondroitin sulfate in the body wall of a sea cucumber. *J. Biol. Chem.* **263**, 18176–18183.

Vieira, R. P., Mulloy, B., and Mourão, P. A. (1991). Structure of a fucose-branched chondroitin sulfate from sea cucumber. Evidence for the presence of 3-O-sulfo-beta-D-glucuronosyl residues. *J. Biol. Chem.* **266**, 13530–13536.

Vilela-Silva, A. C., Werneck, C. C., Valente, A. P., Vacquier, V. D., and Mourão, P. A. (2001). Embryos of the sea urchin *Strongylocentrotus purpuratus* synthesize a dermatan sulfate enriched in 4-O- and 6-O-disulfated galactosamine units. *Glycobiology* **11**, 433–440.

Volpi, N., and Mucci, A. (1988). Characterization of a low-sulfated chondroitin sulfate from the body of *Viviparus ater* (mollusca gastropoda). Modification of its structure by lead pollution. *Glycoconj. J.* **15**, 1071–1078.

Wilson, J. C., Hitchen, P. G., Frank, M., Peak, I. R., Collins, P. M., Morris, H. R., Dell, A., and Grice, I. D. (2005). Identification of a capsular polysaccharide from *Moraxella bovis*. *Carbohydr. Res.* **340**, 765–769.

Yamada, S., Yamane, Y., Sakamoto, K., Tsuda, H., and Sugahara, K. (1998). Structural determination of sulfated tetrasaccharides and hexasaccharides containing a rare disaccharide sequence, -3GalNAc(4,6-disulfate)beta1-4IdoAalpha1-, isolated from por-cine intestinal dermatan sulfate. *Eur. J. Biochem.* **258**, 775–783.

Yamada, S., Van Die, I., Van den Eijnden, D. H., Yokota, A., Kitagawa, H., and Sugahara, K. (1999). Demonstration of glycosaminoglycans in *Caenorhabditis elegans*. *FEBS Lett.* **459**, 327–331.

Yaoita, E., Oguri, K., Okayama, E., Kawasaki, K., Kobayashi, S., Kihara, I., and Okayama, M. (1990). Isolation and characterization of proteoglycans synthesized by cultured mesangial cells. *J. Biol. Chem.* **265**, 522–531.

Zhuo, L., Salustri, A., and Kimata, K. (2003). A physiological function of serum proteogly-can bikunin: The chondroitin sulfate moiety plays a central role. *Glycoconj. J.* **19**, 241–247.

Zierer, M. S., and Mourão, P. A. (2000). A wide diversity of sulfated polysaccharides are synthesized by different species of marine sponges. *Carbohydr. Res.* **328**, 209–216.

Chilkunda D. Nandini* and Kazuyuki Sugahara[†]

Department of Biochemistry
Kobe Pharmaceutical University
Kobe 658–8558, Japan

Role of the Sulfation Pattern of Chondroitin Sulfate in its Biological Activities and in the Binding of Growth Factors

I. Chapter Overview

In recent years chondroitin sulfate (CS) has become a focus of attention by virtue of its important roles in wound healing, promoting neurite outgrowth, axonal regeneration, cell adhesion, cell division, the regulatory roles of growth factors, and so on. Some of these biological activities are at least partly attributable to the interactions of glycosaminoglycans (GAGs) with heparin-binding growth factors. CS chains, with high heterogeneity and variable sulfation patterns, might form distinct domains, which facilitate the growth factors' binding. Here, we review the structural characteristics

* Present address: Department of Pathology and Laboratory Medicine, University of Wisconsin, Madison, WI 53792–8550, USA.
[†] Present address: Graduate School of Life Science, Faculty of Advanced Life Science, Hokkaido University, Sapporo 001–0021, Japan.

Advances in Pharmacology, Volume 53
Copyright 2006, Elsevier Inc. All rights reserved.

1054-3589/06 $35.00
DOI: 10.1016/S1054-3589(05)53012-6

of various CS chains and their binding activity toward growth factors based on available data. Intriguingly, most of the growth factors tested are expressed in the brain. CS variants exhibit typical patterns of binding to growth factors and neurotrophic factors, when tested using the BIAcore or the interaction analysis system (IAsys). Heparan sulfate (HS) and CS chains in a proteoglycan (PG) show synergistic effects by complementing or cooperating with each other in the binding of a growth factor through dynamic interactions. The presence of iduronic acid results in better binding of growth factors. However, for a more efficient binding, a domain consisting of both glucuronic acid and iduronic acid appears to be essential.

II. Introduction

Chondroitin sulfate chains are complex polysaccharides synthesized as GAG side chains of PGs. CS chains are linear polymers comprising glucuronic acid (GlcA) and N-acetyl-D-galactosamine (GalNAc). They are widely distributed in the extracellular matrix (ECM) and at the cell surface. Until recently, the attention in this field has been garnered by HS. However, accumulating evidence suggests pivotal functions of CS in various biological processes (Sugahara and Kitagawa 2000; Sugahara and Yamada, 2000; Sugahara *et al.*, 2003). CS chains have been found in significant amounts in the central nervous system, being implicated in its development (Herndon and Lander, 1990) in addition to wound repair (Trowbridge and Gallo, 2002), infection (Bergefall *et al.*, 2005; Menozzi *et al.*, 2002), growth factors' signaling (Bao *et al.*, 2005a), coagulation (Liaw *et al.*, 2001), and so on apart from other structural roles. In this chapter, we focus on recent advances in the study of CS, with varying structural characteristics, in the binding of growth factors and other biological activities based on recently obtained data.

III. Structures of Typical Disaccharide Units in CS chains

CS chains typically consist of repeating disaccharide units of -4GlcAβ1–3GalNAcβ1-, which can be sulfated on GlcA and/or GalNAc residues. Ordinary CS chains contain monosulfated disaccharide units -4GlcAβ1–3GalNAc(4S) and -4GlcAβ1–3GalNAc(6S), which have been designated as the A unit and C unit, respectively. Such units are present in various proportions in polymer CS chains designated as CS-A, CS-C, or hybrid CS chains, depending on the ratio of the building units. Apart from the earlier mentioned disaccharide units, oversulfated CS chains contain disulfated disaccharide units, such as D, E, H, and K, as exemplified in Fig. 1A (Sugahara and Yamada, 2000). CS chains with iduronic acid (IdoA)-containing disaccharide units are known as CS-B or dermatan sulfate

(DS), which is a stereoisoform of CS, differing at C-5 of hexuronic acid moieties. DS, therefore, consists of disaccharide units iA, iB, iD, and iE, where "i" stands for IdoA along with other conventional disaccharides (Fig. 1B). Unique disaccharides, such as 3-O-sulfated GlcA residues, were detected in squid cartilage CS-E and king crab cartilage CS-K (Kinoshita *et al.*, 1997; Sugahara and Yamada, 2000) and designated as units K, L, and M (Fig. 1C). Fucosylated disaccharide, which is sulfated at the C-4 position, has been designated as unit F.

IV. Structural Variation in CS chains

CS chains vary widely in structure including length, arrangement of disaccharide units, charge density, sulfation pattern, configuration, and so on (Sugahara and Yamada, 2000). Most information regarding structure has been obtained using a combination of techniques involving depolymerization of the CS chain by enzymatic or other hydrolytic methods, HPLC, MALDI-TOF-MS, NMR spectroscopy, gel filtration analysis, and so on. These polysaccharides are found in divergent organisms from worms to humans. Structural elucidation of CS chains has been carried out particularly in marine organisms (Habuchi *et al.*, 1977; Vieira and Mourão, 1988), which were found to exhibit widely varied structural characteristics.

Two oligosaccharides containing glucose were isolated from squid cartilage CS-E (Kinoshita-Toyoda *et al.*, 2004). In that study, squid cartilage CS-E was extensively digested with chondroitinase AC-II, which yielded five highly sulfated novel tetrasaccharides and two odd-numbered oligosaccharides (tri- and pentasaccharides) containing D-Glc. Their structures, determined by fast atom bombardment mass spectrometry and ^{1}H NMR spectroscopy, revealed an internal GlcA(3-O-sulfate) residue for all the novel tetrasaccharide sequences, which rendered the oligosaccharides resistant to the enzyme. The results suggest that GlcA(3-O-sulfate) units are not clustered but rather interspersed in the CS-E polysaccharide chains, being preferentially located in the highly sulfated sequences. The predominant structure (80%) on the nonreducing side of a GlcA(3-O-sulfate) residue was GalNAc(4-O-sulfate), whereas that (59%) on the reducing side was GalNAc(4,6-O-disulfate). The structural variety in the vicinity of the GlcA (3-O-sulfate) residue might represent the substrate specificity of the unidentified chondroitin GlcA 3-O-sulfotransferase, which synthesizes this structure. The results also revealed a trisaccharide and a pentasaccharide sequence, both of which contained a β-D-Glc branch at the C-6 position of the constituent GalNAc residue (Kinoshita-Toyoda *et al.*, 2004).

A

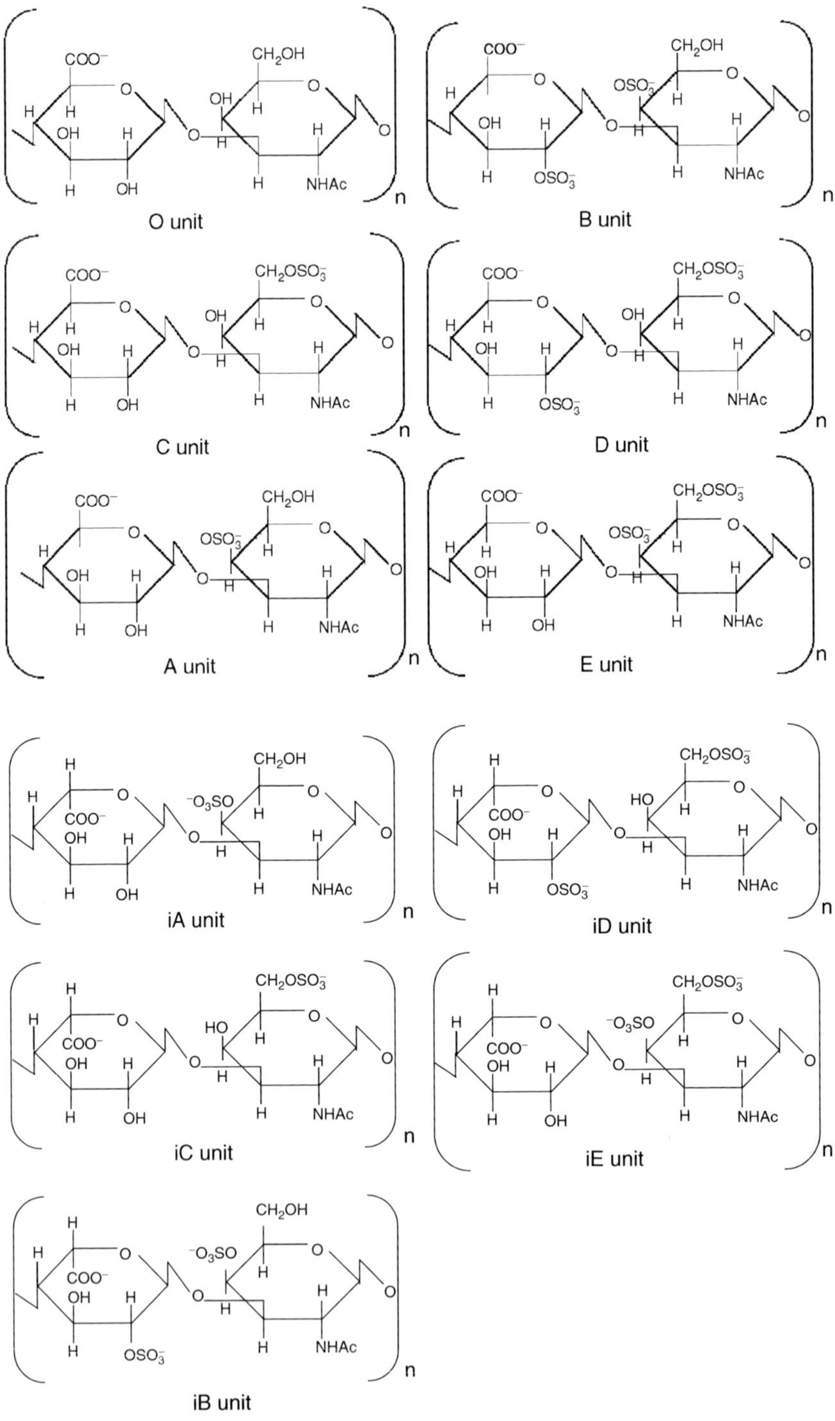

O unit

B unit

C unit

D unit

A unit

E unit

iA unit

iD unit

iC unit

iE unit

iB unit

C

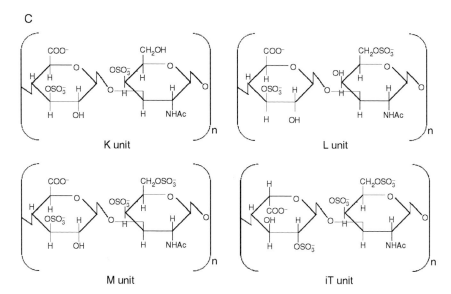

K unit

L unit

M unit

iT unit

FIGURE 1   Structures of disaccharides of CS/DS chains. Disaccharide units predominantly present in CS chains and named based on the sulfation pattern are given in Fig. 1(A), whereas the disaccharide units found in DS or CS/DS hybrid chains are given in Fig. 1(B). "i" in Fig. 1 (B) and (C) represents IdoA. Other minor disaccharide units, which have been identified in various oversulfated CS variants from different sources, are given in Fig. 1(C).

In view of the fact that CS chains are involved in various biological activities, which are brought about presumably by binding to various growth factors, a series of experiments were performed in our laboratory and elsewhere to delineate the essential structural elements in CS isoforms responsible for the binding of growth factors. 6B4-PG/phosphacan is a major PG in the brain and corresponds to the extracellular region of a receptor-type protein-tyrosine phosphatase PTPζ/RPTPβ (Maeda and Noda, 1998; Maeda *et al.*, 1996), which turned out to be identical to DSD-1-PG (Garwood *et al.*, 1999) with neurite outgrowth-promoting activity (Faissner *et al.*, 1994). The CS chains of PTPζ/RPTPβ bind a heparin (Hep)-binding growth factor, pleiotrophin (PTN) (discussed later). Phosphacan was localized immunohistochemically, and it was postulated that the CS chains showed variations during different stages of the brain development (Maeda *et al.*, 2003). Based on the preceding information, phosphacan was purified from different regions of the brain at the different ages and designated as PG-P7, PG-P12, and PG-P20. The disaccharide composition of CS chains was studied based on susceptibility to chondroitinase ABC, and it was observed that PG-P7 had the least amount of A units, the amount of C units decreased drastically from PG-P7 to PG-P20, and D units, which have been implicated in the promotion of neurite outgrowth (Clement *et al.*, 1998; Nadanaka *et al.*, 1998), could only be detected in PG-P20 to the tune of 1.3%. The chain length as well as GlcA content, however, did not show any significant difference (Maeda *et al.*, 2003).

DS, another isomeric variant of CS, was found in the embryonic pig brain, forming a hybrid structure with CS (Bao *et al.*, 2004). To determine the subtle structural variations occurring during the process of development, CS/DS chains were isolated from both embryonic and adult pig brain by extraction with physiological buffers, such as phosphate-buffered saline (PBS), although a significant proportion of cell-surface-bound chains, which were not extracted with PBS, was found. CS/DS chains isolated from embryonic pig brains bore higher proportions of nonsulfated disaccharides than those of adult pig brain. The number of sulfate groups per mole of disaccharide was 0.83–0.84 in the chains of embryonic brain and 0.99 in those of adult brain (Table I), and the two types of chains were similar in molecular size. The main difference was in the amount of IdoA-containing residues; 8–9% in the CS chains extracted from embryonic pig brain compared to less than 1% of all the disaccharides extracted from adult pig brain. The presence of IdoA-containing disaccharides was deduced based on the difference in the resistant oligosaccharides obtained on digestion with chondroitinase AC-I and ABC. Presumably, at least some of the CS/DS chains are derived from phosphacan. These residues had implications for the binding of growth factors as discussed in a later section.

Syndecans are the major cell surface PGs expressed by virtually all epithelial cells. Four kinds of syndecans form a gene family, the transmembrane and cytoplasmic domain being conserved among all of the members (Bernfield *et al.*, 1999, Carey, 1997; Fitzgerald and Bernfield, 1999; Zimmermann and David, 1999). These syndecans show varied expression depending on the cell, tissue, and developmental stage (Kato *et al.*, 1994; Lindahl *et al.*, 1995), suggesting distinct functions for each family member (Kim *et al.*, 1994), although some share activities as has been observed for syndecan-1 and -4 (Bernfield *et al.*, 1999; Carey, 1997; Woods *et al.*, 1998). The majority of GAG chains added to the core proteins of syndecans are of HS type, although syndecan-1 (Rapraeger *et al.*, 1985) and syndecan-4 (Shworak *et al.*, 1994) are modified by CS chains as well. Both the syndecans have been implicated in the promotion of intracellular adhesion and wound healing. Although syndecans-1 and -4 have hybrid structures, information relating to the biological functions attributable to the structure of the CS chains is very limited. The disaccharide composition of the CS chains was studied in our lab after exhaustively digesting the ectodomains of syndecan-1 and -4 with chondroitinase ABC, and the resulting disaccharides were identified using HPLC. The results revealed that syndecan-1 is less sulfated than syndecan-4, with a sulfate to disaccharide ratio of 0.78

TABLE I Disaccharide Composition of Some of the CS Variants Used in Growth Factor Binding Studies

GAG	Biological origin	ΔO[a]	ΔA	ΔC	ΔD	ΔB	ΔE	ΔT	S/Unit
CS-D[c]	Shark skin	ND[b]	36.0	43.0	20.0	ND	1.0	ND	1.21
CS-E[d]	Squid cartilage	8.0	19.0	8.0	ND	ND	56.0	ND	1.53
CS/DS[e]	Hagfish	4.7	38.3	13.5	ND	ND	39.6	3.9	1.43
CS/DS[f]	Shark skin	5.8	55.0	16.6	3.4	8.0	11.2	ND	1.17
CS/DS[g]	Embryonic pig brain	20.0	45.3	32.2	1.5	ND	1.0	ND	0.825
CS/DS[g]	Adult pig brain	4.3	83.0	9.4	1.8	ND	1.5	ND	0.99
CS[b] (Appican)	C6 glioma	1.2	81.2	3.3	ND	ND	14.3	ND	1.13
CS[b] (Appican)	SH-SY5Y neuroblastoma cells	ND	77.5	22.5	ND	ND	ND	ND	1.00
CS[i] (Syndecan-1)	NMuMG cells	29.0	59.0	5.0	ND	ND	7.0	ND	0.78
CS[i] (Syndecan-4)	NMuMG cells	6.0	68.0	17.0	ND	ND	9.0	ND	1.03
CS[j] (DSD-1-PG)	Mouse brain	2.0	68.0	23.0	5.0	ND	ND	ND	1.03

[a] The abbreviations used are ΔO, ΔHexUAα1–3GalNAc; ΔA, ΔHexUA(4-O-sulfate)α1–3GalNAc; ΔC, ΔHexUA(6-O-sulfate)α1–3GalNAc; ΔD, ΔHexUA (2-O-sulfate)α1–3GalNAc(6-O-sulfate); ΔB, ΔHexUA(2-O-sulfate)α1–3GalNAc(4-O-sulfate); ΔE, ΔHexUAα1–3GalNAc(4,6-O-disulfate); ΔT, ΔHexUA (2-O-sulfate)α1–3GalNAc(4,6-O-disulfate).

[b] Not determined.

[c] C. D. Nandini and K. Sugahara, unpublished data.

[d] Note that CS-E includes unusual disulfated and trisulfated disaccharide units containing GlcUA(3S), which are decomposed by chondroitinase ABC and account for up to 10% of all the uronic acid depending on the preparation (Hikino *et al.*, 2003). Hence, the disaccharide composition here was calculated by multiplying the total concentration of disaccharides (mol%) detected by digestion with chondroitinase ABC by a factor of 0.9, and the S/Unit value may be slightly underestimated.

[e] Taken from Nandini *et al.*, 2004.

[f] Taken from Nandini *et al.*, 2005.

[g] Taken from Bao *et al.*, 2004.

[h] Taken from Umehara *et al.*, 2004.

[i] Taken from Deepa *et al.*, 2004.

[j] Taken from Clement *et al.*, 1998.

and1.03, respectively (Table I). In the same vein, syndecan-1 had higher proportions of unsulfated disaccharide and C disaccharide units than syndecan-4, thus pointing to microheterogenity in the CS chain (Deepa *et al.*, 2004). The binding activity of syndecan-1 and -4 toward various growth factors will be discussed in a later section.

CS/DS chains were also isolated from marine sources such as hagfish notochord and shark skin (Nandini *et al.*, 2004, 2005). Notochord is a connective tissue that supports the neural tube and induces the formation of the central nervous system during the development of vertebrates. Earlier, a fraction of isolated CS-H, which was obtained by elution with 3.0 M NaCl on a Dowex column (Anno *et al.*, 1971), was digested, and quite a few of the resulting oligosaccharides were structurally characterized (Ueoka *et al.*, 1999). It showed the presence exclusively of IdoA-containing residues. The CS-H fraction used in subsequent studies was eluted with 2.0 M NaCl and interestingly was a mixture of CS and DS. The digest obtained with chondroitinase ABC showed the presence of large proportions of E (39.6 %) and B (38.3%) units. Digestion with chondroitinase AC-I or B gave rise to a large number of oligosaccharides, suggesting that GlcA-containing and IdoA-containing disaccharide units were distributed throughout the length of the chain. It exhibited a sulfate to disaccharide ratio of 1.43 and a molecular mass of 18 kDa.

Similarly, CS-GAG chains from shark skin were also of a hybrid nature (Nandini *et al.*, 2005) and of a large molecular size (60 kDa). The disaccharide composition revealed a highly complex and heterogeneous structure. The chains were rather unique in that they contained multiple disulfated disaccharide units in appreciable amounts unlike preparations isolated from other marine sources (Anno *et al.*, 1971; Pavão *et al.*, 1995, 1998). The unfractionated CS/DS preparation had a sulfate/disaccharide ratio of 1.08, which was similar to that exemplified by CS/DS-PG (named endocan) secreted from human endothelial cells and circulating in the human bloodstream (Bechard *et al.*, 2001). This finding suggests that CS/DS hybrid chains with a comparable degree of sulfation are indeed present in mammalian systems, which could have wide implications in the development of therapeutics. Another feature observed in shark skin DS is the presence of a unique disaccharide unit, GlcA-containing disulfated disaccharide B unit, which has been hitherto unreported. The functional significance of such units is yet to be ascertained.

V. Epitope Structure Characterized by Monoclonal Antibodies Useful for Immunohistochemistry

To date various monoclonal antibodies, directed against CS variants, have been generated, which has contributed greatly to the localization of CS chains in various tissues. Antibodies, such as CS-56 (Avnur and Geiger, 1984) and MO-225 (Yamagata *et al.*, 1987), have been widely used in detecting CS variants. CS-56 reportedly reacts with CS-A and CS-C (Avnur and Geiger, 1984), but it strongly reacts with CS-D but does not react with variant A, B, or E. In contrast, MO-225 (Yamagata *et al.*, 1987) reacts strongly with CS-D, moderately with CS-C and CS-E, and weakly with CS-A. On the other hand, mAb 473HD recognizes a characteristic CS structure called the DSD-1 epitope, which has neurite outgrowth-promoting activity toward hippocampal neurons (Faissner *et al.*, 1994) and contains the D unit (Clement *et al.*, 1998, 1999; Nadanaka *et al.*, 1998). However, the epitopic structures recognized by these antibodies are poorly characterized.

Attempts have been made to characterize the epitopic structure recognized by the three anti-CS antibodies, CS-56, MO-225, and 473HD (Ito *et al.*, 2005), using size- and structure-defined CS oligosaccharides (Sugahara and Yamada, 2000) obtained from CS-D by employing ELISA and the oligosaccharide microarray method (Fukui *et al.*, 2002). The oligosaccharide fractions to be tested were chemically coupled to the amino group of dipalmitoylphosphatidylethanolamine (DPPE), using their reducing terminal aldehyde groups by reductive amination (Stoll *et al.*, 1988), without disturbing the sulfation pattern-dependent antigenic structures embedded in the CS oligosaccharides. The resultant neoglycolipid probes were immobilized either in microtitre wells on an ELISA plate or onto nitrocellulose membranes to prepare an oligosaccharide microarray. Results obtained by ELISA as well as using the microarray system revealed that the minimum size required for recognition by CS-56 was an octasaccharide, whereas it was a hexasaccharide and larger for MO-225 and 473HD. All the oligosaccharide sequences bound by 473HD, CS-56, and/or MO-225 contained at least a D unit. The unbound oligosaccharide fractions were characterized by an absence of D unit. The preference of these mAbs for CS-D among typical CS variants appears to be attributable to the abundant A–D tetrasaccharide sequence characteristic of CS-D. Additionally, mAb 473HD recognizes DSD-1-PG and nullifies the neuritogenic activity promoted by it. The neuritogenic activity is also abolished by digestion of DSD-1-PG with chondroitinase B, implicating IdoA as one of the active structural elements responsible for the biological activity (Ito *et al.*, 2005). However, the presence of a D unit or IdoA-containing A unit in the epitope recognized by 473HD needs to be unequivocally resolved, since its presence has been hypothesized based on indirect evidence. Further characterization of the epitopic structure will go a long way to furthering the understanding of biological activities attributed to it.

VI. Interactions of Heparin-Binding Growth Factors with CS Chains

The biological activities brought about by CS chains could possibly involve various growth factors, also known as Hep-binding growth factors for their capacity to bind Hep with high affinity. This affinity is due to a high-charge density as well as the presence of structural domains involved in the binding. The importance of CS chains in the binding of growth factors was realized when it was observed that neuronal cell adhesion, mediated by the Hep-binding growth factor, midkine (MK), was specifically inhibited not only by Hep but also by oversulfated squid CS-E (Ueoka et al., 2000). The neuronal cell adhesion was, however, not inhibited by other CS isoforms. It was also demonstrated that pleiotrophin (PTN), another Hep-binding growth factor, bound to 6B4-PG/phosphacan in postnatal day 16 rat brain, and this binding was inhibited by CS-C (Maeda and Noda, 1998; Maeda et al., 1996) presumably due to oversulfated D units contained in CS-C (see in a later section). 6B4-PG/phosphacan is a major PG in the brain and corresponds to the extracellular region of a receptor-like protein-tyrosine phosphatase, PTPζ/RPTPβ, which was found later to be identical to DSD-1-PG (Garwood et al., 1999).

A. Specific Molecular Interactions of Oversulfated CS Variants with Growth Factors

CS variants containing oversulfated disaccharide units, such as E and D, have been reported in bovine brain (Saigo and Egami, 1970), embryonic day 13 (E13) mice (Zou et al., 2003), and E18 rat brain (Ueoka et al., 2000). In embryonic chick brain, small amounts of oversulfated disaccharide units were detected along with A and C units, the proportions of which increased slightly as the development reached completion (Kitagawa et al., 1997). Their expression is developmentally regulated, which is coordinated by sulfotransferases namely chondroitin 4-O-sulfotransferase and chondroitin 6-O-sulfotransferase (Kitagawa et al., 1997). A significant proportion of E unit was observed in appican, which is a PG form of amyloid precursor protein. Appican contained 14.3% E unit (Tsuchida et al., 2001), demonstrating for the first time the presence of E units in a particular brain CSPG.

In view of the above findings, specific molecular interactions of CS-E with various growth factors were examined using real-time analysis with the filter binding assay and validated (Deepa et al., 2002) with the IAsys using an evanescent wave generated by wave guiding to probe the liquid phase. Representative growth factors of the MK family, EGF family, and FGF family were chosen, and the interactions of CS-E with MK, PTN, HB-EGF, FGF-1, FGF-2, FGF-10, FGF-16, and FGF-18 were tested. Among the growth factors taken for testing, all of them except FGF-16 are expressed in the brain during embryonic development. FGF-16, which is expressed in brown adipocytes during embryonic development, was also tested to clarify the generality of the binding of a Hep-binding growth factor to CS-E. Hep was used as a positive control. It was demonstrated that CS-E bound to all the growth factors tested except for FGF-1 in both systems in a dose-dependent manner, suggesting that the binding is highly specific. In both systems, wherein there is a variation in the dynamics of interaction, it was observed that all growth factors, except FGF-1, bound more strongly to CS-E than Hep in the filter binding assay, whereas Hep bound more strongly to the majority of the growth factors tested than CS-E in IAsys. IAsys more closely mimics physiological conditions in which the soluble growth factors interact with CS chains in an immobilized form at the cell surface or in the ECM. On the other hand, complexes measured in the filter binding assay, where both the interacting molecules are in solution, would mimic growth factor–CS complexes released enzymatically from the cell surface or ECM. The affinity of interaction measured in terms of association (k_a), dissociation (k_d), and dissociation equilibrium constants (K_d) showed that the interaction of immobilized CS-E with various growth factors other than FGF-1 was strong and comparable to that of Hep (Table II). FGF-1 bound weakly to CS-E as indicated by its high-K_d value. A CS-E or Hep chain accommodates multiple yet different numbers of various growth factors, probably reflecting distinct overlapping sequences for the binding of multiple growth factors, which are embedded in each sugar chain (Deepa *et al.*, 2002).

Growth factors, such as HB-EGF, showed quick binding and release. The significance of such a pattern of binding requires elucidation. There is a possibility that these low-affinity motifs act as a scaffold to capture the growth factor and then hand it over to other high-affinity motifs and finally direct the growth factor toward the site of interaction with its receptor target at the cell surface (Lander, 1998).

Appican, the CSPG form of the amyloid precursor protein, has been implicated in cell adhesion and neurite outgrowth (Breen *et al.*, 1991; Robakis *et al.*, 1990; Roch *et al.*, 1992). The CS chain of appican with a high proportion of E unit served as an interesting GAG to test the binding growth factors to understand its importance in the brain. The CS chain of appican produced by rat C6 glioma cells was compared with that of SH-SY5Y neuroblastoma cells for its growth factor-binding ability (Umehara *et al.*, 2004). As a first step, ^{3}H-labeled CS fractions were subjected to the nitrocellulose filter binding assay to examine whether the appican CS can bind some of the Hep-binding growth factors expressed in the brain. MK, PTN, FGF-2, and HB-EGF bound to the ^{3}H-labeled CS preparation in a concentration-dependent manner, which was abolished on digestion with chondroitinase ABC, confirming that these interactions are dependent on the CS chain. The interactions were also evaluated using IAsys by immobilizing biotinylated appican CSPG on a sensor chip coated with streptavidin. Both MK and PTN bound to the appican CS when tested at a concentration of 1 μg/ml. To determine the specificity of the binding of MK and PTN to appican CSPG, inhibition experiments were performed using various kinds of CS variants. Strong inhibition occurred only with CS-E, which led to the conclusion that the E disaccharide motif of the CS chain is essential for the binding of MK and PTN to appican CSPG. This was reinforced by the fact

TABLE II Kinetic Parameters of the Interaction of Various Growth Factors with Immobilized Hep and CS-E[a]

Growth factor	Hep			CS-E		
	$k_a\ (M^{-1}S^{-1})$	$k_d\ (s^{-1})$	$K_d\ (nM)$	$k_a\ (M^{-1}S^{-1})$	$k_d\ (s^{-1})$	$K_d\ (nM)$
FGF-2	$(2.4 \pm 0.2) \times 10^5$	$(0.2 \pm 0.06) \times 10^{-2}$	8.6 ± 3.2	$(3.3 \pm 0.3) \times 10^4$	$(0.4 \pm 0.02) \times 10^{-2}$	119.8 ± 14.2
FGF-10	$(1.4 \pm 0.3) \times 10^5$	$(0.2 \pm 0.15) \times 10^{-2}$	17.4 ± 14.4	$(6.5 \pm 2.0) \times 10^4$	$(0.5 \pm 0.07) \times 10^{-2}$	88.6 ± 37.8
FGF-18	$(6.3 \pm 2.9) \times 10^5$	$(0.4 \pm 0.30) \times 10^{-2}$	10.8 ± 9.7	$(5.7 \pm 2.3) \times 10^5$	$(0.3 \pm 0.29) \times 10^{-2}$	8.9 ± 8.7
HB-EGF	$(6.6 \pm 0.4) \times 10^5$	$(0.3 \pm 0.10) \times 10^{-2}$	4.7 ± 3.7	$(2.8 \pm 0.3) \times 10^6$	$(4.2 \pm 0.30) \times 10^{-2}$	16.0 ± 18.4
MK	$(3.5 \pm 1.5) \times 10^4$	$(0.6 \pm 0.08) \times 10^{-2}$	204.0 ± 100.0	$(1.1 \pm 0.3) \times 10^5$	$(0.6 \pm 0.1) \times 10^{-2}$	61.6 ± 25.9
PTN	$(2.6 \pm 0.9) \times 10^5$	$(0.3 \pm 0.20) \times 10^{-2}$	16.1 ± 13.3	$(4.5 \pm 0.4) \times 10^5$	$(0.5 \pm 0.10) \times 10^{-2}$	11.4 ± 3.22

[a]Taken from Deepa et al., 2002.

that appican CSPG produced by SH-SY5Y neuroblastoma cells did not bind either PTN or MK presumably due to the absence of E units (Umehara *et al.*, 2004).

Other oversulfated isoforms of CS also bind growth factors. Namely, CS-D from shark cartilage binds PTN and the CSPGs present in the brain bind PTN with high affinity (Maeda and Noda, 1998; Maeda *et al.*, 1996; Qi *et al.*, 2001). It has been suggested that phosphacan in the brain is composed of several subpopulations of molecules bearing CS chains with different structures, the immunological and compositional structures of which change dramatically during development (Clement *et al.*, 1998; Rauch *et al.*, 1991). Based on the information obtained by immunohistochemical analysis, phosphacan bearing CS chains with structural variations was anticipated and subsequently purified from appropriate regions of whole brain tissue of mice of various ages. The composition is shown in Section III (Maeda *et al.*, 2003). The direct binding of phosphacan with PTN was examined using a BIAcore system, which employs the principle of surface plasmon resonance. Here, PTN was immobilized on the surface of a CM5 sensor chip by amine coupling, where the primary amino groups on the protein were coupled to the carboxymethylated dextran surface. Phosphacan bound to the immobilized PTN with high affinity, which was again dependent on the structure of CS. In other words, PG-P20 displayed high-affinity binding to PTN ($K_d = 0.14$ nM) compared with PG-P7 and PG-P12, which showed fourfold to fivefold lower affinity for PTN than PG-P20. Digestion of phosphacan with chondroitinase ABC resulted in the elimination of the differences in affinity between the three phosphacan preparations and K_d values of 1.4–1.6 nM. This was caused mainly by a decrease in the association rate constants. From these results, it is clear that the presence of CS chains with variable structures influences the binding kinetics. Binding analysis was further carried out with various other GAG species; namely, CS-A, CS-B (DS), CS-C, CS-D, CS-E, and porcine intestinal Hep. CS-E, -D, and -C bound to the immobilized PTN with high affinity. CS-B (DS) also bound, but kinetic parameters were not calculated because of the slow kinetics. The above results indicated that the D unit in CS chains appears to be responsible for the high-affinity binding.

B. Specific Molecular Interactions of Dermatan Sulfate (CS-B) with Growth Factors

Until now, most of the growth factors have required IdoA to bind with GAG (Hileman *et al.*, 1998), with an exception being CS-E (Deepa *et al.*, 2002). CSGAGs isolated from both embryonic and adult pig brains differed in their ability to bind various growth factors (Bao *et al.*, 2004). The binding capacity was greater for CS/DS hybrid chains isolated from embryonic pig brain than those of adult pig brain. Among the growth factors tested, FGF-2,

-10, -18, PTN, and MK bound to CS/DS from embryonic pig brains with high affinity comparable to that of CS-E and Hep (Deepa *et al.*, 2002), whereas FGF-1 and HB-EGF did not show any binding. Digestion with chondroitinase B, which specifically cleaves DS structures containing IdoA residues, markedly reduced the binding activity to the level exhibited by the CS/DS chains of adult pig brain. These results suggest that the activity of brain CS/DS chains to bind various Hep-binding growth factors changes during development and the IdoA residues are involved in the binding.

The critical role of IdoA in the binding to growth factors was further evaluated by determining the binding of growth factors to CS/DS hybrid chains isolated from hagfish notochord (CS-H named after hagfish) (Nandini *et al.*, 2004) and shark skin (Nandini *et al.*, 2005). As in the earlier instances, various Hep-binding growth factors were used to test their binding to the isolated GAGs. Additionally, $VEGF_{165}$, which is a Hep-binding angiogenic growth factor highly specific for endothelial cells, was also tested for its ability to bind the CS-H preparation. All the growth factors tested, except FGF-1, bound to the immobilized CS-H preparation with high affinity. The affinity of the binding was particularly strong for FGF-10, FGF-18, MK, and PTN with K_d values unable to be determined accurately because of negligible dissociation of the growth factors, which is characteristic of such high-affinity binders and may reflect the possibility that CS/DSPGs act as receptors or coreceptors, like HSPGs, to present growth factors to the cell surface (Table III). Although $VEGF_{165}$ bound to a lesser extent, it bound with high affinity as indicated by its low-K_d value (24 nM).

The importance of the CS- and DS-like moieties of CS-H in the binding of growth factors was evaluated after digesting the preparation with either chondroitinase AC-I specific for CS or chondroitinase B specific for DS. CS-H showed significant digestibility with either enzyme. Exogenously added intact CS-H inhibited growth factors from binding to immobilized CS-H to various extents. Whereas CS-H digested with chondroitinase ABC had a negligible inhibitory effect, chondroitinase AC-I and B digests significantly inhibited the growth factors, with the chondroitinase AC-I digest being more inhibitory than the chondroitinase B digest. These results suggested that both the CS- and DS-like moieties were involved in the binding of growth factors and that the chondroitinase AC-I-resistant domains containing DS-like moieties, flanked by CS-like moieties resistant to chondroitinase B, are more closely involved. In other words, IdoA-containing domains play a greater role in the binding of growth factors, with significant contributions by GlcA-containing domains as well.

The DS preparation from shark skin also interacted with various Hep-binding growth factors with high affinity when tested using an IAsys system (Nandini *et al.*, 2005). Earlier, it was observed that DS from porcine skin, which contains mostly IdoA, interacted with PTN with a K_d value of 51 nM (Vacherot *et al.*, 1999) compared to 7.6 nM as shown by DS from shark skin,

TABLE III   Kinetic Parameters for the Interaction of Various Growth Factors with CS/DS Variants

Growth factor	CS-H[a]			SS-DS[c,d]			Pig brain (Embryonic)[e]		
	$k_a\ (M^{-1}S^{-1})$	$k_d\ (s^{-1})$	$K_d{}^b\ (nM)$	$k_a\ (M^{-1}S^{-1})$	$k_d\ (s^{-1})$	$K_d\ (nM)$	$k_a\ (M^{-1}S^{-1})$	$k_d\ (s^{-1})$	$K_d\ (nM)$
FGF-2	$(7.7 \pm 1.4) \times 10^5$	$(2.3 \pm 0.6) \times 10^{-2}$	30.50 ± 7.80	$(2.2 \pm 1.5) \times 10^5$	$(0.1 \pm 0.04) \times 10^{-2}$	13.8 ± 11.1	$(3.85 \pm 0.04) \times 10^5$	$(6.32 \pm 0.35) \times 10^{-3}$	16.4 ± 0.7
FGF-10	$(9.7 \pm 5.1) \times 10^3$	$(4.5 \pm 3.5) \times 10^{-6}$	0.40 ± 0.20	$(1.9 \pm 0.2) \times 10^5$	$(0.2 \pm 0.03) \times 10^{-2}$	8.6 ± 2.3	$(2.19 \pm 0.19) \times 10^5$	$(4.77 \pm 0.47) \times 10^{-3}$	21.8 ± 3.3
FGF-16	$(5.6 \pm 2.1) \times 10^6$	$(6.9 \pm 3.1) \times 10^{-3}$	1.20 ± 0.80	ND^f	ND	ND	ND	ND	ND
FGF-18	$(3.3 \pm 0.6) \times 10^5$	$(7.0 \pm 0.9) \times 10^{-5}$	0.20 ± 0.08	$(31.3 \pm 4.8) \times 10^5$	$(1.2 \pm 0.90) \times 10^{-2}$	4.4 ± 3.6	$(1.55 \pm 0.05) \times 10^6$	$(10.1 \pm 0.09) \times 10^{-2}$	6.5 ± 0.8
HB-EGF	$(1.1 \pm 0.6) \times 10^6$	$(9.1 \pm 0.4) \times 10^{-3}$	10.00 ± 4.00	$(4.7 \pm 0.6) \times 10^5$	$(0.2 \pm 0.10) \times 10^{-2}$	4.5 ± 2.5	ND^g		-
MK	$(8.2 \pm 3.4) \times 10^4$	$(8.9 \pm 2.0) \times 10^{-5}$	1.50 ± 0.90	$(1.0 \pm 0.8) \times 10^5$	$(0.2 \pm 0.04) \times 10^{-2}$	58.5 ± 21.5	$(6.06 \pm 0.61) \times 10^4$	$(3.39 \pm 0.45) \times 10^{-3}$	55.9 ± 8.8
PTN	$(4.2 \pm 0.3) \times 10^5$	$(7.4 \pm 2.5) \times 10^{-5}$	0.17 ± 0.05	$(2.9 \pm 1.5) \times 10^5$	$(0.2 \pm 0.09) \times 10^{-2}$	7.6 ± 5.5	$(6.70 \pm 0.12) \times 10^5$	$(1.48 \pm 0.10) \times 10^{-2}$	22.1 ± 1.1
VEGF$_{165}$	$(7.0 \pm 1.6) \times 10^5$	$(1.7 \pm 0.5) \times 10^{-2}$	24.00 ± 7.00	ND	ND	ND	ND	ND	ND

[a]Taken from Nandini et al., 2004.

[b]K_d value as obtained independently from each k_a and k_d value using the BIAevaluation 3.1 software.

[c]Kinetics determined in IAsys.

[d]Taken from Nandini et al., 2005.

[e]Taken from Bao et al., 2004.

[f]Not determined.

[g]Could not be determined because of slow kinetics of binding.

Note: The apparent k_a, k_d, and K_d values for the interaction of growth factors with immobilized CS-H, SS-DS and embryonic pig brain were determined using the 1:1 languimuir binding with mass transfer model of the BIAevaluation 3.1 software in a BIAcore system or IAsys for SS-DS.

which reinforced the concept that better binding is obtained in a hybrid molecule. The results of the interaction of the DS preparation from shark skin revealed that these chains can accommodate a larger number of growth factors than CS-H, suggesting the importance of the sequence information (Table III) and high-sequence specificity.

C. Binding of Growth Factors to CS Chains in the Presence of HS Chains in a Hybrid Structure

To determine the working combination of CS and HS chains in the binding of growth factors, an elegant experiment was conducted by immobilizing syndecan-1 and -4 PGs from normal murine mammary gland epithelial cells, which are hybrid PGs bearing both CS and HS chains (Deepa *et al.*, 2004). The differences in the disaccharide composition of the CS chains in syndecan-1 and -4 have been discussed in Section IV. The degree of sulfation of the CS chains was higher in syndecan-4 than syndecan-1, and both of them had appreciable proportions of E units. To determine whether the differences in the structure of CS affect the affinity for growth factors, FGF-2, MK, and PTN were tested for binding to immobilized syndecan-1 and -4 using a BIAcore system. Kinetic analyses of the binding indicated that the affinities of the two syndecans were significantly different, presumably reflecting the inherent structural variations in the GAG chains in spite of the fact that they were purified from and synthesized in the same cells.

To delineate the type of GAG chains responsible for the binding, an interaction analysis was carried out by immobilizing individually, syndecans devoid of the CS (designated HS/syndecan) and/or HS chains (designated CS/syndecan). Such syndecans were obtained by digestion with chondroitinase ABC or a mixture of heparinase and heparitinase, respectively. Removal of the CS chains affected the responses to the binding of MK and PTN to syndecan-1 but not the responses of the binding of FGF-2 to syndecan-1. Analysis of the binding affinity revealed that the K_d for the binding of MK and FGF-2 to intact syndecan-1 and HS/syndecan-1 was not significantly different in contrast to the binding of PTN to HS/syndecan-1, which was twofold lower than that for the binding to intact syndecan-1. The k_a and k_d values were lower for the binding of the earlier-mentioned growth factors to HS/syndecan-1 than the intact syndecan-1, which could imply that the presence of CS chains in syndecan-1 results in faster binding and faster release of the growth factors, which would facilitate their transfer to corresponding receptors.

The binding of growth factors to syndecan-4 was unaltered in terms of response in the presence or absence of CS chains. However, alterations in the kinetics of interactions of the growth factors were observed in the absence of CS chains, resulting in a lowering of both the association rates of MK and FGF-2 and the dissociation rates of all three growth factors. These results suggest that the CS chains of syndecan-4 are likely involved in the efficient binding and transfer to a high-affinity receptor of these growth factors. FGF-2 did not bind to CS/syndecan-1 or -4, indicating that HS chains are essential for binding. However, alterations in the kinetics of the binding of FGF-2 to HS/syndecan-4 compared to intact syndecan-4 were observed, which suggest that although FGF-2 cannot interact with the CS chains in the absence of HS chains, it can in the presence thereby showing more efficient binding. It was therefore hypothesized that HS chains, which are located away from where the growth factors bind, may share growth factors with CS chains that are in close proximity to the cell surface receptor, forming a ternary or quarternary complex involving the core protein and then transfer the growth factors to the corresponding receptors. It has been demonstrated (Maeda *et al.*, 1996) that the core protein of phosphacan, the extracellular domain of brain-derived CS-PG PTPζ, together with the CS chain, constitutes the binding sites for PTN.

D. Binding of Neurotrophic Factors to CS Chains

Neurotrophic factors play vital roles as key regulators of cell fate and cell shape in the vertebrate nervous system (Bibel and Barde, 2000). It was earlier observed that CS/DS can act as binding partners for various Hep-binding growth factors. Brain-derived neurotrophic factor (BDNF), which is a representative of the neurotrophin family, glial cell line-derived neuro-trophic factor (GDNF), which is a member of the transforming growth factor β superfamily, and ciliary neurotrophic factor (CNTF), which is a neuropoietic cytokine, were used to test the binding for the possibility that CS or its variant acts as a binding partner. BDNF influences the formation of myelin during nerve regeneration (Kordower *et al.*, 2000; Zhang *et al.*, 2000), and GDNF prevents neurodegeneration during Parkinson's disease. Their binding was compared with that of HS from bovine intestinal mucosa, the structure of which had been characterized earlier (Maccarana *et al.*, 1996). BDNF and GDNF showed significant binding to immobilized HS as well as CS-H, whereas the binding of CNTF to both HS and CS-H was negligible (Nandini *et al.*, 2004). Kinetic analysis revealed that the affinity of BDNF for immobilized CS-H was 360-fold higher than that of HS, whereas the affinity of GDNF for CS-H was 10-fold higher than that of HS, suggest-ing that the interactions are biologically significant (Table IV) with the possible involvement of CS or DS or CS/DS hybrid chains. These results suggest that presumably, CS and HS act in different ways. While HS may transmit the factors as coreceptors to the cell-surface receptors, CS/DS may keep holding the factors when presenting them to receptors or may be enzymatically released as a functional neurotrophic factor–oligosaccharide complex from the PG. The domains responsible for high-affinity binding require further investigation.

TABLE IV Kinetic Parameters[a] for the Binding of Neurotrophic Factors with Immobilized HS, CS-H, and SS-DS

Neurotrophic factor	HS			CS-H			SS-DS		
	$k_a\,(M^{-1}S^{-1})$	$k_d\,(s^{-1})$	$K_D\,(nM)$	$k_a\,(M^{-1}S^{-1})$	$k_d\,(s^{-1})$	$K_D\,(nM)$	$k_a\,(M^{-1}S^{-1})$	$k_d\,(s^{-1})$	$K_D\,(nM)$
BDNF	2.6×10^5	6.7×10^{-2}	254	4.4×10^7	3.0×10^{-2}	0.7	1.7×10^9	61.0	36
GDNF	2.4×10^6	5.8×10^{-2}	24	2.0×10^6	5.2×10^{-3}	2.5	2.5×10^6	2.4×10^{-2}	9.6

[a]Kinetic parameters were obtained by global fitting using a 1:1 Languimuir binding with mass transfer model.

CS/DS chains from shark skin also bound these factors with high affinity, and the binding response was comparable with that of CS-H. Their binding was characterized by higher association and dissociation rates compared to the binding to CS-H perhaps because they were comparatively less sulfated, which might suggest that they can act as a better binding partner than CS-H. The calculated binding capacity of CS/DS chains was also greater than that of CS-H, partly due to the larger chain size.

VII. Influence of Structure on Biological Activities of CS _____

Reports emanating from our laboratory and others have demonstrated the importance of CS and CSPGs in the brain's development (Clement *et al.*, 1999; Garwood *et al.*, 1999; Morgenstern *et al.*, 2002). CSPGs, which constitute a significant population of PGs in the central nervous system, may influence the establishment of boundaries for axonal growth and act as modulators of neuronal outgrowth during the brain's development as well as during regeneration after injury. Various CS variants from marine animals promoted neurite outgrowth *in vitro* (Hikino *et al.*, 2003). This is in contrast to the widely held view that CS chains are intrinsic inhibitory components for axonal growth and the pathfinding of various neurons (Grimpe and Silver, 2004; Ichijo, 2003; Morgenstern *et al.*, 2002). The enzymatic removal of CS chains from CSPGs improves the regeneration of nerve fibers *in vivo* after lesions form in the nigrostriatal tract and injury to the spinal chord (Bradbury *et al.*, 2002; Moon *et al.*, 2001). Additionally, the expression of some CSPG core proteins, particularly neurocan, versican, brevican, and NG2, is highly upregulated following CNS injury (Asher *et al.*, 2000, 2002; Tang *et al.*, 2003; Thon *et al.*, 2000). The role of a CSPG named aggrecan in the brain's development was delineated using an aggercan-deficient model with chicks. A deficiency of aggrecan leads to severely altered phenotypes, which affect cell behavior and neuronal cell markers (Schwartz and Domowicz, 2004). With the aim of looking into the structural relationship as a function of the expression of mRNAs of CS sulfotransferases, a correlation between GAG composition and the levels of the mRNAs encoding sulfotransferases was found (Properzi *et al.*, 2005). Using semiquantitative RT-PCR and *in situ* hybridization, it was observed that the expression of C6ST-l and its sulfated products CS-C and CS-D is selectively upregulated 7 days after cortical injury in the glial cells forming the scar. These results suggest that the sulfation pattern influences the binding properties of CSPGs (Properzi *et al.*, 2005).

That the structure of the CS variant and sulfation pattern play an important role in neuritogenesis was further established by testing for the said activity using CS/DS chains (Hikino *et al.*, 2003) isolated from marine animals (Pavão *et al.*, 1995, 1998; Vilela-Silva *et al.*, 2001). A CS-H fraction, which contained exclusively IdoA-containing disaccharides and was isolated from hagfish notochord, was observed to promote neurite outgrowth in a dose-dependent manner. The neurite outgrowth exhibited by DS preparations containing D units showed a morphology akin to that of CS-D in contrast to DS preparations containing E or iE units, which exhibited a small cell soma and a single long neurite. Neuritogenecity of DSD-1-PG/phosphacan from the mouse brain (Faissner et al., 1994) was presumably dependent on IdoA residues of CS chains and abolished by digestion with chondroitinase B. In contrast, digestion with chondroitinase AC-II or AC-I either did not abolish it or did so only partially. These results suggested that the neuritogenic DSD-1 epitope contains a D unit (Clement et al., 1998; Nadanaka et al., 1998) and an IdoA residue (Hikino et al., 2003).

To further determine the importance of IdoA-containing units in neuritogenesis, the structures of the CS/DS hybrid chains from pig brain were elucidated. It was observed that the CS/DS chains isolated from embryonic pig brain displayed dendritic-like neurite outgrowth in contrast to CS/DS chains isolated from adult pig brain, which exhibited no neuritogenic activity (Bao et al., 2004). Structural studies indicated that embryonic CS/DS chains contain a significant proportion of IdoA as IdoA-GalNAc(4-O-sulfate), thereby irrevocably demonstrating its importance in the promotion of neurite outgrowth. This is in line with the observation that DS has been implicated in a variety of biological processes by the presence of IdoA, whose pyranose ring has the tendency to form various conformations, resulting in an inherent plasticity for interaction with various partners (Ferro et al., 1986; Scott et al., 1995). By contrast, the CS/DS-hybrid chains from adult pig brain contained less than 1% IdoA-containing disaccharides (Bao et al., 2004) and did not promote neurite outgrowth. The importance of the binding of growth factors in promotion of neurite outgrowth was revealed when PTN was identified as one of the ligands responsible for the neurite outgrowth-promoting activity of brain CS/DS (Bao et al., 2005a). Brain CS/DS chains were fractionated based on their affinity for PTN into unbound, low-affinity and high-affinity fractions. The unbound fraction did not promote neurite outgrowth but the low-affinity and high-affinity fractions did, resulting in a distinct morphology, namely dendritic and axonic, respectively, suggesting that the activity in both fractions involves different molecular mechanisms. Further evidence was obtained to suggest a different molecular mechanism. Anti-PTN antibody neutralized the neurite outgrowth-promoting activity of the low-affinity fraction in contrast to that of the high-affinity fraction, which was not neutralized by the antibody.

Bao et al. (2005b) dissected CS/DS hybrid chains from embryonic pig brains by digestion with chondroitinase B and showed that octasaccharides were the minimal size capable of interacting with PTN. Five and eight sequences were purified from fluorescently labeled PTN-bound and -unbound octasaccharide fractions, respectively, by enzymatic digestion followed by PTN-affinity chromatography. The sequencing was accomplished using minute amounts of fluorescently labeled samples by enzymatic digestion in conjunction with HPLC, verifying a critical role for oversulfated D and/or iD disaccharides in the low yet significant affinity for PTN (Table V), which is required for neuritogenesis.

CS/DS chains isolated from hagfish notochord and shark skin also exhibited neurite-outgrowth promoting activity. However, the activity of the CS-H (2.0 M) fraction, which has a hybrid structure, was weaker than that of the CS-H (3.0 M) fraction tested earlier, which contained exclusively IdoA. The morphology of the activated neurons was the same as that exemplified by CS-E, but the neuritogenic activity was weaker. This is in contrast to the neuritogenic activity exhibited by shark skin DS with a comparatively low degree of sulfation. The morphology of the neurons activated by shark skin DS was both axonic and dendritic in nature. These results suggest that the neuritogenic activity might involve the presence of distinct structural domains, the structural elucidation of which would be

TABLE V   A Series of PTN-Bound and -Unbound Octasaccharide Sequences Isolated from CS/DS Hybrid Chains of Embryonic Pig Brains

	PTN-bound octasaccharide			*PTN-unbound octasaccharide*	
Fraction	*Sequence*	*Parent structure*[a]	*Fraction*	*Sequence*	*Parent structure*
F5-b-I	ΔC-C-D-C	iC-C-D-C-iX	F5-ub-a	ΔC-O-C-C	iC-O-C-C-iX
F5-b-II	ΔA-C-D-C	iA-C-D-C-iX	F5-ub-b	ΔA-O-A-C	iA-O-A-C-iX
	or ΔC-A-D-C	iC-A-D-C-iX	F5-ub-c	ΔA-O-A-A	iA-O-A-A-iX
F5-b-III	ΔD-C-D-C	iD-C-D-C-iX	F5-ub-d	ΔC-C-C-C	iC-C-C-C-iX
F5-b-VI	ΔC-D-D-C	iC-D-D-C-iX	F5-ub-e	ΔA-C-C-C	iA-C-C-C-iX
	or ΔC-D-iD-C	iC-C-iD-C-iX	F5-ub-f	ΔC-C-A-C	iC-C-A-C-iX
F5-b-V	ΔE-D-A-D	iE-D-A-D-iX	F5-ub-g	ΔA-C-A-C	iA-C-A-C-IX
	or ΔE-D-iA-D	iE-D-A-D-iX		ΔA-C-C-A	iA-C-C-A-iX
F5-b-VI	ND[b]	ND	F5-ub-h	ΔC-A-A-A	iC-A-A-A-iX

[a]The "i" stands for an L-iduronate residue, and iX represents any disaccharides with an IdoUA residue including iA, iC, iD, iE, iB, or iT, except for iO. For the abbreviations and structures of the disaccharide units, see Fig. 1.

[b]Not determined.

Note: The CS/DS chains were dissected by digestion with chondroitinase B and size fractionated by gel filtration. The isolated octasaccharide fraction was separated into a PTN-bound and a PTN-unbound subfraction using a PTN-affinity column. Each fraction was then separated by anion-exchange HPLC into individual octasaccharides, each of which was sequenced by enzymatic digestion in conjunction with HPLC. The parent decasaccharide sequence corresponding to each isolated octasaccharide is flanked by two iduronate residues and was deduced based on the specificity of chondroitinase B that cleaves GalNAc-iduronate linkages.

helpful in developing therapeutic agents for neuronal diseases and brain injury.

VIII. Perspectives

In coming years, advances in techniques should open up a whole gamut of opportunities to delineate the structural domains responsible for the binding of growth factors. Such studies might help to predict intrinsic mechanisms responsible for biological activities, which in turn would be helpful in developing therapeutics. In addition, recent evidence has revealed that the herpes simplex virus uses cell surface CS-E more efficiently than HS for its infection (Bergefall *et al.*, 2005), suggesting the possibility of developing antiviral sugar drugs. At the same time, with most of the genes encoding glycosyltransferases and sulfotransferases being cloned, elucidation of the functions of CS-variants *in vivo* using molecular biology techniques will offer new insights.

Acknowledgments

The authors thank Prof. K. S. Rangappa, Mysore University, for his critical review of the manuscript during his sabbatical (2005.5–2005.7) at Kobe Pharmaceutical University. This work was supported in part by HAITEKU (2004–2008) from the Japan Private School Promotion Foundation.

References

Anno, K., Seno, N., Mathews, M. B., Yamagata, T., and Suzuki, S. (1971). A new dermatan polysulfate, chondroitin sulfate H, from hagfish notochord. *Biochim. Biophys. Acta* **237**, 173–177.

Asher, R. A., Morgenstern, D. A., Fidler, P. S., Adcock, K. H., Oohira, A., Braistead, J. E., Levine, J. M., Margolis, R. U., Rogers, J. H., and Fawcett, J. W. (2000). Neurocan is upregulated in injured brain and in cytokine-treated astrocytes. *J. Neurosci.* **20**, 2427–2438.

Asher, R. A., Morgenstern, D. A., Shearer, M. C., Adcock, K. H., Pesheva, P., and Fawcett, J. W. (2002). Versican is upregulated in CNS injury and is a product of oligodendrocyte lineage cells. *J. Neurosci.* **22**, 2225–2236.

Avnur, Z., and Geiger, B. (1984). Immunocytochemical localization of native chondroitin-sulfate in tissues and cultured cells using specific monoclonal antibody. *Cell* **38**, 811–822.

Bao, X., Nishimura, S., Mikami, T., Yamada, S., Itoh, N., and Sugahara, K. (2004). Chondroitin sulfate/dermatan sulfate hybrid chains from embryonic pig brain, which contain a higher proportion of L-iduronic acid than those from adult pig brain, exhibit neuritogenic and growth factor binding activities. *J. Biol. Chem.* **279**, 9765–9776.

Bao, X., Mikami, T., Yamada, S., Faissner, A., Muramatsu, T., and Sugahara, K. (2005a). Heparin-binding growth factor, pleiotrophin, mediates neuritogenic activity of embryonic pig brain-derived chondroitin sulfate/dermatan sulfate hybrid chains. *J. Biol. Chem.* **280**, 9180–9191.

Bao, X., Muramatsu, T., and Sugahara, K. (2005b). Demonstration of the pleiotrophin-binding oligosaccharide sequences isolated from chondroitin sulfate/dermatan sulfate hybrid chains of embryonic pig brains. *J. Biol. Chem.* **280**, 35318–35328.

Bechard, D., Gentina, T., Delehedde, M., Scherpereel, A., Lyon, M., Aumercier, M., Vazeux, R., Richet, C., Degand, P., Jude, B., Janin, A., Fernig, D. G., *et al.* (2001). Endocan is a novel chondroitin sulfate/dermatan sulfate proteoglycan that promotes hepatocyte growth factor/scatter factor mitogenic activity. *J. Biol. Chem.* **276**, 48341–48349.

Bergefall, K., Trybala, E., Johanson, M., Uyama, T., Naito, S., Yamada, S., Kitagawa, H., Sugahara, K., and Bergström, T. (2005). Chondroitin sulfate characterized by the E disaccharide unit is a potent inhibitor of herpes simplex virus infectivity and provides binding sites for the virus binding to gro2C cells. *J. Biol. Chem.* in press.

Bernfield, M., Gotte, M., Park, P. W., Reizes, O., Fitzgerald, M. L., Lincecum, J., and Zako, M. (1999). Functions of cell surface heparan sulfate proteoglycans. *Annu. Rev. Biochem.* **68**, 729–777.

Bibel, M., and Barde, Y. A. (2000). Neurotrophins: Key regulators of cell fate and cell shape in the vertebrate nervous system. *Genes Dev.* **14**, 2919–2937.

Bradbury, E. J., Moon, L. D., Popat, R. J., King, V. R., Bennett, G. S., Patel, P. N., Fawcett, J. W., and McMahon, S. B. (2002). Chondroitinase ABC promotes functional recovery after spinal cord injury. *Nature* **416**, 636–640.

Breen, K. C., Bruce, M., and Anderton, B. H. (1991). Beta amyloid precursor protein mediates neuronal cell-cell and cell-surface adhesion. *J. Neurosci. Res.* **28**, 90–100.

Carey, D. J. (1997). Syndecans: Multifunctional cell-surface co-receptors. *Biochem. J.* **327**, 1–16.

Clement, A. M., Nadanaka, S., Masayama, K., Mandl, C., Sugahara, K., and Faissner, A. (1998). The DSD-1-epitope depends on sulfation, correlates with chondroitin sulfate D motifs, and is sufficient to promote neurite outgrowth. *J. Biol. Chem.* **273**, 28444–28453.

Clement, A. M., Sugahara, K., and Faissner, A. (1999). Chondroitin sulfate E promotes neurite outgrowth of rat embryonic day 18 hippocampal neurons. *Neurosci. Lett.* **269**, 125–128.

Deepa, S. S., Umehara, Y., Higashiyama, S., Itoh, N., and Sugahara, K. (2002). Specific molecular interactions of oversulfated chondroitin sulfate E with various heparin-binding growth factors: Implications as a physiological binding partner in the brain and other tissues. *J. Biol. Chem.* **277**, 43707–43716.

Deepa, S. S., Yamada, S., Zako, M., Goldberger, O., and Sugahara, K. (2004). Chondroitin sulfate chains on syndecan-1 and syndecan-4 from normal murine mammary gland epithelial cells are structurally and functionally distinct and cooperate with heparan sulfate chains to bind growth factors: A novel function to control binding of midkine, pleiotrophin, and basic fibroblast growth factor. *J. Biol. Chem.* **279**, 37368–37376.

Faissner, A., Clement, A., Lochter, A., Streit, A., Mandl, C., and Melitta, S. (1994). Isolation of a neural chondroitin sulfate proteoglycan with neurite outgrowth promoting properties. *J. Cell Biol.* **126**, 783–799.

Ferro, D. R., Provasoli, A., Ragami, M., Torri, G., Casu, B., Gatti, G., Jacquinet, J.-C., Sinay, P., Petitou, M., and Choay, J. (1986). Evidence for conformational equilibrium of the sulfated L-iduronate residue in heparin and in synthetic heparin mono- and oligosaccharides: NMR and force-field studies. *J. Am. Chem. Soc.* **108**, 6773–6778.

Fitzgerald, M. L., and Bernfield, M. (1999). *In* "Syndecans in Guidebook to Extracellular Matrix, Anchor and Adhesion Proteins" (T. Kreis, and R. D. Vale, Eds.), pp. 306–311. Oxford University Press, Oxford, UK.

Fukui, S., Feizi, T., Galustian, C., Lawson, A. M., and Chai, W. (2002). Oligosaccharide microarrays for high-throughput detection and specificity assignments of carbohydrate-protein interactions. *Nat. Biotechnol.* **20**, 1011–1017.

Garwood, J., Schnadelbach, O., Clement, A., Schutte, K., Bach, A., and Faissner, A. (1999). DSD-1-proteoglycan is the mouse homolog of phosphacan and displays opposing effects on neurite outgrowth dependent on neuronal lineage. *J. Neurosci.* **19**, 3888–3899.

Grimpe, B., and Silver, J. (2004). A novel DNA enzyme reduces glycosaminoglycan chains in the glial scar and allows microtransplanted dorsal root ganglia axons to regenerate beyond lesions in the spinal cord. *J. Neurosci.* **24**, 1393–1397.

Habuchi, O., Sugiura, K., and Kawai, N. (1977). Glucose branches in chondroitin sulfates from squid cartilage. *J. Biol. Chem.* **252**, 4570–4576.

Herndon, M. E., and Lander, A. D. (1990). A diverse set of developmentally regulated proteoglycans is expressed in the rat central nervous system. *Neuron* **4**, 949–961.

Hikino, M., Mikami, T., Faissner, A., Vilela-Silva, A. C., Pavão, M. S., and Sugahara, K. (2003). Oversulfated dermatan sulfate exhibits neurite outgrowth-promoting activity toward embryonic mouse hippocampal neurons: Implications of dermatan sulfate in neuritogenesis in the brain. *J. Biol. Chem.* **278**, 43744–43754.

Hileman, R. E., Fromm, J. R., Weiler, J. M., and Linhardt, R. J. (1998). Glycosaminoglycan-protein interactions: Definition of consensus sites in glycosaminoglycan binding proteins. *BioEssays* **20**, 156–167.

Ichijo, H. (2003). Roles of proteoglycans in neuronal circuit formation of retinotectal projections. *Connect. Tissue* **35**, 11–17.

Ito, Y., Hikino, M., Yajima, Y., Mikami, T., Sirko, S., Holst, A., Faissner, A., Fukui, S., and Sugahara, K. (2005). Structural characterization of the epitopes of the monoclonal antibodies 473HD, CS-56 and MO-225 specific for chondroitin sulfate D-type using the oligosaccharide library. *Glycobiology* **15**, 593–603.

Kato, M., Wang, H., Bernfield, M., Gallagher, J. T., and Turnbull, J. E. (1994). Cell surface syndecan-1 on distinct cell types differs in fine structure and ligand binding of its heparan sulfate chains. *J. Biol. Chem.* **269**, 18881–18890.

Kim, C. W., Goldberger, O. A., Gallo, R. L., and Bernfield, M. (1994). Members of the syndecan family of heparan sulfate proteoglycans are expressed in distinct cell-, tissue-, and development-specific patterns. *Mol. Biol. Cell* **5**, 797–805.

Kinoshita, A., Yamada, S., Haslam, S. M., Morris, H. R., Dell, A., and Sugahara, K. (1997). Novel tetrasaccharides isolated from squid cartilage chondroitin sulfate E contain unusual sulfated disaccharide units GlcA(3-O-sulfate)beta1–3GalNAc(6-O-sulfate) or GlcA(3-O-sulfate)beta1–3GalNAc. *J. Biol. Chem.* **272**, 19656–19665.

Kinoshita-Toyoda, A., Yamada, S., Haslam, S. M., Khoo, K.-H., Sugiura, M., Morris, H. R., Dell, A., and Sugahara, K. (2004). Structural determination of five 3-O-sulfated glucuronic acid-containing tetersaccharides and two rare glucose-containing oligosac-charides isolated from squid cartilage chondroitin sulfate E. *Biochemistry* **43**, 11063–11074.

Kitagawa, H., Tsutsumi, K., Tone, Y., and Sugahara, K. (1997). Developmental regulation of the sulfation profile of chondroitin sulfate chains in the chicken embryo brain. *J. Biol. Chem.* **272**, 31377–31381.

Kordower, J. H., Emborg, M. E., Bloch, J., Ma, S. Y., Chu, Y., Leventhal, L., McBride, J., Chen, E. Y., Palfi, S., Roitberg, B. Z., Brown, W. D., Holden, J. E., *et al.* (2000). Neurodegeneration prevented by lentiviral vector delivery of GDNF in primate models of Parkinson's disease. *Science* **290**, 767–773.

Lander, A. D. (1998). Proteoglycans: Master regulators of molecular encounter? *Matrix Biol.* **17**, 465–472.

Liaw, P. C., Becker, D. L., Stafford, A. R., Fredenburgh, J. C., and Weitz, J. I. (2001). Molecular basis for the susceptibility of fibrin-bound thrombin to inactivation by heparin cofactor ii in the presence of dermatan sulfate but not heparin. *J. Biol. Chem.* **276**, 20959–20965.

Lindahl, B., Eriksson, L., and Lindahl, U. (1995). Structure of heparan sulphate from human brain, with special regard to Alzheimer's disease. *Biochem. J.* **306**, 177–187.

Maccarana, M., Sakura, Y., Tawada, A., Yoshida, K., and Lindahl, U. (1996). Domain structure of heparan sulfates from bovine organs. *J. Biol. Chem.* **271**, 17804–17810.

Maeda, N., and Noda, M. (1998). Involvement of receptor-like protein tyrosine phosphatase zeta/RPTPbeta and its ligand pleiotrophin/heparin-binding growth-associated molecule (HB-GAM) in neuronal migration. *J. Cell Biol.* **142**, 203–216.

Maeda, N., Nishiwaki, T., Shintani, T., Hamanaka, H., and Noda, M. (1996). 6B4 proteoglycan/phosphacan, an extracellular variant of receptor-like protein-tyrosine phosphatase zeta/RPTPbeta, binds pleiotrophin/heparin-binding growth-associated molecule (HB-GAM). *J. Biol. Chem.* **271**, 21446–21452.

Maeda, N., He, J., Yajima, Y., Mikami, T., Sugahara, K., and Yabe, T. (2003). Heterogeneity of the chondroitin sulfate portion of phosphacan/6B4 proteoglycan regulates its binding affinity for pleiotrophin/heparin binding growth-associated molecule. *J. Biol. Chem.* **278**, 35805–35811.

Menozzi, F. D., Pethe, K., Bifani, P., Soncin, F., Brennan, M. J., and Locht, C. (2002). Enhanced bacterial virulence through exploitation of host glycosaminoglycans. *Mol. Microbiol.* **43**, 1379–1386.

Moon, L. D., Asher, R. A., Rhodes, K. E., and Fawcett, J. W. (2001). Regeneration of CNS axons back to their target following treatment of adult rat brain with chondroitinase ABC. *Nat. Neurosci.* **4**, 465–466.

Morgenstern, D. A., Asher, R. A., and Fawcett, J. W. (2002). Chondroitin sulfate proteoglycans in the CNS injury response. *Prog. Brain Res.* **137**, 313–332.

Nadanaka, S., Clement, A. M., Masayama, K., Faissner, A., and Sugahara, K. (1998). Characteristic hexasaccharide sequences in octasaccharides derived from shark cartilage chondroitin sulfate D with a neurite outgrowth promoting activity. *J. Biol. Chem.* **273**, 3296–3330.

Nandini, C. D., Mikami, T., Ohta, M., Itoh, N., Akiyama-Nambu, F., and Sugahara, K. (2004). Structural and functional characterization of oversulfated chondroitin sulfate/dermatan sulfate hybrid chains from the notochord of hagfish: Neuritogenic activity and binding activities toward growth factors and neurotrophic factors. *J. Biol. Chem.* **279**, 50799–50809.

Nandini, C. D., Itoh, N., and Sugahara, K. (2005). Novel 70-kDa chondroitin sulfate/dermatan sulfate hybrid chains with a unique heterogeneous sulfation pattern from shark skin, which exhibit neuritogenic activity and binding activities for growth factors and neurotrophic factors. *J. Biol. Chem.* **280**, 4058–4069.

Pavão, M. S., Aiello, K. R., Werneck, C. C., Silva, L. C., Valente, A. P., Mulloy, B., Colwell, N. S., Tollefsen, D. M., and Mourão, P. A. (1998). Highly sulfated dermatan sulfates from ascidians: Structure versus anticoagulant activity of these glycosaminoglycans. *J. Biol. Chem.* **273**, 27848–27857.

Pavão, M. S., Mourão, P. A., Mulloy, B., and Tollefsen, D. M. (1995). A unique dermatan sulfate-like glycosaminoglycan from ascidian. Its structure and the effect of its unusual sulfation pattern on anticoagulant activity. *J. Biol. Chem.* **270**, 31027–31036.

Properzi, F., Carulli, D., Asher, R. A., Muir, E., Camargo, L. M., van Kuppevelt, T. H., ten Dam, G. B., Furukawa, Y., Mikami, T., Sugahara, K., Toida, T., Geller, H. M., *et al.* (2005). Chondroitin 6-sulphate synthesis is up-regulated in injured CNS, induced by injury-related cytokines and enhanced in axon-growth inhibitory glia. *Eur. J. Neurosci.* **21**, 378–390.

Qi, M., Ikematsu, S., Maeda, N., Ichihara-Tanaka, K., Sakuma, S., Noda, M., Muramatsu, T., and Kadomatsu, K. (2001). Haptotactic migration induced by midkine: Involvement of protein-tyrosine phosphatase zeta. Mitogen-activated protein kinase, and phosphatidy-linositol 3-kinase. *J. Biol. Chem.* **276**, 15868–15875.

Rapraeger, A., Jalkanen, M., Endo, E., Koda, J., and Bernfield, M. (1985). The cell surface proteoglycan from mouse mammary epithelial cells bears chondroitin sulfate and heparan sulfate glycosaminoglycans. *J. Biol. Chem.* **260**, 11046–11052.

Rauch, U., Gao, P., Janetzko, A., Flaccus, A., Hilgenberg, L., Tekotte, H., Margolis, R. K., and Margolis, R. U. (1991). Isolation and characterization of developmentally regulated chondroitin sulfate and chondroitin/keratan sulfate proteoglycans of brain identified with monoclonal antibodies. *J. Biol. Chem.* **266**, 14785–14801.

Robakis, N. K., Altstiel, L. D., Refolo, L. M., and Anderson, J. P. (1990). Function and metabolism of the protease inhibitor containing Alzheimer amyloid precursors. *In* "Molecular Biology and Genetics of Alzheimer's Disease" (T. Miyatake, D. J. Selkoe, and Y. Ihara, Eds.), pp. 179–188. Elsevier Science, Amsterdam.

Roch, J. M., Shapiro, I. P., Sundsmo, M. P., Otero, D. A., Refolo, L. M., Robakis, N. K., and Saitoh, T. (1992). Bacterial expression, purification, and functional mapping of the amyloid beta/A4 protein precursor. *J. Biol. Chem.* **267**, 2214–2221.

Saigo, K., and Egami, F. (1970). Purification and some properties of acid mucopolysaccharides of bovine brain. *J. Neurochem.* **17**, 633–647.

Schwartz, N. B., and Domowicz, M. (2004). Proteoglycans in brain development. *Glycoconj. J.* **21**, 329–341.

Scott, J. E., Heatley, F., and Wood, B. (1995). Comparison of secondary structures in water of chondroitin-4-sulfate and dermatan sulfate: Implications in the formation of tertiary structures. *Biochemistry* **34**, 15467–15474.

Shworak, N. W., Shirakawa, M., Mulligan, R. C., and Rosenberg, R. D. (1994). Characterization of ryudocan glycosaminoglycan acceptor sites. *J. Biol. Chem.* **269**, 21204–21214.

Stoll, M. S., Mizuochi, T., Childs, R. A., and Feizi, T. (1988). Improved procedure for the construction of neoglycolipids having antigenic and lectin-binding activities, from reducing oligosaccharides. *Biochem. J.* **256**, 661–664.

Sugahara, K., and Kitagawa, H. (2000). Recent advances in the study of the biosynthesis and functions of sulfated glycosaminoglycans. *Curr. Opin. Struct. Biol.* **10**, 518–527.

Sugahara, K., and Yamada, S. (2000). Structure and function of oversulfated chondroitin sulfate variants: Unique sulfation patterns and neuroregulatory activities,. *Trends Glycosci. Glyc.* **12**, 321–349.

Sugahara, K., Mikami, T., Uyama, T., Mizuguchi, S., Nomura, K., and Kitagawa, H. (2003). Recent advances in the structural biology of chondroitin sulfate and dermatan sulfate. *Curr. Opin. Struct. Biol.* **13**, 612–620.

Tang, X., Davies, J. E., and Davies, S. J. (2003). Changes in distribution, cell associations, and protein expression levels of NG2, neurocan, phosphacan, brevican, versican V2, and tenascin-C during acute to chronic maturation of spinal cord scar tissue. *J. Neurosci. Res.* **71**, 427–444.

Thon, N., Haas, C. A., Rauch, U., Merten, T., Fassler, R., Frotscher, M., and Deller, T. (2000). The chondroitin sulphate proteoglycan brevican is upregulated by astrocytes after entorhinal cortex lesions in adult rats. *Eur. J. Neurosci.* **12**, 2547–2558.

Trowbridge, J. M., and Gallo, R. L. (2002). Dermatan sulfate: New functions from an old glycosaminoglycan. *Glycobiology* **12**, 117R–125R.

Tsuchida, K., Shioi, J., Yamada, S., Boghosian, G., Wu, A., Cai, H., Sugahara, K., and Robakis, N. K. (2001). Appican, the proteoglycan form of the amyloid precursor protein, contains chondroitin sulfate E in the repeating disaccharide region and 4-O-sulfated galactose in the linkage region. *J. Biol. Chem.* **276**, 37155–37160.

Ueoka, C., Nadanaka, S., Seno, N., Khoo, K.-H., and Sugahara, K. (1999). Structural determination of novel tetra- and hexasaccharide sequences isolated from chondroitin sulfate H (oversulfated dermatan sulfate) of hagfish notochord. *Glycoconj. J.* **16**, 291–305.

Ueoka, C., Kaneda, N., Okazaki, I., Nadanaka, S., Muramatsu, T., and Sugahara, K. (2000). Neuronal cell adhesion mediated by the heparin-binding neuroregulatory factor midkine, is specifically inhibited by chondroitin sulfate E: Structural and functional implications of over-sulfated chondroitin sulfate. *J. Biol. Chem.* **275**, 37407–37413.

Umehara, Y., Yamada, S., Nishimura, S., Shioi, J., Robakis, N. K., and Sugahara, K. (2004). Chondroitin sulfate of appican, the proteoglycan form of amyloid precursor protein, produced by C6 glioma cells interacts with heparin-binding neuroregulatory factors. *FEBS Lett.* **557**, 233–238.

Vacherot, F., Delbe, J., Heroult, M., Barritault, D., Fernig, D. G., and Courty, J. (1999). Glycosaminoglycans differentially bind HARP and modulate its biological activity. *J. Biol. Chem.* **274**, 7741–7747.

Vieira, R. P., and Mourão, P. A. (1988). Occurrence of a unique fucose-branched chondroitin sulfate in the body wall of a sea cucumber. *J. Biol. Chem.* **263**, 18176–18183.

Vilela-Silva, A. C., Werneck, C. C., Valente, A. P., Vacquier, V. D., and Mourão, P. A. (2001). Embryos of the sea urchin *Strongylocentrotus purpuratus* synthesize a dermatan sulfate enriched in 4-O- and 6-O-disulfated galactosamine units. *Glycobiology* **11**, 433–440.

Woods, A., Oh, E. S., and Couchman, J. R. (1998). Syndecan proteoglycans and cell adhesion. *Matrix Biol.* **17**, 477–483.

Yamagata, M., Kimata, K., Oike, Y., Tani, K., Maeda, N., Yoshida, K., Shimomura, Y., Yoneda, M., and Suzuki, S. (1987). A monoclonal antibody that specifically recognizes a glucuronic acid 2-sulfate-containing determinant in intact chondroitin sulfate chain. *J. Biol. Chem.* **262**, 4146–4152.

Zhang, J. Y., Luo, X. G., Xian, C. J., Liu, Z. H., and Zhou, X. F. (2000). Endogenous BDNF is required for myelination and regeneration of injured sciatic nerve in rodents. *Eur. J. Neurosci.* **12**, 4171–4180.

Zimmermann, P., and David, G. (1999). The syndecans, tuners of transmembrane signaling. *FASEB J.* **13**, S91–S100.

Zou, P., Zou, K., Muramatsu, H., Ichihara-Tanaka, K., Habuchi, O., Ohtake, S., Ikematsu, S., Sakuma, S., and Muramatsu, T. (2003). Glycosaminoglycan structures required for strong binding to midkine, a heparin-binding growth factor. *Glycobiology* **13**, 35–42.

A. D. Theocharis*, I. Tsolakis[†],
G. N. Tzanakakis[§], and Nikos K. Karamanos*

*Laboratory of Biochemistry
Department of Chemistry
University of Patras
26500 Patras
Greece

[†]Department of Surgery
School of Medicine
University of Patras
26500 Patras
Greece

[§]Department of Histology
School of Medicine
University of Crete
71110 Heraklion
Greece

Chondroitin Sulfate as a Key Molecule in the Development of Atherosclerosis and Cancer Progression

I. Chapter Overview

Chondroitin sulfate (CS) is a glycosaminoglycan (GAG) composed of repeating disaccharides of glucuronic acid and N-acetyl-galactosamine, which are variously substituted by sulfate groups. It is covalently attached on several core proteins creating a variety of proteoglycans (PGs) found in extracellular matrix (ECM) and cell membrane but also intracellularly. Chondroitin sulfate interacts with a wide variety of key molecules, such as growth factors, cytokines, chemokines, adhesion molecules and lipoproteins, via specific saccharide domains within the chain. These interactions regulate several biological processes and cell behavior. Several diseases are often associated with a biosynthetic imbalance of chondroitin sulfate

Advances in Pharmacology, Volume 53
Copyright 2006, Elsevier Inc. All rights reserved.

1054-3589/06 $35.00
DOI: 10.1016/S1054-3589(05)53013-8

proteoglycans (CSPGs). Atherosclerosis and cancer are two well-studied diseases in which the abnormal expression and structural modification of CSPGs are seriously implicated. CSPGs are markedly increased in early atherosclerotic lesions, playing important roles in lipid retention, modification, and finally accumulation. Furthermore, CSPGs participate in inflammatory process associated with atherosclerosis and influence arterial smooth muscle cell behavior. They also directly affect elastogenesis and proper formation of ECM. CSPGs are markedly accumulated also in tumor stroma, and its deposition is often correlated to poor prognosis of the disease. CSPGs seem to be implicated in cancer cell growth and progression through direct involvement in cellular functions or by modulating the activity of other effective molecules. This chapter focuses on the molecular involvement of CS in the progression of two main human diseases, cancer and atherosclerosis.

II. Types of CS-Containing Proteoglycans _____

CS is a linear polysaccharide that consists of repeating disaccharide units composed of an *N*-acetyl-galactosamine and a glucuronic acid, which are variously substituted by sulfate groups in several positions. Sulfate groups may occur at C-2 of glucuronic acid and C-4 and C-6 of *N*-acetyl-galactosamine. CS differs in size and disaccharide composition depending on the tissue source or culture conditions. The length and fine structure of the chain are regulated and controlled by different stimuli. Synthesis of CS is initiated by the formation of a tetrasaccharide linker, xylose–galactose–galactose–glucuronic acid, with the xylose covalently bound to a serine or threonine residue on the protein. The biosynthesis of CS chains on distinct core proteins results in the formation of certain CSPGs. CSPGs are major components of ECM of connective tissues and are also found at the surfaces of many cell types and in intracellular secretory granules (Kjellen and Lindahl, 1991; Sugahara *et al.*, 2003).

Several CSPGs of ECM, such as hyalectans (aggrecan, the major PG of cartilage; versican the common PG of noncartilaginous connective tissues and brevican and neurocan, found mainly in brain), have been identified. Decorin and biglycan, which belong to another class of ECMPGs, the small leucine rich proteoglycans (SLRPs), are usually substituted by CS chains (Iozzo, 1998). Cytokine PGs, such as CSF-1 and M-CSF-1, which are released in ECM, have been recognized as part-time CSPGs (Timar *et al.*, 2002). Other matrix PGs like phosphacan, which is the major brain CSPG and corresponds to the extracellular region of a receptor-like protein-tyrosine phosphatase, PTPζ/RPTPβ, have been also discovered, and their biological roles are in focus (Kadomatsu and Muramatsu, 2004).

Proteoglycans of basement membranes perlecan and bamacan are also substituted by CS chains. The presence of heparan sulfate (HS) chains in perlecan suggests that this PG may be a hybrid PG with tissue specific and biosynthetically regulated glycanation (Iozzo, 1998).

Cell-associated PGs are also in some cases hybrids in respect to the type of GAG chains they contain. One of the most studied types of transmembrane PGs is the family of syndecans, which often found to carry HS and/or CS chains (Timar et al., 2002). CD44 is also a part-time transmembrane PG, which is able to carry CS chains in some splice variants. NG2-melanoma associated large CSPG, the human homolog of rat transmembrane CSPG, NG2, consists of a core protein of 250 kDa, which is heavily glycosylated by CS chains (Timar et al., 2002). An unclassified cell associated CSPG is the intact molecule of PTPζ. This is a receptor-type protein tyrosine phosphatase with CS bound chains at the extracellular domain, whereas the intracellular domain exhibits protein tyrosine phosphatase activity. PTPζ plays important biological roles, since it is one of the receptors of midkine and pleiotrophin, two growth factors involved among others in embryogenesis and recently in cancer progression (Kadomatsu and Muramatsu, 2004).

III. CSPGs in the Development of Atherosclerosis

A. CSPGs as Key Players in Lipoprotein Oxidation and Accumulation

Versican is a major ECM CSPG found in normal vessel wall and is markedly accumulated during the development of atherosclerosis, playing important roles in lipid retention, modification, and finally lipid accumulation. It is recognized as a key factor implicated in the development of atherosclerosis. Biglycan and decorin, the hybrid CS/DSPGs, are also found in normal vessel wall and are significantly increased in vascular injury (Wight, 2002; Wight and Merrilees, 2004; Wight et al., 1992). The accumulation of CSPGs in vascular injury is triggered by various growth factors and cytokines, such as TGFβ, PDGF, EGF, bFGF, and IL-1β, which are released in the inflammatory sites, and most of them have mitogenic activity on arterial smooth muscle cells (ASMCs). The migration and proliferation of ASMCs in sites of arterial injury accompanied by the deposition of CSPGs is a hallmark of early atherosclerotic lesions (Wight, 2002; Wight and Merrilees, 2004). A number of studies have shown the close relation of CSPGs with lipoprotein deposits in human atherosclerotic lesions and in lipid induced lesions in experimental animals, suggesting a role for CSPGs in the retention of lipoproteins in the vessel wall. The response to retention hypothesis of atherosclerosis invokes a critical role in atherogenesis for the retention of lipoproteins by matrix PGs. Actually, large CS-lipoprotein complexes have been isolated from human atherosclerotic plaques, and arterial CSPGs interact directly with lipoproteins (Camejo *et al.*, 1998). Furthermore, the small CS/DSPG decorin, which is able to interact with collagen type I that is accumulated in atherosclerotic plaques, also interacts with LDL. It has been, therefore, suggested that decorin acts as a bridge for the retention of lipoproteins in collagen-rich atherosclerotic lesions (Pentikainen *et al.*, 1997). Multiple LDL particles can bind to a single CS chain, and the length of the chain is a determining factor for the binding of LDL. In vascular injury, elongated CS chains have been isolated with enhanced LDL binding properties. Several factors are able to promote CS chain elongation *in vitro* by ASMCs. These factors are the rate of cell proliferation, TGFβ, and oxidized LDL, which cause CS elongation and increase the binding of CSPGs to LDL (Wight and Merrilees, 2004). CS enriched in 6-sulfated units binds LDL more avidly than those enriched in 4-sulfated disaccharides (Cardoso and Mourao, 1994). The overall charge density of the CS chain also influences the interaction of LDL with CS. It has been shown that the binding of LDL with 6-sulfated CS requires the oversulfated regions of the chain (Sambandam *et al.*, 1991). Although the precise structure in CS for LDL binding has yet to be determined, the binding sites in human apoprotein B-100 have been located at residue 3363 (Boren *et al.*, 1998), whereas different binding sites exist in apoprotein B-48 (Flood *et al.*, 2002). Furthermore, it has been shown that 4-sulfated CS prevents Cu^{2+}-induced LDL oxidation, whereas interaction of LDL with 6-sulfated CS increases the susceptibility of lipoproteins to oxidized *in vitro* (Albertini *et al.*, 1997). 6-sulfated CS is markedly increased in early atherosclerotic lesions, suggesting a significant contribution not only to LDL retention but also to modification of LDL in subendothelial layer (Theocharis *et al.*, 2002) (Fig. 1). Actually the binding of LDL to CSPGs makes them more sensitive to structural modifications, such as oxidation and hydrolysis, thereby affecting their potential atherogenecity. CSPGs also affect the intracellular accumulation of lipids. CSPGs-LDL complexes are internilized rapidly by macrophages and ASMCs through both LDL receptor and LDL receptor-related protein pathways (Camejo *et al.*, 1998; Llorente-Cortes *et al.*, 2002). The avidity of this uptake results in intracellular accumulation of lipids and the formation of foam cells, which are found in atheroclerotic plaques.

B. Role of CSPGs in Atherosclerotic Inflammatory Process

The accumulation of CSPGs in the ECM in early atherosclerotic lesions may also influnce the retention of inflammatory cells. CSPGs like versican can bind both to hyaluronan and CD44, stabilizing the CD44-dependent interactions of inflammatory cells with ECM. The interaction of versican with CD44 is mediated through CS chains and the link module domain

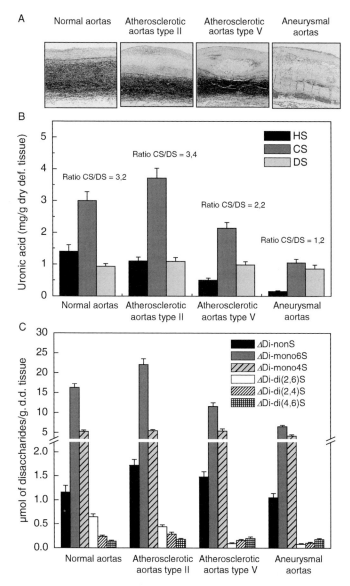

FIGURE I (A) Histochemical examination and evaluation of normal, atherosclerotic type II, atherosclerotic type V, and aneurysmal aortic specimens using Movat's pentachrome staining. Elastic fibers stain black, collagen fibers bright yellow, and PGs/GAGs blue-green, whereas the cytoplasmic contractile apparatus of smooth and striated muscle stains red–orange. (B) Glycosaminoglycan distribution in the corresponding aortic specimens. (C) Disaccharide composition of CS/DS chains isolated from the corresponding aortic specimens (Modified from Theocharis *et al.* 2002, Fig. 1, p. 670, Fig. 3, p. 671, and Table I, p. 672).

present on the amino-terminal region of CD44 (Wight and Merrilees, 2004). Furthermore, CSPGs interact through specific oversulfated sequences in the CS chains with other adhesion molecules present on the surface of inflammatory leukocytes, such as P- and L-selectin, which have been implicated in leucocyte trafficking and inflammatory disease as well as with chemokines (Hirose *et al.*, 2001; Kawashima *et al.*, 1999, 2000, 2002). The adhesion molecules and chemokines preferentially bind the tetrasaccharide GlcA-GalNAc(4S,6S)-GlcA-GalNAc(4S,6S) isolated from squid cartilage CS-E. Thus, CSPGs enriched ECM provides multiple binding sites for inflammatory cells. CSPGs could influence the availability of inflammatory chemokines and further promote inflammation. Versican through its CS chains has been demonstrated that bind several chemokines involved in the recruitment of mononuclear leukocytes. These interactions may sustain the inflammatory response making versican a key molecule of the inflammatory process occurred in atherosclerosis. The CS-containing splice variants of CD44 are also able to interact with interferon γ, regulating some of the biological effects of this cytokine on ASMCs (Hurt-Camejo *et al.*, 1999). The latter suggests a potential role for CSPGs accumulating in atheroslerotic lesions to retain inflammatory cytokines at the surfaces of ASMCs.

C. Versican as an Important Modulator of ASMCs Properties

Versican and hyaluronan aggregates accumulate in the pericellular matrix when ASMCs are stimulated to proliferate and migrate creating a viscoelastic coat around the cells. The accumulation of versican–hyaluronan aggregates is a hallmark in early atherosclerotic lesions. ECM enriched in versican and hyaluronan allows the cells to change shape to prepare their proliferation and migration. In addition, versican acts as an antiadhesive molecule through interactions with hyaluronan at the cell surface (Wight, 2002; Wight and Merrilees, 2004). These properties of versican reside in the CS chains attached on the core protein. It has been demonstrated (Lemire *et al.*, 2002) that the overexpression of V3 isoform of versican, which lacks CS chains, by retroviral transduction in ASMCs promotes adhesion, flattening of the cells, increase in the close contacts, decrease in cell detachment in response to trypsin, reduction of pericellular coats, and inhibition of growth and migration. The effect of V3 expression on these phenotypic changes is thought to be mediated by competition of V3 with V1 for binding to hyaluronan at the cell surface. The exact mechanism through which CS chains involved in cell proliferation is still unknown.

The supramolecular aggregates of versican with hyaluronan and link proteins trap water creating viscoelastic and turgor pressures within the arterial wall. These are considered to create reversibly compressive structures necessary to avoid the deformation of blood vessels by the pulsatile pressures of the circulatory system. In advanced atherosclerotic lesions, a significant stage-related decrease of CSPGs, especially in versican, occurs and is accompanied by a dramatic decrease in aneurysmal aortas (Theocharis and Karamanos, 2002; Theocharis *et al.*, 1999, 2001, 2002) (Fig. 1). This is a result of the decreased number of ASMCs found in advanced lesions, since they are going to apoptosis due to the high-local concentration of oxidants, the limited diffusion of nutrient molecules through thickned intima, or possible direct cytotoxic effect of T lymphocytes present in these lesions. Furthermore, a specific down regulation of the expression of fully glycanated isoform of versican V1 in aneurysmal aortas has been demonstrated. It has been suggested that the elimination of the concentration of versican and the replacement of fully glycanated isoform V0 by limited glycanated isoforms, like V1, in advanced atherosclerotic lesion and in aneurysmal aortic wall create an ECM with lower swelling pressure and decreased viscoelastic properties. These changes may be crucial for the reduction of the aortic wall viscoelastic and compressive properties, and the subsequent deformation and dilatation of the aorta occurred in aortic aneurysm, a disease associated with advanced atherosclerosis.

D. CSPGs as Regulators of ECM Organization and Biomechanical Properties of Aortic Wall

CSPGs are also involved in ECM assembly, providing the vessel wall with specific biomechanical properties. A continuous ECM remodeling takes place during different phases of atherosclerosis as part of tissue injury and inflammatory response. During these phases, a continuous degradation and disassembly of various ECM components is occurred, which is accompanied by reassembly of particular components. Early atherosclerotic lesions are characterized by the deposition of ECM molecules creating a loose and waterly ECM, which permits the cellular proliferation, invasion, and tissue repair. A more fibrous ECM enriched in collagen and assorted glycoproteins then replaces this hydrated ECM in advanced atherosclerotic lesions and aneurysmal aortic wall (Theocharis and Karamanos, 2002; Theocharis *et al.*, 2002; Wight and Merrilees, 2004) (Fig. 1). The newly remodeled ECM is constantly free from mature elastic fibers, a major ECM protein found in media layer of elastic arteries. Elastic fibers are important for the regulation of intimal thickening, ASMCs proliferation, and migration (Brooke *et al.*, 2003). Furthermore, elastic fibers are critical for regulation of the biomechanical properties of the tissue. The elastic fibers in the medial layer totally adsorb the pressure waves of the circulatory system expanding their lamellae. Collagen fibers dominated in all layers of advanced atherosclerotic vessel as well as in aneurysmal aortic wall alter the mechanical properties of the tissue providing vessel wall with stiffness and rigidity, reducing its viscoelastic and compressive properties. Thus, factors regulating the elastic fiber formation are important for controlling vascular lesion formation as well as vessel wall functionality. CS chains predominate in CSPGs in early atherosclerotic lesions seems to be an important factor that inhibits elastic fibers assembly (Hinek *et al.*, 1991). Actually, elastic fibers are depleted in tissues in which versican levels are elevated such as in restenotic lesions. Overexpression of versican isoform V3 that lacks CS chains in ASMCs results in changes in tropoelastin expression and accumulation of elastic fibers in long-term cultures (Merrilees *et al.*, 2002). When transduced cells are seeded into ballon injured rat carotid arteries, a highly structured neointima enriched in elastic lamellae develops. It has been also demonstrated (Hinek *et al.*, 2004) that overexpression of V3 completely reverses impaired elastogenesis in skin fibroblasts from Costello syndrome and Hurler disease. This phenotypic reversal is accompanied by loss of CS from the cell surface and increased levels of elastin binding protein (EBP). It is suggested that induction of elastic fiber production by gene transfer of V3 is mediated by rescue of the tropoelastin chaperone EBP.

Fibroblasts from Costello syndrome and Hurler disease synthesize tropoelastin at a normal rate but are unable to assemble extracellular insoluble elastin. This is also accompanied with low amounts of EBP and is associated with quick lose of EBP into conditioned media, suggesting a deficiency in this recyclable tropoelastin chaperone. Taking together with the observation that β-galactosugars can bind to the galactolectin domain of EBP and to inhibit tropoelastin binding to EBP supports a central regulatory role for CS in elastic fibers assembly. Furthermore, the observation that enzymatic degradation of CS by exogenous added chondroitinase ABC leads to restoration of elastic fibers assembly in cultures of skin fibroblasts derived from patients with Costello syndrome of Hurler disease supports this suggestion (Hinek *et al.*, 2004). The replacement of CS-bearing versican by nonglycanated V3 in versican–hyaluronan–CD44 supramolecular complexes at the cell surface is suggested to be responsible for the rescue of EBP, overexpression of tropoelastin, and proper formation of elastic fibers assembly. Thus, the overexpression of CSPGs, especially that of versican, in early atherosclerotic lesions is probably a negative regulator of elastic fibers formation, development of atherosclerotic lesions, and reduced biomechanical properties of the tissue.

IV. CSPGs in Cancer Development

A. Types, Differential Expression, and Structural Modification of CSPGs in Various Cancer Types

CSPGs are not only important structural molecules for proper ECM assembly but are also functional key molecules regulating several cellular processes (Fig. 2). Abnormal expression and function of PGs have been

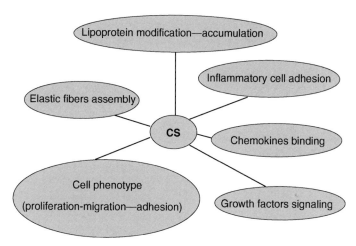

FIGURE 2 Biological functions of CS chains implicated to the development of atherosclerosis and cancer progression.

demonstrated in various types of cancer. The development of newly formed tumor stroma is a characteristic feature of numerous solid tumors. Tumor stroma and tumor fibrotic tissue contain abnormaly higher concentration of PGs than corresponding surrounding tissue. The major types of PGs accumulated in tumor stroma are CSPGs, especially versican and decorin. Proteoglycans accumulated in the tumor stroma exhibit contradictory properties. For example, SLRPs, especially decorin, has proven antiproliferative properties, whereas versican seems to promote tumor growth and spread (Iozzo, 1998; Wegrowski and Maquart, 2004).

Decorin is overexpressed in various malignant tumors such as colorectal carcinoma, colon adenocarcinoma, melanoma, osteosarcoma, basal cell carcinoma. This PG is also expressed in benign tumors with strong fibrotic reaction. In contrast, other malignant tumors are characterized by decreased decorin expression (Wegrowski and Maquart, 2004). Decorin antiproliferative activity is thought partially to be mediated by acting as a natural inhibitor of TGFβ, since decorin core protein binds this growth factor and limits its bioavailability (Yamaguchi et al., 1990). Upregulation of decorin gene expression is associated with growth arrest through upregulation of p21$^{\text{Cip1/WAF1}}$ protein, and therefore, decorin has direct antiprolifeartive properties. Furthermore, decorin acts as a ligand for EGF receptor. In breast cancer, the ectopic expression of decorin induced an inhibition in signaling mediated through EGF receptor (Iozzo, 1998; Wegrowski and Maquart, 2004). In contrast, versican expression is associated with tumor growth, in vitro angiogenesis and cancer cell spread (Wight, 2002). The accumulation of CSPGs in tumor stroma in various malignant tumors is associated with specific posttranslational modifications (Theocharis, 2002; Theocharis and Theocharis, 2002; Theocharis *et al.*, 2000, 2003; Tsara *et al.*, 2002). In colon adenocarcinoma (Theocharis, 2002), decorin and versican accumulation is accompanied by alteration in the type of GAG bound on core proteins. Dermatan sulfate (DS) is the major type of GAG bound on versican and decorin cores and is replaced by CS chains. This alteration is associated with the sulfation pattern of GAG chain, 4-sulfated disaccharides predominated in both PGs in normal tissue are minor consituents of the CS chain in malignant tumors. CS chains are enriched to 6-sulfated disaccharides with elevated amounts of nonsulfated units. Furthermore, CS and remaining DS chains of both PGs have decreased molecular size. Accumulation of versican and decorin in tumor stroma accompanied by posttranslational modifications in the type and sulfation of CS/DS chains of these PGs similar to those observed in colon adenocarcinoma were also observed in pancreatic (Theocharis *et al.*, 2000), gastric (Theocharis *et al.*, 2003), and rectum carcinoma (Theocharis and Theocharis, 2002; Tsara *et al.*, 2002). In contrast to cancer development in gastrointestinal track, the development of laryngeal squamous cell carcinoma follows a different way (Skandalis *et al.*, 2004). Larynx is a complex organ composed of four kinds of cartilage, which comprise the skeletal structure of cartilage and are consisted mainly of collagen type II and aggrecan. The destruction of these cartilages is suggested to be a prerequisite for the spread of endolaryngeal tumors arise from epithelial layer, since cartilages are suggested to behave like natural barriers to the tumor spread. The development of laryngeal squamous cell carcinoma is characterized by a simultaneous destruction of cartilages and decrease of aggrecan, which is accompanied by elevation of matrix PGs versican and decorin in tumor stroma in soft tissue. The accumulation of versican and decorin is not able to balance the marked decrease of aggrecan in this tissue, so a dramatic decrease in CS concentration and to 6-sulfated disaccharide units is observed in laryngeal cancer (Skandalis *et al.* 2004).

B. Structural Alterations of CSPGs Influence the Biology of Cancer Cells

The sulfation pattern of CS and DS is suggested as a key mediator of several biological events. It has been proposed that the increase in the ratio of 6-sulfated to 4-sulfated disaccharides in CS represents a general phenomenon that is occurred in immature tissues, which are containing proliferating and differentiated cells. It has been suggested that influence some developmentally significant events such as cellular adhesion, migration, and neurite outgrowth. As shown by recent studies, the type and the sulfation patterns of versican and decorin present in ECM are of great importance for the migration of the cells through ECM. It has been demonstrated (Perissinotto *et al.*, 2000) that versican promotes the migration of neural crest cells, lining their migratory routes, and both core protein and the GAG side chains mediate this function. Versican purified by the migratory routes of neural crest cells is primarily substituted with 6-sulfated CS. The substitution of versican by DS chains is suggested to be responsible for the repulsion-like effects exerted on the migration of neural crest cells. Identical effects have been documented for aggrecan, which inhibits the migration of neural crest cells. Merle *et al.* (1999) showed that decorin inhibits the migration of MG-63 osteosarcoma cells, and this phenomenon is depended on both core protein and GAG chain and is diferentially mediated by its GAG chains. Particularly, it was demonstrated that decorin bearing DS chain was 20-fold more effective in inhibiting migration of cells than decorin bearing CS chains. These data suggest that fine structural alterations of versican and decorin in tumor stroma may influence directly the biology of cancer cells, contributing to cell growth and migration through a mechanism similar to that observed in neural crest cells and osteosarcoma.

C. Role of CS in Interactions with Growth Factors/Cytokines and Cell Signaling

Studies demonstrated that CS is able to interact with various growth factors that dictate various biological processes during tumor growth and spread (Fig. 2). CS chains interact with heparin binding growth factors, and these interactions are specifically inhibited by CS or DS containing the E disaccharide unit consisted by GlcA-GalNAc(4S, 6S) or the corresponding disaccharide of DS, IdoA-GalNAc(4S, 6S) (Sugahara *et al.*, 2003). CSE isolated from squid cartilage binds several heparin-binding growth factors, including FGF-2, FGF-10, FGF-16, FGF-18 midkine (MK), pleiotrophin (PTN), and heparin binding epidermal growth factor (Deepa *et al.*, 2002; Sugahara *et al.*, 2003). MK and PTN have well-established neuroregulatory activities, promoting neuronal adhesion and migration, survival of hippocampal neurons, and neurite extension (Kadomatsu and Muramatsu, 2004). The interactions of CS-E with MK and PTN as well as with FGF-18 exhibit high affinity comparable to those with heparin. This implies that additionally to HS chains, CS chains containing E units function as coreceptors for these growth factors, similar to the function of DS chains as coreceptor for FGF-2, FGF-7, and HGF (Sugahara *et al.*, 2003). The heparin-binding activity of MK and PTN postulated that HSPGs of cell membrane may be members of the receptor complex of these growth factors. Syndecans, the hybrid HS/CSPGs, are able to bind MK and PTN and is suggested that PTN and *N*-syndecan utilize the contractin-Src pathway for the intracellular signaling in neurite outgrowth (Kadomatsu and Muramatsu, 2004). MK and PTN also bind to CSPG PTPζ with high affinity, and this binding is essential in order to induce nerve-cell migration. PTPζ is a receptor-type protein tyrosine phosphatase of which the extracellular domain bearing CS chains and the intracellular domain exhibit protein tyrosine phosphatase activity. The Kd of PTPζ for MK is 0.56 nM, while chondroitinase digestion increases it to 8.8 nM, indicating that the CS chain is necessary for high affinity. MK and PTPζ utilize PI3-kinase and Erk for osteoblast cell migration and neuronal survival. PTN binds to PTPζ inactivates phosphatase activity of PTPζ and eventually induces tyrosine phosphorylation of β-catenin (Kadomatsu and Muramatsu, 2004). Several studies indicate that MK and PTN are overexpressed in various malignant tumors and may be markers for carcinomas. MK and PTN promote cancer-cell growth and survival. Cell migration activity of MK and PTN has been demonstrated for osteoblastic osteosarcoma cells and seems that N-syndecan and PTPζ are involved in this activity. CS chains play a crucial role in MK-mediated cell migration, and this activity of MK involves PI3-kinase and Erk signaling (Kadomatsu and Muramatsu, 2004). PTN is also an important regulator of angiogenesis, and this function is mediated through PTPζ, involving Src kinase, focal adhesion kinase, PI3-kinase, and Erk signaling (Polykratis *et al.*, 2005).

D. CS as Anticancer Agent

CS can also be used directly as anticancer agent or can be used for efficient drug delivery. CS as well as HS chains exposed to carbodiimide (EDAC) substantially reduced cell viability by induction of apoptosis in myeloma cells and breast cancer cells *in vitro*. The modified CS when injected directly into breast tumors growing in nude mice reduced or abolished cancer-cell growth without causing apparent toxocity to adjacent normal tissues. This new class of CS molecules demonstrates important anticancer activities and may develop as a novel class of therapeutic agents (Pumphrey *et al.*, 2002). Taking into account the observation that CS is overexpressed in several highly metastatic tumors developed the idea to use CS as a target for the selective delivery of anticancer drugs by polyethylene glycol (PEG)-coated liposomes. These liposomes contained a new cationic lipid 3,5-dipentadecycloxybenzamidine hydrochloride (TRX-20) bound preferentially to CS and avidly internalized by highly metastatic tumor cells. When TRX-20 liposomes loaded with cisplatin, they effectively killed the CS-expressing tumor cells *in vitro* and *in vivo*. It is suggested that CS-targeted delivery of anticancer drugs by novel cationic liposomes represents a potentially useful strategy to prevent the local growth and metastasis of tumor cells that have enhanced expression of CS (Lee *et al.*, 2002).

V. Conclusions

In this chapter, we describe that CS chains implicated in several biological functions involved in the development of atherosclerosis and cancer progression. CS plays important role in lipoprotein retention, modification, and internalization in atherosclerosis as well as in the inflammatory process occurred in this disease. ASMCs phenotype, ECM organization, as well as the biomechanical properties of the vessels are also influenced by CS chains, suggesting that CSPGs are key molecules for the development of vascular disease (Fig. 2). Furthermore, an increasing number of recent studies demonstrate marked accumulation of specific CSPGs in the tumor stroma, and CS chains are characterized by specific structural modifications. This general phenomenon demonstrated in various cancer types may suggest a fundamental biological role for CS chains in tumor progression. Although this biological role has not been determined yet, a clear correlation of CSPGs accumulation, especially the deposition of versican, with cancer progression has been demonstrated. Future work will help to clarify the biological functions of CSPGs and their involvement in pathological mechanisms underlying many different human diseases.

References

Albertini, R., Ramos, P., Giessauf, A., Passi, A., DeLuca, G., and Esterbauer, H. (1997). Chondroitin 4-sulfate exhibits inhibitory effect during Cu^{2+} mediated LDL oxidation. *FEBS Lett.* **403,** 154–158.

Boren, J., Olin, K., Lee, I., Chait, A., Wight, T. N., and Innerarity, T. L. (1998). Identification of a principal proteoglycan binding site in LDL: A single point mutation in apoB-100 severely affects proteoglycan interaction without affecting LDL receptor binding. *J. Clin. Invest.* **101,** 2658–2664.

Brooke, B. S., Karnik, S. K., and Li, D. Y. (2003). Extracellular matrix in vascular morphogenesis and disease: Structure versus signal. *Trends Cell Biol.* **13,** 51–56.

Camejo, G., Hurt-Camejo, E., Wiklund, O., and Bondjers, G. (1998). Association of apoB-lipoproteins with arterial proteoglycans: Pathological significance and molecular basis. *Atherosclerosis* **139,** 205–222.

Cardoso, L. E., and Mourao, P. A. (1994). Glycosaminoglycan fraction from human arteries presenting diverse susceptibilities to atherosclerosis have different binding affinities to plasma LDL. *Arterioscler. Thromb.* **14,** 115–124.

Deepa, S. S., Umehara, Y., Higashiyama, S., Itoh, N., and Sugahara, K. (2002). Specific interactions of oversulfated chondroitin sulphate E with various heparin-binding growth factors: Implications as a physiological binding partner. *J. Biol. Chem.* **277,** 43707–43716.

Flood, C., Gustafsson, M., Richardson, P. E., Harvey, S. C., Segrest, J. P., and Boren, J. (2002). Identification of the proteoglycan binding site in apolipoprotein B48. *J. Biol. Chem.* **277,** 32228–32233.

Hinek, A., Mecham, R. P., Keeley, F., and Rabinovitch, M. (1991). Impaired elastin fiber assembly related to reduced 67-kD elastin-binding protein in fetal lamb ductus arteriosus and in cultured aortic smooth muscle cells treated with chondroitin sulfate. *J. Clin. Invest.* **88,** 2083–2094.

Hinek, A., Braun, K. R., Liu, K., Wang, Y., and Wight, T. N. (2004). Retrovirally mediated overexpression of versican V3 reverses impaired elastogenesis and heightened proliferation exhibited by fibroblasts from Costello syndrome and Hurler disease patients. *Am. J. Pathol.* **164,** 119–131.

Hirose, J., Kawashima, H., Yoshie, O., Tashiro, K., and Miyasaka, M. (2001). Versican interacts with chemokines and modulates cellular responces. *J. Biol. Chem.* **276**, 5228–5234.

Hurt-Camejo, E., Rosengren, B., Sartipy, P., Elfsberg, K., Camejo, G., and Svensson, L. (1999). CD44, a cell surface chondroitin sulfate proteoglycan, mediates binding of interferon-γ and some of its biological effects on human vascular smooth muscle cells. *J. Biol. Chem.* **274**, 18957–18964.

Iozzo, R. V. (1998). Matrix proteoglycans: From molecular design to cellular function. *Annu. Rev. Biochem.* **67**, 609–652.

Kadomatsu, K., and Muramatsu, T. (2004). Midkine and pleiotrophin in neural development and cancer. *Cancer Lett.* **204**, 127–143.

Kawashima, H., Li, Y. F., Watanabe, N., Hirose, J., Hirose, M., and Miyasaka, M. (1999). Identification and characterization of ligands for L-selectin in the kidney: Versican, a large chondroitin sulfate proteoglycan, is a ligand for L-selectin. *Int. Immunol.* **11**, 393–405.

Kawashima, H., Hirose, M., Hirose, J., Nagakubo, D., Plaas, A., and Miyasaka, M. (2000). Binding of a large chondroitin sulfate/dermatan sulfate proteoglycan, versican, to L-selectin, P-selectin, and CD44. *J. Biol. Chem.* **275**, 35448–35456.

Kawashima, H., Atarashi, K., Hirose, M., Hirose, J., Yamada, S., Sugahara, K., and Miyasaka, M. (2002). Oversulfated chondroitin/dermatan sulfates containing GlcAβ1/IdoAα1–3GalNAc(4,6-O-disulfate) interact with L- and P-selectin and chemokines. *J. Biol. Chem.* **277**, 12921–12930.

Kjellen, L., and Lindahl, U. (1991). Proteoglycans: Structures and interactions. *Annu. Rev. Biochem.* **60**, 443–475.

Lee, C. M., Tanaka, T., Murai, T., Kondo, M., Kimura, J., Su, W., Kitagawa,, T, Ito, T., Matsuda, H., and Miyasaka, M. (2002). Novel chondroitin sulphate-binding cationic liposomes loaded with cisplatin efficiently suppress the local growth and liver metastasis of tumor cells *in vivo. Cancer Res.* **62**, 4282–4288.

Lemire, J. M., Merrilees, M. J., Braun, K. R., and Wight, T. N. (2002). Overexpression of the V3 variant of versican alters arterial smooth muscle cell adhesion, migration, and proliferation *in vitro. J. Cell. Physiol.* **190**, 38–45.

Llorente-Cortes, V., Otero-Vinas, M., Hurt-Camejo, E., Martinez-Gonzalez, J., and Badimon, L. (2002). Human coronary smooth muscle cells internalize versican-modified LDL through LDL receptor-related protein and LDL receptors. *Arterioscler. Thromb. Vasc. Biol.* **22**, 387–393.

Merle, B., Durussel, L., Delmas, P. D., and Clezardin, P. (1999). Decorin inhibits cell migration through a process requiring its glycosaminoglycan side chain. *J. Cell. Biochem.* **75**, 538–546.

Merrilees, M. J., Lemire, J. M., Fischer, J. W., Kinsella, M. G., Braun, K. R., Clowes, A. W., and Wight, T. N. (2002). Retrovirally mediated overexpression of versican V3 by arterial smooth muscle cells induces tropoelastin synthesis and elastic fiber formation *in vitro* and in neointima after vascular injury. *Circ. Res.* **90**, 481–487.

Pentikainen, M. O., Oorni, K., Lassila, R., and Kovanen, P. T. (1997). The proteoglycan decorin links low density lipoproteins with collagen type I. *J. Biol. Chem.* **272**, 7633–7638.

Perissinotto, D., Iacopetti, P., Bellina, I., Doliana, R., Colombatti, A., Pettway, Z., Bronner-Fraser, M., Shinomura, T., Kimata, K., Morgelin, M., Lofberg, J., and Perris, R. (2000). Avian neural crest cell migration is diversely regulated by the two major hyaluronan-binding proteoglycans PG-M/versican and aggrecan. *Development* **127**, 2823–2842.

Polykratis, A., Katsoris, P., Courty, J., and Papadimitriou, E. (2005). Characterization of heparin affin regulatory peptide signalling in human endothelial cells. *J. Biol. Chem.* **280**, 22454–22461.

Pumphrey, C. Y., Theus, A. M., Li, S., Parrish, R. S., and Sanderson, R. D. (2002). Neoglycans, carbodiimide-modified glycosaminoglycans: A new class of anticancer agents that inhibit cancer cell proliferation and induce apoptosis. *Cancer Res.* **62**, 3722–3728.

Sambandam, T., Baker, J. R., Christner, J. E., and Ekborg, S. L. (1991). Specificity of the low density lipoprotein-glycosaminoglycan interaction. *Arterioscler. Thromb.* **11**, 561–568.

Skandalis, S. S., Theocharis, A. D., Theocharis, D. A., Papadas, T., Vynios, D. H., and Papageorgakopoulou, N. (2004). Matrix proteoglycans are markedly affected in advanced laryngeal squamous cell carcinoma. *Biochim. Biophys. Acta* **1689**, 152–161.

Sugahara, K., Mikami, T., Uyama, T., Mizuguchi, S., Nomura, K., and Kitagawa, H. (2003). Recent advances in the structural biology of chondroitin sulfate and dermatan sulfate. *Curr. Opin. Struct. Biol.* **13**, 612–620.

Theocharis, A. D. (2002). Human colon adenocarcinoma is associated with specific post-translational modifications of versican and decorin. *Biochim. Biophys. Acta* **1588**, 165–172.

Theocharis, A. D., and Karamanos, N. K. (2002). Decreased biglycan expression and differential decorin localization in human abdominal aortic aneurysms. *Atherosclerosis* **165**, 221–230.

Theocharis, A. D., and Theoharis, D. A. (2002). High-performance capillary electrophoretic analysis of hyaluronan and galactosaminoglycan-disaccharides in gastrointestinal carcinomas. Differential disaccharide composition as a possible tool-indicator for malignancies. *Biomed. Chromatogr.* **16**, 157–161.

Theocharis, A. D., Tsolakis, I., Tsegenidis, T., and Karamanos, N. K. (1999). Human abdominal aortic aneurysm is closely associated with compositional and specific structural modifications at the glycosaminoglycan level. *Atherosclerosis* **145**, 359–368.

Theocharis, A. D., Tsara, M. E., Papageorgacopoulou, N., Karavias, D. D., and Theocharis, D. A. (2000). Pancreatic carcinoma is characterized by elevated content of hyaluronan and chondroitin sulfate with altered disaccharide composition. *Biochim. Biophys. Acta* **1502**, 201–206.

Theocharis, A. D., Tsolakis, I., Hjerpe, A., and Karamanos, N. K. (2001). Human abdominal aortic aneurysm is characterized by decreased versican concentration and specific downregulation of versican isoform V0. *Atherosclerosis* **154**, 367–376.

Theocharis, A. D., Theocharis, D. A., DeLuca, G., Hjerpe, A., and Karamanos, N. K. (2002). Compositional and structural alterations of chondroitin and dermatan sulfates during the progression of atherosclerosis and aneurysmal dilatation of the human abdominal aorta. *Biochimie* **84**, 667–674.

Theocharis, A. D., Vynios, D. H., Papageorgakopoulou, N., Skandalis, S. S., and Theocharis, D. A. (2003). Altered content, composition and structure of glycosaminoglycans and proteoglycans in gastric carcinoma. *Int. J. Biochem. Cell Biol.* **35**, 376–390.

Timar, J., Lapis, K., Dudas, J., Sebestyen, A., Kopper, L., and Kovalszky, I. (2002). Proteoglycans and tumor progression: Janus-faced molecules with contradictory functions in cancer. *Semin. Cancer Biol.* **12**, 173–186.

Tsara, M. E., Theocharis, A. D., and Theocharis, D. A. (2002). Compositional and structural alterations of proteoglycans in human rectum carcinoma with special reference to versican and decorin. *Anticancer Res.* **22**, 2893–2898.

Wegrowski, Y., and Maquart, F. X. (2004). Involvement of stromal proteoglycans in tumour progression. *Crit. Rev. Oncol. Hematol.* **49**, 259–268.

Wight, T. N. (2002). Versican: A versatile extracellular matrix proteoglycan in cell biology. *Curr. Opin. Cell Biol.* **14**, 617–623.

Wight, T. N., and Merrilees, M. J. (2004). Proteoglycans in atherosclerosis and restenosis: Key roles for versican. *Circ. Res.* **94**, 1158–1167.

Wight, T. N., Kinsella, M. G., and Owarnstrom, E. E. (1992). The role of proteoglycans in cell adhesion, migration and proliferation. *Curr. Opin. Cell Biol.* **4**, 793–801.

Yamaguchi, Y., Mann, D. M., and Ruoslahti, E. (1990). Negative regulator of transforming growth factor-β by the proteoglycan decorin. *Nature* **346**, 281–284.

Yanusz Wegrowski and François-Xavier Maquart

CNRS UMR 6198, Faculty of Medicine,
IFR-53, 51095 Reims Cedex,
France

Chondroitin Sulfate Proteoglycans in Tumor Progression

I. Chapter Overview

In developing tumor, several chondroitin sulfate proteoglycans (CSPGs) are overexpressed and deposited into extracellular matrix (ECM) during the stromal reaction. The accumulated PGs participate in the organization of ECM and modulate tumor cell behavior. Whereas large CSPGs of the hyalectan (lectican) family, like versican or nervous tissue BEHAB/brevican, carry out protumoral effects by increasing cell motility and migration, the small leucine-rich proteoglycans (SLRP) family, notably decorin and lumican, have antitumoral properties. The CSPGs of cell surface, particularly CD44 or NG2/MAA, synthesized and expressed by tumor cells, stimulate cell growth, migration, and detachment from the substratum, contributing to tumor growth and metastasis. Some fragments of PG core protein (matrikines) and degraded GAGs contribute in local reaction in their own part.

Advances in Pharmacology, Volume 53
Copyright 2006, Elsevier Inc. All rights reserved.

1054-3589/06 $35.00
DOI: 10.1016/S1054-3589(05)53014-X

This chapter discusses the implication of stromal and cell surface CSPGs to the different aspects of tumor growth and metastasis.

II. Introduction

Proteoglycans containing CS chain(s) are ubiquitous components of all extracellular matrices and, probably, all mammals' cell surfaces including erythrocyte membrane (Baggio *et al.*, 1990). CS is synthesized in Golgi compartment by the successive addition of *N*-acetyl-galactosamine and hexuronic acid units (see previous chapters). The synthesis of hexuronic acid is a unique nonredundant pathway controlled by UDP-glucose dehydrogenase (UGDH) (Wegrowski *et al.*, 1998). Mutational inactivation of UGDH is lethal in mammals, stopping embryo development at the step of gastrulation by mesoderm formation failure (Garcia-Garcia and Anderson, 2003). Although GAGs are necessary for the assembling of all extracellular matrices, including tumor stroma, transformed cells of growing and invading tumors keep in touch with ECM of host organ. This matrix contains the intrinsic information to control cell and macromolecular movement (Hornebeck and Birembaut, 2004). CS plays a part in this control. Two well-known examples are: (i) the inhibition of neurite outgrowth by CS (Morgenstern *et al.*, 2002) and (ii) ion exchange exclusion of anionic macromolecules (Jaques, 1991). Recent studies showed that the core protein and fragments of CSPG may also influence the cell behavior. The control of angiogenesis by fragment of perlecan (endorepelin) may serve as an example (Bix and Iozzo, 2005).

Invading tumors synthesize a plethora of macromolecules, including growth factors, chemokines, proteolytic, and glycolytic enzymes for remodeling ECM and facilitate tumor growth. As the PGs are organizers of ECM, they influence the composition of tumor stroma. On the other hand, mesenchymal cells of host organ respond to pathological signals, developing nonimmune defence mechanisms to constrain tumor growth. Once again, PGs play a major role in this struggle. In general, matrix macromolecules and the products of their degradation: GAGs, matrikines, play informative and modulatory roles for mesenchymal host cells and tumor cells (Maquart *et al.*, 2004). Malignant cells escape from this control by modifying cell surface receptors and expressing new molecules which in turn change the cell capacity to adhere to substratum and modify the anchorage-dependent growth, escaping from anoikis (Frisch and Francis, 1994).

Studies of last two decades permitted a great progress in the comprehension of the GAG and PG involvement in the modulation of cell behavior, tumor progression, and metastasis. The recombinant protein approach and the application of monoclonal antibodies revealed interesting features of core protein of CSPG. Previous chapters and different reviews gave a state-of-the-art of stromal and cell surface PGs. The scope of this chapter is to outline the progress of the comprehension of the biological role of CSPG in tumor growth, progression, and invasion during the last decade. Earlier studies have been described in detail in some further reviews (Iida et al., 1996; Iozzo and Cohen, 1994).

III. The Stromal Reaction

Most, if not all, growing solid tumors induce the formation of extracellular stroma, the phenomenon called stromal reaction (Ioachim, 1976). For a long time, ECM was only considered as an architectural support for tumor cells. Recent data, however, indicate that ECM is, in fact, a major component for the regulation of cell activity. The different modules of the proteins that constitute the ECM macromolecules represent, for the cells that enter into contact with them, new signals capable of activating several intracellular signaling pathways, resulting in the modulation of numerous cell functions (Maquart et al., 2004). CSPGs and hyaluronan are necessary to the organization of ECM. They contribute also to cell signaling (Williams and Davies, 2001). Tumor cells can neither proliferate nor migrate without modification of the stroma or without the help of nontumor cells. For example, the migration of the cells is largely supported by CS and hyaluronan.

Extracellular "structural" macromolecules, including CSPG, have a modular architecture. The low-molecular mass "modules," able to influence cell behavior, were recently called "matrikines" (Maquart et al., 2004). The proteolysis and glycolysis of stroma macromolecules may liberate matrikines, which often have properties different to original macromolecule. For instance, the degradation products of hyaluronan inhibit tumor cell growth (Ghatak et al., 2002) whereas macromolecular hyaluronan accelerates cell migration (Adamia et al., 2005).

The concentration of PGs and GAG are higher in tumor stroma that in adjacent host organ stroma (Ricciardelli et al., 1997; Timar et al., 2002) and still more concentrated in tumor growing edge (Nara et al., 1997). Also, the PG's composition is different, and their metabolism accelerated in tumor stroma (Heredia et al., 1996; Papadas et al., 2002; Theocharis and Theocharis, 2002). The PGs may influence tumor cells and host organ fibroblasts, changing their phenotype. For instance, fibroblasts in tumoral zone often acquire a myofibroblastic phenotype (Desmouliere et al., 2004). Except basement membrane, stromal PGs are CS type; heparan sulfate (HS) PGs are fragments of macromolecules shaded from cell surface.

The tumor stromal GAG content and structure were analyzed in details (Nagle, 2004; Shriver et al., 2002; Trowbridge and Gallo, 2002). The composition of GAG is different in tumor as compared to normal tissue, and in general, tumor stroma contains higher concentration of GAGs, indicating an accelerated metabolism. For example, increased galactosaminoglycan (GalAG) deposition characterizes hepatocarcinoma (Kovalszky et al., 1990; Lapis et al., 1990) or cancers of the gastrointestinal tract (Theocharis and Theocharis, 2002). Deposition of GAG is also observed in fibrosis, but their composition and rate of metabolism is more comparable to inflamed tissue. Oversulfation of GAG was reported in fibrosis (Koshiishi et al., 1999) with an increased proportion of dermatan sulfate (DS) (Wegrowski et al., 1999; Yokoyama et al., 1997). In cancer stroma, the ratio CS/HS was found to be increased, partly because of accelerated degradation of HS not only by heparinases/heparitinases (Haimovitz-Friedman et al., 1991) but also by acceleration of CS synthesis. In extreme cases like in mastocytoma, CS replaces HS (Lidholt et al., 1995). The detailed composition of GalAGs of human colon adenocarcinoma was recently published (Daidouji et al., 2002; Theocharis, 2002). In healthy human colon, DS contributes to 90% of GAGs whereas colon adenocarcinoma contains almost 90% of CS with lower-hydrodynamic size. Also the ratio of 4-sulfated to 6-sulfated GAGs is reversed from 4:1 in normal tissue vs. 1:3 in adenocarcinoma. The acceleration of the synthesis of GAG is often accompanied by a substantial increase of nonsulfated disaccharides (Kovalszky et al., 1990). In invading melanoma, the accumulation of CS was associated with the appearance of a higher quantity of CS E, containing 4- and 6-sulfated galactosamine (Smetsers et al., 2004). The accumulation of CS was also noted in prostate tumors (Cardoso et al., 2004). An opposite situation was observed in squamous cell carcinoma, where the loss of CS correlated with the invasion of the tumor into the larynx (Uhlman and Niehans, 1999). The changes of GAG composition may expand to the adjacent, normal tissue as it was observed in the case of renal and liver carcinomas, suggesting the action of soluble factors on adjacent mesenchymal cells (Kovalszky et al., 1990). Such modified macromolecules can modulate tumor cells in different manner.

IV. Tumor Stroma CS/DSPGs

The CSPGs belong to several families. Extracellular PGs include large PGs of the hyalectan family (e.g., agrecan, versican), SLRP, testicans and occasionally substituted with CS, basement membrane PGs (perlecan, agrin). Several collagen types (IX, XII, XIV, and XV) have been shown to exist in CSPG form. Cell surface PGs are divided into three families: transmembrane hyalectans (lecticans), transmembrane syndecans (four genes), and glycosylphosphatidylinositol (GPI)-anchored glypicans (six genes). The nonclassified transmembrane PGs include thrombomodulin, betaglycan, endocan, and NG2/human melanoma PG. Several neural CSPGs have been isolated from brain (Dow and Wang, 1998; Schwartz and Domowicz, 2004). It includes appican, amyloid precursor like protein-2, neuroglycan, neurocan, phosphacan/RPTPbeta/PTPzeta, BEHAB/brevican. Neurocan and brevican shear structural homology with aggrecan and versican of hyalectan family. Numerous excellent reviews describe the properties and characteristics of the PGs (Iozzo, 1998, 1999; Schwartz and Domowicz, 2004). See also the other chapters of this issue.

While some PGs (aggrecan, versican), when synthesized in PG form, are always modified by CS/DS chains, other PGs (e.g., perlecan, syndecans, or glypicans) are either hybrid HS/CS molecules or substituted with HS or CS only. This posttranslational modification of GAG synthesis depends on the concentration and availability of Golgi sugar transferases, which synthesize the GAG nascent chains (Fransson *et al.*, 2000).

The PGs of the same family may share similar tissular/cellular localization. For example, PGs of the SLRP family are located on the collagen fibrils in skin (decorin), cornea (lumican), or tendon (fibromodulin) (Ameye and Young, 2002). The same PG may exist in different spliced forms; the most characteristic are versican and CD44 spliced variants. They were isolated from tumor tissues or from metastases and, at least for the CD44, are associated with the metastatic potential of cells (Naor *et al.*, 2002).

The heterogeneity of GAGs and the existence of more than 50 genes for PGs give a plethora of molecular properties for these macromolecules. Often, the property of an isolated GAG chain is contradictory to those of the same chain attached to the protein core of PGs (Timar *et al.*, 2002). The contradictory properties of PGs vs. GAGs may be seen in tumor progression during stromal reaction (Alaniz *et al.*, 2002; Denholm *et al.*, 2001).

Different PGs have been isolated and characterized from tumor stroma. The expression of SLRP family members was studied in tumors of different origins. Decorin, the most abundant SLRP, is expressed in enhanced level in different malignant tumors like colorectal carcinoma (Tsara *et al.*, 2002), colon adenocarcinoma (Theocharis, 2002), basal cells carcinoma (Hunzelmann *et al.*, 1995), melanoma (Ladanyi *et al.*, 2001), or osteosarcoma (Soderstrom *et al.*, 2002). Numerous benign tumors with strong fibrosing reaction are characterized by enhanced decorin expression and deposition (Berto *et al.*, 2003), especially in central, fibrosing zone. The enhanced expression of decorin during stromal reaction is the result of the hypomethylation of its promoter (Adany and Iozzo, 1991). Other tumors, like lung adenocarcinoma and squamous cell carcinoma (McDoniels-Silvers *et al.*, 2002), hepatocellular carcinoma (Miyasaka *et al.*, 2001), breast carcinoma (Leygue *et al.*, 2000), or ovarian tumors (Nash *et al.*, 2002), are characterized by decreased decorin expression. This may be attributed to intracellular degradation of newly synthesized molecules by illegitimate ubiquitination (Nash *et al.*, 2002). The overexpression of decorin is often accompanied by alterations of the structure of its GAG chain, shifted from DS to CS type (Daidouji *et al.*, 2002). Much less is known about the expression of other SLRP family members. Lumican synthesis is upregulated in pancreatic, colorectal, and breast cancers (Leygue *et al.*, 2000; Lu *et al.*, 2002; Ping Lu *et al.*, 2002) and in stroma of salivary pleiotropic adenoma (Kusafuka *et al.*, 2004). In invasive breast carcinoma, reduced expression of lumican is correlated with cancer progression (Troup *et al.*, 2003). Biglycan is overexpressed in pancreatic cancer (Weber *et al.*, 2001) and hyperplasic thymus (Tomoyasu *et al.*, 1998).

The massive screening techniques based on genomics and proteomics microchips added new knowledge on the expression of SLRP in different tumors. Decorin mRNA expression was observed in pancreatic cancer cells (Blasco *et al.*, 2004) and pancreatic stellate cells (Koninger *et al.*, 2004). Surprisingly, fibromodulin was discovered as tumor-associated antigen in chronic lymphocytic leukemia (Mayr *et al.*, 2005). Several cases of atypical addressing of SLRP were also noted. Lumican accumulated in cytoplasm of the neuroendocrine carcinoma cells (Shinji *et al.*, 2005). Biglycan and decorin were atypically addressed into the nucleus in glioma cells (Liang *et al.*, 1997) and squamous carcinoma cells (Banerjee *et al.*, 2003), respectively.

The implication of SLRP in cancer development has been intensively studied since the discovery of "antioncogenic" effects of decorin. Ectopic expression of decorin retards the growth of many cancer cell lines (Santra *et al.*, 1995) and implanted tumors (Santra *et al.*, 1997). This effect has been observed "at distance" of the decorin expression site. The expression of decorin on the opposite side of the tumor inhibited its growth (Tralhao *et al.*, 2003). Other SLRPs can also contribute to the control of tumor progression. The expression of biglycan by pancreatic cancer cells inhibits cell proliferation by induction of a G1 phase arrest (Weber *et al.*, 2001). Lumican inhibits the anchorage-independent growth of melanoma *in vivo* and *in vitro* (Vuillermoz *et al.*, 2004). The mechanism of tumor growth inhibition by SLRPs may be complex and depend on local cell–protein interaction. The expression of SLRP is often activated during the stromal reaction phase of cancer development (Iozzo, 1995). As these PGs control the formation of the collagen fibrillar network (Iozzo, 1999), the stroma of SLRP-deficient mice could be more permissive for neoplastic progression and formation of metastasis (Ameye and Young, 2002). In addition, it was shown that decorin may regulate tumor angiogenesis. Several SLRPs bind and neutralize growth factors. As growth factors are important molecules for stimulating tumor growth, their neutralization may be an important contribution to cancer therapy. Numerous studies have reported the direct interaction between SLRP and cancer cells. For instance, decorin binds to EGF receptor (Iozzo *et al.*, 1999), downregulates ErbB2 and MAP kinases (Santra *et al.*, 2000) and upregulates p21$^{Cip1/WAF1}$ CDK inhibitor (De Luca *et al.*, 1996), leading to an inhibition of cell proliferation and specific induction of apoptosis in transformed cells (Tralhao *et al.*, 2003). Biglycan and lumican upregulate p27 and downregulate cyclin A and proliferating cell nuclear antigen (Vuillermoz *et al.*, 2004; Weber *et al.*, 2001).

Versican and aggrecan are both high-molecular mass, stromal PGs decorated with CS chains and, in the case of aggrecan, with keratan sulfate (KS) chains also. Like collagen type II, aggrecan is mainly present in cartilaginous matrix. The expression of aggrecan was found enhanced in different tumors of cartilage, including chondroblastoma (Aigner *et al.*, 1999), chondroma (Gottschalk *et al.*, 2001), and chondrosarcoma (Aigner *et al.*, 2002) but decreased in squamous cell carcinoma (Uhlman and Niehans, 1999). The synthesis of aggrecan was also observed in osteosarcoma cells (Liu *et al.*, 1997) and salivary gland adenoma (Zhao *et al.*, 1999), providing an explanation for the formation of pseudo-cartilaginous matrix and calcification, clinically observed in different tumors (Abramovici and Steiner, 2002; Kim *et al.*, 2003).

Versican is expressed in the stroma of several, if not all, human cancers (Isogai *et al.*, 1996), sometimes as the most abundant PG (Tsara *et al.*, 2002). The expression of versican was observed in prostate (Isogai *et al.*, 1996), breast (Suwiwat *et al.*, 2004), lung (Pirinen *et al.*, 2005), ovarian (Voutilainen *et al.*, 2003) cancers and in odontogenic tumors (Ito *et al.*, 2002), several brain tumors (Paulus *et al.*, 1996), melanoma (Touab *et al.*, 2003), pharyngeal squamous cell carcinoma (Pukkila *et al.*, 2004), and keratinocyte tumors (Karvinen *et al.*, 2003). The ECM of glioma contains a small amount of versican, and this PG is absent in squamous cell and *in situ* carcinomas (Karvinen *et al.*, 2003). In general, the most important versican expression was observed in the less differentiated tumors. By immunochemical techniques, versican was localized to peritumoral stroma, and its presence was correlated with hyaluronan expression. Suwiwat *et al.* (2004) analyzed the expression of versican of 86 breast cancers. Versican was expressed on the perifery, and there was no immunostaining in the central part of tumor.

Four isoforms of versican are present in different tissues: V0, V1 V2, and V3 (Cattaruzza *et al.*, 2002). The V3 isoform is deprived of GAG chains. The expression of different isoforms was studied in brain tumors, in melanoma and mesothelioma cells. In brain tumors, only gliomas expressed V2 and V3 isoforms mRNA, with weak immunostaining for the corresponding proteins. More pronounced staining was observed in tumor vessels (Paulus *et al.*, 1996). The aggregation of malignant mesothelioma cells was accompanied by the decreased synthesis of V1 isoform (Syrokou *et al.*, 2002). In melanoma, the expression of V0, V1, and V2 isoforms decreased with cell differentiation (Domenzain *et al.*, 2003) and overexpression of the nonglycosylated V3 isoform correlated with a decreased growth potential of melanoma (Serra *et al.*, 2005) and astrocytoma (Wu *et al.*, 2001).

For diagnosis and prognosis purposes, different cohort studies tried to correlate versican expression with tumor progression and outcome. In breast (Paulus *et al.*, 1996) and nonsmall cell lung cancers (Pirinen *et al.*, 2005), there was a positive correlation between PG expression and the increased risk of relapse or more advanced disease. In prostate cancer, the patients with low-versican expression had better progression-free survival (Ricciardelli *et al.*, 1998). In malignant melanoma dysplastic nevi with severe atypia, versican was a negative prognosis factor, more significant than the characteristic melanoma-associated PG, NG2 (Touab *et al.*, 2003).

The expression of collagenous CS macromolecules is also modulated during tumor development. Collagen type IX is upregulated in ovarian carcinoma (Hibbs *et al.*, 2004). Overexpressed collagen type XIV/undulin and collagen type XVII increased the attachment of the cancer cells to the substratum (Paulus *et al.*, 1993; Tasanen *et al.*, 2004). Collagen type XV and HS collagen type XVIII are restricted to basement membrane zones (Li *et al.*, 2000). In colon adenocarcinoma and ductal breast carcinoma, the loss of collagen type XV from the basement membrane zone was accompanied by its appearance in the interstitium, a phenomenon that may facilitate tumor invasion (Amenta *et al.*, 2000, 2003). The C-terminal NC1 domains of collagens type XV and XVIII, restin and endostatin, respectively, possess strong antiangiogenic properties (Kim and Herbst, 2002). A comprehensive review of the antiangiogenic fragments from different collagens has been recently published (Bix and Iozzo, 2005).

V. Tumor Cell Membrane PGs

The external surface of the mammalian cell is covered with different PGs. The isolation of chemically mutated cells, expressing no GAG chain, demonstrated that this "coat" is not necessary for cell survival. On the contrary, it seems necessary for tissue (organ) formation and, especially, for tumor growth (Esko *et al.*, 1988). The surface PGs are either one transmembrane domain proteins with type I orientation or GPI-anchored proteins. Two families of membrane PGs, syndecans and glypicans, play a fundamental role in tumor progression, but they are mostly studied as HSPGs. Recent reviews described in detail the implication of these macromolecules in tumor biology (Bellin *et al.*, 2002; Filmus, 2001; Sanderson *et al.*, 2004; Wegrowski and Maquart, 2004). The most important CS tranmembrane PGs, broadly distributed in different cell types, are CD44, type III TGF-beta receptor betaglycan, and NG2. This last one is known as high-molecular weight melanoma-associated antigen or cell surface CSPG (HMW-MAA, MSCP, respectively). The minor or restricted full time CSPGs of nonneural origin comprise endothelial cells endocan (Bechard *et al.*, 2001) and thrombomodulin (Parkinson *et al.*, 1992), although thrombomodulin may be substituted with HS chain.

NG2/MAA was identified using monoclonal antibodies for the screening of tumor-associated antigens. It was found to be expressed by most human melanoma cell lines (Wilson *et al.*, 1983). In humans, *NG2/MAA* (CSPG4) gene encodes a 2322 amino acid core protein substituted with one CS chain (Pluschke *et al.*, 1996). It may be expressed as a 450 kDa component containing CS and a 280 kDa glycoprotein by the same cell type (Ross *et al.*, 1983). The extracellular part of molecule is composed of N-terminal globular domain, the central, CS substituted domain, and the juxtamembrane globular domain. The last domain contains proteolytic cleavage sites (Nishiyama *et al.*, 1995). The cytoplasmic C-terminal tail contains the sites of threonine phosphorylation and PZD binding motif, suggesting interactions with other proteic components (Campoli *et al.*, 2004).

NG2 is expressed in numerous embryonic and nondifferentiated cell types, including different mesenchymal cells like immature chondroblasts, osteocytes, smooth muscle cells, mural cells of vasculature, pericytes, and basal keratinocytes (Nishiyama *et al.*, 1991; Ozerdem *et al.*, 2001). It is widely distributed in central and peripheral nervous system, including neuromuscular junction (Petrini *et al.*, 2003). The synthesis of NG2/MAA is generally downregulated in the cells undergoing terminal differentiation. The expression of the molecule was reported in several inflammatory or genetic disorders, for example, muscular dystrophies or Raynaud's syndrome (Petrini *et al.*, 2003), and in many types of tumors. The molecule was mostly studied in melanoma progression, but it is also expressed in different nervous tissue tumors [glioma, astrocytoma, sarcoma, or neuroblastoma (Chekenya *et al.*, 1999)], basal cell and breast carcinomas (Kageshita *et al.*, 1985; Walter-Yohrling *et al.*, 2003), or leukaemia of different origins (Smith *et al.*, 1996). Excellent reviews treat of biology of this PG (Stallcup, 2002 and following issue papers, Campoli *et al.*, 2004).

CD44 (Hermes) is another transmembrane PG, highly involved in cell movement and tumor progression. This molecule was originally discovered as lymphocyte homing receptor (Gallatin *et al.*, 1983). It is an almost ubiquitous adhesive membrane protein. At least 30 different splice products, existing in many cells types, place CD44 as one of the most variable molecule of the cell surface (van Weering, 1994). The standard splicing form (CD44s) is a protein of 37 kDa deprived of GAG chain. The GAG consensus attachment site (SGXG) resides in the variable third exon (v3), so only splice variants containing this region are substituted with GAG chain (Jackson *et al.*, 1995). The full-length molecule exceeds 200 kDa. In keratinocytes CD44 is substituted with HS chain (epican) (Kugelman *et al.*, 1992).

The role of CD44 as prometastatic agent was shown for the first time by Gunthert *et al.* (1991). The authors conferred metastatic potential to carcinoma cells by transfecting them with this molecule. CD44 splice variants are overexpressed in many tumors of epithelial origin (Heider *et al.*, 1993; Wielenga *et al.*, 1993). Overexpression of prometastatic splice variants often accompany the underexpression of the standard form (Pereira *et al.*, 2001). The expression of CD44 isoforms, usually correlated with a high incidence of metastasis, was not seen in all tumors, suggesting the implication of additional phenomena or molecular enhancers. These may include the deregulation of synthesis or shading from membrane, minute expression of some isoforms, interaction with other cell compounds, or changes of substratum composition. The metastatic potential may depend on the complex environment surrounding the primary tumor (Givehchian *et al.*, 1996; Hudson *et al.*, 1996). Recent reviews described in detail the involvement of CD44 in cancer growth and metastasis (Jothy, 2003; Marhaba and Zoller, 2004; Sneath and Mangham, 1998).

Betaglycan is another example of ubiquitous transmembrane CSPG. The core protein of 853 amino acids possesses a short cytoplasmic domain devoid of any signaling motif (Lopez-Casillas *et al.*, 1991). It is a low affinity receptor type III for TGF-beta and the inhibins (Bernard *et al.*, 2002). As TGF-beta is a crucial molecule in tumor development and stromal reaction, the local concentration of this growth factor on betaglycan amplifies the signaling and biological response (Schlessinger *et al.*, 1995). Finally, the CSPG of the endothelium, thrombomodulin, reviewed by Hanly *et al.* (2005) and the discovered endothelial cells CSPG, endocan (Scherpereel *et al.*, 2003) contribute in opposite manner to tumor formation and growth, endocan being protumoral and thrombomodulin antitumoral molecule.

VI. PGs of the Nervous System _____

The nervous tissue is rich in specific species of CSPGs. Neurocan and BEHAB/brevican are specific nervous tissue PGs belonging to the hyalectans/lecticans family, as broadly distributed versican and cartilaginous aggrecan. Brevican exist in long secreted and shorter GPI-anchored N-terminal truncated form of 145 and 80 kDa, respectively. It is a part-time PG (Yamada *et al.*, 1994). Neurocan is a 245 kDa glycoprotein bearing in average three CS chains. The membrane type CSPGs of the nervous tissue comprise NG2 (see in an earlier section), phosphacan/receptor-type protein phosphatase-zeta/beta (RPTP$\zeta\beta$) and neuroglycan C, (NGC, CSPG5) a 539 amino acids (120 kDa) glycoprotein substituted with one CS chain (Yasuda *et al.*, 1998). Soluble appican (Alzheimer amyloid precursor PG) is the splicing variant of amyloid precursor protein (Shioi *et al.*, 1995). An upregulation of the expression of different PGs was observed in nervous tissue tumors. It included brevican in glioma (Nutt *et al.*, 2001) and phosphacan in glioblastoma (Lorente *et al.*, 2005). In general, brain injury, including tumor development, is accompanied by the increase of CS, this last one being strong inhibitor of nerve regeneration and axonal growth. For specific application of CSPG in brain biology, the reader is invited to consult recent reviews (Dow and Wang, 1998; Matsui and Oohira, 2004; Rauch, 2004).

VII. Functions of PGs in Tumor Progression

The formation of tumor is characterized by several steps that are often overlaid: cell transformation by mutation of protooncogenes or antioncogenes, including viral infection, primary growth, alterations of cell adhesion, motility and spreading, cell migration, and, eventually, metastasis formation. For this last case one can add the host-tissue cell response, tumor stroma formation, and angiogenesis, necessary for tumor growth. In all these events, CSPG plays an important part. For instance, early events, like viral infection, may be mediated by CSPG (Olofsson and Bergstrom, 2005). The growth promoting activity of CSPGs can be easily explained by the capacity of CS (and the core protein) to fix different growth factors (Bechard *et al.*, 2001; Wegrowski and Maquart, 2004; Zou *et al.*, 2003). The degradation of CS by the hyaluronidases, HYAL1, HYAL2 (Bertrand *et al.*, 2005; Lokeshwar *et al.*, 2005) liberates oligosaccharides, which potentializes growth factor's activity. The formed oligosacharides may influence cell behavior (Fieber *et al.*, 2004; Rolls *et al.*, 2004). On the other hand, EGF-like motif of the G3 domain of the versican core protein is able to induce EGF receptor signaling, which contributes to the mitogenic activity of this PG in different types of tumor (Cattaruzza *et al.*, 2004; Wu *et al.*, 2001), although antiproliferative activity of G3 region was observed in melanoma cells (Serra *et al.*, 2005).

Many works were devoted to the study of the effect of PGs on cell adhesion, motility, spreading, and invasion. Versican inhibits prostate cancer-cell adhesion to fibronectin but not to laminin (Sakko *et al.*, 2003); cell adhesion via thrombomodulin is abrogated by addition of chondroitin-4 or chondroitin-6-sulfate (Huang *et al.*, 2003). CD44 is a cell adhesion molecule (CAM) that possesses, similarly to hyalectans/lecticans, a globular C-terminal domain adhering to hyaluronan. CD44-hyaluronan interaction, with the concerted action of hyaluronidases, was thought to be a major event of CD44-mediated cell movement, including metastasis. However, the phenomenon may be more complex as numerous matrix molecules are ligands for CD44, including CS itself (Murai *et al.*, 2004). Other receptors for hyaluronan/CS are present on cell membrane, like RHAMM/IHABP (Delpech *et al.*, 1997), LYVE-1 (Jackson, 2003) or annexin 6 (Takagi *et al.*, 2002). NG2 is the example of antiadhesive cell membrane CSPG. It acts by interfering with CD44 (Burg *et al.*, 1998) but increases adhesion to collagen type VI (Tillet *et al.*, 2002) or cooperate with alpha4 beta1 integrin to promote adhesion on fibronectin fragments (Iida *et al.*, 1998; Moyano *et al.*, 1999). The CSPGs involved in tumor progression, CD44 and NG2, induce cell motility (Makagiansar *et al.*, 2004), collagen type IV-dependent cell migration (Chekenya *et al.*, 1999), cell invasion into the ECM and anchorage-independent growth (Burg *et al.*, 1998; Xu and Yu, 2003).

Neoangiogenesis is a host tissue reaction necessary for tumor growth. Different CSPGs contribute to tumor-vessels formation. For example, endothelial cell migration, sprouting, and, especially, invasion into fibrin matrix is mediated by CD44 (Trochon *et al.*, 1996). NG2-positive pericytes form endothelial-free microvessels in growing experimental tumors (Ozerdem and Stallcup, 2003). Formation of microtubes and their endothelialization is inhibited by antiNG2 antibodies and depend of the cooperation of NG2 with PDGF-beta receptor (Ozerdem and Stallcup, 2004). Specifically secreted by endothelial cells, endocan can promote mitogenesis by fixation of hepatocyte growth factor/scatter factor (Bechard *et al.*, 2001). There is no direct evidence on versican implication in angiogenesis. However, recent study of Zheng *et al.* (2004) suggested that the C-terminal globular domain (G3), abundantly expressed in astrocytoma, could accelerate endothelial cell adhesion, proliferation, and migration. The V3 isoform, which contains the G3 domain, is expressed in endothelial cells during neoangiogenesis (Cattaruzza *et al.*, 2002). Sprouting or tubes-forming endothelial cells exceptionally express decorin (Jarvelainen *et al.*, 1992; Schonherr *et al.*, 2001). On the other hand, decorin is also expressed by endothelial cells upon inflammatory stimuli (Nelimarkka *et al.*, 2001) and decorin-deleted mice delayed inflammatory angiogenesis of cornea (Schonherr *et al.*, 2004). However, decorin inhibits tumor cell-mediated angiogenesis (Grant *et al.*, 2002) and endothelial cell migration (Davies Cde *et al.*, 2001). Study of Sulochana *et al.* (2005) identified several decorin-derived peptides that strongly inhibit angiogenesis induced by vascular endothelial growth factor (VEGF) and FGF2. This inhibition depends on the conformational change of a given peptide from an alpha helicoidal to a beta-sheet structure, suggesting that decorin-derived matrikines may have an opposite actions to the native molecule, as it was demonstrated for collagen type XV and XVIII.

The influence of PGs on tumor cell behavior, including angiogenesis, depends on the expression and action of different proteinases systems and proteinases cascades. GAGs influence proteinases activation and activity (Tersariol *et al.*, 2002). The central role in tumor invasion was ascribed to membrane type-1 matrix metalloproteinase (MT1-MMP/MMP-14) (Seiki, 2003), although other metalloproteinases and serine and cysteine proteinases may also play important part (Wegrowski and Maquart, 2004). Active MT1-MMP shed protumoral PGs, including CD44 (Suenaga *et al.*, 2005), betaglycan (Velasco-Loyden *et al.*, 2004), or syndecan-1 (Endo *et al.*, 2003), accelerating tumor invasion (Iida *et al.*, 2004). MT1-MMP colocalizes with CD44 (Murai *et al.*, 2004), and the attachment of CD44 to the substratum contributes to the expression of MMP-2 and MMP-9 (Murray *et al.*, 2004; Wiranowska *et al.*, 2000) and to the displacement of MT1-MMP to the lamellipodia (Mori *et al.*, 2002), facilitating cell migration. MT3-MMP, which colocalizes with NG2, participates in melanoma invasion (Iida *et al.*, 2001). Testican family of CSPGs regulates MT1-MMP activity. Testican 1 is a potent inhibitor of the enzyme (Edgell *et al.*, 2004), and testican 2 abrogates this inhibition (Nakada *et al.*, 2003). Testican 3 suppresses the MT1-MMP-dependent activation of MMP-2 (gelatinase A) (Nakada *et al.*, 2001). Different brain PGs are the substrates of the proteinases of the ADAMTS family (Rauch, 2004).

In general, the large stromal CSPG, of the hyalectans/lecticans family (e.g., versican, brevican) and the cell membrane CSPG (NG2, CD44, endocan) possess protumoral activity, whereas the small stromal PGs of SLRP family (e.g., decorin, lumican) are characterized by antitumoral properties.

VIII. Concluding Remarks

CSPGs are modular macromolecules. Their modules may play different roles in comparison to the whole molecule, when they are liberated as matrikines or produced by alternative splicing (e.g., versican G3 C-terminal part). Aberrantly addressed proteins can amplify the phenomena. For instance, chondroitin synthase 1, secreted by myeloma cells, stimulates osteoclast by activation of the Notch2 receptor via its Fringe domain (Yin, 2005). The discovery of biological functions of the modules provides better knowledge of the regulation of tumor development and angiogenesis and brings novel strategies for selective targeting of tumor development. Different studies on decorin as anticancer protein support this concept.

Much of the studies concerning the implication of GAGs in different aspects of tumor development were done with HS as a leading molecule. However, circulating cells and the "attached" cells undergoing movement express much higher quantity of CS than HS. The expression of CS is often upregulated in these cells, indicating that CS is more connected with cell kinesis, whereas HS is more involved in cell growth. The control of the different GAG expression by modulation of the appropriate enzymes may help in the research of novel antitumoral strategy.

CSPGs play multiple physiological functions. As PGs are necessary for tumor growth and metastasis (Esko *et al.*, 1988) and since one cell type express different PGs, the future studies will have to focus on the elucidation of the complex roles of each PG species in tumor biology and to characterize the complex system of cell membrane and stromal "glycomes" (Feizi, 2000). Further studies should also define the contribution of each component, that is, protein core and GAG chain(s), to the function of the whole PG. In some instances, a PG of a given family can be replaced by another. During angiogenesis, decorin can be replaced by fibromodulin but not by biglycan (Schonherr *et al.*, 2004). The comprehension of such phenomenons merits further studies.

Numerous CSPGs possess protumoral properties. A logical pharmacological strategy would be to search for a directed control, especially an inhibition of their synthesis without affecting the tissue function. As the synthesis of PGs is a complex phenomenon implying a number of enzymes, further studies should define the control points of their metabolism. The inhibition of UDP-glucose dehydrogenase, a key enzyme of GAG synthesis, may constitute an example of the strategy for such a control (Wegrowski *et al.*, 1998).

Acknowledgments

The authors' studies were supported by the grants from La Ligue Contre le Cancer (Comite de la Marne), Centre National de la Recherche Scientifique and Reims University.

References

Abramovici, L., and Steiner, G. C. (2002). Bizarre parosteal osteochondromatous proliferation (Nora's lesion): A retrospective study of 12 cases, 2 arising in long bones. *Hum. Pathol.* **33,** 1205–1210.

Adamia, S., Maxwell, C. A., and Pilarski, L. M. (2005). Hyaluronan and hyaluronan synthases: Potential therapeutic targets in cancer. *Curr. Drug Targets Cardiovasc. Haematol. Disord.* **5,** 3–14.

Adany, R., and Iozzo, R. V. (1991). Hypomethylation of the decorin proteoglycan gene in human colon cancer. *Biochem. J.* **276**(Pt 2), 301–306.

Aigner, T., Loos, S., Inwards, C., Perris, R., Perissinotto, D., Unni, K. K., and Kirchner, T. (1999). Chondroblastoma is an osteoid-forming, but not cartilage-forming neoplasm. *J. Pathol.* **189,** 463–469.

Aigner, T., Muller, S., Neureiter, D., Illstrup, D. M., Kirchner, T., and Bjornsson, J. (2002). Prognostic relevance of cell biologic and biochemical features in conventional chondrosarcomas. *Cancer* **94,** 2273–2281.

Alaniz, L., Cabrera, P. V., Blanco, G., Ernst, G., Rimoldi, G., Alvarez, E., and Hajos, S. E. (2002). Interaction of CD44 with different forms of hyaluronic acid: Its role in adhesion and migration of tumor cells. *Cell Commun. Adhes.* **9,** 117–130.

Amenta, P. S., Briggs, K., Xu, K., Gamboa, E., Jukkola, A. F., Li, D., and Myers, J. C. (2000). Type XV collagen in human colonic adenocarcinomas has a different distribution than other basement membrane zone proteins. *Hum. Pathol.* **31,** 359–366.

Amenta, P. S., Hadad, S., Lee, M. T., Barnard, N., Li, D., and Myers, J. C. (2003). Loss of types XV and XIX collagen precedes basement membrane invasion in ductal carcinoma of the female breast. *J. Pathol.* **199,** 298–308.

Ameye, L., and Young, M. F. (2002). Mice deficient in small leucine-rich proteoglycans: Novel in vivo models for osteoporosis, osteoarthritis, Ehlers-Danlos syndrome, muscular dystrophy, and corneal diseases. *Glycobiology* **12,** 107R–116R.

Baggio, B., Marzaro, G., Gambaro, G., Marchini, F., Williams, H. E., and Borsatti, A. (1990). Glycosaminoglycan content, oxalate self-exchange and protein phosphorylation in erythrocytes of patients with "idiopathic" calcium oxalate nephrolithiasis. *Clin. Sci. Lond.* **79**, 113–116.

Banerjee, A. G., Bhattacharyya, I., Lydiatt, W. M., and Vishwanatha, J. K. (2003). Aberrant expression and localization of decorin in human oral dysplasia and squamous cell carcinoma. *Cancer Res.* **63**, 7769–7776.

Bechard, D., Gentina, T., Delehedde, M., Scherpereel, A., Lyon, M., Aumercier, M., Vazeux, R., Richet, C., Degand, P., Jude, B., Janin, A., Fernig, D. G., *et al.* (2001). Endocan is a novel chondroitin sulfate/dermatan sulfate proteoglycan that promotes hepatocyte growth factor/scatter factor mitogenic activity. *J. Biol. Chem.* **276**, 48341–48349.

Bellin, R., Capila, I., Lincecum, J., Park, P. W., Reizes, O., and Bernfield, M. R. (2002). Unlocking the secrets of syndecans: Transgenic organisms as a potential key. *Glycoconj. J.* **19**, 295–304.

Bernard, D. J., Chapman, S. C., and Woodruff, T. K. (2002). Inhibin binding protein (InhBP/p120), betaglycan, and the continuing search for the inhibin receptor. *Mol. Endocrinol.* **16**, 207–212.

Berto, A. G., Sampaio, L. O., Franco, C. R., Cesar, R. M., Jr., and Michelacci, Y. M. (2003). A comparative analysis of structure and spatial distribution of decorin in human leiomyoma and normal myometrium. *Biochim. Biophys. Acta* **1619**, 98–112.

Bertrand, P., Courel, M. N., Maingonnat, C., Jardin, F., Tilly, H., and Bastard, C. (2005). Expression of HYAL2 mRNA, hyaluronan and hyaluronidase in B-cell non-Hodgkin lymphoma: Relationship with tumor aggressiveness. *Int. J. Cancer* **113**, 207–212.

Bix, G., and Iozzo, R. V. (2005). Matrix revolutions: "Tails" of basement-membrane components with angiostatic functions. *Trends Cell Biol.* **15**, 52–60.

Blasco, F., Penuelas, S., Cascallo, M., Hernandez, J. L., Alemany, C., Masa, M., Calbo, J., Soler, M., Nicolas, M., Perez-Torras, S., Gomez, A., Tarrason, G., *et al.* (2004). Expression profiles of a human pancreatic cancer cell line upon induction of apoptosis search for modulators in cancer therapy. *Oncology* **67**, 277–290.

Burg, M. A., Grako, K. A., and Stallcup, W. B. (1998). Expression of the NG2 proteoglycan enhances the growth and metastatic properties of melanoma cells. *J. Cell. Physiol.* **177**, 299–312.

Campoli, M. R., Chang, C. C., Kageshita, T., Wang, X., McCarthy, J. B., and Ferrone, S. (2004). Human high molecular weight-melanoma-associated antigen (HMW-MAA): A melanoma cell surface chondroitin sulfate proteoglycan (MSCP) with biological and clinical significance. *Crit. Rev. Immunol.* **24**, 267–296.

Cardoso, L. E., Falcao, P. G., and Sampaio, F. J. (2004). Increased and localized accumulation of chondroitin sulphate proteoglycans in the hyperplastic human prostate. *BJU Int.* **93**, 532–538.

Cattaruzza, S., Schiappacassi, M., Kimata, K., Colombatti, A., and Perris, R. (2004). The globular domains of PG-M/versican modulate the proliferation-apoptosis equilibrium and invasive capabilities of tumor cells. *FASEB J.* **18**, 779–781.

Cattaruzza, S., Schiappacassi, M., Ljungberg-Rose, A., Spessotto, P., Perissinotto, D., Morgelin, M., Mucignat, M. T., Colombatti, A., and Perris, R. (2002). Distribution of PG-M/versican variants in human tissues and *de novo* expression of isoform V3 upon endothelial cell activation, migration, and neoangiogenesis *in vitro*. *J. Biol. Chem.* **277**, 47626–47635.

Chekenya, M., Rooprai, H. K., Davies, D., Levine, J. M., Butt, A. M., and Pilkington, G. J. (1999). The NG2 chondroitin sulfate proteoglycan: role in malignant progression of human brain tumours. *Int. J. Dev. Neurosci.* **17**, 421–435.

Daidouji, K., Takagaki, K., Yoshihara, S., Matsuya, H., Sasaki, M., and Endo, M. (2002). Neoplastic changes in saccharide sequence of dermatan sulfate chains derived from human colon cancer. *Dig. Dis. Sci.* **47**, 331–337.

Davies Cde, L., Melder, R. J., Munn, L. L., Mouta-Carreira, C., Jain, R. K., and Boucher, Y. (2001). Decorin inhibits endothelial migration and tube-like structure formation: Role of thrombospondin-1. *Microvasc. Res.* **62**, 26–42.

De Luca, A., Santra, M., Baldi, A., Giordano, A., and Iozzo, R. V. (1996). Decorin-induced growth suppression is associated with up-regulation of p21, an inhibitor of cyclin-dependent kinases. *J. Biol. Chem.* **271**, 18961–18965.

Delpech, B., Girard, N., Olivier, A., Maingonnat, C., van Driessche, G., van Beeumen, J., Bertrand, P., Duval, C., Delpech, A., and Bourguignon, J. (1997). The origin of hyaluronectin in human tumors. *Int. J. Cancer* **72**, 942–948.

Denholm, E. M., Lin, Y. Q., and Silver, P. J. (2001). Anti-tumor activities of chondroitinase AC and chondroitinase B: Inhibition of angiogenesis, proliferation and invasion. *Eur. J. Pharmacol.* **416**, 213–221.

Desmouliere, A., Guyot, C., and Gabbiani, G. (2004). The stroma reaction myofibroblast: A key player in the control of tumor cell behavior. *Int. J. Dev. Biol.* **48**, 509–517.

Domenzain, C., Docampo, M. J., Serra, M., Miquel, L., and Bassols, A. (2003). Differential expression of versican isoforms is a component of the human melanoma cell differentiation process. *Biochim. Biophys. Acta* **1642**, 107–114.

Dow, K. E., and Wang, W. (1998). Cell biology of astrocyte proteoglycans. *Cell. Mol. Life Sci.* **54**, 567–581.

Edgell, C. J., BaSalamah, M. A., and Marr, H. S. (2004). Testican-1: A differentially expressed proteoglycan with protease inhibiting activities. *Int. Rev. Cytol.* **236**, 101–122.

Endo, K., Takino, T., Miyamori, H., Kinsen, H., Yoshizaki, T., Furukawa, M., and Sato, H. (2003). Cleavage of syndecan-1 by membrane type matrix metalloproteinase-1 stimulates cell migration. *J. Biol. Chem.* **278**, 40764–40770.

Esko, J. D., Rostand, K. S., and Weinke, J. L. (1988). Tumor formation dependent on proteoglycan biosynthesis. *Science* **241**, 1092–1096.

Feizi, T. (2000). Progress in deciphering the information content of the "glycome": A crescendo in the closing years of the millennium. *Glycoconj. J.* **17**, 553–565.

Fieber, C., Baumann, P., Vallon, R., Termeer, C., Simon, J. C., Hofmann, M., Angel, P., Herrlich, P., and Sleeman, J. P. (2004). Hyaluronan-oligosaccharide-induced transcription of metalloproteases. *J. Cell Sci.* **117**, 359–367.

Filmus, J. (2001). Glypicans in growth control and cancer. *Glycobiology* **11**, 19R–23R.

Fransson, L. A., Belting, M., Jonsson, M., Mani, K., Moses, J., and Oldberg, A. (2000). Biosynthesis of decorin and glypican. *Matrix Biol.* **19**, 367–376.

Frisch, S. M., and Francis, H. (1994). Disruption of epithelial cell-matrix interactions induces apoptosis. *J. Cell Biol.* **124**, 619–626.

Gallatin, W. M., Weissman, I. L., and Butcher, E. C. (1983). A cell-surface molecule involved in organ-specific homing of lymphocytes. *Nature* **304**, 30–34.

Garcia-Garcia, M. J., and Anderson, K. V. (2003). Essential role of glycosaminoglycans in Fgf signaling during mouse gastrulation. *Cell* **114**, 727–737.

Ghatak, S., Misra, S., and Toole, B. P. (2002). Hyaluronan oligosaccharides inhibit anchorage-independent growth of tumor cells by suppressing the phosphoinositide 3-kinase/Akt cell survival pathway. *J. Biol. Chem.* **277**, 38013–38020.

Givehchian, M., Woerner, S. M., Lacroix, J., Zoller, M., Drings, P., Becker, H., Kayser, K., Ridder, R., and von Knebel Doeberitz, M. (1996). Expression of CD44 splice variants in normal respiratory epithelium and bronchial carcinomas: No evidence for altered CD44 splicing in metastasis. *Oncogene* **12**, 1137–1144.

Gottschalk, D., Fehn, M., Patt, S., Saeger, W., Kirchner, T., and Aigner, T. (2001). Matrix gene expression analysis and cellular phenotyping in chordoma reveals focal differentiation pattern of neoplastic cells mimicking nucleus pulposus development. *Am. J. Pathol.* **158**, 1571–1578.

Grant, D. S., Yenisey, C., Rose, R. W., Tootell, M., Santra, M., and Iozzo, R. V. (2002). Decorin suppresses tumor cell-mediated angiogenesis. *Oncogene* **21**, 4765–4777.

Gunthert, U., Hofmann, M., Rudy, W., Reber, S., Zoller, M., Haussmann, I., Matzku, S., Wenzel, A., Ponta, H., and Herrlich, P. (1991). A new variant of glycoprotein CD44 confers metastatic potential to rat carcinoma cells. *Cell* **65**, 13–24.

Haimovitz-Friedman, A., Falcone, D. J., Eldor, A., Schirrmacher, V., Vlodavsky, I., and Fuks, Z. (1991). Activation of platelet heparitinase by tumor cell-derived factors. *Blood* **78**, 789–796.

Hanly, A. M., Hayanga, A., Winter, D. C., and Bouchier-Hayes, D. J. (2005). Thrombomodulin: Tumour biology and prognostic implications. *Eur. J. Surg. Oncol.* **31**, 217–220.

Heider, K. H., Dammrich, J., Skroch-Angel, P., Muller-Hermelink, H. K., Vollmers, H. P., Herrlich, P., and Ponta, H. (1993). Differential expression of CD44 splice variants in intestinal- and diffuse-type human gastric carcinomas and normal gastric mucosa. *Cancer Res.* **53**, 4197–4203.

Heredia, A., Villena, J., Romaris, M., Molist, A., and Bassols, A. (1996). The effect of TGF-beta 1 on cell proliferation and proteoglycan production in human melanoma cells depends on the degree of cell differentiation. *Cancer Lett.* **109**, 39–47.

Hibbs, K., Skubitz, K. M., Pambuccian, S. E., Casey, R. C., Burleson, K. M., Oegema, T. R., Jr., Thiele, J. J., Grindle, S. M., Bliss, R. L., and Skubitz, A. P. (2004). Differential gene expression in ovarian carcinoma: Identification of potential biomarkers. *Am. J. Pathol.* **165**, 397–414.

Hornebeck, W., and Birembaut, P. (2004). Introduction: Stroma reaction and cancer progression. *Crit. Rev. Oncol. Hematol.* **49**, 177–178.

Huang, H. C., Shi, G. Y., Jiang, S. J., Shi, C. S., Wu, C. M., Yang, H. Y., and Wu, H. L. (2003). Thrombomodulin-mediated cell adhesion: Involvement of its lectin-like domain. *J. Biol. Chem.* **278**, 46750–46759.

Hudson, D. L., Speight, P. M., and Watt, F. M. (1996). Altered expression of CD44 isoforms in squamous-cell carcinomas and cell lines derived from them. *Int. J. Cancer* **66**, 457–463.

Hunzelmann, N., Schonherr, E., Bonnekoh, B., Hartmann, C., Kresse, H., and Krieg, T. (1995). Altered immunohistochemical expression of small proteoglycans in the tumor tissue and stroma of basal cell carcinoma. *J. Invest. Dermatol.* **104**, 509–513.

Iida, J., Meijne, A. M., Knutson, J. R., Furcht, L. T., and McCarthy, J. B. (1996). Cell surface chondroitin sulfate proteoglycans in tumor cell adhesion, motility and invasion. *Semin. Cancer Biol.* **7**, 155–162.

Iida, J., Meijne, A. M., Oegema, T. R., Jr., Yednock, T. A., Kovach, N. L., Furcht, L. T., and McCarthy, J. B. (1998). A role of chondroitin sulfate glycosaminoglycan binding site in alpha4beta1 integrin-mediated melanoma cell adhesion. *J. Biol. Chem.* **273**, 5955–5962.

Iida, J., Pei, D., Kang, T., Simpson, M. A., Herlyn, M., Furcht, L. T., and McCarthy, J. B. (2001). Melanoma chondroitin sulfate proteoglycan regulates matrix metalloproteinase-dependent human melanoma invasion into type I collagen. *J. Biol. Chem.* **276**, 18786–18794.

Iida, J., Wilhelmson, K. L., Price, M. A., Wilson, C. M., Pei, D., Furcht, L. T., and McCarthy, J. B. (2004). Membrane type-1 matrix metalloproteinase promotes human melanoma invasion and growth. *J. Invest. Dermatol.* **122**, 167–176.

Ioachim, H. L. (1976). The stromal reaction of tumors: An expression of immune surveillance. *J. Natl. Cancer Inst.* **57**, 465–475.

Iozzo, R. V. (1995). Tumor stroma as a regulator of neoplastic behavior: Agonistic and antagonistic elements embedded in the same connective tissue. *Lab. Invest.* **73**, 157–160.

Iozzo, R. V. (1998). Matrix proteoglycans: From molecular design to cellular function. *Annu. Rev. Biochem.* **67**, 609–652.

Iozzo, R. V. (1999). The biology of the small leucine-rich proteoglycans: Functional network of interactive proteins. *J. Biol. Chem.* **274**, 18843–18846.

Iozzo, R. V., and Cohen, I. (1994). Altered proteoglycan gene expression and the tumor stroma. *EXS* **70**, 199–214.

Iozzo, R. V., Moscatello, D. K., McQuillan, D. J., and Eichstetter, I. (1999). Decorin is a biological ligand for the epidermal growth factor receptor. *J. Biol. Chem.* **274**, 4489–4492.

Isogai, Z., Shinomura, T., Yamakawa, N., Takeuchi, J., Tsuji, T., Heinegard, D., and Kimata, K. (1996). 2B1 antigen characteristically expressed on extracellular matrices of human malignant tumors is a large chondroitin sulfate proteoglycan, PG-M/versican. *Cancer Res.* **56**, 3902–3908.

Ito, Y., Abiko, Y., Tanaka, Y., Rahemtulla, F., and Kaku, T. (2002). Immunohistochemical localization of large chondroitin sulfate proteoglycan in odontogenic tumor. *Med. Electron Microsc.* **35**, 173–177.

Jackson, D. G. (2003). The lymphatics revisited: New perspectives from the hyaluronan receptor LYVE-1. *Trends Cardiovasc. Med.* **13**, 1–7.

Jackson, D. G., Bell, J. I., Dickinson, R., Timans, J., Shields, J., and Whittle, N. (1995). Proteoglycan forms of the lymphocyte homing receptor CD44 are alternatively spliced variants containing the v3 exon. *J. Cell Biol.* **128**, 673–685.

Jaques, L. B. (1991). Glycosaminoglycans as polyelectrolytes: Rejuvenation of original concepts. *Semin. Thromb. Hemost.* **17**(Suppl 1), 1–4.

Jarvelainen, H. T., Iruela-Arispe, M. L., Kinsella, M. G., Sandell, L. J., Sage, E. H., and Wight, T. N. (1992). Expression of decorin by sprouting bovine aortic endothelial cells exhibiting angiogenesis *in vitro*. *Exp. Cell Res.* **203**, 395–401.

Jothy, S. (2003). CD44 and its partners in metastasis. *Clin. Exp. Metastasis* **20**, 195–201.

Kageshita, T., Johno, M., Ono, T., Arao, T., and Imai, K. (1985). Immunohistological detection of human malignant melanoma using monoclonal antibody to a melanoma-associated antigen. *Arch. Dermatol. Res.* **277**, 334–336.

Karvinen, S., Kosma, V. M., Tammi, M. I., and Tammi, R. (2003). Hyaluronan, CD44 and versican in epidermal keratinocyte tumours. *Br. J. Dermatol.* **148**, 86–94.

Kim, E. S., and Herbst, R. S. (2002). Angiogenesis inhibitors in lung cancer. *Curr. Oncol. Rep.* **4**, 325–333.

Kim, N. R., Suh, Y. L., Shin, H. J., and Park, I. S. (2003). Gliofibroma with extensive calcified deposits. *Clin. Neuropathol.* **22**, 14–22.

Koninger, J., Giese, N. A., di Mola, F. F., Berberat, P., Giese, T., Esposito, I., Bachem, M. G., Buchler, M. W., and Friess, H. (2004). Overexpressed decorin in pancreatic cancer: Potential tumor growth inhibition and attenuation of chemotherapeutic action. *Clin. Cancer Res.* **10**, 4776–4783.

Koshiishi, I., Takenouchi, M., and Imanari, T. (1999). Structural characteristics of oversulfated chondroitin/dermatan sulfates in the fibrous lesions of the liver with cirrhosis. *Arch. Biochem. Biophys.* **370**, 151–155.

Kovalszky, I., Pogany, G., Molnar, G., Jeney, A., Lapis, K., Karacsonyi, S., Szecseny, A., and Iozzo, R. V. (1990). Altered glycosaminoglycan composition in reactive and neoplastic human liver. *Biochem. Biophys. Res. Commun.* **167**, 883–890.

Kugelman, L. C., Ganguly, S., Haggerty, J. G., Weissman, S. M., and Milstone, L. M. (1992). The core protein of epican, a heparan sulfate proteoglycan on keratinocytes, is an alternative form of CD44. *J. Invest. Dermatol.* **99**, 886–891.

Kusafuka, K., Ishiwata, T., Sugisaki, Y., Takemura, T., Kusafuka, M., Hisha, H., and Ikehara, S. (2004). Lumican expression is associated with the formation of mesenchyme-like elements in salivary pleomorphic adenomas. *J. Pathol.* **203**, 953–960.

Ladanyi, A., Gallai, M., Paku, S., Nagy, J. O., Dudas, J., Timar, J., and Kovalszky, I. (2001). Expression of a decorin-like moleculein human melanoma. *Pathol. Oncol. Res.* 7, 260–266.

Lapis, K., Kavalsky, I., Jeney, A., Pogany, G., Molnar, G., Repassy, D., Szecseny, A., and Karacsonyi, S. (1990). Alterations of glycosaminoglycans in human liver and kidney tumors. *Tokai J. Exp. Clin. Med.* 15, 155–165.

Leygue, E., Snell, L., Dotzlaw, H., Troup, S., Hiller-Hitchcock, T., Murphy, L. C., Roughley, P. J., and Watson, P. H. (2000). Lumican and decorin are differentially expressed in human breast carcinoma. *J. Pathol.* 192, 313–320.

Li, D., Clark, C. C., and Myers, J. C. (2000). Basement membrane zone type XV collagen is a disulfide-bonded chondroitin sulfate proteoglycan in human tissues and cultured cells. *J. Biol. Chem.* 275, 22339–22347.

Liang, Y., Haring, M., Roughley, P. J., Margolis, R. K., and Margolis, R. U. (1997). Glypican and biglycan in the nuclei of neurons and glioma cells: Presence of functional nuclear localization signals and dynamic changes in glypican during the cell cycle. *J. Cell Biol.* 139, 851–864.

Lidholt, K., Eriksson, I., and Kjellen, L. (1995). Heparin proteoglycans synthesized by mouse mastocytoma contain chondroitin sulphate. *Biochem. J.* 311(Pt 1), 233–238.

Liu, Y., Watanabe, H., Nifuji, A., Yamada, Y., Olson, E. N., and Noda, M. (1997). Overexpression of a single helix-loop-helix-type transcription factor, scleraxis, enhances aggrecan gene expression in osteoblastic osteosarcoma ROS17/2.8 cells. *J. Biol. Chem.* 272, 29880–29885.

Lokeshwar, V. B., Cerwinka, W. H., and Lokeshwar, B. L. (2005). HYAL1 hyaluronidase: A molecular determinant of bladder tumor growth and invasion. *Cancer Res.* 65, 2243–2250.

Lopez-Casillas, F., Cheifetz, S., Doody, J., Andres, J. L., Lane, W. S., and Massague, J. (1991). Structure and expression of the membrane proteoglycan betaglycan, a component of the TGF-beta receptor system. *Cell* 67, 785–795.

Lorente, G., Nelson, A., Mueller, S., Kuo, J., Urfer, R., Nikolich, K., and Foehr, E. D. (2005). Functional comparison of long and short splice forms of RPTPbeta: Implications for glioblastoma treatment. *Neurooncology* 7, 154–163.

Lu, Y. P., Ishiwata, T., Kawahara, K., Watanabe, M., Naito, Z., Moriyama, Y., Sugisaki, Y., and Asano, G. (2002). Expression of lumican in human colorectal cancer cells. *Pathol. Int.* 52, 519–526.

Makagiansar, I. T., Williams, S., Dahlin-Huppe, K., Fukushi, J., Mustelin, T., and Stallcup, W. B. (2004). Phosphorylation of NG2 proteoglycan by protein kinase C-alpha regulates polarized membrane distribution and cell motility. *J. Biol. Chem.* 279, 55262–55270.

Maquart, F. X., Pasco, S., Ramont, L., Hornebeck, W., and Monboisse, J. C. (2004). An introduction to matrikines: Extracellular matrix-derived peptides which regulate cell activity. Implication in tumor invasion. *Crit. Rev. Oncol. Hematol.* 49, 199–202.

Marhaba, R., and Zoller, M. (2004). CD44 in cancer progression: Adhesion, migration and growth regulation. *J. Mol. Histol.* 35, 211–231.

Matsui, F., and Oohira, A. (2004). Proteoglycans and injury of the central nervous system. *Congenit. Anom. Kyoto* 44, 181–188.

Mayr, C., Bund, D., Schlee, M., Moosmann, A., Kofler, D. M., Hallek, M., and Wendtner, C. M. (2005). Fibromodulin as a novel tumor-associated antigen (TAA) in chronic lymphocytic leukemia (CLL), which allows expansion of specific CD8+ autologous T lymphocytes. *Blood* 105, 1566–1573.

McDoniels-Silvers, A. L., Nimri, C. F., Stoner, G. D., Lubet, R. A., and You, M. (2002). Differential gene expression in human lung adenocarcinomas and squamous cell carcinomas. *Clin. Cancer Res.* 8, 1127–1138.

Miyasaka, Y., Enomoto, N., Nagayama, K., Izumi, N., Marumo, F., Watanabe, M., and Sato, C. (2001). Analysis of differentially expressed genes in human hepatocellular carcinoma using suppression subtractive hybridization. *Br. J. Cancer* 85, 228–234.

Morgenstern, D. A., Asher, R. A., and Fawcett, J. W. (2002). Chondroitin sulphate proteoglycans in the CNS injury response. *Prog. Brain Res.* **137**, 313–332.

Mori, H., Tomari, T., Koshikawa, N., Kajita, M., Itoh, Y., Sato, H., Tojo, H., Yana, I., and Seiki, M. (2002). CD44 directs membrane-type 1 matrix metalloproteinase to lamellipodia by associating with its hemopexin-like domain. *EMBO J.* **21**, 3949–3959.

Moyano, J. V., Carnemolla, B., Albar, J. P., Leprini, A., Gaggero, B., Zardi, L., and Garcia-Pardo, A. (1999). Cooperative role for activated alpha4 beta1 integrin and chondroitin sulfate proteoglycans in cell adhesion to the heparin III domain of fibronectin: Identification of a novel heparin and cell binding sequence in repeat III5. *J. Biol. Chem.* **274**, 135–142.

Murai, T., Miyazaki, Y., Nishinakamura, H., Sugahara, K. N., Miyauchi, T., Sako, Y., Yanagida, T., and Miyasaka, M. (2004). Engagement of CD44 promotes Rac activation and CD44 cleavage during tumor cell migration. *J. Biol. Chem.* **279**, 4541–4550.

Murai, T., Sougawa, N., Kawashima, H., Yamaguchi, K., and Miyasaka, M. (2004). CD44-chondroitin sulfate interactions mediate leukocyte rolling under physiological flow conditions. *Immunol. Lett.* **93**, 163–170.

Murray, D., Morrin, M., and McDonnell, S. (2004). Increased invasion and expression of MMP-9 in human colorectal cell lines by a CD44-dependent mechanism. *Anticancer Res.* **24**, 489–494.

Nagle, R. B. (2004). Role of the extracellular matrix in prostate carcinogenesis. *J. Cell. Biochem.* **91**, 36–40.

Nakada, M., Miyamori, H., Yamashita, J., and Sato, H. (2003). Testican 2 abrogates inhibition of membrane-type matrix metalloproteinases by other testican family proteins. *Cancer Res.* **63**, 3364–3369.

Nakada, M., Yamada, A., Takino, T., Miyamori, H., Takahashi, T., Yamashita, J., and Sato, H. (2001). Suppression of membrane-type 1 matrix metalloproteinase (MMP)-mediated MMP-2 activation and tumor invasion by testican 3 and its splicing variant gene product, N-Tes. *Cancer Res.* **61**, 8896–8902.

Naor, D., Nedvetzki, S., Golan, I., Melnik, L., and Faitelson, Y. (2002). CD44 in cancer. *Crit. Rev. Clin. Lab. Sci.* **39**, 527–579.

Nara, Y., Kato, Y., Torii, Y., Tsuji, Y., Nakagaki, S., Goto, S., Isobe, H., Nakashima, N., and Takeuchi, J. (1997). Immunohistochemical localization of extracellular matrix components in human breast tumours with special reference to PG-M/versican. *Histochem. J.* **29**, 21–30.

Nash, M. A., Deavers, M. T., and Freedman, R. S. (2002). The expression of decorin in human ovarian tumors. *Clin. Cancer Res.* **8**, 1754–1760.

Nelimarkka, L., Salminen, H., Kuopio, T., Nikkari, S., Ekfors, T., Laine, J., Pelliniemi, L., and Jarvelainen, H. (2001). Decorin is produced by capillary endothelial cells in inflammation-associated angiogenesis. *Am. J. Pathol.* **158**, 345–353.

Nishiyama, A., Dahlin, K. J., Prince, J. T., Johnstone, S. R., and Stallcup, W. B. (1991). The primary structure of NG2, a novel membrane-spanning proteoglycan. *J. Cell Biol.* **114**, 359–371.

Nishiyama, A., Lin, X. H., and Stallcup, W. B. (1995). Generation of truncated forms of the NG2 proteoglycan by cell surface proteolysis. *Mol. Biol. Cell* **6**, 1819–1832.

Nutt, C. L., Matthews, R. T., and Hockfield, S. (2001). Glial tumor invasion: A role for the upregulation and cleavage of BEHAB/brevican. *Neuroscientist* **7**, 113–122.

Olofsson, S., and Bergstrom, T. (2005). Glycoconjugate glycans as viral receptors. *Ann. Med.* **37**, 154–172.

Ozerdem, U., Grako, K. A., Dahlin-Huppe, K., Monosov, E., and Stallcup, W. B. (2001). NG2 proteoglycan is expressed exclusively by mural cells during vascular morphogenesis. *Dev. Dyn.* **222**, 218–227.

Ozerdem, U., and Stallcup, W. B. (2003). Early contribution of pericytes to angiogenic sprouting and tube formation. *Angiogenesis* **6**, 241–249.

Ozerdem, U., and Stallcup, W. B. (2004). Pathological angiogenesis is reduced by targeting pericytes via the NG2 proteoglycan. *Angiogenesis* 7, 269–276.

Papadas, T. A., Stylianou, M., Mastronikolis, N. S., Papageorgakopoulou, N., Skandalis, S., Goumas, P., Theocharis, D. A., and Vynios, D. H. (2002). Alterations in the content and composition of glycosaminoglycans in human laryngeal carcinoma. *Acta Otolaryngol.* **122**, 330–337.

Parkinson, J. F., Koyama, T., Bang, N. U., and Preissner, K. T. (1992). Thrombomodulin: An anticoagulant cell surface proteoglycan with physiologically relevant glycosaminoglycan moiety. *Adv. Exp. Med. Biol.* **313**, 177–188.

Paulus, W., Baur, I., Dours-Zimmermann, M. T., and Zimmermann, D. R. (1996). Differential expression of versican isoforms in brain tumors. *J. Neuropathol. Exp. Neurol.* **55**, 528–533.

Paulus, W., Baur, I., Schuppan, D., and Roggendorf, W. (1993). Characterization of integrin receptors in normal and neoplastic human brain. *Am. J. Pathol.* **143**, 154–163.

Pereira, P. A., Rubenthiran, U., Kaneko, M., Jothy, S., and Smith, A. J. (2001). CD44s expression mitigates the phenotype of human colorectal cancer hepatic metastases. *Anticancer Res.* **21**, 2713–2717.

Petrini, S., Tessa, A., Carrozzo, R., Verardo, M., Pierini, R., Rizza, T., and Bertini, E. (2003). Human melanoma/NG2 chondroitin sulfate proteoglycan is expressed in the sarcolemma of postnatal human skeletal myofibers: Abnormal expression in merosin-negative and Duchenne muscular dystrophies. *Mol. Cell. Neurosci.* **23**, 219–231.

Ping Lu, Y., Ishiwata, T., and Asano, G. (2002). Lumican expression in alpha cells of islets in pancreas and pancreatic cancer cells. *J. Pathol.* **196**, 324–330.

Pirinen, R., Leinonen, T., Bohm, J., Johansson, R., Ropponen, K., Kumpulainen, E., and Kosma, V. M. (2005). Versican in nonsmall cell lung cancer: Relation to hyaluronan, clinicopathologic factors, and prognosis. *Hum. Pathol.* **36**, 44–50.

Pluschke, G., Vanek, M., Evans, A., Dittmar, T., Schmid, P., Itin, P., Filardo, E. J., and Reisfeld, R. A. (1996). Molecular cloning of a human melanoma-associated chondroitin sulfate proteoglycan. *Proc. Natl. Acad. Sci. USA* **93**, 9710–9715.

Pukkila, M. J., Kosunen, A. S., Virtaniemi, J. A., Kumpulainen, E. J., Johansson, R. T., Kellokoski, J. K., Nuutinen, J., and Kosma, V. M. (2004). Versican expression in pharyngeal squamous cell carcinoma: An immunohistochemical study. *J. Clin. Pathol.* **57**, 735–739.

Rauch, U. (2004). Extracellular matrix components associated with remodeling processes in brain. *Cell Mol. Life Sci.* **61**, 2031–2045.

Ricciardelli, C., Mayne, K., Sykes, P. J., Raymond, W. A., McCaul, K., Marshall, V. R., and Horsfall, D. J. (1998). Elevated levels of versican but not decorin predict disease progression in early-stage prostate cancer. *Clin. Cancer Res.* **4**, 963–971.

Ricciardelli, C., Mayne, K., Sykes, P. J., Raymond, W. A., McCaul, K., Marshall, V. R., Tilley, W. D., Skinner, J. M., and Horsfall, D. J. (1997). Elevated stromal chondroitin sulfate glycosaminoglycan predicts progression in early-stage prostate cancer. *Clin. Cancer Res.* **3**, 983–992.

Rolls, A., Avidan, H., Cahalon, L., Schori, H., Bakalash, S., Litvak, V., Lev, S., Lider, O., and Schwartz, M. (2004). A disaccharide derived from chondroitin sulphate proteoglycan promotes central nervous system repair in rats and mice. *Eur. J. Neurosci.* **20**, 1973–1983.

Ross, A. H., Cossu, G., Herlyn, M., Bell, J. R., Steplewski, Z., and Koprowski, H. (1983). Isolation and chemical characterization of a melanoma-associated proteoglycan antigen. *Arch. Biochem. Biophys.* **225**, 370–383.

Sakko, A. J., Ricciardelli, C., Mayne, K., Suwiwat, S., LeBaron, R. G., Marshall, V. R., Tilley, W. D., and Horsfall, D. J. (2003). Modulation of prostate cancer cell attachment to matrix by versican. *Cancer Res.* **63**, 4786–4791.

Sanderson, R. D., Yang, Y., Suva, L. J., and Kelly, T. (2004). Heparan sulfate proteoglycans and heparanase–partners in osteolytic tumor growth and metastasis. *Matrix Biol.* **23**, 341–352.

Santra, M., Eichstetter, I., and Iozzo, R. V. (2000). An anti-oncogenic role for decorin. Down-regulation of ErbB2 leads to growth suppression and cytodifferentiation of mammary carcinoma cells. *J. Biol. Chem.* **275**, 35153–35161.

Santra, M., Mann, D. M., Mercer, E. W., Skorski, T., Calabretta, B., and Iozzo, R. V. (1997). Ectopic expression of decorin protein core causes a generalized growth suppression in neoplastic cells of various histogenetic origin and requires endogenous p21, an inhibitor of cyclin-dependent kinases. *J. Clin. Invest.* **100**, 149–157.

Santra, M., Skorski, T., Calabretta, B., Lattime, E. C., and Iozzo, R. V. (1995). *De novo* decorin gene expression suppresses the malignant phenotype in human colon cancer cells. *Proc. Natl. Acad. Sci. USA* **92**, 7016–7020.

Scherpereel, A., Gentina, T., Grigoriu, B., Senechal, S., Janin, A., Tsicopoulos, A., Plenat, F., Bechard, D., Tonnel, A. B., and Lassalle, P. (2003). Overexpression of endocan induces tumor formation. *Cancer Res.* **63**, 6084–6089.

Schlessinger, J., Lax, I., and Lemmon, M. (1995). Regulation of growth factor activation by proteoglycans: What is the role of the low affinity receptors? *Cell* **83**, 357–360.

Schonherr, E., Levkau, B., Schaefer, L., Kresse, H., and Walsh, K. (2001). Decorin-mediated signal transduction in endothelial cells: Involvement of Akt/protein kinase B in up-regulation of p21(WAF1/CIP1) but not p27(KIP1). *J. Biol. Chem.* **276**, 40687–40692.

Schonherr, E., Sunderkotter, C., Schaefer, L., Thanos, S., Grassel, S., Oldberg, A., Iozzo, R. V., Young, M. F., and Kresse, H. (2004). Decorin deficiency leads to impaired angiogenesis in injured mouse cornea. *J. Vasc. Res.* **41**, 499–508.

Schwartz, N. B., and Domowicz, M. (2004). Proteoglycans in brain development. *Glycoconj. J.* **21**, 329–341.

Seiki, M. (2003). Membrane-type 1 matrix metalloproteinase: A key enzyme for tumor invasion. *Cancer Lett.* **194**, 1–11.

Serra, M., Miquel, L., Domenzain, C., Docampo, M. J., Fabra, A., Wight, T. N., and Bassols, A. (2005). V3 versican isoform expression alters the phenotype of melanoma cells and their tumorigenic potential. *Int. J. Cancer* **114**, 879–886.

Shinji, S., Tajiri, T., Ishiwata, T., Seya, T., Tanaka, N., and Naito, Z. (2005). Different expression levels of lumican in human carcinoid tumor and neuroendocrine cell carcinoma. *Int. J. Oncol.* **26**, 873–880.

Shioi, J., Pangalos, M. N., Ripellino, J. A., Vassilacopoulou, D., Mytilineou, C., Margolis, R. U., and Robakis, N. K. (1995). The Alzheimer amyloid precursor proteoglycan (appican) is present in brain and is produced by astrocytes but not by neurons in primary neural cultures. *J. Biol. Chem.* **270**, 11839–11844.

Shriver, Z., Liu, D., and Sasisekharan, R. (2002). Emerging views of heparan sulfate glycosaminoglycan structure/activity relationships modulating dynamic biological functions. *Trends Cardiovasc. Med.* **12**, 71–77.

Smetsers, T. F., van de Westerlo, E. M., ten Dam, G. B., Overes, I. M., Schalkwijk, J., van Muijen, G. N., and van Kuppevelt, T. H. (2004). Human single-chain antibodies reactive with native chondroitin sulfate detect chondroitin sulfate alterations in melanoma and psoriasis. *J. Invest. Dermatol.* **122**, 707–716.

Smith, F. O., Rauch, C., Williams, D. E., March, C. J., Arthur, D., Hilden, J., Lampkin, B. C., Buckley, J. D., Buckley, C. V., Woods, W. G., Dinndorf, P. A., Sorensen, P., *et al.* (1996). The human homologue of rat NG2, a chondroitin sulfate proteoglycan, is not expressed on the cell surface of normal hematopoietic cells but is expressed by acute myeloid leukemia blasts from poor-prognosis patients with abnormalities of chromosome band 11q23. *Blood* **87**, 1123–1133.

Sneath, R. J., and Mangham, D. C. (1998). The normal structure and function of CD44 and its role in neoplasia. *Mol. Pathol.* **51**, 191–200.

Soderstrom, M., Bohling, T., Ekfors, T., Nelimarkka, L., Aro, H. T., and Vuorio, E. (2002). Molecular profiling of human chondrosarcomas for matrix production and cancer markers. *Int. J. Cancer* **100**, 144–151.

Stallcup, W. B. (2002). The NG2 proteoglycan: Past insights and future prospects. *J. Neurocytol.* **31**, 423–435.

Suenaga, N., Mori, H., Itoh, Y., and Seiki, M. (2005). CD44 binding through the hemopexin-like domain is critical for its shedding by membrane-type 1 matrix metalloproteinase. *Oncogene* **24**, 859–868.

Sulochana, K. N., Fan, H., Jois, S., Subramanian, V., Sun, F., Manjunatha Kini, R., and Ge, R. (2005). Peptides derived from human decorin leucine rich repeat 5 inhibit angiogenesis. *J. Biol. Chem* **280**, 27935–27948.

Suwiwat, S., Ricciardelli, C., Tammi, R., Tammi, M., Auvinen, P., Kosma, V. M., LeBaron, R. G., Raymond, W. A., Tilley, W. D., and Horsfall, D. J. (2004). Expression of extracellular matrix components versican, chondroitin sulfate, tenascin, and hyaluronan, and their association with disease outcome in node-negative breast cancer. *Clin. Cancer Res.* **10**, 2491–2498.

Syrokou, A., Dobra, K., Tzanakakis, G. N., Hjerpe, A., and Karamanos, N. K. (2002). Synthesis and expression of mRNA encoding for different versican splice variants is related to the aggregation of human epithelial mesothelioma cells. *Anticancer Res.* **22**, 4157–4162.

Takagi, H., Asano, Y., Yamakawa, N., Matsumoto, I., and Kimata, K. (2002). Annexin 6 is a putative cell surface receptor for chondroitin sulfate chains. *J. Cell Sci.* **115**, 3309–3318.

Tasanen, K., Tunggal, L., Chometon, G., Bruckner-Tuderman, L., and Aumailley, M. (2004). Keratinocytes from patients lacking collagen XVII display a migratory phenotype. *Am. J. Pathol.* **164**, 2027–2038.

Tersariol, I. L., Pimenta, D. C., Chagas, J. R., and Almeida, P. C. (2002). Proteinase activity regulation by glycosaminoglycans. *Braz. J. Med. Biol. Res.* **35**, 135–144.

Theocharis, A. D. (2002). Human colon adenocarcinoma is associated with specific post-translational modifications of versican and decorin. *Biochim. Biophys. Acta* **1588**, 165–172.

Theocharis, A. D., and Theocharis, D. A. (2002). High-performance capillary electrophoretic analysis of hyaluronan and galactosaminoglycan-disaccharides in gastrointestinal carcinomas. Differential disaccharide composition as a possible tool-indicator for malignancies. *Biomed. Chromatogr.* **16**, 157–161.

Tillet, E., Gential, B., Garrone, R., and Stallcup, W. B. (2002). NG2 proteoglycan mediates beta1 integrin-independent cell adhesion and spreading on collagen VI. *J. Cell. Biochem.* **86**, 726–736.

Timar, J., Lapis, K., Dudas, J., Sebestyen, A., Kopper, L., and Kovalszky, I. (2002). Proteoglycans and tumor progression: Janus-faced molecules with contradictory functions in cancer. *Semin. Cancer Biol.* **12**, 173–186.

Tomoyasu, H., Kikuchi, A., and Kamo, I. (1998). Identification of haemopoietic biglycan in hyperplastic thymus associated with myasthenia gravis. *J. Neuroimmunol.* **89**, 59–63.

Touab, M., Arumi-Uria, M., Barranco, C., and Bassols, A. (2003). Expression of the proteoglycans versican and mel-CSPG in dysplastic nevi. *Am. J. Clin. Pathol.* **119**, 587–593.

Tralhao, J. G., Schaefer, L., Micegova, M., Evaristo, C., Schonherr, E., Kayal, S., Veiga-Fernandes, H., Danel, C., Iozzo, R. V., Kresse, H., and Lemarchand, P. (2003). In vivo selective and distant killing of cancer cells using adenovirus-mediated decorin gene transfer. *FASEB J.* **17**, 464–466.

Trochon, V., Mabilat, C., Bertrand, P., Legrand, Y., Smadja-Joffe, F., Soria, C., Delpech, B., and Lu, H. (1996). Evidence of involvement of CD44 in endothelial cell proliferation, migration and angiogenesis *in vitro*. *Int. J. Cancer* **66**, 664–668.

Troup, S., Njue, C., Kliewer, E. V., Parisien, M., Roskelley, C., Chakravarti, S., Roughley, P. J., Murphy, L. C., and Watson, P. H. (2003). Reduced expression of the small leucine-rich proteoglycans, lumican, and decorin is associated with poor outcome in node-negative invasive breast cancer. *Clin. Cancer Res.* **9**, 207–214.

Trowbridge, J. M., and Gallo, R. L. (2002). Dermatan sulfate: New functions from an old glycosaminoglycan. *Glycobiology* **12**, 117R–125R.

Tsara, M. E., Theocharis, A. D., and Theocharis, D. A. (2002). Compositional and structural alterations of proteoglycans in human rectum carcinoma with special reference to versican and decorin. *Anticancer Res.* **22**, 2893–2898.

Uhlman, D. L., and Niehans, G. A. (1999). Immunohistochemical study of chondroitin-6-sulphate and tenascin in the larynx: A loss of chondroitin-6-sulphate expression accompanies squamous cell carcinoma invasion. *J. Pathol.* **189**, 470–474.

van Weering, D. H. J., Bass, P. D., and Bos, J. L. (1994). A PCR based method for the analysis of human CD44 splice products. *PCR Methods Appl.* **3**, 100–1006.

Velasco-Loyden, G., Arribas, J., and Lopez-Casillas, F. (2004). The shedding of betaglycan is regulated by pervanadate and mediated by membrane type matrix metalloprotease-1. *J. Biol. Chem.* **279**, 7721–7733.

Voutilainen, K., Anttila, M., Sillanpaa, S., Tammi, R., Tammi, M., Saarikoski, S., and Kosma, V. M. (2003). Versican in epithelial ovarian cancer: Relation to hyaluronan, clinicopathologic factors and prognosis. *Int. J. Cancer* **107**, 359–364.

Vuillermoz, B., Khoruzhenko, A., D'Onofrio, M. F., Ramont, L., Venteo, L., Perreau, C., Antonicelli, F., Maquart, F. X., and Wegrowski, Y. (2004). The small leucine-rich proteoglycan lumican inhibits melanoma progression. *Exp. Cell Res.* **296**, 294–306.

Walter-Yohrling, J., Cao, X., Callahan, M., Weber, W., Morgenbesser, S., Madden, S. L., Wang, C., and Teicher, B. A. (2003). Identification of genes expressed in malignant cells that promote invasion. *Cancer Res.* **63**, 8939–8947.

Weber, C. K., Sommer, G., Michl, P., Fensterer, H., Weimer, M., Gansauge, F., Leder, G., Adler, G., and Gress, T. M. (2001). Biglycan is overexpressed in pancreatic cancer and induces G1-arrest in pancreatic cancer cell lines. *Gastroenterology* **121**, 657–667.

Wegrowski, Y., Bellon, G., Quereux, C., and Maquart, F. X. (1999). Biochemical alterations of uterine leiomyoma extracellular matrix in type IV Ehlers-Danlos syndrome. *Am. J. Obstet. Gynecol.* **180**, 1032–1034.

Wegrowski, Y., and Maquart, F. X. (2004). Involvement of stromal proteoglycans in tumour progression. *Crit. Rev. Oncol. Hematol.* **49**, 259–268.

Wegrowski, Y., Perreau, C., Bontemps, Y., and Maquart, F. X. (1998). Uridine diphosphoglucose dehydrogenase regulates proteoglycan expression: cDNA cloning and antisense study. *Biochem. Biophys. Res. Commun.* **250**, 206–211.

Wielenga, V. J., Heider, K. H., Offerhaus, G. J., Adolf, G. R., van den Berg, F. M., Ponta, H., Herrlich, P., and Pals, S. T. (1993). Expression of CD44 variant proteins in human colorectal cancer is related to tumor progression. *Cancer Res.* **53**, 4754–4756.

Williams, S. J., and Davies, G. J. (2001). Protein–carbohydrate interactions: Learning lessons from nature. *Trends Biotechnol.* **19**, 356–362.

Wilson, B. S., Ruberto, G., and Ferrone, S. (1983). Immunochemical characterization of a human high molecular weight–melanoma associated antigen identified with monoclonal antibodies. *Cancer Immunol. Immunother.* **14**, 196–201.

Wiranowska, M., Rojiani, A. M., Gottschall, P. E., Moscinski, L. C., Johnson, J., and Saporta, S. (2000). CD44 expression and MMP-2 secretion by mouse glioma cells: Effect of interferon and anti-CD44 antibody. *Anticancer Res.* **20**, 4301–4306.

Wu, Y., Zhang, Y., Cao, L., Chen, L., Lee, V., Zheng, P. S., Kiani, C., Adams, M. E., Ang, L. C., Paiwand, F., and Yang, B. B. (2001). Identification of the motif in versican G3 domain that plays a dominant-negative effect on astrocytoma cell proliferation through inhibiting versican secretion and binding. *J. Biol. Chem.* **276**, 14178–14186.

Xu, Y., and Yu, Q. (2003). E-cadherin negatively regulates CD44-hyaluronan interaction and CD44-mediated tumor invasion and branching morphogenesis. *J. Biol. Chem.* **278**, 8661–8668.

Yamada, H., Watanabe, K., Shimonaka, M., and Yamaguchi, Y. (1994). Molecular cloning of brevican, a novel brain proteoglycan of the aggrecan/versican family. *J. Biol. Chem.* **269**, 10119–10126.

Yasuda, Y., Tokita, Y., Aono, S., Matsui, F., Ono, T., Sonta, S., Watanabe, E., Nakanishi, Y., and Oohira, A. (1998). Cloning and chromosomal mapping of the human gene of neuroglycan C (NGC), a neural transmembrane chondroitin sulfate proteoglycan with an EGF module. *Neurosci. Res.* **32**, 313–322.

Yin, L. (2005). Chondroitin synthase 1 is a key molecule in myeloma cell-osteoclast interactions. *J. Biol. Chem.* **280**, 15666–15672.

Yokoyama, Y., Ishikawa, O., and Miyachi, Y. (1997). Disaccharide analysis of skin glycosaminoglycan in localized scleroderma. *Dermatology* **194**, 329–333.

Zhao, M., Takata, T., Kudo, Y., Sato, S., Ogawa, I., Wakida, K., Uchida, T., and Nikai, H. (1999). Biosynthesis of glycosaminoglycans and aggrecan by tumor cells in salivary pleomorphic adenoma: Ultrastructural evidence. *J. Oral Pathol. Med.* **28**, 442–450.

Zheng, P. S., Wen, J., Ang, L. C., Sheng, W., Viloria-Petit, A., Wang, Y., Wu, Y., Kerbel, R. S., and Yang, B. B. (2004). Versican/PG-M G3 domain promotes tumor growth and angiogenesis. *FASEB J.* **18**, 754–756.

Zou, P., Zou, K., Muramatsu, H., Ichihara-Tanaka, K., Habuchi, O., Ohtake, S., Ikematsu, S., Sakuma, S., and Muramatsu, T. (2003). Glycosaminoglycan structures required for strong binding to midkine, a heparin-binding growth factor. *Glycobiology* **13**, 35–42.

Sachiko Aono and Atsuhiko Oohira

Department of Perinatology
Institute for Developmental Research
Aichi Human Service Center
Aichi 480-0392, Japan

Chondroitin Sulfate Proteoglycans in the Brain

I. Chapter Overview

Chondroitin sulfate proteoglycans (CSPGs) play important roles in the morphogenesis and maintenance of various tissues including the central nervous system (CNS) through interactions of their core proteins and/or chondroitin sulfate (CS) chains with cell adhesion molecules, extracellular matrix (ECM) molecules, and growth factors. In this chapter, we summarize studies on functions of CSPGs in the neurogenetic, developing, and mature CNS, focusing on molecular interactions. In particular, we discuss the roles of CSPGs in perineuronal nets (PNNs) found in the mature brain. We also describe the results obtained using gene-targeting technology in studies of brain-specific CSPGs such as neurocan, phosphacan, and neuroglycan C. However, CSPGs are also involved in the pathology of neuronal diseases and lesions. The expression of CSPGs is upregulated in glial scars formed in response to injuries to the mature CNS, and at increased levels, CSPGs are

Advances in Pharmacology, Volume 53
Copyright 2006, Elsevier Inc. All rights reserved.

1054-3589/06 $35.00
DOI: 10.1016/S1054-3589(05)53015-1

generally considered to inhibit axonal regeneration in the CNS. Finally, we describe the response of the immature CNS to neuronal degeneration in terms of the expression of brain-specific CSPGs. Thus, we conclude that CSPGs can act as functional molecules in the CNS at all stages of development under both physiological and pathological conditions.

II. Introduction

In the 1960s, proteoglycans (PGs) were reported as important structural components of the ECM of cartilage and as molecules specific to the tissue. Now they are generally considered one of the major constituents of ECM of various tissues, including the brain (Höök *et al.*, 1984). Numerous studies performed since the 1990s have taught us that PGs function as not only structural elements supporting cells but also components regulating various cellular events related to the development of the CNS.

A great variety of PGs exist in the developing as well as mature brain. Bandtlow and Zimmerman (2000) have drawn up a list of PGs observed in the CNS. In the CNS, the majority of PGs carry side chains composed of either CS or heparan sulfate (HS). These PGs are designated CSPGs and HSPGs, respectively. HS is the major sulfated glycosaminoglycan (GAG) (about 25% of all GAG) in the fetal rat brain but accounts for only approximately 10% of all the GAG in the postnatal brain. On the other hand, CS is a minor GAG (about 10% of all GAG) in the fetal rat brain, but becomes the major GAG around 20 days after birth (Oohira *et al.*, 1986). Considering these observations, CSPGs function in the developing and mature brain in a manner different from HSPGs.

A significant amount of evidence that CSPGs function in the pathogenesis of neuronal diseases and lesions as well as in the development of the CNS has been accumulated (Fawcett and Asher, 1999; Matsui and Oohira, 2004; Morgenstern *et al.*, 2002; Properzi *et al.*, 2003; Rhodes and Fawcett, 2004). When the CNS is injured, the expression of several CSPGs is upregulated in glial scars formed around the site of the damage. These CSPGs are considered to inhibit axonal regeneration in glial scars, and overcoming this inhibitory effect has important implications in terms of repairing the CNS.

In this chapter, we focus on the CSPG molecules and discuss their putative functions in the development of the CNS under both physiological and pathological conditions.

III. Species and Structures of CSPGs Specific to the CNS

As shown in Table I, numerous CSPGs are expressed in the CNS. Among them, brevican (Yamada *et al.*, 1994), glycosylphophatidylinosito1 (GPI)-anchored brevican (Seidenbecher *et al.*, 1995), neurocan (Rauch *et al.*,

TABLE I Major Chondroitin Sulfate Proteoglycans Expressed in the Central Nervous System (CNS)

Name	Core protein size[a]	Type	Cellular origin
Brevican[b]	145	S	Glial cells/neurons
GPI-brevican[b]	140/125	GPI	Glial cells
Versican V0	~550	S	
Versican V1	~500	S	
Versican V2[b]	400	S	Oligodendrocytes
Aggrecan	370	S	Neurons
Neurocan[b]	245	S	Neurons/astrocytes
Phosphacan[b]	300	S	Glial cells/neurons
RPTPβ	380	M	
Neuroglycan C-I[b]	120	M	Neurons
Neuroglycan C-III[b]	>120	M	Neurons
Neuroglycan C-IV[b]	<120	M	Neurons
NG2	300	M	O2A glial progenitor cells
Appicans	96–130	M	Astroytes/microglia
L-APLP2S	100/110	M	Astroytes/microglia
Testican/SPOCK		S	Neurons

[a]Core protein size (kDa) estimated by sodium dodecylsulfate-polyacrylamide gel electrophoresis.
[b]Proteoglycans specific to the CNS.
S, secretary PG; GPI, glycosylphophatidylinositol-anchored PG; M, transmembrane PG.

1992), versican V2 (Dours-Zimmermann and Zimmerman, 1994), phosphacan (Maeda et al., 1992; Maurel et al., 1994), receptor-type protein tyrosine phosphatase β (RPTPβ) (Krueger and Saito, 1992; Levy et al., 1993), and neuroglycan C (NGC) (Watanabe et al., 1995) have been reported as PGs specific to the CNS (Bandtlow and Zimmermann, 2000). In this chapter, we focus on CSPGs specific to the CNS.

As shown in Fig. 1A, brevican, neurocan, and versican are members of the hyalectan (Iozzo and Murdoch, 1996) or lectican (Ruoslahti, 1996) family along with aggrecan (Domowicz et al., 1995; Krueger et al., 1992). Hyalectans except for GPI-anchored brevican are secreted molecules that take part in the formation of ECM. They are highly similar at the NH$_2$-terminal, which has an immunoglubulin (IgG)-like domain followed by a hyaluronan (HA) binding tandem repeat, and at the COOH-terminal, which includes epidermal growth factor (EGF)-like repeats, a lectin-like domain, and a complement regulatory protein (CRP)-like domain (Bandtlow and Zimmermann, 2000). Brevican has two splice variants, brevican and GPI-anchored brevican, and both are expressed in the CNS (Seidenbecher et al., 1995). Versican V2 among four versican splice variants (V0, V1, V2, and V3) is specific to the CNS and localizes to oligodendrocytes (Niederöst et al., 1999). No splice variants have been reported for neurocan (Rauch

A

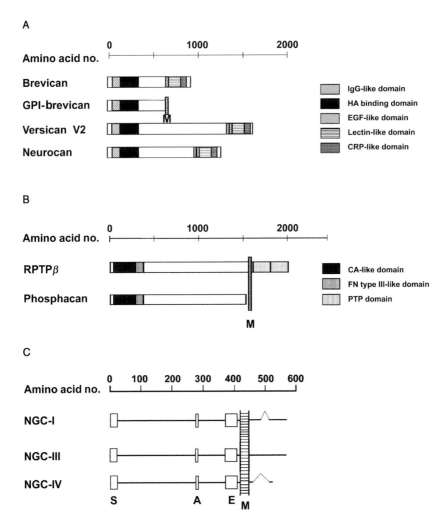

FIGURE 1 Schematic representation of the structures of CSPGs specific to the CNS. (A) Hyalectan family; (B) splice variants of receptor-type protein tyrosine phosphatase β (RPTPβ); (C) splice variants of neuroglycan C (NGC). GPI-brevican, glycosylphophatidylinositol-anchored brevican; IgG, immunoglobulin; HA, hyalruonan; EGF, epithelium growth factor; CRP, complement regulatory protein; CA, carbonic anhydrase; FN, fibronectin; PTP, protein tyrosine phosphatase; M, membrane; S, signal peptide; A, acidic domain; E, EGF-like domain.

et al., 1991), however, a developmentally regulated proteolysis of neurocan in the middle of its GAG attachment domain produces two PG fragments, neurocan-N and neurocan-C, the N- and C-terminal halves of neurocan, respectively (Matsui *et al.*, 1994; Rauch *et al.*, 1992).

RPTPβ, a membrane CSPG, has an N-terminal carbonic anhydrase (CA)-like domain followed by a fibronectin (FN) type III-like domain and a cytoplasmic phosphatase domain (Fig. 1B). Phosphacan, a secreted CSPG, consists of the entire extracellular domain of RPTPβ (Maeda *et al.*, 1994; Maurel *et al.*, 1994). Short RPTPβ has a large deletion in the extracellular domain of RPTPβ (Garwood *et al.*, 1999). The shortest splice variant does not bear CS chains (Sakurai *et al.*, 1996). These four RPTPβ transcripts are generated by the alternative splicing of a single gene (Levy *et al.*, 1993).

NGC is a transmembrane-type CSPG that is exclusively expressed in the CNS (Aono *et al.*, 2006; Watanabe *et al.*, 1995; Yasuda *et al.*, 1998). Most NGC molecules in the mature cerebellum and retina but not in the immature counterparts exist in a non-PG form without CS, indicating that NGC is a part-time PG (Aono *et al.*, 2000a,b; Inatani *et al.*, 2000). NGC has four splice variants; NGC-I, -II, and -III (Aono *et al.*, 2000a) and NGC-IV (Aono *et al.*, 2006). Its core protein consists of an N-terminal domain to which a single CS chain attaches (Aono *et al.*, 2004), an acidic domain, an EGF domain (Kinugasa *et al.*, 2004), a membrane-spanning segment, and a cytoplasmic domain variable in the splice variants (Fig. 1C).

IV. CSPGs in the Neurogenetic Stage

At embryonic day 13, the rat brain is rich in neural stem cells and expresses two sulfated GAGs, CS and HS (Oohira *et al.*, 1986). HS is considered to regulate FGF-mediated cell proliferation by forming a ternary complex with FGF-2 and FGF receptor 1 (Schlessinger *et al.*, 2000). Actually, Nurcombe *et al.* (1993) have reported that an HSPG preparation from the early embryonic mouse telencephalon promotes the FGF-2-mediated proliferation of neuroepithelial cells, in which HSPGs, such as glypican-4 (Hagihara *et al.*, 2000), syndecan-1 (Ford-Perriss *et al.*, 2003), and perlecan-related molecule (Joseph *et al.*, 1996), are expressed.

Many molecular species of CSPG are expressed in the CNS (Table I) and have been shown to be involved in various cellular events in the formation and maintenance of the neural network (Bandtlow and Zimmermann, 2000; Oohira *et al.*, 2000b). However, very few studies have been done on the structure and function of CS/CSPGs in the brain primordium. In 2004, Kabos *et al.* reported that neural precursor cells synthesized and secreted some CSPGs including the hyalectan family. Brain-specific CSPGs, such as neurocan, phosphacan/ RPTPβ, and NGC, are detected in the surroundings of neural stem/progenitor cells in the ventricular zone of the rat telencephalon at embryonic day 14 (Ida *et al.*, 2006). A CS preparation from the telencephalon of embryonic day-14-old rat promotes the FGF-2-mediated proliferation of neural stem/progenitor cells. Zou *et al.* (2003) have reported that the mouse brain synthesizes CS rich in a highly sulfated disaccharide unit, E unit, at embryonic day 13 and that midkine, which is known as a heparin-binding growth factor, binds strongly to the E-unit-rich CS.

These observations suggest that CSPGs are involved in the proliferation of neural stem cells together with some growth factors.

V. CSPGs in the Developing Brain

A complicated neural network in the brain is formed through various cellular events including mitogenesis, migration, differentiation, axonal out-growth, and synaptogenesis. These cellular events occur during the develop-ment of the brain in a spatially and temporally regulated manner and are regulated by various cell–cell and cell–substratum interactions. It is now considered that various molecules, such as ECM constituents, neurotrophic factors, and cell surface glycoonjugates including PGs, are involved in these cellular events (Bandtlow and Zimmerman, 2000; Margolis and Margolis, 1997; Oohira et al., 1994, 1998, 2000b; Small et al., 1996).

Striking and distinctive changes in concentration in the hyalectan family are observed in the developing rat brain (Milev et al., 1998). The concentra-tions of versican V2 and brevican increase steadily during the brain's devel-opment up to adulthood, while the concentration of neurocan reaches a peak in the early postnatal period and declines thereafter. These observa-tions indicate that neurocan is a major hyalectan in the developing mamma-lian brain. Intact neurocan is observed in pre- and early postnatal brains, while it is hardly detectable in the mature brain (Matsui et al., 1994; Rauch et al., 1992).

Phosphacan/RPTPβ and neurocan are major CSPGs in the developing mammalian brain and are involved in the modulation of cell adhesion and neurite outgrowth (Faissner et al., 1994; Inatani et al., 2001; Maeda and Noda, 1996; McKeon et al., 1999; Sango et al., 2003). In the CNS, these CSPGs can either promote or inhibit neurite outgrowth depending on neuro-nal cell types and experimental conditions. Phosphacan has outgrowth-pro-moting effects on mesencepharic and hippocampal neurons (Faissner et al., 1994), while phosphacan and neurocan inhibit neurite outgrowth or are repulsive substrata for cortical neurons, retinal ganglion cells, DRG neurons, and some regenerating neurons after CNS injury (Inatani et al., 2001; Maeda and Noda, 1996; McKeon et al., 1999; Sango et al., 2003). GAGs themselves serve as a modulator for neurite outgrowth (Clement et al., 1999; Hikino et al., 2003; Oohira et al., 2000a) and probably for cell adhesion.

Major ligands of neurocan and phosphacan/RPTPβ have been reviewed by Oohira et al. (2000b). The interactions of N-CAM, Ng-CAM/L1, pleiotrophin, amphoterin, and bFGF with neurocan and the interactions of TAG-1, pleiotrophin, midkine, amphoterin, and bFGF with phosphacan are affected by the CS moiety of the core proteins.

Although NGC is less abundant than neurocan and phosphacan in the developing brain, it shows various unique characteristics in the developing CNS. The expression of NGC is developmentally regulated: NGC is detected in the rat brain at embryonic day 14 (Ida *et al.*, 2006). The amount of NGC increases to reach a maximum around postnatal day 20 and then decreases (Watanabe *et al.*, 1995). NGC is a novel part-time PG that changes its structure from a PG form to a non-PG form during the development of the cerebellum (Aono *et al.*, 2000a,b) and retina (Inatani *et al.*, 2000). The ectodomain of NGC is phosphorylated both intracellulary and pericellularly by casein kinase II-like protein kinase (Yamauchi *et al.*, 2002). The structure of the carbohydrate moiety of NGC is developmentally regulated and differs from that of neurocan or phosphacan (Shuo *et al.*, 2004).

Some evidence that NGC is involved in neuritogenesis and/or synaptogenesis has been accumulated. Schumacher *et al.* (1997) have reported that CALEB, a chicken NGC homolog, is implicated in neurite formation. The expression of CALEB mRNA is dynamically upregulated after damage to the optic nerve (Schumacher *et al.*, 2001). Immunostaining of cultured neuronal cells with anti-NGC antibody demonstrated that NGC was concentrated in dendritic filopodia (Inatani *et al.*, 2000), which are considered to develop into neurites or postsynaptic spines. It was found that a recombinant NGC ectodomain significantly stimulated neurite outgrowth of primary cultured neurons from the rat cerebral cortex (unpublished observation).

Although neither interactive partners of NGC at dendritic filopodia and growth cones nor signaling pathways related to the elongation of neurites by NGC have been identified yet, some binding proteins have been reported. An acidic amino acid cluster of CALEB mediates the binding of CALEB to the fibrinogen-like globe within tenascin-C or tenasin-R (Schumacher *et al.*, 2001). The interactions of CALEB and tenascin-C and -R seem to be regulated during development (Schumacher and Stübe, 2003). NGC/CALEB also interacts with the Golgi-associated protein PIST via the juxtamembrane cytoplasmic peptide segment of NGC/CALEB (Hassel *et al.*, 2003). The interaction may play a role in the intracellular transport of NGC/CALEB.

Jüttner *et al.* (2005) have reported that synapses display higher paired-pulse ratios, less depression during prolonged repetitive activation, and a lower release probability at early but not mature postnatal stages in NGC/CALEB-deficient mice.

These observations indicate that CSPGs specific to the CNS take some part in neurite outgrowth and synaptogenesis in the developing brain.

VI. CSPGs in the Mature Brain

Perineuronal nets are reticular networks observed on the surface of cell bodies and proximal dendrites of certain neurons in the adult mammalian CNS (Blümcke *et al.*, 1995; Celio and Blümcke, 1994; Celio *et al.*, 1998;

Matsui *et al.*, 1998). Versican V2 is a major CSPG in the mature brain (Schmalfeldt *et al.*, 1998) and detected in PNNs along with brevican (Brückner *et al.*, 1998). In the adult brain, these hyalectans are thought to interact with HA and tenascin-R to form a ternary complex between neurons and glia, to interact with carbohydrate and protein ligands in the ECM, and to act as linkers of these ECM molecules (Yamaguchi, 2000). Bral2/Hapln4, a brain link protein colocalized with brevican in the PNNs, is involved in the formation of PNNs (Bekku *et al.*, 2003). Neurocan (Matsui *et al.*, 1998) and phosphacan (Wintergerst *et al.*, 1996) are also observed in PNNs.

Bral1/Hapln2, another brain link protein, is suggested to stabilize the binding between HA and hyalectans (Hirakawa *et al.*, 2000), and it colocalizes with versican V2 at the nodes of Ranvier of the mature brain (Oohashi *et al.*, 2002). Versican V2 is a major inhibitor of axonal growth in the ECM of the mature CNS, prevents excessive axonal growth during late phases of development, and participates in the structural stabilization of the mature CNS (Schmalfeldt *et al.*, 2000).

Brevican also inhibits neurite outgrowth from cerebellar granule neurons *in vitro* (Yamada *et al.*, 1997). This PG is located on the surface of neuroglial sheaths of cerebellar glomeruli and is suggested to control the infiltration of axons and dendrites into the mature glomeruli. This inhibitory activity requires CS chains.

Studies suggest a functional role for CSPG in synaptic plasticity in the adult CNS. In young animals, monocular deprivation leads to a shift in ocular dominance, whereas in adults after the critical period there is no such shift. The organization of neurocan into PNNs coincides with the end of the critical period. Pizzorusso *et al.* (2002) have reported that the mature ECM is inhibitory for experience-dependent plasticity, and degradation of neurocan reactivates cortical plasticity in the visual cortex.

Upregulated expressions of the NGC protein and mRNA are observed in the corticolimbic circuitry in parallel with behavioral changes after withdrawal from chronic cocaine treatment in the adult rat (Toda *et al.*, 2002). These observations seem to suggest that NGC is also involved in synaptic plasticity.

Studies using gene-targeting technology indicate that CSPGs are related to synaptic activities. Late-phase hippocampal long-term potentiation (LTP) is reduced in neurocan-deficient mice (Zhou *et al.*, 2001). Brevican-deficient mice display impaired hippocampal CA1 LTP but show no obvious deficits in learning and memory (Brakebusch *et al.*, 2002). Phosphacan/RPTPβ-deficient mice show normal LTP and learning abilities in the Morris water maze task, whereas adult mutant mice exhibit enhanced LTP and impairment in the task (Niisato *et al.*, 2005).

These observations indicate that CSPGs participate not only in structural stabilization but also in synaptic plasticity and synaptic activities in the mature CNS.

VII. CSPGs and CNS Injuries

It is well known that axonal regeneration is unsuccessful in the injured adult CNS and that a glial scar formed at the site of the damage prevents the regeneration. In the glial scar, many inhibitory molecules including CSPGs are found (Fawcett and Asher, 1999; Matsui *et al.*, 2004; Morgenstern *et al.*, 2002; Properzi *et al.*, 2003; Rhodes and Fawcett, 2004). Some CSPGs whose expression is upregulated markedly in response to injuries to the CNS are considered to be involved in the pathogenesis and/or repair of neuronal damage. Omitting CS chains/CSPGs from the affected site promotes axonal regeneration in the mature CNS (Bradbury *et al.*, 2002).

Matsui *et al.* (2005) have reported that the amounts of neurocan, phosphacan, and NGC decrease in the rat brain following neonatal hypoxia-ischemia. Qi *et al.* (2003) have reported that the expression of neurocan mRNA is not upregulated in the transected juvenile spinal cord. The immature CNS with high plasticity seems to respond to neuronal degeneration in a manner different from the mature CNS.

Acknowledgments

We thank all of our colleagues and the collaborators who have contributed so much dedicated effort and thought to our work. Research conducted at the authors' laboratory was supported in part by Grants-in-Aid for Scientific Research from the Ministry of Education, Science, Culture, and Sports of Japan, by the Japan Society for the Promotion of Science, and by a grant from the Mizutani Foundation for Glycoscience.

References

Aono, S., Keino, H., Ono, T., Yasuda, Y., Tokita, Y., Matsui, F., Taniguchi, M., Sonta, S., and Oohira, A. (2000a). Genomic organization and expression pattern of mouse neuroglycan C in the cerebellar development. *J. Biol. Chem.* 275, 337–342.

Aono, S., Keino, H., Tokita, Y., Yamauchi, S., and Oohira, A. (2000b). Neuroglycan C, a part-time proteoglycan, in the central nervous system. *Connect. Tissue* 32, 45–48.

Aono, S., Tokita, Y., Shuo, T., Yamauchi, S., Matsui, F., Nakanishi, K., Hirano, K., Sano, M., and Oohira, A. (2004). Glycosylation site for chondroitin sulfate on the neural part-time proteoglycan, neuroglycan C. *J. Biol. Chem.* 279, 46536–46541.

Aono, S., Tokita, Y., Yasuda, Y., Hirano, K., Yamauchi, S., Shuo, T., Matsui, F., Keino, H., Kashiwai, A., Kawamura, N., Shimada, A., Kishikawa, M., *et al.* (2006). Expression and identification of a new splice variant of neuroglycan a transmembrane chondroitin sulfate proteoglycan, in the human brain. *J. Neurosci. Res.* 83, 110–118.

Bandtlow, C. E., and Zimmermann, D. R. (2000). Proteoglycans in the developing brain: New conceptual insights for old proteins. *Physiol. Rev.* 80, 1267–1290.

Bekku, Y., Su, W.-D., Hirakawa, S., Fässler, R., Ohtsuka, A., Kang, J. S., Sanders, J., Murakami, T., Ninomiya, Y., and Oohashi, T. (2003). Molecular cloning of Bral2, a novel brain-specific link protein, and immunohistochemical colocalization with brevican in perineuronal nets. *Mol. Cell. Neurosci.* **24**, 148–159.

Blümcke, I., Eggli, P., and Celio, M. R. (1995). Relationship between astrocytic processes and "perineuronal nets" in rat neocortex. *Glia* **15**, 131–140.

Bradbury, E. J., Moon, L. D. F., Popat, R. J., King, V. R., Bennett, G. S., Patel, P. N., Fawcett, J. W., and McMahon, S. B. (2002). Chondroitinase ABC promotes functional recovery after spinal cord injury. *Nature* **416**, 636–640.

Brakebusch, C., Seidenbecher, C. I., Asztely, F., Rauch, U., Matthies, H., Meyer, H., Krug, M., Böckers, T. M., Zhou, X., Kreutz, M. R., Montag, D., Gundelfinger, E. D., *et al.* (2002). Brevican-deficient mice display impaired hippocampal CA1 long-term potentiation but show no obvious deficits in learning and memory. *Mol. Cell. Biol.* **22**, 7417–7427.

Brückner, G., Bringmann, A., Härtig, W., Köppe, G., Delpech, B., and Brauer, K. (1998). Acute and long-lasting changes in extracellular-matrix chondroitin-sulphate proteoglycans induced by injection of chondroitinase ABC in the adult rat brain. *Exp. Brain Res.* **121**, 300–310.

Celio, M. R., and Blümcke, I. (1994). Perineuronal nets: A specialized form of extracellular matrix in the adult nervous system. *Brain Res. Brain Res. Rev.* **19**, 128–145.

Celio, M. R., Spreafico, R., De Biasi, S., and Vitellaro-Zuccarello, L. (1998). Perineuronal nets: Past and present. *Trends Neurosci.* **21**, 510–515.

Clement, A. M., Sugahara, K., and Faissner, A. (1999). Chondroitin sulfate E promotes neurite outgrowth of rat embryonic day 18 hippocampal neurons. *Neurosci. Lett.* **269**, 125–128.

Domowicz, M., Li, H., Hennig, A., Henry, J., Vertel, B. M., and Schwartz, N. B. (1995). The biochemically and immunologically distinct CSPG of notochord is a product of the aggrecan gene. *Dev. Biol.* **171**, 655–664.

Dours-Zimmermann, M. T., and Zimmermann, D. R. (1994). A novel glycosaminoglycan attachment domain identified in two alternative splice variants of human versican. *J. Biol. Chem.* **269**, 32992–32998.

Faissner, A., Clement, A., Lochter, A., Streit, A., Mandl, C., and Schachner, M. (1994). Isolation of a neural chondroitin sulfate proteoglycan with neurite outgrowth promoting properties. *J. Cell Biol.* **126**, 783–799.

Fawcett, J. W., and Asher, R. A. (1999). The glial scar and central nervous system repair. *Brain Res. Bull.* **49**, 377–391.

Ford-Perriss, M., Turner, K., Guimond, S., Apedaile, A., Haubeck, H.-D., Turnbull, J., and Murphy, M. (2003). Localisation of specific heparan sulfate proteoglycans during the proliferative phase of brain development. *Dev. Dyn.* **227**, 170–184.

Garwood, J., Schnädelbach, O., Clement, A., Schütte, K., Bach, A., and Faissner, A. (1999). DSD-1-proteoglycan is the mouse homolog of phosphacan and displays opposing effects on neurite outgrowth dependent on neuronal lineage. *J. Neurosci.* **19**, 3888–3899.

Hagihara, K., Watanabe, K., Chun, J., and Yamaguchi, Y. (2000). Glypican-4 is an FGF2-binding heparan sulfate proteoglycan expressed in neural precursor cells. *Dev. Dyn.* **219**, 353–367.

Hassel, B., Schreff, M., Stübe, E.-M., Blaich, U., and Schumacher, S. (2003). CALEB/NGC interacts with the Golgi-associated protein PIST. *J. Biol. Chem.* **278**, 40136–40143.

Hikino, M., Mikami, T., Faissner, A., Vilela-Silva, A.-C. E. S., Pavao, M. S. G., and Sugahara, K. (2003). Oversulfated dermatan sulfate exhibits neurite outgrowth-promoting activity toward embryonic mouse hippocampal neurons: Implications of dermatan sulfate in neuritogenesis in the brain. *J. Biol. Chem.* **278**, 43744–43754.

Hirakawa, S., Oohashi, T., Su, W.-D., Yoshioka, H., Murakami, T., Arata, J., and Ninomiya, Y. (2000). The brain link protein-1 (BRAL1): cDNA cloning, genomic structure, and characterization as a novel link protein expressed in adult brain. *Biochem. Biophys. Res. Commun.* **276**, 982–989.

Höök, M., Kjellén, L., Johansson, S., and Robinson, J. (1984). Cell-surface glycosaminoglycans. *Annu. Rev. Biochem.* **53,** 847–869.

Ida, M., Shuo, T., Hirano, K., Tokita, Y., Nakanishi, K., Matsui, F., Aono, S., Fujita, H., Fujiwara, Y., Kaji, T., and Oohira, A. (2006). Identification and functions of chondroitin sulfate in the milieu of neural stem cells. *J. Biol. Chem.* **281,** 5982–5991.

Inatani, M., Tanihara, H., Oohira, A., Otori, Y., Nishida, A., Honjo, M., Kido, N., and Honda, Y. (2000). Neuroglycan C, a neural tissue-specific transmembrane chondroitin sulfate proteoglycan, in retinal neural network formation. *Invest. Ophthalmol. Vis. Sci.* **41,** 4338–4346.

Inatani, M., Honjo, M., Otori, Y., Oohira, A., Kido, N., Tano, Y., Honda, Y., and Tanihara, H. (2001). Inhibitory effects of neurocan and phosphacan on neurite outgrowth from retinal ganglion cells in culture. *Invest. Ophthalmol. Vis. Sci.* **42,** 1930–1938.

Iozzo, R. V., and Murdoch, A. D. (1996). Proteoglycans of the extracellular environment: Clues from the gene and protein side offer novel perspectives in molecular diversity and function. *FASEB J.* **10,** 598–614.

Joseph, S. J., Ford, M. D., Barth, C., Portbury, S., Bartlett, P. F., Nurcombe, V., and Greferath, U. (1996). A proteoglycan that activates fibroblast growth factors during early neuronal development is a perlecan variant. *Development* **122,** 3443–3452.

Jüttner, R., Moré, M. I., Das, D., Babich, A., Meier, J., Henning, M., Erdmann, B., Müller, E.-C., Otto, A., Grantyn, R., and Rathjen, F. G. (2005). Impaired synapse function during postnatal development in the absence of CALEB, an EGF-like protein processed by neuronal activity. *Neuron* **46,** 233–245.

Kabos, P., Matundan, H., Zandian, M., Bertolotto, C., Robinson, M. L., Davy, B. E., Yu, J. S., and Krueger, R. C., Jr. (2004). Neural precursors express multiple chondroitin sulfate proteoglycans, including the lectican family. *Biochem. Biophys. Res. Commun.* **318,** 955–963.

Kinugasa, Y., Ishiguro, H., Tokita, Y., Oohira, A., Ohmoto, H., and Higashiyama, S. (2004). Neuroglycan C, a novel member of the neuregulin family. *Biochem. Biophys. Res. Commun.* **321,** 1045–1049.

Krueger, N. X., and Saito, H. (1992). A human transmembrane protein-tyrosine-phosphatase, PTPζ, is expressed in brain and has an N-terminal receptor domain homologous to carbonic anhydrases. *Proc. Natl. Acad. Sci. USA* **89,** 7417–7421.

Krueger, R. C., Jr., Hennig, A. K., and Schwartz, N. B. (1992). Two immunologically and developmentally distinct chondroitin sulfate proteolglycans in embryonic chick brain. *J. Biol. Chem.* **267,** 12149–12161.

Levy, J. B., Canoll, P. D., Silvennoinen, O., Barnea, G., Morse, B., Honegger, A. M., Huang, J.-T., Cannizzaro, L. A., Park, S.-H., Druck, T., Huebner, K., Sap, J., *et al.* (1993). The cloning of a receptor-type protein tyrosine phosphatase expressed in the central nervous system. *J. Biol. Chem.* **268,** 10573–10581.

Maeda, N., and Noda, M. (1996). 6B4 proteoglycan/phosphacan is a repulsive substratum but promotes morphological differentiation of cortical neurons. *Development* **122,** 647–658.

Maeda, N., Matsui, F., and Oohira, A. (1992). A chondroitin sulfate proteoglycan that is developmentally regulated in the cerebellar mossy fiber system. *Dev. Biol.* **151,** 564–574.

Maeda, N., Hamanaka, H., Shintani, T., Nishiwaki, T., and Noda, M. (1994). Multiple receptor-like protein tyrosine phosphatases in the form of chondroitin sulfate proteoglycan. *FEBS Lett.* **354,** 67–70.

Margolis, R. U., and Margolis, R. K. (1997). Chondroitin sulfate proteoglycans as mediators of axon growth and pathfinding. *Cell Tissue Res.* **290,** 343–348.

Matsui, F., and Oohira, A. (2004). Proteoglycans and injury of the central nervous system. *Congenit. Anom. (Kyoto)* **44,** 181–188.

Matsui, F., Watanabe, E., and Oohira, A. (1994). Immunological identification of two proteoglycan fragments derived from neurocan, a brain-specific chondroitin sulfate proteoglycan. *Neurochem. Int.* **25**, 425–431.

Matsui, F., Nishizuka, M., Yasuda, Y., Aono, S., Watanabe, E., and Oohira, A. (1998). Occurrence of a N-terminal proteolytic fragment of neurocan, not a C-terminal half, in a perineuronal net in the adult rat cerebrum. *Brain Res.* **790**, 45–51.

Matsui, F., Kakizawa, H., Nishizuka, M., Hirano, K., Shuo, T., Ida, M., Tokita, Y., Aono, S., Keino, H., and Oohira, A. (2005). Changes in the amounts of chondroitin sulfate proteoglycans in rat brain following neonatal hypoxia-ischemia. *J. Neurosci. Res.* **81**, 837–845.

Maurel, P., Rauch, U., Flad, M., Margolis, R. K., and Margolis, R. U. (1994). Phosphacan, a chondroitin sulfate proteoglycan of brain that interacts with neurons and neural cell-adhesion molecules, is an extracellular variant of a receptor-type protein tyrosine phosphatase. *Proc. Natl. Acad. Sci. USA* **91**, 2512–2516.

McKeon, R. J., Jurynec, M. J., and Buck, C. R. (1999). The chondroitin sulfate proteoglycans neurocan and phosphacan are expressed by reactive astrocytes in the chronic CNS glial scar. *J. Neurosci.* **19**, 10778–10788.

Milev, P., Maurel, P., Chiba, A., Mevissen, M., Popp, S., Yamaguchi, Y., Margolis, R. K., and Margolis, R. U. (1998). Differential regulation of expression of hyaluronan-binding proteoglycans in developing brain: Aggrecan, versican, neurocan, and brevican. *Biochem. Biophys. Res. Commun.* **247**, 207–212.

Morgenstern, D. A., Asher, R. A., and Fawcett, J. W. (2002). Chondroitin sulphate proteoglycans in the CNS injury response. *Prog. Brain Res.* **137**, 313–332.

Niederöst, B. P., Zimmermann, D. R., Schwab, M. E., and Bandtlow, C. E. (1999). Bovine CNS myelin contains neurite growth-inhibitory activity associated with chondroitin sulfate proteoglycans. *J. Neurosci.* **19**, 8979–8989.

Niisato, K., Fujikawa, A., Komai, S., Shintani, T., Watanabe, E., Sakaguchi, G., Katsuura, G., Manabe, T., and Noda, M. (2005). Age-dependent enhancement of hippocampal long-term potentiation and impairment of spatial learning through the Rho-associated kinase pathway in protein tyrosine phosphatase receptor type ζ-deficient mice. *J. Neurosci.* **25**, 1081–1088.

Nurcombe, V., Ford, M. D., Wildschut, J. A., and Bartlett, P. F. (1993). Developmental regulation of neural response to FGF-1 and FGF-2 by heparan sulfate proteoglycan. *Science* **260**, 103–106.

Oohashi, T., Hirakawa, S., Bekku, Y., Rauch, U., Zimmermann, D. R., Su, W.-D., Ohtsuka, A., Murakami, T., and Ninomiya, Y. (2002). Bral1, a brain-specific link protein, colocalizing with the versican V2 isoform at the nodes of Ranvier in developing and adult mouse central nervous systems. *Mol. Cell Neurosci.* **19**, 43–57.

Oohira, A., Matsui, F., Matsuda, M., and Shoji, R. (1986). Developmental change in the glycosaminoglycan composition of the rat brain. *J. Neurochem.* **47**, 588–593.

Oohira, A., Katoh-Semba, R., Watanabe, E., and Matsui, F. (1994). Brain development and multiple molecular species of proteoglycan. *Neurosci. Res.* **20**, 195–207.

Oohira, A., Aono, S., Matsui, F., Yasuda, Y., and Tokita, Y. (1998). Transmembrane chondroitin sulfate proteoglycans in the developing brain: Involvement in signal transduction as well as in cell adhesion. *Connect. Tissue* **30**, 49–56.

Oohira, A., Kushima, Y., Tokita, Y., Sugiura, N., Sakurai, K., Suzuki, S., and Kimata, K. (2000a). Effects of lipid-derivatized glycosaminoglycans (GAGs), a novel probe for functional analyses of GAGs, on cell-to-substratum adhesion and neurite elongation in primary cultures of fetal rat hippocampal neurons. *Arch. Biochem. Biophys.* **378**, 78–83.

Oohira, A., Matsui, F., Tokita, Y., Yamauchi, S., and Aono, S. (2000b). Molecular interactions of neural chondroitin sulfate proteoglycans in the brain development. *Arch. Biochem. Biophys.* **374**, 24–34.

Pizzorusso, T., Medini, P., Berardi, N., Chierzi, S., Fawcett, J. W., and Maffei, L. (2002). Reactivation of ocular dominance plasticity in the adult visual cortex. *Science* **298**, 1248–1251.

Properzi, F., Asher, R. A., and Fawcett, J. W. (2003). Chondroitin sulphate proteoglycans in the central nervous system: Changes and synthesis after injury. *Biochem. Soc. Trans.* **31**, 335–336.

Qi, M.-L., Wakabayashi, Y., Enomoto, M., and Shinomiya, K. (2003). Changes in neurocan expression in the distal spinal cord stump following complete cord transection: A comparison between infant and adult rats. *Neurosci. Res.* **45**, 181–188.

Rauch, U., Gao, P., Janetzko, A., Flaccus, A., Hilgenberg, L., Tekotte, H., Margolis, R. K., and Margolis, R. U. (1991). Isolation and characterization of developmentally regulated chondroitin sulfate and chondroitin/keratan sulfate proteoglycans of brain identified with monoclonal antibodies. *J. Biol. Chem.* **266**, 14785–14801.

Rauch, U., Karthikeyan, L., Maurel, P., Margolis, R. U., and Margolis, R. K. (1992). Cloning and primary structure of neurocan, a developmentally regulated, aggregating chondroitin sulfate proteoglycan of brain. *J. Biol. Chem.* **267**, 19536–19547.

Rhodes, K. E., and Fawcett, J. W. (2004). Chondroitin sulphate proteoglycans: Preventing plasticity or protecting the CNS? *J. Anat.* **204**, 33–48.

Ruoslahti, E. (1996). Brain extracellular matrix. *Glycobiology* **6**, 489–492.

Sakurai, T., Friedlander, D. R., and Grumet, M. (1996). Expression of polypeptide variants of receptor-type protein tyrosine phosphatase β: The secreted form, phosphacan, increases dramatically during embryonic development and modulates glial cell behavior *in vitro*. *J. Neurosci. Res.* **43**, 694–706.

Sango, K., Oohira, A., Ajiki, K., Tokashiki, A., Horie, M., and Kawano, H. (2003). Phosphacan and neurocan are repulsive substrata for adhesion and neurite extension of adult rat dorsal root ganglion neurons *in vitro*. *Exp. Neurol.* **182**, 1–11.

Schlessinger, J., Plotnikov, A. N., Ibrahimi, O. A., Eliseenkova, A. V., Yeh, B. K., Yayon, A., Linhardt, R. J., and Mohammadi, M. (2000). Crystal structure of a ternary FGF-FGFR-heparin complex reveals a dual role for heparin in FGFR binding and dimerization. *Mol. Cell* **6**, 743–750.

Schmalfeldt, M., Bandtlow, C. E., Dours-Zimmermann, M. T., Winterhalter, K. H., and Zimmermann, D. R. (2000). Brain derived versican V2 is a potent inhibitor of axonal growth. *J. Cell Sci.* **113**, 807–816.

Schmalfeldt, M., Dours-Zimmermann, M. T., Winterhalter, K. H., and Zimmermann, D. R. (1998). Versican V2 is a major extracellular matrix component of the mature bovine brain. *J. Biol. Chem.* **273**, 15758–15764.

Schumacher, S., and Stübe, E.-M. (2003). Regulated binding of the fibrinogen-like domains of tenascin-R and tenascin-C to the neural EGF family member CALEB. *J. Neurochem.* **87**, 1213–1223.

Schumacher, S., Volkmer, H., Buck, F., Otto, A., Tárnok, A., Roth, S., and Rathjen, F. G. (1997). Chicken acidic leucine-rich EGF-like domain containing brain protein (CALEB), a neural member of the EGF family of differentiation factors, is implicated in neurite formation. *J. Cell Biol.* **136**, 895–906.

Schumacher, S., Jung, M., Nörenberg, U., Dorner, A., Chiquet-Ehrismann, R., Stuermer, C. A., and Rathjen, F. G. (2001). CALEB binds via its acidic stretch to the fibrinogen-like domain of tenascin-C or tenascin-R and its expression is dynamically regulated after optic nerve lesion. *J. Biol. Chem.* **276**, 7337–7345.

Seidenbecher, C. I., Richter, K., Rauch, U., Fässler, R., Garner, C. C., and Gundelfinger, E. D. (1995). Brevican, a chondroitin sulfate proteoglycan of rat brain, occurs as secreted and cell surface glycosylphosphatidylinositol-anchored isoforms. *J. Biol. Chem.* **270**, 27206–27212.

Shuo, T., Aono, S., Matsui, F., Tokita, Y., Maeda, H., Shimada, K., and Oohira, A. (2004). Developmental changes in the biochemical and immunological characters of the carbohydrate moiety of neuroglycan C, a brain-specific chondroitin sulfate proteoglycan. *Glycoconj. J.* **20**, 267–278.

Small, D. H., Mok, S. S., Williamson, T. G., and Nurcombe, V. (1996). Role of proteoglycans in neural development, regeneration, and the aging brain. *J. Neurochem.* **67**, 889–899.

Toda, S., McGinty, J. F., and Kalivas, P. W. (2002). Repeated cocaine administration alters the expression of genes in corticolimbic circuitry after a 3-week withdrawal: A DNA macroarray study. *J. Neurochem.* **82**, 1290–1299.

Watanabe, E., Maeda, N., Matsui, F., Kushima, Y., Noda, M., and Oohira, A. (1995). Neuroglycan C, a novel membrane-spanning chondroitin sulfate proteoglycan that is restricted to the brain. *J. Biol. Chem.* **270**, 26876–26882.

Wintergerst, E. S., Faissner, A., and Celio, M. R. (1996). The proteoglycan DSD-1-PG occurs in perineuronal nets around parvalbumin-immunoreactive interneurons of the rat cerebral cortex. *Int. J. Dev. Neurosci.* **14**, 249–255.

Yamada, H., Watanabe, K., Shimonaka, M., and Yamaguchi, Y. (1994). Molecular cloning of brevican, a novel brain proteoglycan of the aggrecan/versican family. *J. Biol. Chem.* **269**, 10119–10126.

Yamada, H., Fredette, B., Shitara, K., Hagihara, K., Miura, R., Ranscht, B., Stallcup, W. B., and Yamaguchi, Y. (1997). The brain chondroitin sulfate proteoglycan brevican associates with astrocytes ensheathing cerebellar glomeruli and inhibits neurite outgrowth from granule neurons. *J. Neurosci.* **17**, 7784–7795.

Yamaguchi, Y. (2000). Lecticans: Organizers of the brain extracellular matrix. *Cell Mol. Life Sci.* **57**, 276–289.

Yamauchi, S., Tokita, Y., Aono, S., Matsui, F., Shuo, T., Ito, H., Kato, K., Kasahara, K., and Oohira, A. (2002). Phosphorylation of neuroglycan C, a brain-specific transmembrane chondroitin sulfate proteoglycan, and its localization in the lipid rafts. *J. Biol. Chem.* **277**, 20583–20590.

Yasuda, Y., Tokita, Y., Aono, S., Matsui, F., Ono, T., Sonta, S., Watanabe, E., Nakanishi, Y., and Oohira, A. (1998). Cloning and chromosomal mapping of the human gene of neuroglycan C (NGC), a neural transmembrane chondroitin sulfate proteoglycan with an EGF module. *Neurosci. Res.* **32**, 313–322.

Zhou, X.-H., Brakebusch, C., Matthies, H., Oohashi, T., Hirsch, E., Moser, M., Krug, M., Seidenbecher, C. I., Boeckers, T. M., Rauch, U., Buettner, R., Gundelfinger, E. D., *et al.* (2001). Neurocan is dispensable for brain development. *Mol. Cell Biol.* **21**, 5970–5978.

Zou, P., Zou, K., Muramatsu, H., Ichihara-Tanaka, K., Habuchi, O., Ohtake, S., Ikematsu, S., Sakuma, S., and Muramatsu, T. (2003). Glycosaminoglycan structures required for strong binding to midkine, a heparin-binding growth factor. *Glycobiology* **13**, 35–42.

Uwe Rauch* and Joachim Kappler[†]

*Department of Experimental Pathology
Universitet Lund, Lund, Sweden

[†]Physiologisch-Chemisches Institut
Rheinische Friedrich-Wilhelms-Universität Bonn 53115 Bonn
Germany

Chondroitin/Dermatan Sulfates in the Central Nervous System: Their Structures and Functions in Health and Disease

I. Chapter Overview

The central nervous system (CNS) is a rich and complex source of proteins modified with chondroitin/dermatan sulfate (CS/DS) chains. During brain development, a particularly high content of CSs has been revealed. Their finely tuned expression patterns in relation to axonal fiber tracts suggest important functions. Chondroitin sulfate proteoglycans (CSPGs), which have been identified in the brain, are brevican, neurocan, versican, aggrecan, decorin, biglycan, testican-1, phosphacan, NG2, appican, APLP2, and neuroglycan-C. The analysis of developmental changes in the overall composition of CS revealed in several species a decrease of 6-sulfated and unsulfated residues, with a concomitant increase of 4-sulfation. *In vitro*, CSPG-associated mechanisms can modulate neuritogenesis either positively or negatively, and the physiological role of CS moieties appears to depend on the proteoglycan (PG) core protein, the substrate,

Advances in Pharmacology, Volume 53
Copyright 2006, Elsevier Inc. All rights reserved.

1054-3589/06 $35.00
DOI: 10.1016/S1054-3589(05)53016-3

the type of cells, and their stage of development. *In vivo*, application of CS, CSPGs, or chondroitinase has been shown to affect neuronal development, function, and plasticity. As components of perineuronal nets aggrecan, brevican, phosphacan, and neurocans N-terminal fragment regulate synaptic plasticity. Binding partners of CSPGs include growth factors and neurotrophic factors as well as structural components of cells or the extracellular matrix (ECM). Chondroitin sulfate proteoglycans have been implicated in response to traumatic lesions and in the course of various diseases affecting the CNS, as degenerative processes, inflammatory diseases, and epilepsy. Their inhibitory effect on axon regeneration after spinal cord injury renders the manipulation of their level a promising therapeutic strategy.

II. Introduction

The CNS is a rich and probably most complex source of proteins modified with CS/DS chains. This heterogeneity arises from the possibility to modify a large number of distinct core proteins with different variants of CS ranging from unsulfated to oversulfated forms[1]. The development of the brain is not only characterized by cellular migration and differentiation but, in contrast to most other tissues, also by neurite formation, dendritic and axonal elongation, fasciculation, and guidance. Especially at these stages, a high content of CS has been revealed, indicating that the presence of CSPGs as such is of paramount importance.

III. Structures and Expression Patterns of CSPGs in the CNS

A. PGs Carrying CS in the Brain

Cell membrane and secreted CSPGs, which have been detected in brain and characterized by identification of their core protein sequence, are summarized in Table I. Some of the molecules listed in Table I, like brevican, can be considered as "part time PGs", core proteins, which are not always modified with a glycosaminoglycan (GAG) chain. There are probably many other proteins, which can occasionally be modified with GAG chains but are usually not considered as PGs, like tenascin-R (Probstmeier

---

[1] In the following text they will be often simply named CS chains, since a differential analysis of the susceptibility of these chains to chondroitinase ABC, AC, and B, combined with a detailed size analysis of the digestion products as, for example, the analysis by Bao *et al.* (2004), is only rarely routinely performed and more crude methods of analysis, like a test of their filtration properties through membranes with pore sizes calibrated for proteins, might underestimate the content of iduronic acid residues, should they occur isolated rather than clustered.

TABLE I Secreted and Cell Surface CSPGs Which Have been Observed in the CNS

Name used in review	Other name(s)	Location	Approximate size (extra+intracellular)	CS-chains	KO mice	Observed peculiarities	Reference
Brevican	BEHAB	GPI bound/ secreted	650/900 aa*	0–1	Viable	Impaired LTP	Brakebusch et al., 2002
Neurocan		Secreted	1250 aa	2–3	Viable	Impaired L-LTP	Zhou et al., 2001
Versican	PG-M	Secreted	1600(V2), 2400(V1), 3300(V0)aa	2–3, 8–9, 10–12	Embryonic letal	No heart development	Mjaatvedt et al., 1998
Aggrecan		Secreted	2000 aa	up to 100	Perinatal letal	No cartilage	Watanabe et al., 1994
Decorin		Secreted	350 aa	1!	Viable	Impaired collagen fibrils	Ameye and Young, 2002
Biglycan		Secreted	350 aa	2!	Viable	Osteoporosis	Ameye and Young, 2002
Testican		Secreted	450 aa	1–2	Viable	Not reported	Edgell et al., 2004
Phosphacan/ PTP-beta	DSD-1/RPTPz	Secreted/ transmembrane	1600/1600+650 aa	3–5	Viable	Impaired remyelination	Harroch et al., 2002
NG2		Transmembrane	2200+100 aa	1–2	Viable	Impaired PDGF response	Grako et al., 1999
Appican	APP	Transmembrane	650+50 aa	0–1	Viable	Decreased locomotion	Zheng et al., 1995
APLP2		Transmembrane	650+50 aa	0–1	Viable	Not reported	Von-Koch et al., 1997
Neuroglycan C	CALEB	Transmembrane	400+100 aa	0–1	Not reported		

*aa, amino acids.

Brevican and phosphacan/phosphotyrosinphosphatase (PTP)-beta can be expressed as secreted and membrane bound variants by alternative splicing. Size values of transmembrane molecules with a cytoplasmic C-terminal tail, are separated into extracellular and intracellular protein regions. CS-chain numbers of more than one are approximations based on the number of suitable attachment motifs.

et al., 2000) and laminins (Sasaki *et al.*, 2001, 2002). Furthermore, the recombinant production of PGs in mammalian cells can lead to misclassifications of certain core proteins. Testican-2, for example, is recombinantly produced as CSPG but carries only heparan sulfate in brain (Schnepp *et al.*, 2005).

The interaction of the lecticans (aggrecan, versican, neurocan, and brevican) with hyaluronan can be stabilized by link proteins, some of which are brain specific molecules (Bekku *et al.*, 2003; Rauch *et al.*, 2004). Lecticans are mainly distinguished by the length of their mucin-like central region and the number of GAG attachment sites within this region (Fig. 1). The term "mucin-like" is used to indicate that these protein regions show no significant homology to established protein domains with a defined tertiary structure, usually lack cysteins, and can be enriched in serines, threonines, and prolines but are not like real mucins completely dominated by these amino acids. Regions with such a character, which are also evident in phosphacan, neuroglycan C, and NG2 appear to be preferred sites of CS chain attachments (Fig. 1).

B. Developmental Changes and Structural Analysis of CS in the Brain

Developmental changes of GAGs have been analyzed in rodent, pig, and embryonic chicken brain. During postnatal rat brain development the concentration of CS related to the lipid-free dry weight of brain tissue has a peak value of about 4.5 μmol disaccharide units/g 1 week after birth. The amount decreases within a few days to 80% and during the following 3 weeks gradually to about 60% of this value, to remain after the age of 1 month at a relatively constant value of about 2.5 μmol/g (Margolis *et al.*, 1975a,b). A peak value of sulfated GAGs about 1 week after birth, which is followed by a sharper decrease, followed by a slight gradual increase has also been found in mouse cerebrum and cerebellum (Burkart and Wiesmann, 1987). The turnover of sulfated GAGs during their peak production period is as high as 90% in 24 h (Burkart and Wiesmann, 1987). This might reflect a high degree of remodeling of the ECM at this developmental stage. However, in pulse/chase studies only the degradation of the PGs, which have been produced during the pulse period, can be determined. Thus, the high turnover of these newly synthesized PGs might also indicate a production of an excess of PGs and consecutive degradation of those molecules, which had no chance to be integrated into ECM superstructures. Many CSPGs, which are so abundant in brain at this developmental stage, might constitute a pool of molecules, not necessarily used to build higher order matrix structures. They might have to fulfill not a structural but possibly a dynamic function, which is not understood as yet. The amount of these CSPGs may be important to regulate the volume of the

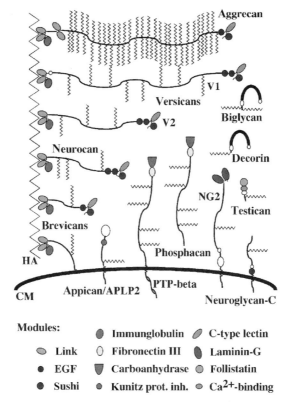

FIGURE 1 Secreted and cell surface CSPGs, which have been observed in the central nervous system. Schematic presentation of the PGs with common ECM modules represented in color. The interactions of the N-terminal domains of the lecticans with haluronan (HA) are indicated at the left side. The anchorage of cell surface bound PGs to the cell membrane (CM) via GPI moieties (brevican) or transmembrane domains is indicated at the bottom. Protein parts, which contain cysteins and may represent less established extracellular protein modules, are indicated as white globules. Regions lacking cysteins, which might have a mucine-like character, are indicated as black lines. Bolder lines in decorin and biglycan represent leucine rich repeats. Zigzag-lines represent transmembrane domains (small), CS chains (medium), and HA (big). (See Color Insert.)

extracellular space in the developing brain. It has been noticed that in rat brain the decrease of CS during postnatal brain development coincides with a reduction of the fraction of the total brain volume occupied by the ECM, which decreases from about 40% to 20% of the total brain volume (Sykova, 2001).

An analysis of the composition of CS of 1 week old rat brain revealed 29% unsulfated, 51% 4-sulfated, and 19% 6-sulfated disaccharides, while less than 0.5% unsulfated, 96% 4-sulfated, and 2.5% 6-sulfated disaccharides were found in adult brain (Flaccus *et al.*, 1991). The amount of disulfated disaccharides remained 1% at both investigated time points. The significant decrease in 6-sulfated disaccharides during postnatal rat brain development has been confirmed and correlated with the decline of the expression of C6-sulfotransferase-1 in brain (Properzi *et al.*, 2005). Also in embryonic chicken brain, the overall content of CS and the relative amount of 6-sulfated disaccharides decreases, from about 60% at day 6 to about 45% at day 17 (Kitagawa *et al.*, 1997). A very detailed structural examination with a special emphasis on the iduronic acid content has been performed with CS isolated from embryonic and adult pig brain (Bao *et al.*, 2004). Consistent with the data obtained from rodent brain, this analysis revealed a decrease of unsulfated chondroitin from about 20% to 5% and a decrease of chondroitin-6-sulfate from about 33% to 10%, comparing embryonic and adult chondroitinase ABC digestion products, respectively. Digestion with chondroitinase AC and chondroitinase B revealed that embryonic CS contains a significant portion of DS, with 8–9% disaccharides containing iduronic acid units, whereas such units accounted for less than 1% of the adult CS.

Although significant at embryonic stages, in comparison to other tissues the iduronic acid substitution of brain CS appears rather sparse, since CS chains of small PGs of the decorin type secreted by skin fibroblasts can have 87% of their uronic acid residues isomerized to iduronic acid (Rauch *et al.*, 1986). This low amount of DS in brain tissue could be associated with the observation that patients with a lysosomal storage disease, Maroteaux-Lamy disease that solely affects the depolymerization of CS, are not significantly affected by mental deficits but can exhibit severe dwarfism and other abnormalities. These patients are lacking *N*-acetyl-galactosamine-4-sulfate sulfatase activity. Interestingly, their urine contains DS but not iduronic acid free CS, which is apart from the exoglycosylytic pathway also susceptible to endoglycosylytic degradation by mammalian hyaluronidases, while regions rich in iduronic acid resists hyaluronidase activity (Coster *et al.*, 1975).

C. Developmental Changes of CS Chains Attached to Particular Core Proteins

Developmental changes of the sulfate substitution of the CS chains of neurocan, phosphacan, a keratan sulfate (KS)-modified phosphacan variant, and neuroglycan C isolated from mouse and rat brain have been reported (Hikino *et al.*, 2003; Maeda *et al.*, 2003; Rauch *et al.*, 1991; Shuo *et al.*, 2004). The results are summarized in Table II. As for brain CS, in general, a decrease in 6-sulfation is also evident for each individual PG investigated. While all values in Table II were derived from PGs isolated

TABLE II CS Compositions of Individual PGs Isolated with Monoclonal Antibodies from Brain Tissue

Source, age	mAb	0-S,	4-S, (CS-A)	6-S, (CS-C)	2,6-diS (CS-D)	4,6-diS (CS-E)
Neurocan						
Rat brain, 7d	1D1	–	80	20	–	–
Rat brain, 10d	1G2	10.2	63	24.5	0.8	1.5
Rat brain, adult	1D1	–	97	<3	–	–
Phosphacan						
Mouse brain, postnatal	DSD-1	2	68	23	5	–
Rat brain, 7d	3F8	–	67	33	–	–
Rat cortex, 7d	6B4	4.3	63.6	32.1	–	–
Rat brain, 10d	6B4	11.7	64.5	21.9	0.8	1.1
Rat cortex, 12d	6B4	2.7	83.2	14.1	–	–
Rat brain, 20d	6B4	6.9	85.8	6.0	1.3	–
Rat brain, adult	3F8	–	96	<4	–	–
Phosphacan-KS						
Rat brain, 7d	3H1	–	>99	<1	–	–
Rat brain, adult	3H1	–	>99	<1	–	–
Neuroglycan C						
Rat brain, 10d	C5	8.4	76.9	10	0.7	4.0
Rat brain, adult	C5	6.2	89	2.1	0.2	2.5

The antibody used for isolation is indicated in the first column. Note that 3H1 recognizes a carbohydrate (KS) epitope. All values represent percent values of the total amount of analyzed disaccharides. The spectrum of those might vary between different analytical protocols. Data were compiled from: (Hikino et al., 2003; Maeda et al., 2003; Rauch et al., 1991; Shuo et al., 2004).

with the aid of monoclonal antibodies from brain, a significant fraction of 14.3% of the oversulfated (4,6-disulfated) E motif in the GAG chains of recombinant appican was produced by C6 glioma (Tsuchida et al., 2001). Oversulfated disaccharides as well as human brain derived appican have been implicated in the support of neurite outgrowth (Salinero et al., 2000).

D. Immunocytochemical Expression Patterns of CS and CSPGs in the Developing Brain

During development of the rodent forebrain, CSPGs are distributed throughout the proliferative zone that initially comprises the thin wall of the telencephalic vesicle (Bandtlow and Zimmermann, 2000). Later, chondroitin, CS-C, and the neurocan core protein become most prominent in the preplate, which contains growing processes of preplate neurons. Subsequently, when cortical plate neurons subdivide the preplate, these molecules are present in the marginal zone and the subplate. Later, labeling of CSPGs declines rapidly concomitant with the differentiation of the cortex (Kappler et al., 1997).

Interestingly, axons of preplate and cortical plate neurons extend obliquely across the CSPG-rich subplate to enter the CSPG-poor intermediate zone. In the upper intermediate zone, they abruptly change their direction to run in parallel to the subplate zone. Adjacent to this path, the thalamic afferent axons extend within the CSPG-rich subplate. Cortical neurons and their efferent axons express the neural cell adhesion molecules TAG-1 and highly polysialylated NCAM, while thalamocortical axons in the subplate express L1. Thus, CSPGs in the subplate may regulate the segregation of these tracts (Bandtlow and Zimmermann, 2000). Other PGs, which display a different laminar pattern as decorin (Kappler et al., 1998) or a nonlaminar expression pattern, like phosphacan, may play different roles in the cerebral cortex (Miller et al., 1995).

CS and CSPGs are also present in the developing cerebellum (Meyer-Puttlitz et al., 1996), spinal cord (Katoh-Semba et al., 1998; Meyer-Puttlitz et al., 1996), and in different sensory systems. In the spinal cord, neurocan and phosphacan may guide axonal growth from the dorsal root ganglia. In the developing mouse retina, CSPGs follow a centrifugal, receding gradient, which correlates with the sequence of axogenesis (Chung et al., 2000a; Leung et al., 2004). In the optic chiasm, CS forms boundaries in the vicinity of decussating axons (Chung et al., 2000b) and may be involved in active sorting of dorsal retinal axons from ventral retinal axons (Chung et al., 2000a; Leung et al., 2004). In the mouse olfactory system, neurocan is detected in primary olfactory axons as they extend toward the telencephalon and contact the olfactory bulb (Clarris et al., 2000).

E. Perineuronal Nets

"Perineuronal nets" enwrap cell bodies and proximal dendrites of certain neurons in the adult mammalian CNS and may represent a supportive and protective scaffolding (Celio and Blümcke, 1994). These ECM structures are confined to the space interposed between glial processes and the nerve cells. PGs within perineuronal nets may entrap the tissue fluid and form a perineuronal gel layer, which protects the synapses as a "perisynaptic barrier" (Murakami and Ohtsuka, 2003). While axon terminals on the principal neurons in the superior olivary nuclei contain CS-A and CS-C (Atoji et al., 1995), CS-D was found in the broad ECM around them (Atoji et al., 1997). A prominent individual CSPGs identified in perineuronal nets is aggrecan (Matthews et al., 2002), and a major function of perineuronal nets appears to be the stabilization of synaptic connections at the expense of plasticity (Pizzorusso et al., 2002). A negative correlation has been noticed between their presence and the susceptibility of neurons to Alzheimer's disease or oxidative stress (Morawski et al., 2004).

IV. Physiological Functions of CSPGs

A. Cell Culture Studies

1. Neuritogenesis

CSPGs inhibit neuritogenesis of dorsal root ganglia neurons, retinal neurons, and forebrain neurons on laminin substrata (Silver and Miller, 2004). Furthermore, CS and CSPG preparations were found to inhibit neuritogenesis in assays performed with many other neuron types on different substrates (Bandtlow and Zimmermann, 2000). While in some cases elimination of the CS chains reduced or abolished the inhibitory activity, in other cases the core proteins themselves were inhibitory as well (Ughrin et al., 2003). Many of these studies used laminin as an adhesive and outgrowth promoting substrate. However, since laminin itself may carry CS moieties (Sasaki et al., 2002), exogenous CSPGs may also interfere with interactions mediated by such chains.

On the other hand, CS and DS promote neurite growth of embryonic rat brain neurons on polyornithine (Lafont et al., 1992), and synthetic DS-like oligosaccharides mimic these morphological effects (Lafont et al., 1994). CS promotes axon growth of thalamic neurons (Fernaud-Espinosa et al., 1994), while CS-E and oversulfated DS also promote neurite outgrowth of hippocampal neurons (Hikino et al., 2003). The CS/DS hybrid epitope of phosphacan is sufficient to promote neurite outgrowth.

In summary, CSPG-associated mechanisms can modulate neuritogenesis in vitro either positively or negatively depending on the PG core protein, the substrate, the type of cells, and their stage of development. Furthermore, differentially localized inhibitory or stimulatory CS-binding molecules may be involved (Emerling and Lander, 1996; Kantor *et al.*, 2004).

2. Signal Transduction Mechanisms and Neuron Survival

CSPGs activate signal transduction pathways, which regulate the actin cytoskeleton. CSPG was found to induce a transient rise in cytosolic calcium levels in neurons (Snow *et al.*, 1994). This might contribute to the activation of protein kinase C, which mediates inhibitory activities of CSPGs (Sivasankaran *et al.*, 2004). Downstream signaling seems to involve Rho and ROCK, since inhibition of these proteins stimulates neurite growth on CSPGs (Dergham *et al.*, 2002). Moreover, the inhibitory activity of a CSPG mixture on retina ganglion cell axon growth is blocked by the application of C3 transferase, and specific inhibitors of Rho kinase (Monnier *et al.*, 2003). In agreement with the observation that the Rho signaling pathway plays a role in neuronal survival (Kobayashi *et al.*, 2004), CSPGs and even CS/DS can promote the survival of neurons (Junghans *et al.*, 1995; Kappler *et al.*, 1997).

B. Analysis of CS Chains and PG Function *In Vivo*

I. Knockout Models

Basic observations reported from CSPG deletions have been included in Table I. Most complete eliminations of brain CSPGs revealed only subtle changes. Brain development is apparently normal in mice deficient in chondroitin-6-sulfotransferase, despite of a disappearance of the CS-D (2,6-disulfated) motif (Uchimura *et al.*, 2002).

2. Effects of Chondroitinase on CNS Development

CSPGs of perineuronal nets appear to be involved in the control of synaptic plasticity. *In vivo* treatment with chondroitinase ABC was able to eliminate perineuronal nets and to reactivate ocular dominance plasticity in the adult visual cortex of rats (Pizzorusso *et al.*, 2002). In the optic chiasm, chondroitinase treatment of brain slice preparations reduced dramatically the uncrossed component that normally passes to the ipsilateral optic tract (Chung *et al.*, 2000a) and interfered with the age-related axon order in the optic tract (Leung *et al.*, 2003).

3. Effects of CS or PG Application *In Vivo*

Application of exogenous CS to the ventricular surfaces of intact retinas in organ culture induces complete inversion of retinal ganglion cell bodies and their axons within the retinal neuroepithelium, that is, both the cell body and nerve fiber layers were repolarized to the opposite side of the neuroe-pithelium (Brittis and Silver, 1994). Furthermore, CS and biglycan influence neuronal function in adult animals when injected into the nucleus basalis magnocellularis of the ventral pallidum of adult rats (Hasenöhrl *et al.*, 1995; Huston *et al.*, 2000) leading to long lasting improvements of memory and learning, even in behaviorally impaired old animals (Huston *et al.*, 2000).

C. Binding Partners of CSPGs

CSPG has been shown to interact with many different soluble and membrane-associated molecules. These interactions have been reviewed (Bandtlow and Zimmermann, 2000). Binding of a variety of growth factors and cytokines to oversulfated CS/DS has been described. Midkine and pleiotrophin interact with oversulfated CS/DS hybrid chains purified from embryonic pig brain (Bao *et al.*, 2004, 2005) and CS from hagfish notochord (CS-H) (Nandini *et al.*, 2004). FGF2, FGF10, and FGF18 interact with embryonic pig brain CS/DS (Bao *et al.*, 2004). Furthermore, FGF2, FGF10, FGF16, and FGF18 interact with CS-H (Nandini *et al.*, 2004). Glial-derived neurotrophic factor, brain-derived neurotrophic factor, VEGF165, and HB-EGF interact with CS-H (Nandini *et al.*, 2005). More-over, collapsin response mediator proteins (CRMPs) from neonatal rat brain were found to bind to CS with high affinity, and CRMP-specific antisera coprecipitated CS from brain extracts (Franken *et al.*, 2003).

V. CSPGs in CNS Diseases

A. Traumatic Lesions

After CNS injuries, the formation of scar tissue by a variety of cell types expressing multiple axon growth inhibitory molecules is thought to present a physical and molecular barrier to axon regeneration (Silver and Miller, 2004). CSPG molecules have been shown to be present in this glial scar. After transection, fibers of the adult rat postcommissural fornix sprout over short distances but fail to traverse the lesion site terminating in close vicinity to the wound. Here, CSPG labeling is confined to the immediate vicinity of the lesion site. CSPGs form a homogeneous meshwork around the wound. Regrowing fornix fibers invade and elongate within this CSPG-rich region up to the lesion site, where they terminate (Lips *et al.*, 1995). In this lesion model, upregulation of decorin and biglycan was shown (Stichel *et al.*, 1995). The rapid upregulation of decorin in astrocytes within a wide area around the lesion was followed by a massive appearance of biglycan that remained restricted to the transection site associated with sheet-like struc-tures. Similar glial scarring, which is accompanied by CSPG expression, has been reported after axotomy of the nigrostriatal tract (Moon *et al.*, 2002), after stab wounds and knife lesions of the cerebral cortex (Asher *et al.*, 2000, 2002; Matsui *et al.*, 2002; Vorisek *et al.*, 2002), after transection of the entorhinal cortex (Deller *et al.*, 2000; Haas *et al.*, 1999; Thon *et al.*, 2000), and after lesions of the spinal cord (Camand *et al.*, 2004; Inman and Steward, 2003; Jones *et al.*, 2002, 2003a,b; Lemons *et al.*, 1999; Tang *et al.*, 2003). In none of these central lesion models, an effective regeneration of lesioned fiber tracts has been observed. Local treatment of the lesion zones with chondroitinase ABC promoted the regeneration of neurites in the spinal cord (Bradbury *et al.*, 2002; Caggiano *et al.*, 2005; Yick *et al.*, 2003, 2004). However, it should not be neglected that treatment with chondroitinase ABC leads to the formation of disaccharide fragments, which can exert neurotrophic effects that may contribute to the positive effects on neurite growth *in vivo* (Rolls *et al.*, 2004). In a different approach, targeting the mRNA of xylosyltransferase-1 reduces specifically GAG chains. Applied to the injured spinal cord, a strong reduction of the GAG chains in the lesion zone allowed axons to regenerate around the core of the lesion (Grimpe and Silver, 2004). Thus, CS moieties are necessary parts of structures, which inhibit axon regeneration after spinal core lesions. Different CSPG-binding molecules may contribute to the inhibitory properties of parts of the glial scar toward central neurites (Emerling and Lander, 1996).

Consequences of CSPG-associated inhibitory mechanisms are the activation of protein kinase C isoforms, and Rho and ROCK (Sivasankaran *et al.*, 2004). Thus, treatment with a PKC inhibitor, Go6976 (Sivasankaran *et al.*, 2004), C3 transferase to inactivate Rho, or Y27632 to inhibit ROCK stimulated axon regeneration and functional recovery after spinal cord injury (Dergham *et al.*, 2002).

B. Degenerative, Inflammatory, and Epileptic Lesions

In Alzheimer's disease, DS and CS localize to the characteristic lesions (i.e., senile/neuritic plaques, cerebrovascular amyloid deposits, and neurofibrillary tangles) (Snow *et al.*, 1992), and CS-A and DS were shown to be potent enhancers of amyloid fibrillogenesis (Castillo *et al.*, 1999).

In the autoimmune disease, multiple sclerosis glial scar tissue consists in active lesions of a central plaque region surrounded by a zone of reactive astrocytes at its edge, which is prominently stained with a monoclonal antibody against DSPG, 3-B-3 (Sobel and Ahmed, 2001), versican, aggrecan, and neurocan. On the other hand, phosphacan was distributed more uniformly (Sobel and Ahmed, 2001) and the phosphacan/PTPbeta mRNA was found to be expressed at high levels in cells with oligodendrocyte morphology (Harroch *et al.*, 2002).

In epilepsy, alterations in the occurrence of CSPGs were observed. In mesial temporal lobe epilepsy, markedly increased CS levels have been observed in dissected tissue and cerebrospinal fluid (Perosa *et al.*, 2002a, b). An increase of CS could be observed also in animal experiments after the occurrence of seizures in models of pilocarpine (Naffah-Mazzacoratti *et al.*, 1999) and domoate (Heck *et al.*, 2004) induced epileptic states.

VI. Conclusions

Chondroitin and low-sulfated CS are very likely rather unsocial molecules, which create a noninterfering or only weakly interacting, quasi-isolating environment. An important prerequisite for any complex wiring system is certainly a sufficient isolation and segregation of connections from each other. Few molecules have been identified which bind specifically to low or medium sulfated CS chains, and these represent the vast majority of CS chains in the brain. However, low and medium sulfated CS can display a considerable heterogeneity. Epimerization gives rise to DS, and alterations in sulfation give rise to chondroitin, CS-A, and CS-C. Unless molecules have been identified, which bind under physiological conditions to at least a significant subfraction, low or medium sulfated CS chains could be considered as molecules mainly designed to be repellent, which renders them bad substrates for attachment and migration in two-dimensional *in vitro* assay systems. Fortunately, the central nervous system is not a two-dimensional environment.

Oversulfated CS/DS motifs have been isolated from developing brain (Bao *et al.*, 2004, 2005; Zou *et al.*, 2003), which are able to interact with a variety of different cytokines with high affinities and may modulate the activity of these cytokines.

The effects of CS moieties critically depend on their context, which is specified to a major extent by the core proteins to which they are attached. A major function of core proteins is probably to determine the distribution of CS chains by immobilizing them specifically to the appropriate positions. Attached to specific PG core proteins, oversulfated CS/DS moieties could be strategically localized, modulating diffusion gradients, and neurotrophic signaling of growth factors.

Taken together, the heterogeneity of CS structures and of core proteins makes CSPGs versatile molecules, which are able to act both as barrier molecules and "master regulators of molecular encounter" (Lander, 1998). The interesting effects observed after alteration of CSPG function with the CS-degrading enzymes in CNS lesion models will stimulate the pharmacological interest in these molecules in the future.

References

Ameye, L., and Young, M. F. (2002). Mice deficient in small leucine-rich proteoglycans: Novel *in vivo* models for osteoporosis, osteoarthritis, Ehlers-Danlos syndrome, muscular dystrophy, and corneal diseases. *Glycobiology* **12**, 107R–116R.

Asher, R. A., Morgenstern, D. A., Fidler, P. S., Adcock, K. H., Oohira, A., Braistead, J. E., Levine, J. M., Margolis, R. U., Rogers, J. H., and Fawcett, J. W. (2000). Neurocan is upregulated in injured brain and in cytokine-treated astrocytes. *J. Neurosci.* **20**, 2427–2438.

Asher, R. A., Morgenstern, D. A., Shearer, M. C., Adcock, K. H., Pesheva, P., and Fawcett, J. W. (2002). Versican is upregulated in CNS injury and is a product of oligodendrocyte lineage cells. *J. Neurosci.* **22**, 2225–2236.

Atoji, Y., Yamamoto, Y., and Suzuki, Y. (1995). The presence of chondroitin sulfate A and C within axon terminals in the superior olivary nuclei of the adult dog. *Neurosci Lett.* **189**, 39–42.

Atoji, Y., Yamamoto, Y., Suzuki, Y., Matsui, F., and Oohira, A. (1997). Immunohistochemical localization of neurocan in the lower auditory nuclei of the dog. *Hear. Res.* **110**, 200–208.

Bandtlow, C. E., and Zimmermann, D. R. (2000). Proteoglycans in the developing brain: New conceptual insights for old proteins. *Physiol. Rev.* **80**, 1267–1290.

Bao, X., Nishimura, S., Mikami, T., Yamada, S., Itoh, N., and Sugahara, K. (2004). Chondroitin sulfate/dermatan sulfate hybrid chains from embryonic pig brain, which contain a higher proportion of L-iduronic acid than those from adult pig brain, exhibit neuritogenic and growth factor binding activities. *J. Biol. Chem.* **279**, 9765–9776.

Bao, X., Mikami, T., Yamada, S., Faissner, A., Muramatsu, T., and Sugahara, K. (2005). Heparin-binding growth factor, pleiotrophin, mediates neuritogenic activity of embryonic pig brain-derived chondroitin sulfate/dermatan sulfate hybrid chains. *J. Biol. Chem.* **280**, 9180–9191.

Bekku, Y., Su, W. D., Hirakawa, S., Fässler, R., Ohtsuka, A., Kang, J. S., Sanders, J., Murakami, T., Ninomiya, Y., and Oohashi, T. (2003). Molecular cloning of Bral2, a novel brain-specific link protein, and immunohistochemical colocalization with brevican in perineuronal nets. *Mol. Cell Neurosci.* **24**, 148–159.

Bradbury, E. J., Moon, L. D., Popat, R. J., King, V. R., Bennett, G. S., Patel, P. N., Fawcett, J. W., and McMahon, S. B. (2002). Chondroitinase ABC promotes functional recovery after spinal cord injury. *Nature* **416**, 636–640.

Brakebusch, C., Seidenbecher, C. I., Asztely, F., Rauch, U., Matthies, H., Meyer, H., Krug, M., Bockers, T. M., Zhou, X., Kreutz, M. R., Montag, D., Gundelfinger, E. D., *et al.* (2002). Brevican-deficient mice display impaired hippocampal CA1 long-term potentiation but show no obvious deficits in learning and memory. *Mol. Cell Biol.* **22**, 7417–7427.

Brittis, P. A., and Silver, J. (1994). Exogenous glycosaminoglycans induce complete inversion of retinal ganglion cell bodies and their axons within the retinal neuroepithelium. *Proc. Natl. Acad. Sci. USA* **91**, 7539–7542.

Burkart, T., and Wiesmann, U. N. (1987). Sulfated glycosaminoglycans (GAG) in the developing mouse brain. Quantitative aspects on the metabolism of total and individual sulfated GAG *in vivo. Dev. Biol.* **120**, 447–456.

Caggiano, A. O., Zimber, M. P., Ganguly, A., Blight, A. R., and Gruskin, E. A. (2005). Chondroitinase ABCI improves locomotion and bladder function following contusion injury of the rat spinal cord. *J. Neurotrauma* **22**, 226–239.

Camand, E., Morel, M. P., Faissner, A., Sotelo, C., and Dusart, I. (2004). Long-term changes in the molecular composition of the glial scar and progressive increase of serotoninergic fibre sprouting after hemisection of the mouse spinal cord. *Eur. J. Neurosci.* **20**, 1161–1176.

Castillo, G. M., Lukito, W., Wight, T. N., and Snow, A. D. (1999). The sulfate moieties of glycosaminoglycans are critical for the enhancement of beta-amyloid protein fibril formation. *J. Neurochem.* **72**, 1681–1687.

Celio, M. R., and Blümcke, I. (1994). Perineuronal nets: A specialized form of extracellular matrix in the adult nervous system. *Brain Res. Brain Res. Rev.* **19**, 128–145.

Chung, K. Y., Taylor, J. S., Shum, D. K., and Chan, S. O. (2000a). Axon routing at the optic chiasm after enzymatic removal of chondroitin sulfate in mouse embryos. *Development* **127**, 2673–2683.

Chung, K. Y., Shum, D. K., and Chan, S. O. (2000b). Expression of chondroitin sulfate proteoglycans in the chiasm of mouse embryos. *J. Comp. Neurol.* **417**, 153–163.

Clarris, H. J., Rauch, U., and Key, B. (2000). Dynamic spatiotemporal expression patterns of neurocan and phosphacan indicate diverse roles in the developing and adult mouse olfactory system. *J. Comp. Neurol.* **423**, 99–111.

Coster, L., Malmstrom, A., Sjoberg, I., and Fransson, L. (1975). The co-polymeric structure of pig skin dermatan sulphate: Distribution of L-iduronic acid sulphate residues in co-polymeric chains. *Biochem. J.* **145**, 379–389.

Deller, T., Haas, C. A., and Frotscher, M. (2000). Reorganization of the rat fascia dentata after a unilateral entorhinal cortex lesion. Role of the extracellular matrix. *Ann. N.Y. Acad. Sci.* **911**, 207–220.

Dergham, P., Ellezam, B., Essagian, C., Avedissian, H., Lubell, W. D., and McKerracher, L. (2002). Rho signaling pathway targeted to promote spinal cord repair. *J. Neurosci.* **22**, 6570–6577.

Edgell, C. J., BaSalamah, M. A., and Marr, H. S. (2004). Testican-1: A differentially expressed proteoglycan with protease inhibiting activities. *Int. Rev. Cytol.* **236**, 101–122.

Emerling, D. E., and Lander, A. D. (1996). Inhibitors and promoters of thalamic neuron adhesion and outgrowth in embryonic neocortex: Functional association with chondroitin sulfate. *Neuron* **17**, 1089–1100.

Fernaud-Espinosa, I., Nieto-Sampedro, M., and Bovolenta, P. (1994). Differential effects of glycosaminoglycans on neurite outgrowth from hippocampal and thalamic neurones. *J. Cell Sci.* **107**, 1437–1448.

Flaccus, A., Janetzko, A., Tekotte, H., Margolis, R. K., and Margolis, R. U. (1991). Immunocytochemical localization of chondroitin and chondroitin 4- and 6-sulfates in developing rat cerebellum. *J. Neurochem.* **56**, 1608–1615.

Franken, S., Junghans, U., Rosslenbroich, V., Baader, S. L., Hoffmann, R., Gieselmann, V., Viebahn, C., and Kappler, J. (2003). Collapsin response mediator proteins of neonatal rat brain interact with chondroitin sulfate. *J. Biol. Chem.* **278**, 3241–3250.

Grako, K. A., Ochiya, T., Barritt, D., Nishiyama, A., and Stallcup, W. B. (1999). PDGF (alpha)-receptor is unresponsive to PDGF-AA in aortic smooth muscle cells from the NG2 knockout mouse. *J. Cell Sci.* **112**, 905–915.

Grimpe, B., and Silver, J. (2004). A novel DNA enzyme reduces glycosaminoglycan chains in the glial scar and allows microtransplanted dorsal root ganglia axons to regenerate beyond lesions in the spinal cord. *J. Neurosci.* **24**, 1393–1397.

Haas, C. A., Rauch, U., Thon, N., Merten, T., and Deller, T. (1999). Entorhinal cortex lesion in adult rats induces the expression of the neuronal chondroitin sulfate proteoglycan neurocan in reactive astrocytes. *J. Neurosci.* **19**, 9953–9963.

Harroch, S., Furtado, G. C., Brueck, W., Rosenbluth, J., Lafaille, J., Chao, M., Buxbaum, J. D., and Schlessinger, J. (2002). A critical role for the protein tyrosine phosphatase receptor type Z in functional recovery from demyelinating lesions. *Nat. Genet.* **32**, 411–414.

Hasenöhrl, R. U., Frisch, C., Junghans, U., Muller, H. W., and Huston, J. P. (1995). Facilitation of learning following injection of the chondroitin sulfate proteoglycan biglycan into the vicinity of the nucleus basalis magnocellularis. *Behav. Brain Res.* **70**, 59–67.

Heck, N., Garwood, J., Loeffler, J. P., Larmet, Y., and Faissner, A. (2004). Differential upregulation of extracellular matrix molecules associated with the appearance of granule cell dispersion and mossy fiber sprouting during epileptogenesis in a murine model of temporal lobe epilepsy. *Neuroscience* **129**, 309–324.

Hikino, M., Mikami, T., Faissner, A., Vilela-Silva, A. C., Pavao, M. S., and Sugahara, K. (2003). Oversulfated dermatan sulfate exhibits neurite outgrowth-promoting activity toward embryonic mouse hippocampal neurons: Implications of dermatan sulfate in neuritogenesis in the brain. *J. Biol. Chem.* **278**, 43744–43754.

Huston, J. P., Weth, K., De Souza Silva, A., Junghans, U., Müller, H. W., and Hasenöhrl, R. U. (2000). Facilitation of learning and long-term ventral pallidal-cortical cholinergic activation by proteoglycan biglycan and chondroitin sulfate C. *Neuroscience* **100**, 355–361.

Inman, D. M., and Steward, O. (2003). Ascending sensory, but not other long-tract axons, regenerate into the connective tissue matrix that forms at the site of a spinal cord injury in mice. *J. Comp. Neurol.* **462**, 431–449.

Jones, L. L., Margolis, R. U., and Tuszynski, M. H. (2003a). The chondroitin sulfate proteoglycans neurocan, brevican, phosphacan, and versican are differentially regulated following spinal cord injury. *Exp. Neurol.* **182**, 399–411.

Jones, L. L., Sajed, D., and Tuszynski, M. H. (2003b). Axonal regeneration through regions of chondroitin sulfate proteoglycan deposition after spinal cord injury: A balance of permissiveness and inhibition. *J. Neurosci.* **23**, 9276–9288.

Jones, L. L., Yamaguchi, Y., Stallcup, W. B., and Tuszynski, M. H. (2002). NG2 is a major chondroitin sulfate proteoglycan produced after spinal cord injury and is expressed by macrophages and oligodendrocyte progenitors. *J. Neurosci.* **22**, 2792–2803.

Junghans, U., Koops, A., Westmeyer, A., Kappler, J., Meyer, H. E., and Müller, H. W. (1995). Purification of a meningeal cell-derived chondroitin sulphate proteoglycan with neurotrophic activity for brain neurons and its identification as biglycan. *Eur. J. Neurosci.* **7**, 2341–2350.

Kantor, D. B., Chivatakarn, O., Peer, K. L., Oster, S. F., Inatani, M., Hansen, M. J., Flanagan, J. G., Yamaguchi, Y., Sretavan, D. W., Giger, R. J., and Kolodkin, A. L. (2004). Semaphorin 5A is a bifunctional axon guidance cue regulated by heparan and chondroitin sulfate proteoglycans. *Neuron* **44**, 961–975.

Kappler, J., Junghans, U., Koops, A., Stichel, C. C., Hausser, H. J., Kresse, H., and Müller, H. W. (1997). Chondroitin/dermatan sulphate promotes the survival of neurons from rat embryonic neocortex. *Eur. J. Neurosci.* **9**, 306–318.

Kappler, J., Stichel, C. C., Gleichmann, M., Gillen, C., Junghans, U., Kresse, H., and Müller, H. W. (1998). Developmental regulation of decorin expression in postnatal rat brain. *Brain Res.* **793**, 328–332.

Katoh-Semba, R., Matsuda, M., Watanabe, E., Maeda, N., and Oohira, A. (1998). Two types of brain chondroitin sulfate proteoglycan: Their distribution and possible functions in the rat embryo. *Neurosci. Res.* **31**, 273–282.

Kitagawa, H., Tsutsumi, K., Tone, Y., and Sugahara, K. (1997). Developmental regulation of the sulfation profile of chondroitin sulfate chains in the chicken embryo brain. *J. Biol. Chem.* **272**, 31377–31381.

Kobayashi, K., Takahashi, M., Matsushita, N., Miyazaki, J., Koike, M., Yaginuma, H., Osumi, N., Kaibuchi, K., and Kobayashi, K. (2004). Survival of developing motor neurons mediated by Rho GTPase signaling pathway through Rho-kinase. *J. Neurosci.* **24**, 3480–3488.

Lafont, F., Rouget, M., Triller, A., Prochiantz, A., and Rousselet, A. (1992). *In vitro* control of neuronal polarity by glycosaminoglycans. *Development* **114**, 17–29.

Lafont, F., Prochiantz, A., Valenza, C., Petitou, M., Pascal, M., Rouget, M., and Rousselet, A. (1994). Defined glycosaminoglycan motifs have opposite effects on neuronal polarity *in vitro*. *Dev. Biol.* **165**, 453–468.

Lemons, M. L., Howland, D. R., and Anderson, D. K. (1999). Chondroitin sulfate proteoglycan immunoreactivity increases following spinal cord injury and transplantation. *Exp. Neurol.* **160**, 51–65.

Lander, A. D. (1998). Proteoglycans: Master regulators of molecular encounter? *Matrix Biol.* **17**, 465–472.

Leung, K. M., Taylor, J. S., and Chan, S. O. (2003). Enzymatic removal of chondroitin sulphates abolishes the age-related axon order in the optic tract of mouse embryos. *Eur. J. Neurosci.* **17**, 1755–1767.

Leung, K. M., Margolis, R. U., and Chan, S. O. (2004). Expression of phosphacan and neurocan during early development of mouse retinofugal pathway. *Brain Res. Dev. Brain Res.* **152**, 1–10.

Lips, K., Stichel, C. C., and Müller, H. W. (1995). Restricted appearance of tenascin and chondroitin sulphate proteoglycans after transection and sprouting of adult rat postcommissural fornix. *J. Neurocytol.* **24**, 449–464.

Maeda, N., He, J., Yajima, Y., Mikami, T., Sugahara, K., and Yabe, T. (2003). Heterogeneity of the chondroitin sulfate portion of phosphacan/6B4 proteoglycan regulates its binding affinity for pleiotrophin/heparin binding growth-associated molecule. *J. Biol. Chem.* **278**, 35805–35811.

Margolis, R. K., Margolis, R. U., Preti, C., and Lai, D. (1975a). Distribution and metabolism of glycoproteins and glycosaminoglycans in subcellular fractions of brain. *Biochemistry* **14**, 4797–4804.

Margolis, R. U., Margolis, R. K., Chang, L. B., and Preti, C. (1975b). Glycosaminoglycans of brain during development. *Biochemistry* **14**, 85–88.

Matsui, F., Kawashima, S., Shuo, T., Yamauchi, S., Tokita, Y., Aono, S., Keino, H., and Oohira, A. (2002). Transient expression of juvenile-type neurocan by reactive astrocytes in adult rat brains injured by kainate-induced seizures as well as surgical incision. *Neuroscience* **112**, 773–781.

Matthews, R. T., Kelly, G. M., Zerillo, C. A., Gray, G., Tiemeyer, M., and Hockfield, S. (2002). Aggrecan glycoforms contribute to the molecular heterogeneity of perineuronal nets. *J. Neurosci.* **22**, 7536–7547.

Meyer-Puttlitz, B., Junker, E., Margolis, R. U., and Margolis, R. K. (1996). Chondroitin sulfate proteoglycans in the developing central nervous system. II. Immunocytochemical localization of neurocan and phosphacan. *J. Comp. Neurol.* **366**, 44–54.

Miller, B., Sheppard, A. M., Bicknese, A. R., and Pearlman, A. L. (1995). Chondroitin sulfate proteoglycans in the developing cerebral cortex: The distribution of neurocan distinguishes forming afferent and efferent axonal pathways. *J. Comp. Neurol.* **355**, 615–628.

Mjaatvedt, C. H., Yamamura, H., Capehart, A. A., Turner, D., and Markwald, R. R. (1998). The Cspg2 gene, disrupted in the hdf mutant, is required for right cardiac chamber and endocardial cushion formation. *Dev. Biol.* **202**, 56–66.

Monnier, P. P., Sierra, A., Schwab, J. M., Henke-Fahle, S., and Mueller, B. K. (2003). The Rho/ROCK pathway mediates neurite growth-inhibitory activity associated with the chondroitin sulfate proteoglycans of the CNS glial scar. *Mol. Cell Neurosci.* **22**, 319–330.

Moon, L. D., Asher, R. A., Rhodes, K. E., and Fawcett, J. W. (2002). Relationship between sprouting axons, proteoglycans and glial cells following unilateral nigrostriatal axotomy in the adult rat. *Neuroscience* **109**, 101–117.

Morawski, M., Bruckner, M. K., Riederer, P., Bruckner, G., and Arendt, T. (2004). Perineuronal nets potentially protect against oxidative stress. *Exp. Neurol.* **188**, 309–315.

Murakami, T., and Ohtsuka, A. (2003). Perisynaptic barrier of proteoglycans in the mature brain and spinal cord. *Arch. Histol. Cytol.* **66**, 195–207.

Naffah-Mazzacoratti, M. G., Arganaraz, G. A., Porcionatto, M. A., Scorza, F. A., Amado, D., Silva, R., Bellissimo, M. I., Nader, H. B., and Cavalheiro, E. A. (1999). Selective alterations of glycosaminoglycans synthesis and proteoglycan expression in rat cortex and hippocampus in pilocarpine-induced epilepsy. *Brain Res. Bull.* **50**, 229–239.

Nandini, C. D., Itoh, N., and Sugahara, K. (2005). Novel 70-kDa chondroitin sulfate/dermatan sulfate hybrid chains with a unique heterogeneous sulfation pattern from shark skin, which exhibit neuritogenic activity and binding activities for growth factors and neurotrophic factors. *J. Biol. Chem.* **280**, 4058–4069.

Nandini, C. D., Mikami, T., Ohta, M., Itoh, N., Akiyama-Nambu, F., and Sugahara, K. (2004). Structural and functional characterization of oversulfated chondroitin sulfate/dermatan sulfate hybrid chains from the notochord of hagfish. Neuritogenic and binding activities for growth factors and neurotrophic factors. *J. Biol. Chem.* **279**, 50799–50809.

Perosa, S. R., Porcionatto, M. A., Cukiert, A., Martins, J. R., Amado, D., Nader, H. B., Cavalheiro, E. A., Leite, J. P., and Naffah-Mazzacoratti, M. G. (2002a). Extracellular matrix components are altered in the hippocampus, cortex, and cerebrospinal fluid of patients with mesial temporal lobe epilepsy. *Epilepsia* **43**(Suppl 5), 159–161.

Perosa, S. R., Porcionatto, M. A., Cukiert, A., Martins, J. R., Passeroti, C. C., Amado, D., Matas, S. L., Nader, H. B., Cavalheiro, E. A., Leite, J. P., and Naffah-Mazzacoratti, M. G. (2002b). Glycosaminoglycan levels and proteoglycan expression are altered in the hippocampus of patients with mesial temporal lobe epilepsy. *Brain Res. Bull.* **58**, 509–516.

Pizzorusso, T., Medini, P., Berardi, N., Chierzi, S., Fawcett, J. W., and Maffei, L. (2002). Reactivation of ocular dominance plasticity in the adult visual cortex. *Science* **298**, 1248–1251.

Probstmeier, R., Stichel, C. C., Müller, H. W., Asou, H., and Pesheva, P. (2000). Chondroitin sulfates expressed on oligodendrocyte-derived tenascin-R are involved in neural cell recognition. Functional implications during CNS development and regeneration. *J. Neurosci. Res.* **60**, 21–36.

Properzi, F., Carulli, D., Asher, R. A., Muir, E., Camargo, L. M., van Kuppevelt, T. H., ten Dam, G. B., Furukawa, Y., Mikami, T., Sugahara, K., Toida, T., Geller, H. M., and Fawcett, J. W. (2005). Chondroitin 6-sulphate synthesis is up-regulated in injured CNS, induced by injury-related cytokines and enhanced in axon-growth inhibitory glia. *Eur. J. Neurosci.* **21**, 378–390.

Rauch, U., Glössl, J., and Kresse, H. (1986). Comparison of small proteoglycans from skin fibroblasts and vascular smooth-muscle cells. *Biochem. J.* **238**, 465–474.

Rauch, U., Gao, P., Janetzko, A., Flaccus, A., Hilgenberg, L., Tekotte, H., Margolis, R. K., and Margolis, R. U. (1991). Isolation and characterization of developmentally regulated chondroitin sulfate and chondroitin/keratan sulfate proteoglycans of brain identified with monoclonal antibodies. *J. Biol. Chem.* **266**, 14785–14801.

Rauch, U., Hirakawa, S., Oohashi, T., Kappler, J., and Roos, G. (2004). Cartilage link protein interacts with neurocan, which shows hyaluronan binding characteristics different from CD44 and TSG-6. *Matrix Biol.* **22**, 629–639.

Rolls, A., Avidan, H., Cahalon, L., Schori, H., Bakalash, S., Litvak, V., Lev, S., Lider, O., and Schwartz, M. (2004). A disaccharide derived from chondroitin sulphate proteoglycan promotes central nervous system repair in rats and mice. *Eur. J. Neurosci.* **20**, 1973–1983.

Salinero, O., Moreno-Flores, M. T., and Wandosell, F. (2000). Increasing neurite outgrowth capacity of beta-amyloid precursor protein proteoglycan in Alzheimer's disease. *J. Neurosci. Res.* **60**, 87–97.

Sasaki, T., Mann, K., and Timpl, R. (2001). Modification of the laminin alpha 4 chain by chondroitin sulfate attachment to its N-terminal domain. *FEBS Lett.* **505**, 173–178.

Sasaki, T., Mann, K., Miner, J. H., Miosge, N., and Timpl, R. (2002). Domain IV of mouse laminin beta1 and beta2 chains. *Eur. J. Biochem.* **269**, 431–442.

Schnepp, A., Komp Lindgren, P., Hulsmann, H., Kroger, S., Paulsson, M., and Hartmann, U. (2005). Mouse testican-2: Expression, glycosylation and effects on neurite outgrowth. *J. Biol. Chem.* **280,** 11274–11280.

Shuo, T., Aono, S., Matsui, F., Tokita, Y., Maeda, H., Shimada, K., and Oohira, A. (2004). Developmental changes in the biochemical and immunological characters of the carbohydrate moiety of neuroglycan C, a brain-specific chondroitin sulfate proteoglycan. *Glycoconj. J.* **20,** 267–278.

Silver, J., and Miller, J. H. (2004). Regeneration beyond the glial scar. *Nat. Rev. Neurosci.* **5,** 146–156.

Sivasankaran, R., Pei, J., Wang, K. C., Zhang, Y. P., Shields, C. B., Xu, X. M., and He, Z. (2004). PKC mediates inhibitory effects of myelin and chondroitin sulfate proteoglycans on axonal regeneration. *Nat. Neurosci.* **7,** 261–268.

Snow, A. D., Mar, H., Nochlin, D., Kresse, H., and Wight, T. N. (1992). Peripheral distribution of dermatan sulfate proteoglycans (decorin) in amyloid-containing plaques and their presence in neurofibrillary tangles of Alzheimer's disease. *J. Histochem. Cytochem.* **40,** 105–113.

Snow, D. M., Atkinson, P. B., Hassinger, T. D., Letourneau, P. C., and Kater, S. B. (1994). Chondroitin sulfate proteoglycan elevates cytoplasmic calcium in DRG neurons. *Dev. Biol.* **166,** 87–100.

Sobel, R. A., and Ahmed, A. S. (2001). White matter extracellular matrix chondroitin sulfate/dermatan sulfate proteoglycans in multiple sclerosis. *J. Neuropathol. Exp. Neurol.* **60,** 1198–1207.

Stichel, C. C., Kappler, J., Junghans, U., Koops, A., Kresse, H., and Muller, H. W. (1995). Differential expression of the small chondroitin/dermatan sulfate proteoglycans decorin and biglycan after injury of the adult rat brain. *Brain Res.* **704,** 263–274.

Sykova, E. (2001). Glial diffusion barriers during aging and pathological states. *Prog. Brain Res.* **132,** 339–363.

Tang, X., Davies, J. E., and Davies, S. J. (2003). Changes in distribution, cell associations, and protein expression levels of NG2, neurocan, phosphacan, brevican, versican V2, and tenascin-C during acute to chronic maturation of spinal cord scar tissue. *J. Neurosci. Res.* **71,** 427–444.

Thon, N., Haas, C. A., Rauch, U., Merten, T., Fässler, R., Frotscher, M., and Deller, T. (2000). The chondroitin sulphate proteoglycan brevican is upregulated by astrocytes after entorhinal cortex lesions in adult rats. *Eur. J. Neurosci.* **12,** 2547–2558.

Tsuchida, K., Shioi, J., Yamada, S., Boghosian, G., Wu, A., Cai, H., Sugahara, K., and Robakis, N. K. (2001). Appican, the proteoglycan form of the amyloid precursor protein, contains chondroitin sulfate E in the repeating disaccharide region and 4-O-sulfated galactose in the linkage region. *J. Biol. Chem.* **276,** 37155–37160.

Uchimura, K., Kadomatsu, K., Nishimura, H., Muramatsu, H., Nakamura, E., Kurosawa, N., Habuchi, O., El-Fasakhany, F. M., Yoshikai, Y., and Muramatsu, T. (2002). Functional analysis of the chondroitin 6-sulfotransferase gene in relation to lymphocyte subpopulations, brain development, and oversulfated chondroitin sulfates. *J. Biol. Chem.* **277,** 1443–1450.

Ughrin, Y. M., Chen, Z. J., and Levine, J. M. (2003). Multiple regions of the NG2 proteoglycan inhibit neurite growth and induce growth cone collapse. *J. Neurosci.* **23,** 175–186.

von-Koch, C. S., Zheng, H., Chen, H., Trumbauer, M., Thinakaran, G., van der Ploeg, L. H., Price, D. L., and Sisodia, S. S. (1997). Generation of APLP2 KO mice and early postnatal lethality in APLP2/APP double KO mice. *Neurobiol. Aging* **18,** 661–669.

Vorisek, I., Hajek, M., Tintera, J., Nicolay, K., and Sykova, E. (2002). Water ADC, extracellular space volume, and tortuosity in the rat cortex after traumatic injury. *Magn. Reson. Med.* **48,** 994–1003.

Watanabe, H., Kimata, K., Line, S., Strong, D., Gao, L. Y., Kozak, C. A., and Yamada, Y. (1994). Mouse cartilage matrix deficiency (cmd) caused by a 7 bp deletion in the aggrecan gene. *Nat. Genet.* **7**, 154–157.

Yick, L. W., Cheung, P. T., So, K. F., and Wu, W. (2003). Axonal regeneration of Clarke's neurons beyond the spinal cord injury scar after treatment with chondroitinase ABC. *Exp. Neurol.* **182**, 160–168.

Yick, L. W., So, K. F., Cheung, P. T., and Wu, W. T. (2004). Lithium chloride reinforces the regeneration-promoting effect of chondroitinase ABC on rubrospinal neurons after spinal cord injury. *J. Neurotrauma* **21**, 932–943.

Zheng, H., Jiang, M., Trumbauer, M. E., Sirinathsinghji, D. J., Hopkins, R., Smith, D. W., Heavens, R. P., Dawson, G. R., Boyce, S., Conner, M. W., Stevens, K. A., Slunt, H. H., *et al.* (1995). Beta-amyloid precursor protein-deficient mice show reactive gliosis and decreased locomotor activity. *Cell* **81**, 525–531.

Zhou, X. H., Brakebusch, C., Matthies, H., Oohashi, T., Hirsch, E., Moser, M., Krug, M., Seidenbecher, C. I., Boeckers, T. M., Rauch, U., Buettner, R., Gundelfinger, E. D., *et al.* (2001). Neurocan is dispensable for brain development. *Mol. Cell Biol.* **21**, 5970–5978.

Zou, P., Zou, K., Muramatsu, H., Ichihara-Tanaka, K., Habuchi, O., Ohtake, S., Ikematsu, S., Sakuma, S., and Muramatsu, T. (2003). Glycosaminoglycan structures required for strong binding to midkine, a heparin-binding growth factor. *Glycobiology* **13**, 35–42.

Asya Rolls and Michal Schwartz

Department of Neurobiology
The Weizmann Institute of Science
76100 Rehovot, Israel

Chondroitin Sulfate Proteoglycan and its Degradation Products in CNS Repair

I. Chapter Overview

Increased levels of chondroitin sulfate proteoglycan (CSPG) character-ize responses to various types of tissue injury both in the periphery and in the central nervous system (CNS). In the periphery, CSPG secretion following insult has been associated with the repair process, while in the CNS, it is mainly thought to inhibit regeneration. Central nervous system repair is a highly complicated process; neural tissue has low tolerance to any deviation from homeostasis, and it is characterized with intensive perpetuating tissue damage. Despite its reputation as an inhibitor of CNS recovery, several recent studies suggested that CSPG might have beneficial features in the context of the injured CNS. For example, CSPG promotes neuronal survival

In the memory of Prof. Ofer Lider, a man who loved life, science, and the matrix between them.

Advances in Pharmacology, Volume 53
Copyright 2006, Elsevier Inc. All rights reserved.
1054-3589/06 $35.00
DOI: 10.1016/S1054-3589(05)53017-5

and seals the injury site, thereby blocking the leakage of neurotoxic compounds from the damaged site to the healthy neighboring tissue. Additionally, CSPG spatially restricts the immune response to the injured loci by promoting the adhesion of immune cells and binding of relevant cytokines. Moreover, the degradation products of CSPG (i.e., CSPG-derived disaccharides) were also demonstrated to be highly effective in promoting axonal growth, microglial activation, and controlling T-cell functions. Thus, these CSPG-degradation products are not wasteful derivatives of an unneeded molecule but rather carry great therapeutic potential. The variety of the features characterizing CSPG in the context of CNS might indicate that the crucial factor leading to the adverse effect of CSPG is not its mere presence but rather an outcome caused by the lack of synchrony between its degradation and the requirements of the tissue in the process of repair. Revisiting the therapeutic potential of CSPG and its degradation products might lead to a better understanding of the endogenous repair mechanisms and potential pharmacological applications related to this molecule.

II. Introduction

Proteoglycans (PGs) are a diverse group of molecules composed of repeated disaccharide glycosaminoglycan (GAG) chains, linked to a central core protein. PGs are defined by both their core protein and their carbohydrate constituents. CSPG is the major type of PG expressed in the CNS, and the mammalian brain contains many different types of CSPGs. During development, CSPG exhibits a complex pattern of expression: generally, regions with very high CSPG expression are confined to barrier zones that are refractory to axon growth (Brittis et al., 1992; Snow et al., 1991; Steindler et al., 1990), although some types of CSPGs (e.g., phosphacan) are expressed along fiber pathways and in regions where axon growth occurs (Maeda and Noda, 1996; Maeda et al., 1992; Oohira et al., 1994). CSPGs are therefore considered to be neural-growth modulators having selective repulsive activities on subsets of neurons, restricting their growth at specific locations (Maeda and Noda, 1996; Oohira et al., 1994).

CNS injury commonly results in devastating tissue damage and is characterized by poor regenerative capacity. One of the major characteristics of the injured CNS tissue is the significant increase in the production of CSPG (Levine, 1994; McKeon et al., 1991; Pindzola et al., 1993). The intense expression of CSPG at the injury site, along with the well-documented growth inhibitory nature of this molecule (Chen et al., 2002; Matsui and Oohira, 2004; Properzi et al., 2003), has led to the common perception of CSPG as one of the major factors leading to the phenomenon of limited CNS regeneration. Other lines of evidence indicate that CSPG has a role in inducing inflammation in the CNS (Fitch and Silver, 1997). Since the common wisdom considered immune activation in the CNS as generally destructive, this was considered as further validation to the deleterious effect of CSPG on CNS repair.

In this chapter, we will try to provide a broad view of the variety of features characterizing CSPG and examine their effects on CNS repair. Along with studies suggesting an inhibitory effect of CSPG on axonal growth, we will present other findings describing different features of CSPG, which can actually support CNS healing. We will also examine the effects of CSPG on immune activation in light of the current view of a controlled immune response as supportive of CNS repair (Kipnis and Schwartz, 2005). To complete the picture of the beneficial and destructive features of CSPG in the CNS repair process, we will also summarize recent data indicating the potential role of CSPG degradation products on CNS recovery. Finally, we will discuss the therapeutic potential of CSPG and its degradation products.

III. CSPG in Wound Healing

CSPG, as well as other PGs, are found to be prominent molecules during wound healing through their influential role in cell–cell and cell–matrix interactions. The healing process is a multifactorial reaction, which can be broadly classified into five overlapping phases including inflammation, granular tissue formation, reepithelialization, matrix production, and remodeling. In general, GAGs are overexpressed during the early stages of wound healing and return to their normal levels during the remodeling phase, although these molecules were reported to play an essential role at every stage of wound healing. Various PGs, including CSPG, play a structural role in the wound healing process; by forming cross-links between collagen and the PGs, they regulate the three-dimensional organization of collagen and tissue replantation. Moreover, the interaction between PGs and collagen provides adequate strength to the tissue, and by blocking the cleavage sites of collagen, PGs may inhibit the action of collagenase and collagen degradation (Parthiba and Gupta, 2000).

Various PGs are known to be involved in cell functions by regulating growth factor and cytokine activity (Villena and Brandan, 2004). Most of the growth factors and cytokines that are involved in wound healing are immobilized at the cell surface and in the ECM through PG binding (Ramsden and Rider, 1992; Ruoslahti and Yamaguchi, 1991). Presenting a ligand in an extracellular matrix (ECM)-binding form offers multiple advantages to cells. Tethering the ligand within a region of space inhibits ligand spreading, and creates elevated local concentration of effective molecules. Unlike soluble ligands, access to the bound compound is limited to cells within or migrating into the ECM protein-containing region. This feature is especially important with compounds that could be harmful at excessive levels such as in the case of TNF-α, which is neuroprotective in low levels, but cytotoxic when expressed at higher concentrations. In addition, tethering of such ligands at highly effective local concentration endows them with unique biochemical properties, generally boosting the natural potential of these factors. Moreover, the binding to ECM can be a means to expose cryptic determinants needed for their signaling.

Another important aspect of CSPG, as well as of other PGs, is their role in the immune response. On the one hand, various cells of the immune system, such as leukocytes and macrophages produce CSPG (Jones and Tuszynski, 2002; Makatsori et al., 2003). On the other hand, CSPG production is regulated, among other factors, by immune components such as the cytokines IL-1, IL-4, and TNF-α (Sorensson et al., 2003; Wegrowski et al., 1995). CSPG directly affects various cells of the immune system including T cell, B cells, natural killer (NK) cells, dendritic cells (DCs), macrophages and microglia in terms of cell motility, differentiation, proliferation, and cytokine secretion (Aoyama et al., 2005; Delfino et al., 1994; Garnier et al., 2003; Kwakkenbos et al., 2005; MacDermott et al., 1985; Rachmilewitz and Tykocinski, 1998; Wrenshall et al., 1999; Yang et al., 2002). Thus, for example, it was reported that CSPG promotes DCs maturation (Yang et al., 2002), induces secretion of Th1-type cytokines (IFN-γ, IL-2, and IL-12) by OVA-sensitized spleenocytes, and suppresses secretion of Th2-type cytokines (IL-5 and IL-10) from those cells (Sakai et al., 2002).

Angiogenesis is another crucial factor required for efficient repair. The formation of new blood vessels promotes recovery and supports the immune response. The role of CSPG in promoting angiogenesis (Denholm et al., 2001) supports the general line of evidences indicating that CSPG is a major player promoting the recovery process.

IV. General Aspects of CNS Repair

The CNS has limited regenerative capacity in adulthood. One of the major factors contributing to this phenomenon is the high availability of growth inhibitory molecules in the region of CNS injury. Some such factors, such as myelin debris (Domeniconi and Filbin, 2005; Fouad et al., 2001; Fournier et al., 2002; Grados-Munro and Fournier, 2003; He and Koprivica, 2004; Kastin and Fan, 2005; Teng and Tang, 2005), are a consequence of the insulted neural tissue, while others, such as CSPG, are synthesized de novo by various CNS cell types.

Additionally, the CNS is characterized by perpetuating degeneration processes, in which toxic compounds generated at the injured site cause further damage to the neurons spared from the primary insult. Among those factors are physiological compounds that exceed their normal levels such as glutamate and nitric oxide (Fig. 1).

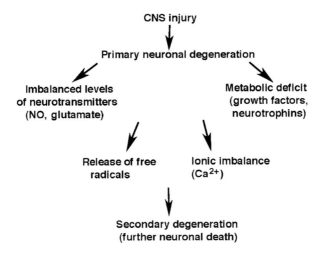

FIGURE I   Perpetuating degeneration processes in the injured CNS. The direct damage to neurons triggers a series of event resulting in additional death of neurons that were able to escape the primary insult.

Repair mechanisms (regeneration and neurogenesis) are limited in the CNS. However, almost paradoxically, the CNS has a limited source of protective mechanisms such as the immune response that is available and protective to other tissues but is highly constrained in the context of the CNS. The mechanisms used by the innate immune response, such as the secretion of nitric oxide or phagocytosis of damaged cells by microglia/macrophages, can be destructive in the CNS if not properly controlled (Fig. 2). Moreover, the CNS is actually an immune privileged site. Taken together, these observations have led to the common wisdom of viewing the interaction between the immune and the CNS as a detriment to healing. In recent years, however, studies indicate that a well-balanced immune response is crucial for CNS repair. It was shown that animals suffering from immune deficiency have reduced CNS repair capacity, and boosting the immune response has been proven to augment healing in several models of CNS injury (Kipnis *et al.*, 2001; Schori *et al.*, 2001). The immune response in the CNS is a highly complicated reaction mediated by both cells resident in the CNS, such as microglia, and other cells that infiltrate the CNS following the insult. Microglia are the local macrophages of the CNS. They act as stand-by cells in the service of both the immune and the nervous systems. In healthy CNS, these cells are quiescent, but in the event of injury to axons or cell bodies, provided that their activity is well controlled, they can be activated to buffer harmful compounds, clear debris from the damaged site, and secrete neurotrophic factors. In the absence of controlled activation, these cells acquire a destructive phenotype associated with increased

Neurotoxic effects (innate immunity)	Neuroprotective effects (adaptive immunity)
Excessive nitric oxide secretion	Neurotrophic-factor secretion
Uncontrolled phagocytosis	Debris removal
Intense TNF-alpha secretion	Antigen presentation
	Buffering toxicity
	Growth-factor secretion

FIGURE 2   The different phenotypes of activated microglia. Activated microglia result in different phenotypes depending on the type of activation/milieu. Neurotoxic features characterize the activation of these cells by microorganisms. Neuroprotective features usually characterize activation of microglia by controlled levels of IFN-γ or IL-4.

levels of TNF-α and nitric oxide secretion, accelerating the damage to the tissue. Thus, T cell-activated microglia can be protective to neural tissue via the secretion of neurotrophic factors and buffering toxicity (Butovsky *et al.*, 2005; Shaked *et al.*, 2005) (Fig. 2). In section VB , we will discuss the role of CSPG in this dialog.

V. CSPG in CNS Repair

In the CNS, CSPG is intensively secreted following injury. Major depositions of this molecule are commonly observed around the lesion site, where the glial scar forms. The glial scar contains astrocytes, oligodendrocyte precursor cells, microglia, and meningeal cells. Several of these cell types including astrocytes, microglia/macrophages, and even neurons, secrete or express CSPG on their membranes.

A. The Inhibitory Effect of CSPG on Axonal Growth

The growth inhibitory effect of CSPG on neurons has been widely discussed in the past years. In fact, CSPG inhibition is considered to be a major impediment to regeneration observed in the injured CNS. Evidence of the growth inhibitory nature of CSPG comes from various findings: the lack of axonal elongation on CSPG both *in vivo* and *in vitro* (Asher *et al.*, 2002; Dou and Levine, 1994; Friedlander *et al.*, 1994; Schmalfeldt *et al.*, 2000; Smith-Thomas *et al.*, 1994; Yamada *et al.*, 1997); the observations that enzymatic degradation of CSPG promotes axonal growth through the glial scar (Bradbury *et al.*, 2002; Chau *et al.*, 2004; McKeon *et al.*, 1991; Moon *et al.*, 2001; Tropea *et al.*, 2003; Yick *et al.*, 2000), and the physiological role of CSPG during development in creating boundaries for the growing axons.

CSPG expression is high in areas that are refractory to axonal growth such as the roof plate in the spinal cord (Snow *et al.*, 1991), the peripheral region of the retina near the pupil (Brittis *et al.*, 1992). Most of the growth inhibitory function of CSPG is mediated through its sugar chains or their core proteins. The sulfation pattern directly influences the binding properties and function of CSPGs; however, the specific sulfation pattern required for the inhibitory activity of these molecules on axon growth is yet unknown.

B. The Effects of CSPG on the Immune Response

The interaction between immune components and CSPG has far-reaching implications on the regulation of CNS repair. The classic notion, which views the immune response as merely destructive in the context of the CNS, regards the interaction between the immune components and CSPG as yet another evidence of the destructive role of CSPG. However, in light of the recent indications that CNS repair can benefit from a well-balanced immune response, a reexamination of this interaction is required. Thus, for example, our studies have suggested that when CSPG is used as a matrix, it activates microglia (Rolls *et al.*, 2004a). CSPG was also found by us to act in synergy with low levels of interferon (IFN)-γ in inducing microglia to express MHC class-II molecules and to secrete the neurotrophic factors NGF, NT4/5, and NT3. Such a synergy allows the benefit of IFN-γ activation to be augmented without the cost of inducing the killing mechanism (TNF-α, nitric oxide) (Shaked *et al.*, 2005) that is associated with higher levels of IFN-γ (Rolls *et al.*, 2004a). Moreover, we recently found a correlation *in vivo* between MHC class-II-expressing microglia/macrophages and major depositions of CSPG at the site of CNS injury (A. R. unpublished data). Other studies indicate that cultured macrophages secrete factors capable of robustly digesting PGs in an *in vitro* model of the glial scar (Horn *et al.*, 2004), possibly suggesting a regulatory interaction between CSPG and macrophages/microglia in the recovering CNS.

C. CSPG Isolates the Damaged Site

When considering the repair process in the CNS, one of the major requirements is the effective sealing of the injury site to prevent the diffusion of mediators of damage to the surrounding healthy tissue. In this regard, the production of CSPG in the margins of the lesion can be crucial due to its physical properties. Studies indicate that the diffusion rate through CSPG is significantly lower compared to other matrices. A study that examined the diffusion parameters in rat cortex following a cortical stab wound indicated that an increase in CSPG levels was associated with a decrease in the diffusion parameters, making the tissue less permissive and indicating that

CSPG deposition can impose diffusion barriers (Roitbak and Sykova, 1999; Sykova, 2001).

D. CSPG in Neural Survival

Another aspect worth noting in the context of CNS repair is the effect of CSPG on neuronal survival. Some CSPG types were shown to markedly enhance neuronal survival. For example, astrocytes synthesize and release the small CSPG molecule, biglycan, which was found to support survival of neocortical neurons *in vitro*, possibly via the activation of tyrosine kinases (Koops *et al.*, 1996). Additionally, CSPG was reported to be neuroprotective from nitric oxide-mediated death of cultured neonatal retinal ganglion cells (Nichel *et al.*, 1995). A similar neuroprotective effect of CSPG on neuronal survival was observed in beta-amyloid toxicity. The beta-amyloid peptide in its aggregated form is toxic to neurons both *in vitro* and *in vivo*. The aggregated form of a fragment of the beta 1–42 peptide, believed to be responsible for this toxicity, is able to form senile plaques. Various PGs, including CSPG, are localized throughout the senile plaques found in Alzheimer's patients. Studies indicate that both heparan sulfate proteoglycan (HSPG) and CSPG prevent neurite fragmentation and toxicity normally induced by the aggregated beta-amyloid peptide (Woods *et al.*, 1995). In other studies, intraocular injections of CS type C resulted in a significant salvage of axotomized ganglion cells (Huxlin *et al.*, 1995b). Moreover, normal brain development is associated with massive cell death programmed as part of brain establishment. *In vivo* injection of CSPG into the eyes of rat pups during the postnatal part of the period of naturally occurring ganglion cell death prevents, in a dose- and time-dependent manner, the death of a significant number of the ganglion cells that are normally lost (Huxlin *et al.*, 1995a). In the embryonic stages of rat neocortical development, CSPG are mainly located in specific brain layers. CSPG expression is maintained after birth and even extends to postnatal day 7; expression is downregulated by postnatal day 21, concomitant with the period of naturally occurring cell death. The latter observation is consistent with a putative role of CSPG in the control of neuron survival during cortical shaping and formation (Kappler *et al.*, 1997).

It therefore seems that CSPG has a very complicated role in CNS repair (Fig. 3); although it is deleterious to axonal growth, it is also beneficial in some other respects to regeneration. It might therefore be more instructive to examine the beneficial or inhibitory effect of CSPG on CNS repair not in a global way but in the context of each phase in the repair process. Thus, CSPG expression might be pivotal in the initial phases following injury for promoting neuronal survival, limiting the spread of damage and localizing the immune response; however, its presence in the latter stages might be destructive due to its inhibitory effect on regenerating axons.

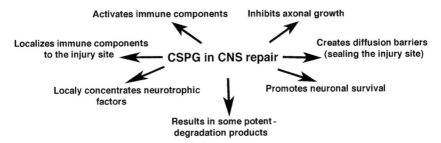

FIGURE 3 Effects of CSPG on CNS repair. CSPGs are characterized by various effects on the different aspects of CNS repair.

VI. Degradation Products

A. CSPG-Degrading Enzymes

The expression patterns of CSPG in the injured CNS are characterized by a transient increase immediately following the insult and a relative decrease in its levels about 10–14 days following injury (Jones *et al.*, 2003). Nevertheless, in some cases, the levels of CSPG remain elevated for months or even years. The specific enzymes responsible for the observed decline in CSPG levels have not been fully characterized. Broadly, GAGs can be depolymerized enzymatically either by eliminative cleavage with lyases or by hydrolytic cleavage with hydrolases. Often, these enzymes are specific for residues in the polysaccharide chain bearing certain modifications. They elicit sequence-specific interactions with the GAG chains, which seem to be dependent on the conformational flexibility of each specific sequence. This difference in enzymatic mechanism yields mixtures of chemically distinct GAG oligosaccharides generated from their parent molecules.

B. The Effects of CSPG-Degradation Products on Neuronal Tissue

Some of these CSPG derivatives demonstrate completely different properties from those of the intact molecule. Several GAG derivatives demonstrate growth-promoting features. For example, octasaccharides derived from CS D induce neurite outgrowth (Nadanaka *et al.*, 1998). We demonstrated that a disaccharide derived from CSPG promotes axonal growth in both PC12 and in primary hippocampal cultures (Rolls *et al.*, 2004b). When the CSPG-derived disaccharide is added to cultures of PC12 cells, it exhibits a neuroprotective effect from glutamate- or nitric oxide-induced toxicity. *In vivo* studies indicate that CSPG-derived disaccharide can protect neurons in several rodent models such as glutamate-induced toxicity (Rolls *et al.*, 2004b) in the eye or elevated intraocular pressure

(Bakalash *et al.*, 2005). The neuroprotective effect of this compound is mediated via the activation of intracellular signaling in the neural cells and the direct activation of microglia to a neuroprotective phenotype.

C. The Effects of CSPG-Degradation Products on Immune Components

Various GAG derivatives were reported to affect the inflammatory response. Some possess anti-inflammatory features while others seem to induce inflammation. For example, CSPG-derived disaccharides modulate T cell-mediated responses, limiting their motility and activation by reducing the levels of TNF-α and IFN-γ from these cells (Rolls *et al.*, 2006). Heparin-derived disaccharides affect both T cells and macrophages, limiting cytokine secretion (Cahalon *et al.*, 1997). However, on the other hand, low-molecular mass fragments of hyaluronan (HA) demonstrate proinflammatory potential. *In vivo* CSPG-derived disaccharides were shown to attenuate experimental autoimmune encephalomyelitis (EAE) (Rolls *et al.*, 2006) in mice and to relieve experimental autoimmune uveitis (EAU) in rats, both induced by activated T cells. Moreover, CSPG-derived disaccharides reduce DTH response in mice (Rolls *et al.*, 2006). The DTH response is mediated by T cells, mainly of T_{H1} type. The phenomenon of degradation products that exhibit properties different from their parent compound has been observed before: IL-2-degradation products were reported to have anti-inflammatory effects, in contrast to the proinflammatory properties of intact IL-2 (Ariel *et al.*, 1998), and it was therefore suggested that degradation products might have a regulatory role.

VII. Pharmacological Implications

In this chapter, we discussed the different aspects of CSPG in CNS repair. Although recent evidences indicate that CSPG can contribute to the recovery, many treatments were designed in order to overcome its growth inhibitory effects. Here, we discuss the most common treatments in this field. We also provide an overview on the therapeutic applications and possible uses of the CSPG-degrading products (Fig. 4).

A. Balancing CSPG

I. Preventing CSPG Formation

Treatments were developed to prevent the deposition of CSPG, including suppression of CSPG-core protein synthesis and suppression of GAG-chain synthesis by DNA degrading enzymes. Decorin is a compound that suppresses the synthesis of several CSPG types by inhibiting the activity of

* **Preventing CSPG expression**
DNA-degrading enzymes
Prevention of GAG sulfation

* **Degrading CSPG**
Chondroitinase ABC
Hyaluronidase

* **Controlling intracellular growth-associated signals**
Rho inactivation (C3-transferase, PKC-inhibitor)
cdc42 activation (CA cdc42)
Rac-1 activation (CA-Rac-1)

* **CSPG-degradation products promoting axonal growth**
CSPG-derived saccharides

FIGURE 4   Therapeutic intervention to overcome the inhibitory effect of CSPG. Classification of the different approaches directed to overcome the inhibitory effects of CSPG on axonal growth. The different treatments in each category are listed.

transforming growth factor β (Yamaguchi *et al.*, 1990) and the growth-factors receptor tyrosine kinase, known to promote synthesis of PG (Asher *et al.*, 2000). Decorin administration to injured sites in the adult-rat spinal cord promotes axon growth. The DNA-degrading enzymes are another example of a treatment designed to suppress CSPG deposition; they were designed to target and degrade mRNA encoding an enzyme (xylosyltransferase-1), which initiates GAGs synthesis on core proteins. When such enzymes are infused around injured sites, they reduce the expression of CSPG and promote neuronal regeneration (Grimpe and Silver, 2004).

2. Degrading CSPG

One of the most common approaches to overcome the growth inhibition imposed by CSPG is the degradation of CSPG by specific enzymes. Local application of chondroitinase ABC (ChABC) at the injury site upregulates a regeneration-associated protein, GAP43, in injured neurons and promotes regeneration of both ascending-sensory projections and descending-corticospinal tract axons. ChABC treatment also restores postsynaptic activity below the lesion after electrical stimulation of corticospinal neurons and promotes functional recovery of locomotor and proprioceptive behaviors (Bradbury *et al.*, 2002). Such treatments with ChABC were reported to be effective in several *in vivo* models such as spinal-cord injury (Bradbury *et al.*, 2002), sciatic nerve transection (Zuo *et al.*, 2002), and nerve grafts (Krekoski *et al.*, 2001). It was further demonstrated that CSPG degradation reactivates visual cortical plasticity in mature rats (Pizzorusso *et al.*, 2002).

Not all enzymatic treatments result in increased recovery despite complete degradation and elimination of the CSPG molecule, as determined by immunohistochemical analysis, such as in the case of CSPG degradation of by hyaluronidase (Moon *et al.*, 2003). This may indicate that the effectiveness of the enzymatic treatment derives not only from the elimination of CSPG but also from the generation of specific degradation products that contribute to the repair.

3. Overcoming Inhibitory Intracellular Signaling Associated with CSPG

A different approach was designed to overcome the inhibitory effect of CSPG by affecting intracellular-signaling pathways to either counteract the inhibitory signal imposed by CSPG or to activate alternative pathways inducing growth in neurons. For example, the Rho/ROCK pathway mediates signals from CSPG and other inhibitory molecules (Monnier *et al.*, 2003; Tufvesson and Westergren-Thorsson, 2003). The activation of Rho is mediated by PKC. Therefore, a PKC inhibitor was infused to injured-adult rat spinal cords to suppress the Rho/ROCK pathway. This treatment promoted regeneration of dorsal column axons but not of corticospinal tract cells (Sivasankaran *et al.*, 2004). C3 transferase is another example of a molecule designed to inactivate Rho and thereby induce axonal growth of neurons cultured on CSPG (Dergham *et al.*, 2002). Other members of the Rhofamily of small GTPases, cdc-42 and Rac-1, induce axonal growth upon activation. Treatments designed to promote their activation resulted in increased number of neurites growing on CSPG (Jain *et al.*, 2004). The fact that the growth inhibitory effect of CSPG on neurons can be overcome by direct activation of intracellular mechanisms promoting axonal growth may indicate that CSPG does not impose a mechanical barrier to regeneration but rather affects its intracellular signaling.

B. Benefiting from CSPG-Degradation Products

I. Competing with CSPG

Degradation products of CSPG, mostly oligosaccharides, were tested as treatments in different models of CNS insult. The main use of the degradation products has been in cases in which CSPG depositions were reported to contribute to pathology, such as in the case of Alzheimer's disease, in which PGs and GAGs facilitate amyloid fibril formation and stabilize the plaque aggregates at the earliest stage of fibril formation. Monosaccharides and disaccharides were used to compete with the intact CSPG and heparin for amyloid-beta binding, thereby decreasing plaque formation (Gupta-Bansal *et al.*, 1995).

2. Affecting Cell Signaling

Other CSPG-derived compounds were demonstrated to directly activate intracellular mechanisms and affect cell behavior. Disaccharides derived from CSPG (CSPG-DS) can directly induce axonal growth and neuronal survival, activating the PKCα and PYK2 intracellular-signaling pathways (Rolls *et al.*, 2004b). Microglial activation to a neuroprotective phenotype was also observed following CSPG-DS treatment, which was associated with ERK1/2 and PYK2 activation (Rolls *et al.*, 2004b). The systemic or local application of CSPG-DS in the eye toxicity model (when the toxic factors are either excessive levels of glutamate or aggregated beta-amyloid) was demonstrated to be neuroprotective, resulting in enhanced neuronal survival and increased functional recovery. These effects were achieved without degrading the intact CSPG, and it is therefore possible that application of the disaccharides helps to maintain the balance between the intact and degraded CSPG forms, without the need for additional CSPG degradation.

VIII. Conclusions

CSPG levels are elevated in various pathological conditions both in the CNS and in the periphery, where these compounds are associated mainly with wound repair processes. In the CNS, although the expression of CSPG is observed during normal development (Schwartz and Domowicz, 2004), by adulthood, the expression of CSPG is detected mainly under injurious conditions (Properzi *et al.*, 2003) and in several other pathologies such as Alzheimer's and MS. CSPGs are generally thought to be inhibitory for CNS repair. One of the reasons for this perception is their growth inhibitory properties and their association with recruitment of immune components such as macrophages/microglia and T cells. Here, we suggest that CSPGs are actually needed for the CNS repair process. Yet, the regulation of CSPG production and clearance under the conditions following injury might not be optimal. According to this view, the destructive effect of this group of molecules may be a result of their excessive expression or unbalanced degradation kinetics, factors that could limit their effectiveness. The reparative functions of these molecules, either by sealing off the injury site, generating diffusion barriers, promoting neuronal survival or activation and localization of the immune response, can be lost, following treatments focused on the elimination of CSPG. The observations that the degradation products of CSPG yield potent protective and therapeutic compounds without the need for CSPG degradation might offer the possibility of exploiting this group of compounds for novel pharmacological treatments for acute and chronic degenerative conditions in the CNS.

References

Aoyama, E., Yoshihara, R., Tai, A., Yamamoto, I., and Gohda, E. (2005). PKC- and PI3K-dependent but ERK-independent proliferation of murine splenic B cells stimulated by chondroitin sulfate B. *Immunol. Lett.* **99**, 80–84.

Ariel, A., Hershkoviz, R., Avron, A., Franitza, S., Hardan, I., Cahalon, L., Fridkin, M., and Lider, O. (1998). IL-2 induces T cell adherence to extracellular matrix: Inhibition of adherence and migration by IL-2 peptides generated by leukocyte elastase. *J. Immunol.* **161**, 2465–2472.

Asher, R. A., Morgenstern, D. A., Shearer, M. C., Adcock, K. H., Pesheva, P., and Fawcett, J. W. (2002). Versican is upregulated in CNS injury and is a produci of oligodendrocyte lineage cells. *J. Neurosci.* **22**, 2225–2236.

Asher, R. A., Morgenstern, D. A., Fidler, P. S., Adcock, K. H., Oohira, A., Braistead, J. E., Levine, J. M., Margolis, R. U., Rogers, J. H., and Fawcett, J. W. (2000). Neurocan is upregulated in injured brain and in cytokine-treated astrocytes. *J. Neurosci.* **20**, 2427–2438.

Bakalash, S., Rolls, A., Cahalon, L., and Chwartz, M. (2005). Controlling inflammation and neurodegeneration: The dual action of chondroitin sulfate proteoglycan degradation product. *Invest. Ophthalmol. Vis. Sci.* **46**, E-Abstract 1289.

Bradbury, E. J., Moon, L. D., Popat, R. J., King, V. R., Bennett, G. S., Palei, P. N., Fawcett, J. W., and McMahon, S. B. (2002). Chondroitinase ABC promotes functional recovery after spinal cord injury. *Nature* **416**, 636–640.

Brittis, P. A., Canning, D. R., and Silver, J. (1992). Chondroitin sulfate as a regulator of neuronal patterning in the retina. *Science* **255**, 733–736.

Butovsky, O., Talpalar, A. E., Ben-Yaakov, K., and Schwartz, M. (2005). Activation of microglia by aggregated beta-amyloid or lipopolysaccharide impairs MHC-II expression and renders them cytotoxic whereas IFN-gamma and IL-4 render them protective. *Mol. Cell Neurosci.* **29**(3), 381–393.

Cahalon, L., Lider, O., Schor, H., Avron, A., Gilat, D., Hershkoviz, R., Margalit, R., Eshel, A., Shoseyev, O., and Cohen, I. R. (1997). Heparin disaccharides inhibit tumor necrosis factor-alpha production by macrophages and arrest immune inflammation in rodents. *Int. Immunol.* **9**, 1517–1522.

Chau, C. H., Shum, D. K., Li, H., Pei, J., Lui, Y. Y., Wirthlin, L., Chan, Y. S., and Xu, X. M. (2004). Chondroitinase ABC enhances axonal regrowth through Schwann cell-seeded guidance channels after spinal cord injury. *FASEB J.* **18**, 194–196.

Chen, Z. J., Negra, M., Levine, A., Ughrin, Y., and Levine, J. M. (2002). Oligodendrocyte precursor cells: Reactive cells that inhibit axon growth and regeneration. *J. Neurocytol.* **31**, 481–495.

Delfino, D. V., Patrene, K. D., DeLeo, A. B., DeLeo, R., Herberman, R. B., and Boggs, S. S. (1994). Role of CD44 in the development of natural killer cells from precursore in long-term cultures of mouse bone marrow. *J. Immunol.* **152**, 5171–5179.

Denholm, E. M., Lin, Y. Q., and Silver, P. J. (2001). Anti-tumor activities of chondroitinase AC and chondroitinase B: Inhibition of angiogenesis, proliferation and invasion. *Eur. J. Pharmacol.* **416**, 213–221.

Dergham, P., Ellezam, B., Essagian, C., Avedissian, H., Lubell, W. D., and McKerracher, L. (2002). Rho signaling pathway targeted to promote spinal cord repair. *J. Neurosci.* **22**, 6570–6577.

Domeniconi, M., and Filbin, M. T. (2005). Overcoming inhibitors in myelin to promote axonal regeneration. *J. Neurol. Sci.* **233**, 43–47.

Dou, C. L., and Levine, J. M. (1994). Inhibition of neurite growth by the NG2 chondroitin sulfate proteoglycan. *J. Neurosci.* **14**, 7616–7628.

Fitch, M. T., and Silver, J. (1997). Activated macrophages and the blood-brain barrier: Inflammation after CNS injury leads to increases in putative inhibitory molecules. *Exp. Neurol.* **148**, 587–603.

Fouad, K., Dietz, V., and Schwab, M. E. (2001). Improving axonal growth and functional recovery after experimental spinal cord injury by neutralizing myelin associated inhibitors. *Brain Res. Rev.* **36**, 204–212.

Fournier, A. E., GrandPre, T., Gould, G., Wang, X., and Strittmatter, S. M. (2002). Nogo and the Nogo-66 receptor. *Prog. Brain Res.* **137**, 361–369.

Friedlander, D. R., Milev, P., Karthikeyan, L., Margolis, R. K., Margolis, R. U., and Grumet, M. (1994). The neuronal chondroitin sulfate proteoglycan neurocan binds to the neural cell adhesion molecules Ng-CAM/Ll/NILE and N-CAM, and inhibits neuronal adhesion and neurite outgrowth. *J. Cell Biol.* **125**, 669–680.

Garnier, P., Gibbs, R. V., and Rider, C. C. (2003). A role for chondroitin sulphate B in the activity of interleukin 12 in stimulating gamma-interferon secretion. *Immunol. Lett.* **85**, 53–58.

Grados-Munro, E. M., and Fournier, A. E. (2003). Myelin-associated inhibitors of axon regeneration. *J. Neurosci. Res.* **74**, 479–485.

Grimpe, B., and Silver, J. (2004). A novel DNA enzyme reduces glycosaminoglycan chains in the glial scar and allows microtransplanted dorsal root ganglia axons to regenerate beyond lesions in the spinal cord. *J. Neurosci.* **24**, 1393–1397.

Gupta-Bansal, R., Frederickson, R. C., and Brunden, K. R. (1995). Proteoglycan-mediated inhibition of A beta proteolysis: A potential cause of senile plaque accumulation. *J. Biol. Chem.* **270**, 18666–18671.

He, Z., and Koprivica, V. (2004). The Nogo signaling pathway for regeneration block. *Annu. Rev. Neurosci.* **27**, 341–368.

Horn, K. P., Steinmetz, M. P., Tom, V. J., and Miller, J. H. (2004). Soluble macrophages-derived factors digest proteoglycan and enhance neurite outgrowth in an *in vitro* model of the glial scar. Society for Neuroscience, Program No. 43.17.

Huxlin, K. R., Carr, R., Schulz, M., Sefton, A. J., and Bennett, M. R. (1995). Trophic effect of collicular proteoglycan on neonatal rat retinal ganglion cells in situ. *Brain. Res. Dev.* **84**, 77–88.

Huxlin, K. R., Dreher, B., Schulz, M., Sefton, A. J., and Bennett, M. R. (1995). Effect of collicular proteoglycan on the survival of adult rat retinal ganglion cells following axotomy. *Eur. J. Neurosci.* **7**, 96–107.

Jain, A., Brady-Kalnay, S. M., and Bellamkonda, R. V. (2004). Modulation of Rho GTPase activity alleviates chondroitin sulfate proteoglycan-dependent inhibition of neurite extension. *J. Neurosci. Res.* **77**, 299–307.

Jones, L. L., and Tuszynski, M. H. (2002). Spinal cord injury elicits expression of keratan sulfate proteoglycans by macrophages, reactive microglia, and oligodendrocyte progenitors. *J. Neurosci.* **22**, 4611–4624.

Jones, L. L., Margolis, R. U., and Tuszynski, M. H. (2003). The chondroitin sulfate proteoglycans neurocan, brevican, phosphocan, and versican are differentially regulated following spinal cord injury. *Exp. Neurol.* **182**(2), 399–411.

Kappler, J., Junghans, U., Koops, A., Stichel, C. C., Hausser, H. J., Kresse, H., and Muller, H. W. (1997). Chondroitin/dermatan sulphate promotes the survival of neurons from rat embryonic neocortex. *Eur. J. Neurosci.* **9**, 306–318.

Kastin, A. J., and Fan, W. (2005). Targeting neurite growth inhibitors to induce CNS regeneration. *Curr. Pharm. Des.* **11**, 1247–1253.

Kipnis, J., Yoles, E., Schori, H., Hauben, E., Shaked, I., and Schwartz, M. (2001). Neuronal survival after CNS insult is determined by a genetically encoded autoimmune response. *J. Neurosci.* **21**(13), 4564–4571.

Kipnis, J., and Schwartz, M. (2005). Controlled autoimmunity in CNS maintenance and repair: Naturally occurring CD4+ CD25+ regulatory T-cells at the crossroads of health and disease. *Neuromolecular Med.* **7**(3), 197–206.

Koops, A., Kappler, J., Junghans, U., Kuhn, G., Kresse, H., and Muller, H. W. (1996). Cultured astrocytes express biglycan, a chondroitin/dermatan sulfate proteoglycan supporting the survival of neocortical neurons. *Brain Res. Mol.* **41**, 65–73.

Krekoski, C. A., Neubauer, D., Zuo, J., and Muir, D. (2001). Axonal regeneration into acellular nerve grafts is enhanced by degradation of chondroitin sulfate proteoglycan. *J. Neurosci.* **21**, 6206–6213.

Kwakkenbos, M. J., Pouwels, W., Matmati, M., Stacey, M., Lin, H. H., Gordon, S., van Lier, R. A., and Hamann, J. (2005). Expression of the largest CD97 and EMR2 isoforms on leukocytes facilitates a specific interaction with chondroitin sulfate on B cells. *J. Leukoc. Biol.* **77**, 112–119.

Levine, J. M. (1994). Increased expression of the NG2 chondroitin-sulfate proteoglycan after brain injury. *J. Neurosci.* **14**, 4716–4730.

Lider, O., Mekori, Y. A., Miller, T., Bar-Tana, R., Vlodavsky, I., Baharav, E., Cohen, I. R., and Naparstek, Y. (1990). Inhibition of T lymphocyte heparanase by heparin prevents T cell migration and T cell-mediated immunity. *Eur. J. Immunol.* **20**, 493–499.

MacDermott, R. P., Schmidt, R. E., Caulfield, J. P., Hein, A., Bartley, G. T., Ritz, J., Schlossman, S. F., Austen, K. F., and Stevens, R. L. (1985). Proteoglycans in cell-mediated cytotoxicity: Identification, localization, and exocytosis of a chondroitin sulfate proteoglycan from human cloned natural killer cells during target cell lysis. *J. Exp. Med.* **162**, 1771–1787.

Maeda, N., and Noda, M. (1996). 6B4 proteoglycan/phosphacan is a repulsive substratum but promotes morphological differentiation of cortical neurons. *Development* **122**, 647–658.

Maeda, N., Matsui, F., and Oohira, A. (1992). A chondroitin sulfate proteoglycan that is developmentally regulated in the cerebellar mossy fiber System. *Dev. Biol.* **151**, 564–574.

Makatsori, E., Lamari, F. N., Theocharis, A. D., Anagnostides, S., Hjerpe, A., Tsegenidis, T., and Karamanos, N. K. (2003). Large matrix proteoglycans, versican and perlecan, are expressed and secreted by human leukemic monocytes. *Anticancer Res.* **23**, 3303–3309.

Matsui, F., and Oohira, A. (2004). Proteoglycans and injury of the central nervous system. *Congenit. Anom. (Kyoto)* **44**, 181–188.

McKeon, R. J., Schreiber, R. C., Rudge, J. S., and Silver, J. (1991). Reduction of neurite outgrowth in a model of glial scarring following CNS injury is correlated with the expression of inhibitory molecules on reactive astrocytes. *J. Neurosci.* **11**, 3398–3411.

Monnier, P. P., Sierra, A., Schwab, J. M., Henke-Fahle, S., and Mueller, B. K. (2003). The Rho/ROCK pathway mediates neurite growth-inhibitory activity associated with the chondroitin sulfate proteoglycans of the CNS glial scar. *Mol. Cell. Neurosci.* **22**, 319–330.

Moon, L. D., Asher, R. A., and Fawcett, J. W. (2003). Limited growth of severed CNS axons after treatment of adult rat brain with hyaluronidase. *J. Neurosci. Res.* **71**, 23–37.

Moon, L. D., Asher, R. A., Rhodes, K. E., and Fawcett, J. W. (2001). Regeneration of CNS axons back to their target following treatment of adult rat brain with chondroitinase ABC. *Nat. Neurosci.* **4**, 465–466.

Nadanaka, S., Clement, A., Masayama, K., Faissner, A., and Sugahara, K. (1998). Characteristic hexasaccharide sequences in octasaccharides derived from shark cartilage chondroitin sulfate D with a neurite outgrowth promoting activity. *J. Biol. Chem.* **273**, 3296–3307.

Nichel, K. A., Schulz, M. W., and Bennett, M. R. (1995). Nitric oxide-mediated death of cultured neonatal retinal ganglion cells: Neuroprotective properties of glutamate and chondroitin sulfate proteoglycan. *Brain Res.* **697**, 1–16.

Oohira, A., Katoh-Semba, R., Watanabe, E., and Matsui, F. (1994). Brain development and multiple molecular species of proteoglycan. *Neurosci. Res.* **20**, 195–207.

Pindzola, R. R., Doller, C., and Silver, J. (1993). Putative inhibitory extracellular matrix molecules at the dorsal root entry zone of the spinal cord during development and after root and sciatic nerve lesions. *Dev. Biol.* **156**, 34–48.

Pizzorusso, T., Medini, P., Berardi, N., Chierzi, S., Fawcett, J. W., and Maffei, L. (2002). Reactivation of ocular dominance plasticity in the adult visual cortex. *Science* **298**, 1248–1251.

Pratibha, V., and Gupta, P. D. (2000). Cutaneous wound healing: Significance of proteoglycans in scar formation. *Curr. Sci.* **78**(6).

Properzi, F., Asher, R. A., and Fawcett, J. W. (2003). Chondroitin sulphate proteoglycans in the central nervous system: Changes and synthesis after injury. *Biochem. Soc. Trans.* **31**, 335–336.

Rachmilewitz, J., and Tykocinski, M. L. (1998). Differential effects of chondroitin sulfates A and B on monocyte and B-cell activation: Evidence for B-cell activation via a CD44-dependent pathway. *Blood* **92**, 223–229.

Ramsden, L., and Rider, C. C. (1992). Selective and differential binding of interleukin (IL)-1 alpha, IL-1 beta, IL-2 and IL-6 to glycosaminoglycans. *Eur. J. Immunol.* **22**, 3027–3031.

Roitbak, T., and Sykova, E. (1999). Diffusion barriers evoked in the rat cortex by reactive astrogliosis. *Glia* **28**, 40–48.

Rolls, A., Avidan, H., Cahalon, L., Schori, H., Bakalash, S., and Lider, O. (2004a). Chondroitin sulfate proteoglycan a SOS molecule in CNS repair.. Society for Neuroscience, Program No. 24.5.2004.

Rolls, A., Avidan, H., Cahalon, L., Schori, H., Bakalash, S., Litvak, V., Lev, S., Lider, O., and Schwartz, M. (2004b). A disaccharide derived from chondroitin sulphate proteoglycan promotes central nervous system repair in rats and mice. *Eur. J. Neurosci.* **20**, 1973–1983.

Rolls, A., Cahalon, L., Bakalash, S., Avidan, H., Lider, O., and Schwartz, M. (2006). A sulfated disaccharide derived from chondroitin sulfate proteoglycan protects against inflammation–associated neurodegeneration. *FASEB J.* **20**(3), 547–549.

Ruoslahti, E., and Yamaguchi, Y. (1991). Proteoglycans as modulators of growth factor activities. *Cell* **64**, 867–869.

Sakai, S., Akiyama, H., Harikai, N., Toyoda, H., Toida, T., Maitani, T., and Imanari, T. (2002). Effect of chondroitin sulfate on murine splenocytes sensitized with ovalbumin. *Immunol. Lett.* **84**, 211–216.

Schmalfeldt, M., Bandtlow, C. E., Dours-Zimmermann, M. T., Winterhalter, K. H., and Zimmermann, D. R. (2000). Brain derived versican V2 is a potent inhibitor of axonal growth. *J. Cell Sci.* **113**, 807–816.

Schori, H., Kipnis, J., Yoles, E., WoldeMussie, E., Ruiz, G., Wheeler, L. A., and Schwartz, M. (2001). Vaccination for protection of retinal ganglion cells against death from glutamate toxicity and ocular hypertension: Implications for glaucoma. *Proc. Natl. Acad. Sci. USA* **98**(6), 3398–3403.

Schwartz, M. (2001). Vaccination for protection of retinal ganglion cells against death from glutamate cytotoxicity and ocular hypertension: Implications for glaucoma. *Proc. Natl. Acad. Sci. USA* **98**(6), 3398–3403.

Schwartz, M., and Moalem, G. (2001). Beneficial immune activity after CNS injury: Prospects for vaccination. *J. Neuroimmunol.* **113**, 185–192.

Schwartz, N. B., and Domowicz, M. (2004). Proteoglycans in brain development. *Glycoconj. J.* **21**, 329–341.

Shaked, I., Tchoresh, D., Gersner, R., Meiri, G., Mordechai, S., Xiao, X., Kart, R. P., and Schwartz, M. (2005). Protective autoimmunity: Interferon-gamma enables microglia to remove glutamate without evoking inflammatory mediators. *J. Neurochem.* **92**, 997–1009.

Sivasankaran, R., Pei, J., Wang, K. C., Zhang, Y. P., Shields, C. B., Xu, X. M., and He, Z. (2004). PKC mediates inhibitory effects of myelin and chondroitin sulfate proteoglycans on axonal regeneration. *Nat. Neurosci.* **7**, 261–268.

Smith-Thomas, L. C., Fok-Seang, J., Stevens, J., Du, J. S., Muir, E., Faissner, A., Geller, H. M., Rogers, J. H., and Fawcett, J. W. (1994). An inhibitor of neurite outgrowth produced by astrocytes. *J. Cell Sci.* **107**, 1687–1695.

Snow, D. M., Watanabe, M., Letourneau, P. C., and Silver, J. (1991). A chondroitin sulfate proteoglycan may influence the direction of retinal ganglion cell outgrowth. *Development* **113**, 1473–1485.

Sorensson, J., Bjornson, A., Ohlson, M., Ballermann, B. J., and Haraldsson, B. (2003). Synthesis of sulfated proteoglycans by bovine glomerular endothelial cells in culture. *Am. J. Physiol. Renal Physiol.* **284**, F373–F380.

Steindler, D. A., O'Brien, T. F., Laywell, E., Harrington, K., Faissner, A., and Schachner, M. (1990). Boundaries during normal and abnormal brain development: *In vivo* and *in vitro* studies of glia and glycoconjugates. *Exp. Neurol.* **109**, 35–56.

Sykova, E. (2001). Glial diffusion barriers during aging and pathological states. *Prog. Brain. Res.* **132**, 339–363.

Teng, F. Y., and Tang, B. L. (2005). Nogo signaling and non-physical injury-induced nervous system pathology. *J. Neurosci. Res.* **79**, 273–278.

Tropea, D., Calco, M., and Maffei, L. (2003). Synergistic effects of brain-derived neurotrophic factor and chondroitinase ABC on retinal fiber sprouting after denervation of the superici colliculus in aduli rats. *J. Neurosci.* **23**, 7034–7044.

Tufvesson, E., and Westergren-Thorsson, G. (2003). Biglycan and decorin induce morphological and cytoskeletal changes involving signalling by the small GTPases RhoA and Rac1 resulting in lung fibroblast migration. *J. Cell Sci.* **116**, 4857–4864.

Villena, J., and Brandan, E. (2004). Dermatan sulfate exerts an enhanced growth factor response on skeletal muscle satellite cell proliferation and migration. *J. Cell. Physiol.* **198**, 169–178.

Wegrowski, Y., Paltot, V., Gillery, P., Kalis, B., Randoux, A., and Maquart, F. X. (1995). Stimulation of sulphated glycosaminoglycan and decorin production in adult dermal fibroblasts by recombinant human interleukin-4. *Biochem. J.* **307**, 673–678.

Woods, A. G., Cribbs, D. H., Whittemore, E. R., and Cotman, C. W. (1995). Heparan sulfate and chondroitin sulfate glycosaminoglycan attenuate beta-amyloid (25–35) induced neurodegeneration in cultured hippocampal neurons. *Brain Res.* **697**, 53–62.

Wrenshall, L. E., Stevens, R. B., Cerra, F. B., and Platt, J. L. (1999). Modulation of macrophage and B cell function by glycosaminoglycans. *J. Leukoc. Biol.* **66**, 391–400.

Yamada, H., Predette, B., Shitara, K., Hagihara, K., Miura, R., Ranscht, B., Stallcup, W. B., and Yamaguchi, Y. (1997). The brain chondroitin sulfate proteoglycan brevican associates with astrocytes ensheathing cerebellar glomeruli and inhibits neurite outgrowth from granule neurons. *J. Neurosci.* **17**, 7784–7795.

Yamaguchi, Y., Mann, D. M., and Ruoslahti, E. (1990). Negative regulation of transforming growth factor-beta by the proteoglycan decorin. *Nature* **346**, 281–284.

Yang, R., Yan, Z., Chen, F., Hansson, G. K., and Kiessling, R. (2002). Hyaluronic acid and chondroitin sulphate A rapidly promote differentiation of immature DC with upregulation of costimulatory and antigen-presenting molecules, and enhancement of NF-kappaB and protein kinase activity. *Scand. J. Immunol.* **55**, 2–13.

Yick, L. W., Wu, W., So, K. F., Yip, H. K., and Shum, D. K. (2000). Chondroitinase ABC promotes axonal regeneration of Clarke's neurons after spinal cord injury. *Neuroreport* **11**, 1063–1067.

Zuo, J., Neubauer, D., Graham, J., Krekoski, C. A., Ferguson, T. A., and Muir, D. (2002). Regeneration of axons after nerve transection repair is enhanced by degradation of chondroitin sulfate proteoglycan. *Exp. Neurol.* **176**(1), 221–228.

D. Channe Gowda

Department of Biochemistry and Molecular Biology
Pennsylvania State University College of Medicine
Hershey, Pennsylvania 17033

Role of Chondroitin-4-Sulfate in Pregnancy-Associated Malaria

I. Chapter Overview

Many pathogenic microorganisms use glycosaminoglycans (GAGs) as receptor for cell- or tissue-specific invasion, causing infection. In the case of pregnancy-associated malaria, *Plasmodium falciparum*-infected red blood cells (IRBCs) adhere in the placenta, leading to a number of clinical manifestations. A uniquely low-sulfated extracellular chondroitin sulfate proteoglycan (CSPG) localized in the intervillous space of the placenta is the receptor for the IRBC adherence. Chondroitin-4-sulfate (C4S) chains of the CSPG specifically mediate the IRBC adherence, and the optimal IRBC binding involves a C4S dodecasaccharide motif comprising two 4-sulfated and four nonsulfated disaccharides. The sulfate and hydroxyl groups at C-4 of N-acetylgalactosamine (GalNAc) and the carboxyl group of uronic acid are critical for the IRBC adhesion, whereas the N-acetyl group of GalNAc is not involved. *P. falciparum* erythrocyte membrane protein-1, a member of

Advances in Pharmacology, Volume 53
Copyright 2006, Elsevier Inc. All rights reserved.

1054-3589/06 $35.00
DOI: 10.1016/S1054-3589(05)53018-7

the parasite *var* gene family of proteins that is expressed on the surface of IRBCs, has been proposed as the ligand for IRBC adherence. In malaria endemic areas, pregnant women produce IRBC antiadhesion antibodies in a pregnancy stage-specific manner, which protect against placental malaria. A comprehensive understanding of the structural interactions involved in IRBC adherence to placental CSPG would be valuable in designing C4S oligosaccharides or mimetic peptide therapeutics for the treatment of placental malaria. While many pathogens are known to use heparan sulfate (HS) as a receptor for attachment to host cells or tissues, the involvement of CSPG in pathogen adhesion is very rare. As far as we are aware, the adherence of *P. falciparum* IRBCs in the placenta is the only unequivocally established case in which CSPG is involved in the interactions of pathogens with the host.

II. Glycosaminoglycans as Receptor for Microbial Adhesion and Invasion of Host Cells and Tissues _____

Accumulated evidence indicates that during evolution, many microorganisms (pathogenic bacteria, viruses, and parasites) have adapted to exploit the GAG chains of proteoglycans (PGs) of specific cells and tissues for efficient invasion, propagation, and survival in the host (Rostand and Esko, 1997; Wadstrom and Ljungh, 1999). Of the several GAG types present in animal cells and tissues, the majority of the GAG-recognizing microorganisms use HS chains of heparan sulfate proteoglycans (HSPGs) as receptor for infecting the hosts. The HS chains of animal cells differ considerably with regard to the sulfate content and relative amount of glucuronic acid (GlcA) and iduronic acid, leading to cell-specific HS structural features. Thus, animals express HS chains of diverse structural features that are differentially recognized by adhesive proteins on the surface of various microbes for attachment and invasion of host cells. For example, herpes simplex virus (HSV) adheres to the HS chains of the host cells through the interaction of viral surface glycoproteins, glycoprotein B (gpB) and glycoprotein C (gpC), using different HS structural motifs (Herold *et al.*, 1995). *P. falciparum* sporozoites invade hepatocytes by binding to heparin-like motifs of the HS chains that are enriched with N-sulfated glucosamine and 2-sulfated uronic acid (Pinzon-Ortiz *et al.*, 2001; Pradel *et al.*, 2002). Other microorganisms that are reported to use HS chains for entry into host include *Haemophilus influenzae*, human immunodeficiency virus, cytomegalovirus, dengue virus, *Trypanosoma cruzi*, *Leishmania donovani*, *Bordetella pertussis*, *Borrelia burgdorfeii*, *Helicobactor pylori*, *Neisseria gonorrhoeae*, *Chlamydia trachomatis*, *Leishmania* amastigotes, *Staphylococcus aureus*, *S. mutans*, and *S. pyogenes* (Frick *et al.*, 2003; Lima *et al.*, 2002; Pradel *et al.*, 2002; Rostand and Esko, 1997; Wadstrom and Ljungh,

1999). *Toxoplasma gondii* has been reported to bind a variety of GAGs, which include heparin, C4S, and chondroitin 6-sulfate (C6S) (Carruthers *et al.*, 2000). However, the broad GAG-recognition specificity of *T. gondii* is not firmly established.

In contrast to a large number of diverse types of microorganisms that have been shown to use HS chains of HSPGs as receptor for the adhesion and invasion of host cells, only a limited number of microbes appear to use chondroitin sulfate (CS). Hitherto there have been no reports regarding microorganisms using dermatan sulfate (DS) as a receptor. Subsets of HSV and *T. gondii* have been reported to use the CS chains of CSPGs as the host cell receptor (Banfield *et al.*, 1995; Carruthers *et al.*, 2000), but the receptor specificity has not been unequivocally established. The blood stage *P. falciparum* has been shown to use the CS chains of CSPGs for IRBC adherence in the host (discussed in a later section), and to date, this is the only microorganism that has been conclusively shown to use the CS chains for adhesion in the host. Hyaluronic acid (HA) has also been suggested as a receptor for *P. falciparum* adherence (Beeson and Brown, 2004; Chai *et al.*, 2001). However, this finding has been controversial (Valiyaveettil *et al.*, 2001), and further studies are required to determine if HA is also a receptor. As far as we are aware, there are no other reports regarding microorganisms using HA as a receptor for adhesion to host tissues.

III. Structural Features and Occurrence of Chondroitin Sulfates

The focus of this chapter is to discuss the role of CS in the adherence of *P. falciparum*-IRBCs in the human placenta, which leads to pregnancy-associated malaria. As discussed in detail in chapter 3, CS consists of a repeating disaccharide moiety made up of GlcA and GalNAc with variable number of sulfate groups on GalNAc residue (Bhavanadan and Davidson, 1992; Kjellen and Lindahl, 1991). The CS chains of most animal CSPGs belong to two groups: (i) C4S also called chondroitin sulfate A (CSA) with sulfate group at C4 of GalNAc and (ii) C6S also known as chondroitin sulfate C (CSC) with sulfate group at C6 of GalNAc. However, the sulfation of GalNAc residues of CS during biosynthesis is usually not complete, and the CS chains of many animal cells are sulfated to variable degrees, resulting in the formation of partially sulfated CS chains. For example, while most of the GalNAc residues of the sturgeon notochord CS are sulfated, only ~15% of the GalNAc in the CS chains of a subpopulation of bovine corneal CSPG is sulfated (Muthusamy *et al.*, 2004a). In the CS chains of most animal cell and tissue CSPGs, 70–80% of the GalNAc are sulfated at C4 or C6. The CS chains of certain animal tissues contain sulfate groups at C4 of some GalNAc residues and at C6 of others, forming copolymeric structures. For example, ~53% and ~39% of the GalNAc residues in the CS chains of bovine tracheal CSPG have sulfate groups at C4 and C6, respectively, and the remainder of the GalNAc is nonsulfated (Alkhalil *et al.*, 2000). On the other hand, the CS chains of some animal-tissue CSPGs are oversulfated. For instance, ~60% of the GalNAc residue of the squid cartilage CS (CS E) are sulfated at both C4 and C6. In shark cartilage CS (CS D), ~23% of the disaccharide moieties contain sulfate groups at both C2 of GlcA and C6 of GalNAc (Alkhalil *et al.*, 2000).

IV. Malaria Infection and Parasite Interaction with the Host

Malaria is a deadly infectious disease in the tropical and subtropical regions of the world. Despite the availability of various drugs for treatment, malaria continues to be a leading cause of deaths. In addition to causing 2–3 millions deaths annually, the disease contributes enormously to the socioeconomic burden of the people living in the endemic areas (Gilles and Warrell, 1997; Sachs and Malany, 2002; Sherman, 1998). Malaria is also a major health problem for travelers, military personnel, business people, and diplomats from nonmalarial regions entering endemic areas (Sachs and Malany, 2002). In recent years, the spread of drug-resistant parasites and insecticide-resistant mosquitoes is exacerbating the problem (Greenwood and Mutabingwa, 2002). Therefore, novel therapeutics and/or a vaccine are needed to combat malaria effectively. A comprehensive understanding of the parasite biology and parasite–host interactions is likely to facilitate such efforts.

The parasitic protozoan of the genus *Plasmodium* is the causative agent of malaria (Gilles and Warrell, 1997; Sherman, 1998). More than a hundred *Plasmodium* species are present in nature, which infect various animals, including human, monkeys, rodents, birds, and reptiles. However, malaria in human is caused by four species, *P. falciparum*, *P. vivax*, *P. malaraie*, and *P. ovale*. Of these, *P. falciparum* is the most virulent and responsible for more than 90% of malaria fatalities (Gilles and Warrell, 1997; Sherman, 1998). The mode of infection and developmental stages are similar for all four human malaria parasites. The parasites enter the host in the form of sporozoites during a bite by infected mosquitoes and selectively infect liver cells. Infection at the liver stage is largely asymptomatic, and over a period of time the parasites mature and differentiate into merozoites. Each infected liver cell releases tens of thousands of merozoites, which specifically invade red blood cells. In the blood stage, the parasite multiplies every 48 h, each infected erythrocyte releasing 8–24 merozoites, which go on to infect other erythrocytes (Gilles and Warrell, 1997). Multiplication of the blood-stage parasites leads to massive destruction of red blood cells and stimulation of host innate immune system to produce proinflammatory mediators. These events collectively contribute to severe anemia, periodic fever and chills, metabolic acidosis, and many organ-related pathological conditions (Gilles and Warrell, 1997; Miller *et al.*, 2002; Sherman, 1998). Since most of the events of parasite–host interactions are common to all four human malaria parasite species, why only *P. falciparum* but not other three species causes fatal forms of disease remains poorly understood. However, accumulated evidence indicates that adherence of parasite IRBCs to the microvascular endothelial surface, a distinctive feature of *P. falciparum* compared to the other three human parasite species, may play a key role (Miller *et al.*, 2002; Weatherall *et al.*, 2002). Extensive accumulation of the IRBCs in the microvascular capillaries of vital organs causes capillary blockage with deprivation of oxygen and nutrients and production of toxic levels of proinflammatory cytokines (Miller *et al.*, 2002). These events damage the endothelial cell lining, causing organ dysfunction and severe organ-related pathological conditions such as coma, pulmonary edema, respiratory distress, liver dysfunction, and renal failure (Heddini, 2002; Hommel, 1993; Weatherall *et al.*, 2002).

Sequestration of IRBCs in the microvascular capillaries of the host organs is an adaptive mechanism for the efficient survival of the parasite in the harsh environment of the host. This mechanism provides the parasite several survival advantages: (i) by avoiding clearance of the IRBCs by the spleen, (ii) establishing a low oxygen environment that is conducive for its growth, (iii) efficient multiplication under decreased blood flow, and (iv) evading the host defense by inducing effective immune suppression locally. Abolition of IRBC adherence is likely to allow the host to effectively clear infection, preventing the development of malaria pathology. Therefore, understanding the IRBC-adherence mechanism and structural interactions involved in the adherence could offer strategies for the development of therapeutics and/or a vaccine for malaria.

P. falciparum has evolved to use several host receptors on the vascular endothelial surface for IRBC adherence and effective survival by evading the host immune responses. The identified host receptors involved in IRBC adherence include, CD36, intercellular adhesion molecule-1, vascular cell adhesion molecule-1, E-selectin, platelet endothelial cell adhesion molecule-1/CD31, and thrombospondin on vascular endothelial cell surface (Baruch *et al.*, 1996; Chaiyaroj *et al.*, 1994; Heddini *et al.*, 2001; Ockenhouse *et al.*, 1992; Pasloske and Howard, 1994; Treutiger *et al.*, 1997; Udomsangpetch *et al.*, 1997). IRBCs have also been reported to bind to complement receptor, HS, and C4S (Chaiyaroj *et al.*, 1996; Robert *et al.*, 1995; Rogerson *et al.*, 1995; Rowe *et al.*, 1997; Vogt, *et al.*, 2003). It is believed that the adherent proteins expressed on the surfaces of IRBCs are members of antigenic *var* gene family of proteins that are collectively called *P. falciparum* erythrocyte membrane protein 1 (PfEMP1) (Baruch *et al.*, 1995, 1996; Borst *et al.*, 1995; Gardner *et al.*, 1996; Noviyanti and Brown, 2003; Smith *et al.*, 1995, 2000a,b, 2001; Su *et al.*, 1995). The *P. falciparum* genome has a repertoire of ~60 distinct *var* genes, which are variably expressed in different parasite strains. In infected individuals, the parasite, through its ability to express divergent PfEMP1s from the *var* gene repertoire, can adhere to various organs and multiply, causing organ-related illness. However, over a period of time, the host produces anti-adhesive antibodies against the adherent PfEMP1, inhibiting IRBC adhesion and aiding the clearance of infection (Bull and Marsh, 2002; Bull *et al.*, 1998; Giha *et al.*, 2000). Thus, in immune-protected people, the IRBCs cannot adhere to the vascular capillaries, thereby limiting parasite growth. To over-come this host's immune-defensive mechanism, the parasite switches to other adherent phenotypes by expressing PfEMP1s with different receptor specificity through the use of its *var* gene repertoire (Gatton, *et al.*, 2003; Giha *et al.*, 1999; Jensen *et al.*, 2004; Paget-McNicol *et al.*, 2002; Peters *et al.*, 2002). This ability of the parasite to express varying PfEMP1 for which the host has not yet developed adhesion inhibitory antibodies enables it to selectively adhere through a different receptor and efficiently survive in the host.

V. Adherence of *P. falciparum*-Infected Erythrocytes in the Placenta and Pregnancy-Associated Malaria

In malaria endemic areas, women are highly susceptible to *P. falciparum* malaria during pregnancy, especially those who are pregnant for the first time (Brabin 1983; Brabin and Rogerson, 2001; Duffy and Desowitz, 2001; Steketee *et al.*, 1988). This phenomenon occurs, even though women in general, like men, have protective immunity acquired during adulthood (Artavanis-Tsakonas *et al.*, 2003; Baird, 1995; Day and Marsh, 1991; Hviid, 1998; Riley *et al.*, 1994; Roberts, 2003). The reason for the suscepti-bility of pregnant women is that the development of the placenta provides a new receptor for *P. falciparum* adherence that is not expressed on the vascular endothelial surface (Duffy, 2001; Fried, 2001). Therefore, indivi-duals other than pregnant women are not exposed at significant levels to this parasite subtype. In the absence of the phenotype-specific protective immu-nity, the antigenically distinct *P. falciparum* selectively adhere to the placenta and multiplies, leading to the massive accumulation of IRBCs in the inter-villous space (Beeson *et al.*, 2002; Brabin *et al.*, 2004; Fried and Duffy, 1998; Miller and Smith, 1998). In response to this IRBC sequestration (Fig. 1), macrophages infiltrate the placenta in large numbers and release toxic levels of proinflammatory cytokines (Brabin *et al.*, 2004; Menendez *et al.*, 2000; Ordi *et al.*, 2001; Rogerson *et al.*, 2003). These events affect the normal functions of the placenta, causing placental malaria, which is characterized by a number of clinical manifestations that include low-birth weight, still birth, abortion, premature delivery, and maternal morbidity and mortality

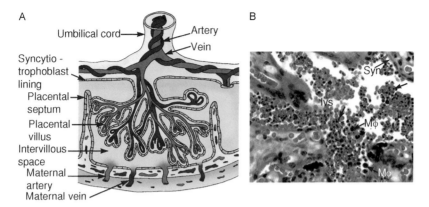

FIGURE 1 (A) Schematic diagram of a portion of human placenta. (B) Photograph of a tissue section of *P. falciparum*-infected placenta fixed with 10% formaldehyde and stained with hemotoxylin and eosin. IVS, intervillous space; Syn, syncytiotrophoblast lining; Mϕ, macrophage/mococytes; arrows, IRBCs. (See Color Insert.)

(Brabin *et al.*, 2004; Crocker *et al.*, 2004; Ismail *et al.*, 2000; McGregor *et al.*, 1983; Menendez, 1995; Menendez *et al.*, 2000; Ordi *et al.*, 2001; Rogerson *et al.*, 2003; Steketee *et al.*, 2001; Walter *et al.*, 1982). Over successive pregnancies, women develop placental parasite-specific immunity and acquire resistance to placental malaria (Duffy, 2001). Therefore, in endemic areas, the multigravidae are at relatively low risk of developing placental malaria.

VI. C4S Mediates the Adherence of *P. falciparum* IRBCs in Human Placenta

The adherence of IRBCs in the placenta of *P. falciparum*-infected women, the observed low levels of parasitemia in the peripheral blood despite the accumulation of IRBCs at high density in the placenta, and the pregnancy-associated malarial complications have been known for more than 100 years (Duffy, 2001). Nevertheless, until recently, the underlying mechanism for IRBC adherence in the placenta was unknown. Since almost all adults in endemic areas, where *P. falciparum* infection occurs on a daily or weekly basis, people are generally resistant to developing severe illness. Thus, the susceptibility of women to placental malaria had been attributed to immune suppression during pregnancy (Duffy, 2001). However, this notion does not explain the observed decrease in susceptibility to placental malaria with increasing gravidity (Brabin, 1983).

In 1995, Rogerson *et al.* discovered that a population of *P. falciparum* laboratory strains can adhere to CHO cells and that the binding is mediated by C4S. The CHO cell-adherent IRBCs were unable to bind CHO cell mutants deficient in the expression of C4S, and the IRBC binding to CHO cells was inhibited by C4S but not by C6S, DS, HS, or heparin (Rogerson *et al.*, 1995). Treatment of CHO cells with chondroitinase ABC but not heparitinase caused a drastic reduction in IRBC binding. It was further found that a minor population of IRBCs isolated from the peripheral blood of infected persons bound to immobilized C4S (Chaiyaroj *et al.*, 1996), suggesting that the C4S-IRBC binding is biologically relevant. During the same period, Robert *et al.* (1995) showed that IRBCs of *P. falciparum* laboratory strains could bind *in vitro* cultured human lung endothelial cells and *Saimiri* monkey brain microvascular endothelial cells in a C4S-depenedent manner. The binding of IRBCs to the endothelial cells was inhibited by C4S but not by C6S, DS, HS, HA, or keratan sulfate (KS) (Robert *et al.*, 1995). The binding was also abolished on treatment of endothelial cells with chondroitinase ABC and chondroitinase AC II. These two independent studies clearly established that a subpopulation of *P. falciparum* IRBCs could bind to C4S. A year later, Fried and Duffy (1996) discovered the biological relevance of IRBC binding to C4S by demonstrating C4S-dependent adherence of IRBC in the placenta of *P. falciparum*-infected pregnant women.

By testing various extracellular matrix (ECM) molecules, including C4S, DS, fucoidin, fibronectin, laminin, fibrinogen, and different collagen types immobilized on plastic surface, Fried and Duffy (1996) found that the IRBCs isolated from *P. falciparum*-infected placentas could bind to C4S but not to other molecules tested, such as C6S, DS, and heparin. The placental IRBCs could adhere to tissue sections of uninfected placentas, and the binding was inhibited by soluble C4S but not by DS. Treatment of the placental tissue sections with chondroitinase ABC abolished IRBC binding. Furthermore, the placental IRBC isolates were unable to bind to CD36, the major receptor for IRBC adherence in vascular capillaries in males and nonpregnant women. On the other hand, IRBCs from the peripheral blood of nonpregnant women were unable to bind to the immobilized C4S and instead adhered to CD36 (Fried and Duffy, 1996). Thus, it was demonstrated that IRBC adherence in the placenta and vascular capillaries is mediated by distinct host receptors, namely C4S and endothelial cell adhesion molecules, respectively. Subsequently, several investigators substantiated the adherence of IRBCs to C4S (Achur *et al.*, 2000; Beeson *et al.*, 1998; Cooke *et al.*, 1996; Duffy and Fried, 1999; Gysin *et al.*, 1997; Gowda and Ockenhouse, 1999; Maubert *et al.*, 1997, 2000; Pouvelle *et al.*, 1998; Rogerson and Brown, 1997). The IRBCs were also shown to adhere to immobilized C4S under shear stress conditions similar to those of physiological blood flow in postcapillary venules, demonstrating that the C4S-dependent binding of IRBCs is physiologically relevant (Cooke *et al.*, 1996; Rogerson *et al.*, 1997).

It has also been shown that a minor population of IRBCs from the peripheral blood of *P. falciparum*-infected individuals (particularly those from Thailand), presumably regardless of gender, could bind to immobilized C4S (Chaiyaroj *et al.*, 1996). However, the IRBCs do not adhere significantly to vascular endothelia because CSPGs are rarely present on the vascular endothelial surface *in vivo* even though *in vitro* cultured endothelial cells synthesize significant levels of CSPGs as components of the ECM and cell surface. Therefore, C4S-adherent *P. falciparum* phenotypes are unable to selectively accumulate in males and nonpregnant women. This explains why protective immunity to malaria that is developed by people in endemic areas during their childhood years does not include antibodies that prevent C4S-IRBC adhesion and immunity against C4S-adherent phenotype.

VII. Uniquely Low-Sulfated Extracellular CSPG is the Major Receptor for IRBC Adherence in Human Placenta _____

To identify the CSPG that mediates IRBC adherence in the human placenta, Achur *et al.* (2000) have purified and structurally characterized the CSPGs and other related PGs of human placenta. It has been found that human placenta contains three distinct types of CSPGs: (i) a uniquely low-sulfated extracellular aggrecan family CSPG; (ii) several cell-associated CSPGs; (iii) tissue-matrix PGs containing copolymeric DS/CS chains (Achur *et al.*, 2000). These three CSPG types account, respectively, for 24%, 2%, and 74% of the total CSPGs in the placenta.

The CS chains of extracellular CSPG are extremely low sulfated; on an average, only one in twelve of the disaccharide residues are 4-sulfated. The level of sulfation in the CS chains of placental CSPG from different individuals varies considerably; 4–12% of 4-sulfated and 86–98% of nonsulfated disaccharide residues (Achur *et al.*, 2000). The cell-associated CSPGs comprise a mixture of several distinct PGs, including low-abundance syndecan and the CSPG form of thrombomodulin in cytotrophoblasts, syncytiotrophoblasts, and fetal villous blood capillary endothelial cells (Achur *et al.*, 2000; Gowda *et al.* unpublished observations). Since these CSPGs are distributed in several cell types of the placenta, it is likely that only very low amounts of CSPGs are present on the syncytiotrophoblast surface. The CS chains of these CSPGs are moderately sulfated; 27–33% are 4-sulfated, 13–15% 6-sulfated, and 52–60% nonsulfated disaccharide residues. Tissue matrix PGs include mainly decorin and biglycan with DS/CS copolymeric chains (Achur *et al.*, 2000). These matrix DS/CSPGs are localized in the stromal tissue and blood vessel walls but are absent in the intervillous space or on the syncytiotrophoblast cells. Therefore, these DS/CSPGs are not accessible for IRBC interactions.

The IRBC-binding ability of the purified placental CSPG was assessed by an *in vitro* cytoadherence assay (Fig. 2). Of the two CSPG types of the human placenta that are accessible for IRBC interactions, the extracellular CSPG and cell surface CSPGs, it is the former, despite being extremely low sulfated, that efficiently binds IRBCs in a concentration-dependent manner (Achur *et al.*, 2000). Treatment of the CSPG-coated plates with chondroitinase ABC or testicular hyaluronidase completely abolished the IRBC binding, whereas treatment with *Streptomyces hyalurolyticus* hyaluronidase or heparitinase had no effect, indicating that the CS chains of the CSPG mediate the IRBC adhesion. Consistent with this conclusion, the IRBC binding to the CSPG is efficiently inhibited by C4S, and the inhibition is dose dependent (Fig. 3). In contrast, C6S, HA, HS, heparin, dextran sulfate, or pentosan polysulfate are noninhibitory. From these data, it is evident that the placental IRBCs have strict specificity to C4S. The cell-associated CSPGs of the placenta can also bind IRBCs, but their IRBC-binding capacity is significantly lower than that of the extracellular low-sulfated CSPG (Achur *et al.*, 2000). Therefore, the low-sulfated CSPG, being accessible for IRBCs and able to strongly bind IRBCs, functions as the major receptors for IRBC adherence in the placenta (also see discussion in a later section).

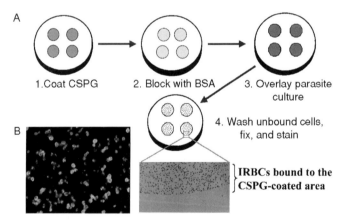

FIGURE 2 (A) Schematic diagram illustrating the various steps of the *in vitro* cytoadherence assay used for assessing the binding of IRBCs to CSPG coated onto plastic Petri dishes. The CSPG solutions (10–15 µl at 10–400 ng/ml in PBS) are spotted as 4 mm spots, blocked with 2% BSA in PBS, overlaid with parasite culture. The unbound cells washed off with PBS, and bound cells are fixed, stained with Giemsa, and photographed under a microscope. (B) Photograph under a microscope, showing the binding of IRBCs prestained with SYBR Green to CSPG-coated plates. (See Color Insert.)

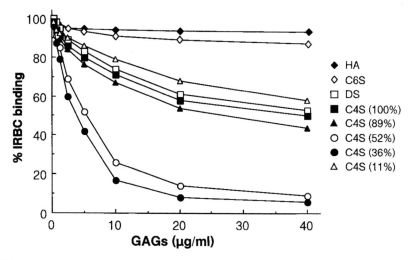

FIGURE 3 Inhibition of IRBC binding to the human placental low-sulfated CSPG coated onto plastic plates by various GAGs. The assay was performed as described by Alkhalil *et al.* (2000). The level of 4-sulfated disaccharides in the partially sulfated C4S is indicated in the parenthesis; the reminder represents nonsulfated disaccharides.

VIII. CSPG Receptor for IRBC Adhesion is Localized in the Intervillous Space of the Placenta

In *P. falciparum*-infected placentas, the IRBCs sequester predominantly in the intervillous space (Fig. 1). Immunohistochemical analysis of the placental tissue sections, using antibodies specific to the core proteins of the placental PGs, showed strong staining in the intervillous space and weak but significant staining on the syncytiotrophoblast surface (Muthusamy *et al.*, 2004b). The staining was abolished upon prior treatment of the tissue sections with chondroitinase ABC. Immunohistochemical analysis using monoclonal antibodies against the unsaturated disaccharide motifs, formed on the core saccharides at the GAG chain-attachment sites, upon treatment of CSPG with chondroitinase ABC, showed that anti-Δdi-4S antibody but not anti-Δdi-6S antibody could strongly stain the intervillous space and to a lesser degree the syncytiotrophoblast surface (Muthusamy *et al.*, 2004b). Mild washing of the unfixed, frozen placental tissue sections with isotonic buffers completely washed off the low-sulfated CSPG with concomitant abolition of the antibody staining in the intervillous space. Based on these data, it was concluded that the low-sulfated CSPG is localized mainly in the intervillous space. Firm evidence for the intervillous space CSPG being the placental IRBC receptor came from colocalization of the CSPG and IRBC adherence (Muthusamy *et al.*, 2004b). Analysis of IRBC binding to the fixed placental tissue sections showed that IRBCs adhered at high density in the intervillous space and at low levels on the syncytiotrophoblasts. The IRBC adherence was C4S dependent, since the tissue sections pretreated with chondroitinase ABC were unable to bind IRBCs and the adherence of IRBCs was inhibited by soluble C4S. This *ex vivo* IRBC adherence pattern closely resembled the distribution pattern of low-sulfated CSPGs in the placenta as observed by immunohistochemical analysis. Dual immunofluorescence staining of the endogenous RBCs and the low-sulfated CSPG and *ex vivo* IRBC adherence on the same tissue section using prestained IRBCs with SYBR Green colocalized the low-sulfated CSPG and the adhered IRBCs, mainly in the intervillous space and at low levels on the syncytiotrophoblasts (Muthusamy *et al.*, 2004b). The distribution patterns of CSPG and *ex vivo*-adhered IRBCs were similar to the pattern of IRBC adherence in *P. falciparum*-infected placentas, that is, predominantly in the intervillous space and at low but significant levels on the syncytiotrophoblast lining (Fig. 1B). Thus, it has been established that the low-sulfated CSPG is localized to intervillous space and is the major receptors for IRBC adherence in human placenta.

IX. Structural Requirement for the IRBC Adherence to Human Placental CSPG Receptor

The structural interactions involved in IRBC adhesion to the CS chains of the placental CSPG receptor have been determined by inhibition analysis using CS with varying sulfation pattern (Alkhalil *et al.*, 2000; Beeson *et al.*, 1998; Chai *et al.*, 2002; Fried *et al.*, 2000; Fusai *et al.*, 2000; Maubert *et al.*, 1997). A comparative analysis of a fully sulfated C4S from sturgeon notochord and two C4S/C6S copolymers from bovine trachea and whale cartilage was carried out. The two C4S/C6S tested were about 2.5-fold more efficient in inhibiting IRBC adhesion to placental CSPG compared to the fully 4-sulfated CS (Alkhalil *et al.*, 2000). This is despite the fact that the C4S/C6S copolymers have significant levels of 6-sulfate groups. Since the C4 hydroxyl groups of the 6-sulfated GalNAc residues in the bovine tracheal and whale cartilage C4S/C6S are not substituted, it appears that the 6-sulfated disaccharides with free hydroxyl groups at C4 of GalNAc essentially function as non-4-sulfated disaccharide residues in binding IRBCs (Alkhalil *et al.*, 2000). Based on these data, it was inferred that the IRBC adhesion involves the participation of both 4-sulfated and non-4-sulfated disaccharides of the C4S chains (Alkhalil *et al.*, 2000). When the 6-sulfate groups of the bovine tracheal and whale cartilage CS were completely removed by regioselective 6-O-desulation, the inhibitory capacities of the CS were significantly increased (Alkhalil *et al.*, 2000; Fried *et al.*, 2000), suggesting that either the C6 sulfate groups sterically interfere with IRBC binding to a certain degree or the C6 hydroxyl groups of GalNAc are involved in binding.

To determine the level of 4-sulfate groups required for optimal IRBC binding by partially sulfated C4S, Alkhalil *et al.* (2000) prepared a series of partially sulfated C4S containing 3–89% sulfate groups and measured their ability to bind IRBCs. Of these C4S tested, only those that had 30–52% 4-sulfate groups could maximally inhibit IRBC binding to placental CSPG, whereas C4S containing 3–11% or >80% sulfate groups were less inhibitory (Fig. 3, and not shown).

Gowda and coworkers (unpublished results) have studied the role of various functional groups of CS in IRBC binding to placental CSPG. To assess the role of N-acetyl groups in IRBC binding, the acetyl groups of bovine tracheal CS were replaced by the N-propionyl, N-butyryl, N-hexanoyl, or N-benzoyl groups and tested for inhibition of IRBC binding to placental CSPG. The inhibitory capacity of each derivative was similar to that of the unmodified bovine tracheal CS, demonstrating that the N-acetyl groups of the GalNAc residues of C4S are not involved in IRBC adherence. Conversion of more than >65% of the carboxyl groups of the bovine tracheal CS into primary hydroxyl groups resulted in the complete loss of inhibitory activity, whereas the CS in which ~15% carboxyl groups were reduced was almost fully active. The CS in which ~50% carboxyl groups were reduced has retained only 30–40% of the inhibitory activity. Gowda and coworkers (unpublished results) also studied the inhibitory activities of partially sulfated C4S (carboxyl groups equatorially disposed) with sulfate content ranging from 30–60% and compared with those of DS (carboxyl groups axially oriented) with similar sulfate content. In each case, the inhibitory activity of DS was about 50% less than the C4S with similar sulfate content. Thus, it was demonstrated that the carboxyl groups of C4S are critical for IRBC binding.

X. Minimum C4S Structural Motif Involved in the IRBC Adherence to Placental CSPG

To determine the minimum C4S-chain length involved in IRBC binding, oligosaccharides of varying sizes, prepared by enzymatic digestion of CS, have been tested for the inhibition of IRBC binding. Using oligosaccharides formed by chondroitinase ABC digestion of bovine tracheal CS, Beeson *et al.* (1998) reported that a tetradecasaccharide is the minimum structural motif required, whereas Pouvelle *et al.* (1998) found that oligosaccharides with eighteen or nineteen disaccharides were required for efficient inhibition of IRBC adherence. However, Alkhalil *et al.* (2000) tested oligosaccharides of various sizes, prepared by testicular hyaluronidase digestion of CS from three different sources, and showed that a dodecasaccharide (six disaccharide units) is the minimum motif required for maximum inhibition of

IRBC adherence to the placental CSPG (Fig. 4). Subsequently, Chai *et al.* (2002) confirmed that the dodecasaccharide is the minimum chain length needed for IRBC binding. Furthermore, Alkhalil *et al.* (2000), by evaluating the inhibitory activity of C4S dodecasaccharides containing different sulfate contents, demonstrated that oligosaccharides with two or three sulfate groups have higher inhibitory capacity than those with either one or more than three sulfate groups. In contrast to this finding, Chai *et al.* (2002) reported that five sulfate groups are required for the maximal interaction of C4S dodecasaccharides with IRBCs. However, it is not clear whether the dodecasaccharide used by Chai *et al.* (2002) was exclusively 4-sulfated or it contained one or more 6-sulfated groups in addition to the 4-sulfate groups. Since bovine tracheal CS was used in their study, it is possible that the tested oligosaccharides contained significant levels of 6-sulfate groups and the actual 4-sulfate content is considerably low. This controversy was addressed, and it was found that two or three 4-sulfate groups within the dodecasaccharide minimal structural motif are sufficient for optimal binding of IRBCs (Achur and Gowda, unpublished results).

The requirement of a C4S motif with six disaccharides for efficient binding suggests that a conformational structure is involved in IRBC adherence. In solution, C4S exists as a left-handed, single stranded helix with three disaccharides per turn (Cael *et al.*, 1978). Therefore, the dodecasaccharide motif of C4S corresponds to two turns of the helical conformation. Since 4-sulfated and 4-nonsulfated disaccharides in the ratios of 1:1–1:2 are required for efficient interaction with IRBCs, it appears that a specific distribution

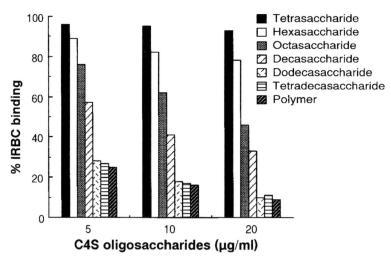

FIGURE 4   Inhibition of IRBC binding to the human placental low-sulfated CSPG coated onto plastic plates by C4S oligosaccharides of varying sizes. The assay was performed as described by Alkhalil *et al.* (2000).

pattern of the sulfate groups in a conformational structure involving the interaction of several structural elements within each turn of the two helices of the dodecasaccharide motif is involved in IRBC binding.

XI. Distribution of Sulfated Disaccharide Residues in the CS Chains of Placental CSPG

Given that a minimum of two 4-sulfate groups in a dodecasaccharide motif of the C4S is required for optimal binding of IRBCs and that the CS chains of placental CSPG contain only 2–14% sulfate groups (Achur et al., 2003; Alkhalil et al., 2000), it is clear that the sulfate groups in the placental CS chains are clustered at certain regions at a density of at least two 4-sulfated disaccharides per dodecasaccharide motif. To determine whether this is the case, Achur et al. (2003) have studied the distribution of sulfate groups in the CS chains of the placental CSPG receptor. The CS chains of placental CSPGs were prepared and digested with Streptococcus dysgalactiae hyaluronidase, an endo-β-N-acetylhexosaminyl lyase that preferentially acts on the nonsulfated regions of the partially sulfated CS chains. The enzyme converted 80–90% of the CS chains into nonsulfated di- and tetrasaccharides and the remainder into larger oligosaccharides (Achur et al., 2003). Size and disaccharide compositional analyses indicated that the majority of larger oligosaccharides were 6–14 disaccharide moieties in length, consisting of 20–28% 4-sulfated and 72–80% nonsulfated disaccharide repeating residues. These results indicated that the majority of sulfate groups in the CS chains of the placental CSPGs are distributed such that certain regions of the polysaccharide have ~28% 4-sulfated disaccharide units and the other regions contain a few or no sulfate groups. IRBC-adhesion inhibition analysis demonstrated that the oligosaccharides corresponding to the sulfate group-clustered domains of the placental CS chains could efficiently inhibit IRBC binding to placental CSPG. The inhibitory capacity of the oligosaccharides of the placental CS chain was comparable to that of the C4S with 36% 4-sulfated disaccharides. Together, the above results indicate that the sulfate groups in the CS chains of placental CSPGs are uniquely distributed and that these sulfate-clustered domains provide the necessary structural elements for the efficient adhesion of IRBCs, even though the CS chains have overall a low degree of sulfation (Achur et al., 2003).

XII. Low-Sulfated Placental CSPG is Expressed Throughout the Second and Third Trimester

In malaria endemic areas, the prevalence of P. falciparum infection in pregnant women peaks during 13–20 weeks of gestation (Brabin, 1983). This peak prevalence corresponds to the period when IRBCs accumulate heavily in the placenta. These observations imply that receptors for IRBC adhesion in the placenta are expressed early during the pregnancy. Agbor-Enoh *et al.* (2003) have studied the expression pattern of CSPG in the intervillous space of the placenta during the course of pregnancy. The extracellular CSPG has been purified from placentas at 16, 24, 28, 33, and 38 weeks of gestation, structurally characterized and IRBC-adherence characteristics studied. The low-sulfated CSPG was found to be present in the intervillous space at all gestational ages studied. The level of CSPG expressed per unit tissue weight was similar in placentas of various gestational ages and were comparable to the levels of low-sulfated CSPG in the term placentas. The structural features of the CS chains of the CSPG purified from placentas of different gestational ages were similar to those of the term placentas, comprising 4–10% 4-sulfated and 96–90% nonsulfated disaccharide moieties (Agbor-Enoh *et al.*, 2003). The molecular size of the CSPG decreases with increased gestational age. However, the IRBC-binding capacity of the CSPGs isolated from placentas of different gestational ages was similar to that of the CSPG purified from term placentas. These results indicate that the low-sulfated CSPG is available for IRBC adherence in the placenta during the entire second and third trimesters of gestation. However, the observed peak prevalence of placental malaria corresponds to the period when the host immune response is still developing, and the parasites grow unhindered.

XIII. Presence of C4S-IRBC Antiadhesion Antibodies in Pregnant Women in Malaria Endemic Areas

In malaria endemic areas, the rate of *P. falciparum* infection in pregnant women starts declining in the weeks following the peak-prevalence period (Brabin, 1983; Zhou *et al.*, 2002). Given that the CSPG receptor for IRBC adherence is expressed at high levels throughout the second and third trimesters (Agbor-Enoh *et al.*, 2003) and that placenta rapidly develops during these periods, the observed decline in parasite prevalence after 20 weeks of gestation is not due to a decrease in the level of the CSPG receptor in the placenta. Moreover, in malaria endemic areas, nonpregnant women have acquired protective immunity to *P. falciparum* malaria and thus are resistant to severe malaria in a manner similar to their male counterparts (Brabin, 1983). However, women during pregnancy are generally at higher risk of malaria, and the risk is greatest during the first pregnancy, deceasing with subsequent pregnancies (Brabin, 1983). Fried *et al.* (1998) have shown that sera from pregnant women from different malaria endemic countries (Kenya, Malawi and Thailand) inhibit IRBC adherence to immobilized C4S and to placental tissue sections. These investigators also found that the C4S-IRBC adherence inhibitory antibodies were absent in males and women who were not previously pregnant. Antiadhesion antibodies were also absent in the sera of people from malaria-free regions. Subsequently, several studies (Beeson *et al.*, 1999, 2004; Gysin *et al.*, 1999; Maubert *et al.*, 1999; O'Neil-Dune *et al.*, 2001; Ricke *et al.*, 2000; Staalsoe *et al.*, 2001), using sera from different endemic regions, showed that most pregnant women have IRBC-C4S adhesion inhibitory antibodies at term, and the antibodies are produced in a gender-specific manner, substantiating the findings of Fried *et al.* (1998).

In pregnant women, the antiC4S-IRBC adhesion antibodies are produced differentially in a gravidity status-specific manner. It appears that in highly endemic areas, the majority of pregnant women at term contain antiadhesion antibodies, and the adhesion inhibitory activity of sera from certain primigravidae at term is comparable to that of sera from multigravidae (O'Neil-Dunne *et al.*, 2001). This observation appears to contradict, at first glance, the finding that primigravidae are highly susceptible while multigravidae are relatively resistant to placental malaria. However, as discussed below, the differential disposition of primigravidae and multigravidae to placental malaria appears to be related to, at least in part, the efficiency with which the antibodies are produced during the early stage of pregnancy. O'Neil-Dunne *et al.* (2001) have showed that antibodies are usually absent in all pregnant women prior to 12 weeks of gestation, regardless of gravidity, and that antibodies are produced during pregnancy in the majority of *P. falciparum*-infected pregnant women. Analysis of sera from pregnant women at different stages of pregnancy showed that primigravidae and multigravidae differentially produce antiadhesion antibodies during pregnancy. Primigravidae lacked antibodies prior to 20 weeks of pregnancy and began producing antibodies during 20–24 weeks of gestation. In contrast, multigravidae lacked antibodies until 12 weeks of pregnancy and produced antibodies during 12–16 weeks of gestation, significantly earlier than primigravidae. After 20 weeks of gestation, there was no significant difference in the levels of antibodies between primigravidae and multigravidae. This pregnancy stage-dependent differential antibody response is likely due to the pre-existing memory of an antiadhesion antibody response in multigravidae acquired during earlier pregnancies and the lack of such a memory response in primigravidae. The differential kinetics of this antibody response appears, at least in part, to contribute to the gravidity-dependent differential susceptibilities to pregnancy-associated malaria.

The differences in kinetics of the antiadhesion antibody responses also explain the previously observed difference in the prevalence of *P. falciparum* infection during pregnancy in primigravidae and multigravidae (Brabin, 1983). In highly endemic areas, peak prevalence of *P. falciparum* infection occurs during 13–16 weeks of pregnancy both in primigravidae and multigravidae. Thereafter, the prevalence of parasites rapidly declines in multigravidae but persists, at peak levels, until around 20 weeks in primigravidae (Brabin, 1983). However, the rate of parasite clearance during the third trimester is similar in these two groups. Therefore, the peak prevalence of parasite infection and the differential recovery during the second trimester of primigravidae and multigravidae correspond to the periods when both populations lacked antiadhesion antibodies. The subsequent comparable rate of recovery from infection during the third trimester relates to the similar levels of antibodies in either group.

The sera from pregnant women in different geographical areas can inhibit C4S-IRBC adherence, regardless of whether IRBCs are from C4S-adherent laboratory cultured parasites or from infected placenta of women in different endemic areas. This indicates the expression of a common, well-conserved parasite adhesive protein or a limited set of variant adhesive proteins in genetically different strains of the C4S-adherent parasites. The ability of antibodies to inhibit IRBC adherence shows a causal relationship between IRBC adherence in the placenta and placental pathology. Consistent with this conclusion, it has been reported that antiadhesion antibodies are associated with normal birth weight and better survival of the newborns (Beeson et al., 2004; Duffy and Fried, 2003a; Staalsoe et al., 2004; Taylor et al., 2004). These findings and other accumulated evidence support the idea that the C4S-IRBC adherence step is an effective target for the development of therapeutics and/or a vaccine.

XIV. P. falciparum Adhesive Protein that Mediates IRBC Adherence to the Placental CSPG

Although information on the P. falciparum adhesive protein expressed on the IRBC surface that mediates C4S-dependent binding of IRBCs in human placenta represents an important aspect of placental malaria, discussion about the parasite protein is beyond the scope of this chapter. The readers are referred to recently published reviews (Beeson and Brown, 2002; Duffy and Fried, 2003b; Gowda et al., 2004; Rowe and Kyes, 2004; Scherf et al., 2001; Sherman et al., 2003; Smith and Deitisch, 2004).

XV. Conclusions

After the discovery in 1996 that a subpopulation of P. falciparum IRBCs binds C4S and this phenomenon is involved in IRBC adherence in human placenta, various studies have conclusively demonstrated that placental IRBC adherence is mediated by C4S. These include: (i) identification, structural characterization, and localization of the placental low-sulfated CSPG and its ability to efficiently bind IRBCs; (ii) comprehensive studies on the structure and IRBC binding activity of C4S; (iii) the discovery that pregnant women produce C4S-IRBC antiadhesion antibodies in a gender- and gravidity-specific manner and that the presence of high levels of these antibodies provide protection against placental malaria-associated poor pregnancy outcomes.

Regarding the C4S structure–activity relationship, several critical C4S structural elements involved in IRBC binding are known, but much more remains to be understood. For example, although it is known that a C4S dodecasaccharide with two 4-sulfate groups is the motif involved in IRBC adherence, the precise location of 4-sulfated disaccharide moieties within the oligosaccharide is not known. Fifteen different structures are possible for a dodecasaccharide with two 4-sulfated and four non-4-sulfated disaccharide moieties variously distributed. Determining which one of those structures can maximally bind IRBCs is challenging. For example, separation of the various oligosaccharides from a mixture of dodecasaccharides formed by enzymatic degradations of C4S is almost impossible. An alternative synthetic approach will also be a daunting task. However, the knowledge that has already been gained regarding the structural interactions involved in IRBC binding offers valuable insight into efforts aimed at developing novel therapeutics based on C4S oligosaccharides or peptide mimetics for treating pregnancy-associated malaria.

Compared to the definitive information known about the CSPG receptor and many C4S structural interactions involved in IRBC adhesion, the identity of the parasite-adhesive protein remains unclear. Although it is widely believed that PfEMP1 encoded by one or more *var* genes mediates IRBC binding to placental CSPG, unequivocal evidence is lacking. It is possible that PfEMP1 is the parasite adhesive protein, but direct biochemical evidence is needed to conclusively show that PfEMP1 is the CSPG ligand on the IRBC surface. Considering the intensity of ongoing efforts in various laboratories around the world, it is hoped that definitive answers will be soon forthcoming, thus offering strategies for the development of therapeutics and/or a vaccine for pregnancy-associated malaria.

Acknowledgments

I would like to thank Dr Abdulnaser Alkhalil and Deborah Tomazin for the artwork, Figs. 2 and 1A, respectively, Drs Rajeshwara Achur and Arivalagan Muthusamy for their help in the preparation of Figs. 1, 3, and 4 and manuscript, Dr Diane Taylor, Georgetown University, for a photograph of the malaria-infected placental tissue section (Fig. 1B), National Institute of Allergy and Infectious Diseases, National Institutes of Health for grant support AI 45086 for the work done in my laboratory.

References

Achur, R. N., Valiyaveettil, M., Alkhalil, A., Ockenhouse, C. F., and Gowda, D. C. (2000). Characterization of proteoglycans of human placenta and identification of unique chondroitin sulfate proteoglycans of the intervillous spaces that mediate the adherence of *Plasmodium falciparum*-infected erythrocytes to the placenta. *J. Biol. Chem.* **275**, 40344–40356.

Achur, R. N., Valiyaveettil, M., and Gowda, D. C. (2003). The low sulfated chondroitin sulfate proteoglycans of human placenta have sulfate group-clustered domains that can efficiently bind *Plasmodium falciparum*-infected erythrocytes. *J. Biol. Chem.* **278**, 11705–11713.

Agbor-Enoh, S. T., Achur, R. N., Valiyaveettil, M., Taylor, D. W., and Gowda, D. C. (2003). Chondroitin sulfate proteoglycan expression and binding of *Plasmodium falciparum*-infected erythrocytes in the human placenta during pregnancy. *Infect. Immun.* **71**, 2455–2461.

Alkhalil, A., Achur, R. N., Valiyaveettil, M., Ockenhouse, C. F., and Gowda, D. C. (2000). Structural requirements for the adherence of *Plasmodium falciparum*-infected erythrocytes to chondroitin sulfate proteoglycans of human placenta. *J. Biol. Chem.* **275**, 40357–40364.

Artavanis-Tsakonas, K., Tongren, J. E., and Riley, E. M. (2003). The war between the malaria parasite and the immune system: Immunity, immunoregulation and immunopathology. *Clin. Exp. Immunol.* **133**, 145–152.

Baird, J. K. (1995). Host age as a determinant of naturally acquired immunity to *Plasmodium falciparum* malaria. *Parasitol. Today* **11**, 105–111.

Banfield, B. W., Leduc, Y., Esford, L., Schubert, K., and Tufaro, F. (1995). Evidence for an interaction of herpes simplex virus with chondroitin sulfate proteoglycans during infection. *J. Virol.* **69**, 3290–3298.

Baruch, D. I., Gormely, J. A., Ma, C., Howard, R. J., and Pasloske, B. L. (1996). *Plasmodium falciparum* erythrocyte membrane protein 1 is a parasitized erythrocyte receptor for adherence to CD36, thrombospondin, and intercellular adhesion molecule-1. *Proc. Natl. Acad. Sci. USA* **93**, 3497–3502.

Baruch, D. I., Pasloske, B. L., Singh, H. B., Bi, X., Ma, X. C., Feldman, M., Taraschi, T. F., and Howard, R. J. (1995). Cloning the *P. falciparum* gene encoding PfEMP1, a malarial variant antigen and adherence receptor on the surface of parasitized human erythrocytes. *Cell* **82**, 77–87.

Beeson, J. G., and Brown, G. V. (2002). Pathogenesis of *Plasmodium falciparum* malaria: The roles of parasite adhesion and antigenic variation. *Cell. Mol. Life Sci.* **59**, 258–271.

Beeson, J. G., and Brown, G. V. (2004). *Plasmodium falciparum*-infected erythrocytes demonstrate dual specificity for adhesion to hyaluronic acid and chondroitin sulfate A and have distinct adhesive properties. *J. Infect. Dis.* **189**, 169–179.

Beeson, J. G., Amin, N., Kanjala, M., and Rogerson, S. J. (2002). Selective accumulation of mature asexual stages of *Plasmodium falciparum*-infected erythrocytes in the placenta. *Infect. Immun.* **70**, 5412–5415.

Beeson, J. G., Brown, G. V., Molyneux, M. E., Mhango, C., Dzinjalamala, F., and Rogerson, S. J. (1999). *Plasmodium falciparum* isolates from infected pregnant women and children are associated with distinct adhesive and antigenic properties. *J. Infect. Dis.* **180**, 464–472.

Beeson, J. G., Chai, W., Rogerson, S. J., Lawson, A. M., and Brown, G. V. (1998). Inhibition of binding of malaria-infected erythrocytes by a tetradecasaccharide fraction from chondroitin sulfate A. *Infect. Immun.* **66**, 3397–3402.

Beeson, J. G., Mann, E. J., Elliott, S. R., Lema, V. M., Tadesse, E., Molyneux, M. E., Brown, G. V., and Rogerson, S. J. (2004). Antibodies to variant surface antigens of *Plasmodium falciparum*-infected erythrocytes and adhesion inhibitory antibodies are associated with placental malaria and have overlapping and distinct targets. *J. Infect. Dis.* **189**, 540–551.

Bhavanadan, V. P., and Davidson, E. A. (1992). Proteoglycans: Structure, synthesis, function. *In* "Glycoconjugates" (H. J. Allen and E. C. Kissilus, Eds.), pp. 167–202. Marcel Dekker, Inc., New York.

Borst, P., Bitter, W., McCulloch, R., Van Leeuwen, F., and Rudenko, G. (1995). Antigenic variation in malaria. *Cell* **82**, 1–4.

Brabin, B. J. (1983). An analysis of malaria in pregnancy in Africa. *Bull. WHO* **61**, 1005–1016.

Brabin, B., and Rogerson, S. (2001). The epidemiology and outcome of maternal malaria. *In* "Malaria in Pregnancy: Deadly Parasite, Susceptible Host" (P. E. Duffy and M. Fried, Eds.), pp. 27–51. Taylor and Francis, New York, NY.

Brabin, B. J., Romagosa, C., Abdelgalil, S., Menendez, C., Verhoeff, F. H., McGready, R., Fletcher, K. A., Owens, S., D'Alessandro, U., Nosten, F., Fischer, P. R., and Ordi, J. (2004). The sick placenta-the role of malaria. *Placenta* **25**, 359–378.

Bull, P. C., and Marsh, K. (2002). The role of antibodies to *Plasmodium falciparum*-infected-erythrocyte surface antigens in naturally acquired immunity to malaria. *Trends Microbiol.* **10**, 55–58.

Bull, P. C., Lowe, B. S., Kortok, M., Molyneux, C. S., Newbold, C. I., Marsh, K., Parasite Giha, H. A., Staalsoe, T., Dodoo, D., Roper, C., Satti, G. M., Arnot, D. E., *et al.* (1998). Overlapping antigens on the infected red cell surface are targets for naturally acquired immunity to malaria. *Nat. Med.* **4**, 358–360.

Cael, J. J., Winter, W. T., and Arnott, S. (1978). Calcium chondroitin 4-sulfate: Modular conformation and organization of polysaccharide chains in proteoglycan. *J. Mol. Biol.* **125**, 21–42.

Carruthers, V. B., Håkansson, S., Giddings, O. K., and Sibley, L. D. (2000). *Toxoplasma gondii* uses sulfated proteoglycans for substrate and host cell attachment. *Infect. Immun.* **68**, 4005–4011.

Chai, W., Beeson, J. G., Kogelberg, H., Brown, G. V., and Lawson, A. M. (2001). Inhibition of adhesion of *Plasmodium falciparum*-infected erythrocytes by structurally defined hyaluronic acid dodecasaccharides. *Infect. Immun.* **69**, 420–425.

Chai, W., Beeson, J. G., and Lawson, A. M. (2002). The structural motif in chondroitin sulfate for adhesion of *Plasmodium falciparum*-infected erythrocytes comprises disaccharide units of 4-*O*-sulfated and non-sulfated *N*-acetylgalactosamine linked to glucuronic acid. *J. Biol. Chem.* **277**, 22438–22446.

Chaiyaroj, S. C., Angkasekwinai, P., Buranakiti, A., Looareesuwan, S., Rogerson, S. J., and Brown, G. V. (1996). Cytoadherence characteristics of *Plasmodium falciparum* isolates from Thailand: Evidence for chondroitin sulfate A as a cytoadherence receptor. *Am. J. Trop. Med. Hyg.* **55**, 76–80.

Chaiyaroj, S. C., Coppel, R. L., Novakovic, S., and Brown, G. V. (1994). Multiple ligands for cytoadherence are present on the surface of *P. falciparum*-infected erythrocytes. *Proc. Natl. Acad. Sci. USA* **91**, 10805–10808.

Cooke, B. M., Rogerson, S. J., Brown, G. V., and Coppel, R. L. (1996). Adhesion of malaria-infected red blood cells to chondroitin sulfate A under flow conditions. *Blood* **88**, 4040–4044.

Crocker, I. P., Tanner, O. M., Myers, J. E., Bulmer, J. N., Walraven, G., and Baker, P. N. (2004). Syncytiotrophoblast degradation and the pathophysiology of the malaria-infected placenta. *Placenta* **25**, 2732–2782.

Day, K. P., and Marsh, K. (1991). Naturally acquired immunity to *Plasmodium falciparum*. *Parasitol. Today* **7**, 68–71.

Duffy, P. E. (2001). Immunity to malaria during pregnancy: Different host, different parasite. *In* "Malaria in Pregnancy: Deadly Parasite, Susceptible Host" (P. E. Duffy and M. Fried, Eds.), pp. 71–125. Taylor and Francis, New York, NY.

Duffy, P. E., and Desowitz, R. S. (2001). Pregnancy malaria throughout history: Dangerous labors. *In* "Malaria in Pregnancy: Deadly parasite, Susceptible Host" (P. E. Duffy and M. Fried, Eds.), pp. 1–25. Taylor and Francis, New York, NY.

Duffy, P. E., and Fried, M. (1999). Malaria during pregnancy: Parasites, antibodies and chondroitin sulphate A. *Biochem. Soc. Trans.* **27**, 478–482.

Duffy, P. E., and Fried, M. (2003a). Antibodies that inhibit *P. falciparum* adhesion to chondroitin sulfate A are associated with increased birth weight and the gestational age of newborns. *Infect. Immun.* **71**, 6620–6623.

Duffy, P. E., and Fried, M. (2003b). *Plasmodium falciparum* adherence in the placenta. *Curr. Opin. Microbiol.* **6**, 371–376.

Fried, M. (2001). Parasite adhesion and its role in placental malaria: Hideout of the parasite. *In* "Malaria in Pregnancy: Deadly Parasite, Susceptible Host" (P. E. Duffy and M. Fried, Eds.), pp. 159–187. Taylor and Francis, New York, NY.

Frick, I. M., Schmidtchen, A., and Sjobring, U. (2003). Interactions between M proteins of *Streptococcus pyogenes* and glycosaminoglycans promote bacterial adhesion to host cells. *Eur. J. Biochem.* **270**, 2303–2311.

Fried, M., and Duffy, P. E. (1996). Adherence of *Plasmodium falciparum* to chondroitin sulfate A in the human placenta. *Science* **271**, 1502–1504.

Fried, M., and Duffy, P. E. (1998). Maternal malaria and parasite adhesion. *J. Mol. Med.* **76**, 162–171.

Fried, M., Lauder, R. M., and Duffy, P. E. (2000). *Plasmodium falciparum*: Adhesion of placental isolates modulated by the sulfation characteristics of the glycosaminoglycan receptor. *Exp. Parasitol.* **95**, 75–78.

Fried, M., Nosten, F., Brockman, A., Brabin, B. J., and Duffy, P. E. (1998). Maternal antibodies block malaria. *Nature* **395**, 851–852.

Fusai, T., Parzy, D., Spillmann, D., Eustacchio, F., Pouvelle, B., Lepolard, C., Scherf, A., and Gysin, J. (2000). Characterisation of the chondroitin sulphate of Saimiri brain microvascular endothelial cells involved in *Plasmodium falciparum* cytoadhesion. *Mol. Biochem. Parasitol.* **108**, 25–37.

Gardner, J. P., Pinches, R. A., Roberts, D. J., and Newbold, C. I. (1996). Variant antigens and endothelial receptor adhesion in *Plasmodium falciparum*. *Proc. Natl. Acad. Sci. USA* **93**, 3503–3508.

Gatton, M. L., Peters, J. M., Fowler, E. V., and Cheng, Q. (2003). Switching rates of *Plasmodium falciparum var* genes: Faster than we thought? *Trends Parasitol.* **19**, 202–208.

Greenwood, B., and Mutabingwa, T. (2002). Malaria in 2002. *Nature* **415**, 670–672.

Giha, H. A., Staalsoe, T., Dodoo, D., Roper, C., Satti, G. M., Arnot, D. E., Hviid, L., and Theander, T. G. (2000). Antibodies to variable *Plasmodium falciparum*-infected erythrocyte surface antigens are associated with protection from novel malaria infections. *Immunol. Lett.* **7**, 117–126.

Giha, H. A., Staalsoe, T., Dodoo, D., Elhassan, I. M., Roper, C., Satti, G. M., Arnot, D. E., Hviid, L., and Theander, T. G. (1999). Overlapping antigenic repertoires of variant antigens expressed on the surface of erythrocytes infected by *Plasmodium falciparum*. *Parasitology* **119**(Part 1), 7–17.

Gilles, H. M. and Warrell, D. A. (Eds.) (1997). "Bruce-Chawatt's Essential Malariology", pp. 1–340. Arnold Publishers, London.

Gowda, D. C., and Ockenhouse, C. F. (1999). Adherence of *Plasmodium falciparum*-infected erythrocytes to chondroitin sulfate. *Bioscience Rep.* **19**, 261–271.

Gowda, D. C., Achur, R., Muthusamy, A., and Takagaki, K. (2004). Unusually low-sulfated chondroitin sulfate of human placenta and its role in placental malaria. *Trends Glycosci. Glycotech.* **16**, 407–420.

Gysin, J., Pouvelle, B., Fievet, N., Scherf, A., and Lepolard, C. (1999). *Ex vivo* desequestration of *P. falciparum*-infected erythrocytes from human placenta by CSA. *Infect. Immun.* **67**, 6596–6602.

Gysin, J., Pouvelle, B., Tonqueze, M. L., Edelman, L., and Boffa, M.-C. (1997). Chondroitin sulfate of thrombomodulin is an adhesion receptor for *Plasmodium falciparum*-infected erythrocytes. *Mol. Biochem. Parasitol.* **88**, 267–271.

Heddini, A. (2002). Malaria pathogenesis: A jigsaw with an increasing number of pieces. *Int. J. Parasitol.* **32**, 1587–1598.

Heddini, A., Pettersson, F., Kai, O., Shafi, J., Obiero, J., Chen, Q., Barragan, A., Wahlgren, M., and Marsh, K. (2001). Fresh isolates from children with severe *Plasmodium falciparum* malaria bind to multiple receptors. *Infect. Immun.* **69**, 5849–5856.

Herold, B. C., Gerber, S. I., Polonsky, T., Belval, B. J., Shaklee, P. N., and Holme, K. (1995). Identification of structural features of heparin required for inhibition of herpes simplex virus type 1 binding. *Virology* **206**, 1108–1116.

Hommel, M. (1993). Amplification of cytoadherence in cerebral malaria: Towards a more rational explanation of disease. *Ann. Trop. Med. Parasitol.* **87**, 627–635.

Hviid, L. (1998). Clinical disease, immunity and protection against *Plasmodium falciparum* malaria in populations living in endemic areas. *Expert Rev. Mol. Med.* **24**, 1–10.

Ismail, M. R., Ordi, J., Menendez, C., Ventura, P. J., Aponte, J. J., Kahigwa, E., Hirt, R., Cardesa, A., and Alonso, P. L. (2000). Placental pathology in malaria: A histological, immunohistochemical, and quantitative study. *Hum. Pathol.* **31**, 85–93.

Jensen, A. T., Magistrado, P., Sharp, S., Joergensen, L., Lavstsen, T., Chiucchiuini, A., Salanti, A., Vestergaard, L. S., Lusingu, J. P., Hermsen, R., Sauerwein, R., Christensen, J., *et al.* (2004). *Plasmodium falciparum* associated with severe childhood malaria preferentially expresses PfEMP1 encoded by group A *var* genes. *J. Exp. Med.* **199**, 1179–1190.

Kjellen, L., and Lindahl, U. (1991). Proteoglycans: Structures and interactions. *Annu. Rev. Biochem.* **60**, 443–475.

Lima, A. P., Almeida, P. C., Tersariol, I. L., Schmitz, V., Schmaier, A. H., Juliano, L., Hirata, I. Y., Muller-Esterl, W., Chagas, J. R., and Scharfstein, J. (2002). Heparan sulfate modulates kinin release by *Trypanosoma cruzi* through the activity of cruzipain. *J. Biol. Chem.* **277**, 5875–5881.

Maubert, B., Fievet, N., Tami, G., Cot, M., Boudin, C., and Deloron,, P. (1999). Development of antibodies against chondroitin sulfate A-adherent *P. falciparum* in pregnant women. *Infect. Immun.* **67**, 5367–5371.

Maubert, B., Guilbert, L. J., and Deloron, P. (1997). Cytoadherence of *Plasmodium falciparum* to intercellular adhesion molecule 1 and chondroitin-4-sulfate expressed by the syncytio-trophoblast in the human placenta. *Infect. Immun.* **65**, 1251–1257.

Maubert, B., Fievet, N., Tami, G., Boudin, C., and Deloron, P. (2000). Cytoadherence of *Plasmodium falciparum*-infected erythrocytes in the human placenta. *Parasite Immunol.* **22**, 191–199.

McGregor, I. A., Wilson, M. E., and Billewicz, W. Z. (1983). Malaria infection of the placenta in The Gambia, West Africa; its incidence and relationship to still birth, birth weight and placental weight. *Trans. R. Soc. Trop. Med. Hyg.* **77**, 232–244.

Menendez, C. (1995). Malaria during pregnancy: A priority area of malaria research and control. *Parasitol. Today* **11**, 178–183.

Menendez, C., Ordi, J., Ismail, M. R., Ventura, P. J., Aponte, J. J., Kahigwa, E., Font, F., and Alonso, P. L. (2000). The impact of placental malaria on gestational age and birth weight. *J. Infect. Dis.* **181**, 1740–1745.

Miller, L. H., and Smith, J. D. (1998). Motherhood and malaria. *Nat. Med.* **4**, 1244–1245.

Miller, L. H., Baruch, D. I., Marsh, K., and Doumbo, O. K. (2002). The pathogenic basis of malaria. *Nature* **415**, 673–679.

Muthusamy, A., Achur, R. N., Valiyaveettil, M., and Gowda, D. C. (2004a). *Plasmodium falciparum*: Adherence of the parasite-infected erythrocytes to chondroitin sulfate proteoglycans bearing structurally distinct chondroitin sulfate chains. *Exp. Parasitol.* **107**, 183–188.

Muthusamy, A., Achur, R. N., Bhavanandan, V. P., Fouda, G. G., Taylor, D. W., and Gowda, D. C. (2004b). *Plasmodium falciparum*-infected erythrocytes adhere both in the intervillous space and on the villous surface of human placenta by binding to the low-sulfated chondroitin sulfate proteoglycan receptor. *Am. J. Pathol.* **164**, 2013–2025.

Noviyanti, R., and Brown, G. V. (2003). Phenotypic switching and *var* gene transcription in *Plasmodium falciparum*. *Adv. Exp. Med. Biol.* **531**, 149–159.

Ockenhouse, C. F., Tegoshi, T., Maeno, Y., Benjamin, C., Ho, M., Kan, K. E., Thway, Y., Win, K., Aikawa, M., and Lobb, R. R. (1992). Human vascular endothelial cell adhesion receptors for *Plasmodium falciparum*-infected erythrocytes: Roles for endothelial leukocyte adhesion molecule 1 and vascular cell adhesion molecule 1. *J. Exp. Med.* **176**, 1183–1189.

O'Neil-Dunne, I., Achur, R. N., Agbor-Enoh, S. T., Valiyaveettil, M., Naik, R. S., Ockenhouse, C. F., Zhou, A., Megnekou, R., Leke, R., Taylor, D. W., and Gowda, D. C. (2001). Gravidity-dependent production of antibodies that inhibit the binding of *Plasmodium falciparum*-infected erythrocytes to placental chondroitin sulfate proteoglycan during pregnancy. *Infect. Immun.* **69**, 7487–7492.

Ordi, J., Menendez, C., Ismail, M. R., Ventura, P. J., Palacin, A., Kahigwa, E., Ferrer, B., Cardesa, A., and Alonso, P. L. (2001). Placental malaria is associated with cell-mediated inflammatory responses with selective absence of natural killer cells. *J. Infect. Dis.* **183**, 1100–1107.

Pasloske, B. L., and Howard, R. J. (1994). Malaria, the red cell, and the endothelium. *Annu. Rev. Med.* **45**, 283–295.

Paget-McNicol, S., Gatton, M., Hastings, I., and Saul, A. (2002). The *Plasmodium falciparum var* gene switching rate, switching mechanism and patterns of parasite recrudescence described by mathematical modeling. *Parasitology* **124**(Part 3), 225–235.

Peters, J., Fowler, E., Gatton, M., Chen, N., Saul, A., and Cheng, Q. (2002). High diversity and rapid changeover of expressed *var* genes during the acute phase of *Plasmodium falciparum* infections in human volunteers. *Proc. Natl. Acad. Sci. USA* **99**, 10689–10694.

Pinzon-Ortiz, C., Friedman, J., Esko, J., and Sinnis, P. (2001). The binding of the circumsporozoite protein to cell surface heparan sulfate proteoglycans is required for plasmodium sporozoite attachment to target cells. *J. Biol. Chem.* **276**, 26784–26791.

Pouvelle, B., Fusai, T., Lepolard, C., and Gysin, J. (1998). Biological and biochemical characteristics of cytoadhesion of *Plasmodium falciparum*-infected erythrocytes to chondroitin-4-sulfate. *Infect. Immun.* **66**, 4950–4956.

Pradel, G., Garapaty, S., and Frevert, U. (2002). Proteoglycans mediate malaria sporozoite targeting to the liver. *Mol. Microbiol.* **45**, 637–651.

Ricke, C. H., Staalsoe, T., Koram, K., Akanmori, B. D., Riley, E. M., Theander, T. G., and Hviid, L. (2000). Plasma antibodies from malaria-exposed pregnant women recognize variant surface antigens on *Plasmodium falciparum*-infected erythrocytes in a parity-dependent manner and block parasite adhesion to chondroitin sulfate A. *J. Immunol.* **165**, 3309–3316.

Riley, E. M., Hviid, L., and Theander, T. G. (1994). Malaria. *In* "Parasite Infections and the Immune System" (F. Kierszenbaum, Ed.), pp. 119–143. Academic Press, New York, NY.

Roberts, D. J. (2003). Understanding naturally acquired immunity to *Plasmodium falciparum* malaria. *Infect. Immun.* **71**, 589–590.

Robert, C., Pouvelle, B., Meyer, P., Muanza, K., Fujioka, H., Aikawa, M., Scherf, A., and Gysin, J. (1995). Chondroitin-4-sulphate (proteoglycan), a receptor for *Plasmodium falciparum*-infected erythrocyte adherence on brain microvascular endothelial cells. *Res. Immunol.* **146**, 383–393.

Rogerson, S. J., and Brown, G. V. (1997). Chondroitin sulfate A as an adherence receptor for *Plasmodium falciparum* infected erythrocytes. *Parasitol. Today* **13**, 70–75.

Rogerson, S. J., Chiayaroj, S. C., Ng, K., Reeder, J. C., and Brown, G. V. (1995). Chondroitin sulfate A is a cell surface receptor for *Plasmodium falciparum*-infected erythrocytes. *J. Exp. Med.* **182**, 15–20.

Rogerson, S. J., Novakovic, S., Cooke, B. M., and Brown, G. V. (1997). *Plasmodium falciparum*-infected erythrocytes adhere to the proteoglycan thrombomodulin in static and flow-based systems. *Exp. Parasitol.* **86**, 8–18.

Rogerson, S. J., Pollina, E., Getachew, A., Tadesse, E., Lema, V. M., and Molyneux, M. E. (2003). Placental monocyte infiltrates in response to *Plasmodium falciparum* malaria infection and their association with adverse pregnancy outcomes. *Am. J. Trop. Med. Hyg.* **68**, 115–119.

Rostand, K. S., and Esko, J. D. (1997). Microbial adherence to and invasion through proteoglycans. *Infect. Immun.* **65**, 1–8.

Rowe, J. A., and Kyes, S. A. (2004). The role of *Plasmodium falciparum var* genes in malaria in pregnancy. *Mol. Microbiol.* **53**, 1011–1019.

Rowe, J. A., Moulds, J. M., Newbold, C. I., and Miller, L. H. (1997). *P. falciparum* rosetting mediated by a parasite-variant erythrocyte membrane protein and complement-receptor 1. *Nature* **388**, 292–295.

Sachs, J., and Malany, P. (2002). The economic and social burden of malaria. *Nature* **415**, 680–685.

Scherf, A., Pouvelle, B., Buffet, P. A., and Gysin, J. (2001). Molecular mechanisms of *Plasmodium falciparum* placental adhesion. *Cell. Microbiol.* **3**, 125–131.

Sherman, I. W. (Ed.) (1998). "Malaria: Parasite Biology, Pathogenesis, and Protection", pp. 1–575. ASM Press, Washington, DC.

Sherman, I. W., Eda, S., and Winograd, E. (2003). Cytoadherence and sequestration in *Plasmodium falciparum*: Defining the ties that bind. *Microbes Infect.* **5**, 897–909.

Smith, J. D., and Deitisch, K. W. (2004). Pregnancy-associated malaria and the prospects for syndrome-specific antimalaria vaccines. *J. Exp. Med.* **200**, 1093–1097.

Smith, J. D., Chitnis, C. E., Craig, A. G., Roberts, D. J., Hudson-Taylor, D. E., Peterson, D. S., Pinches, R., Newbold, C. I., and Miller, L. H. (1995). Switches in expression of *Plasmodium falciparum var* genes correlate with changes in antigenic and cytoadherent phenotypes of infected erythrocytes. *Cell* **82**, 101–110.

Smith, J. D., Subramanian, G., Gamain, B., Baruch, D. I., and Miller, L. H. (2000a). Classification of adhesive domains in the *Plasmodium falciparum* erythrocyte membrane protein 1 family. *Mol. Biochem. Parasitol.* **110**, 293–310.

Smith, J. D., Craig, A. G., Kriek, N., Hudson-Taylor, D., Kyes, S., Fagen, T., Pinches, R., Baruch, D. I., Newbold, C. I., and Miller, L. H. (2000b). Identification of a *Plasmodium falciparum* intercellular adhesion molecule-1 binding domain: A parasite adhesion trait implicated in cerebral malaria. *Proc. Natl. Acad. Sci. USA* **97**, 1766–1771.

Smith, J. D., Gamain, B., Baruch, D. I., and Kyes, S. (2001). Decoding the language of *var* genes and *Plasmodium falciparum* sequestration. *Trends Parasitol.* **17**, 538–545.

Staalsoe, T., Megnekou, R., Fievet, N., Ricke, C. H., Zornig, H. D., Leke, R., Taylor, D. W., Deloron, P., and Hviid, L. (2001). Acquisition and decay of antibodies to pregnancy-associated variant antigens on the surface of *Plasmodium falciparum*-infected erythrocytes that protect against placental parasitemia. *J. Infect. Dis.* **184**, 618–626.

Staalsoe, T., Shulman, C. E., Bulmer, J. N., Kawuondo, K., Marsh, K., and Hviid, L. (2004). Variant surface antigen-specific IgG and protection against clinical consequences of pregnancy-associated *Plasmodium falciparum* malaria. *Lancet* **363**, 283–289.

Steketee, R. W., Breman, J. G., Paluku, K. M., Moore, M., Roy, J., and Ma-Disu, M. (1988). Malaria infection in pregnant women in Zaire: The effects and the potential for intervention. *Ann. Trop. Med. Parasitol.* **82**, 113–120.

Steketee, R. W., Nahlen, B. L., Parise, M. E., and Menendez, C. (2001). The burden of malaria in pregnancy in malaria-endemic areas. *Am. J. Trop. Med. Hyg.* **64**(Suppl 1–2), 28–35.

Su, X. Z., Heatwole, V. M., Wertheimer, S. P., Guinet, F., Herrfeldt, J. A., Peterson, D. S., Ravetch, J. A., and Wellems, T. E. (1995). The large diverse gene family *var* encodes proteins involved in cytoadherence and antigenic variation of *Plasmodium falciparum*-infected erythrocytes. *Cell* **82**, 89–100.

Taylor, D. W., Zhou, A., Marsillio, L. E., Thuta, L. W., Leke, E. B., Branch, O., Gowda, D. C., Long, C., and Leke, R. F. G. (2004). Antibodies that inhibit the binding of *Plasmodium falciparum*-infected erythrocytes to CSA and to the C-terminus of merozoite protein 1 (MSP1–19) correlate with reduced placental malaria in Cameroonian women. *Infect. Immun.* **72**, 1603–1607.

Treutiger, C. J., Heddini, A., Fernadez, V., Muller, W. A., and Wahlgren, M. (1997). PECAM-1/CD-31, an endothelial receptor for binding *Plasmodium falciparum*-infected erythrocytes. *Nat. Med.* **3**, 1405–1408.

Udomsangpetch, R., Reinhardt, P. H., Schollaardt, T., Elliott, J. F., Kubes, P., and Ho, M. (1997). Promiscuity of clinical *Plasmodium falciparum* isolates for multiple adhesion molecules under flow conditions. *J. Immunol.* **158**, 4358–4364.

Valiyaveettil, M., Achur, R. N., Alkhalil, A., Ockenhouse, C. F., and Gowda, D. C. (2001). *Plasmodium falciparum* cytoadherence to human placenta: Evaluation of hyaluronic acid and chondroitin 4-sulfate for binding of infected erythrocytes. *Exp. Parasitol.* **99**, 57–65.

Vogt, A. M., Barragan, A., Chen, Q., Kironde, F., Spillmann, D., and Wahlgren, M. (2003). Heparan sulfate on endothelial cells mediates the binding of *Plasmodium falciparum*-infected erythrocytes via the DBL1alpha domain of PfEMP1. *Blood* **101**, 2405–2411.

Wadstrom, T., and Ljungh, L. (1999). Glycosaminoglycan-binding microbial proteins on tissue adhesion and invasion: Key events in microbial pathogenicity. *J. Med. Microbiol.* **48**, 223–233.

Walter, P. R., Garin, Y., and Blot, P. (1982). Placental pathologic changes in malaria: A histologic and ultrastructural study. *Am. J. Pathol.* **109**, 330–342.

Weatherall, D. J., Miller, L. H., Baruch, D. I., Marsh, K., Doumbo, O. K., Casals-Pascual, C., and Roberts, D. J. (2002). Malaria and the red cell. *Hematology (Am. Soc. Hematol. Educ. Program)*, 35–57.

Zhou, A., Megnekou, R., Leke, R., Fogako, J., Metenou, S., Trock, B., Taylor, D. W., and Leke, R. F. (2002). Prevalence of *Plasmodium falciparum* infection in pregnant Cameroonian women. *Am. J. Trop. Med. Hyg.* **67**, 566–570.

PART III

Pharmacological Activities of Chondroitin Sulfate

Toshihiko Toida*, Shinobu Sakai*, Hiroshi Akiyama[†], and Robert J. Linhardt[‡]

*Graduate School of Pharmaceutical Sciences
Chiba University
Chiba 263-8522, Japan

[†]National Institute of Health Sciences
Tokyo 158-8501, Japan

[‡]Department of Chemistry and Chemical Biology
Biology and Chemical and Biological Engineering
Rensselaer Polytechnic Institute
Troy, New York 12180

Immunological Activity of Chondroitin Sulfate

I. Chapter Overview

The use of chondroitin sulfate (CS) for the symptomatic treatment of osteoarthritis (OA) has become very popular; however, it has also been the subject of controversy for several reasons. First, the nutraceutical industry is less regulated than the pharmaceutical industry and thus, the nutraceutical CS often suffers from poor quality control. Second, the bioavailability of orally administered CS is not generally accepted. Third, the mechanism of the effect of CS for treatment of OA remains unclear. There is abundant *in vitro* and *in vivo* evidence from animal and human clinical studies demonstrating the efficacy and safety of CS. This chapter focuses on the immunological activity of structurally regulated CSs. The mechanism of this immunological activity appears to be through CS binding to receptors related to cytokine production in lymphocytes such as splenocytes.

Advances in Pharmacology, Volume 53
1054-3589/06 $35.00
DOI: 10.1016/S1054-3589(05)53019-9

II. Introduction

Most important pharmaceuticals have their origin in natural products, such as herbs and antibiotics, however, many physicians are deeply skeptical about the use of natural remedies. This skepticism is based on the concerns about the lack of scientific evidences of their efficacy. A new class has emerged called nutraceuticals, which are nutritional supplements with presumed pharmaceutical properties and efficacy. Because these substances are relatively unregulated, there is no requirement for rigorous scientific evidences before marketing. This lack of regulation also poses severe problems with purity and quality control. Glucosamine and CS sales alone in Japan are estimated at several billion JPY (several hundred million US dollars) in retail sales. Furthermore, the combination of glucosamine and CS is a very popular nutraceutical in the USA. While there is no scientific evidence on the efficacy of glucosamine and CS in the treatment of joint disease, the market of this nutraceutical product continues to grow. Self-medicating patients represent the driving force making nutraceutical products bestsellers throughout the world. Glucosamine and CS have been widely studied in tissue culture, animal models of arthritis, veterinary clinical trials, and human comparative or placebo controlled trials. All published studies suggest a positive effect, and no trial has shown significant side effects. Based on the absence of conclusive data, the National Institute of Health has started *"NIH Glucosamine/Chondroitin Arthritis Intervention Trial (GAIT)"* (http://www.niams.nih.gov/ne/press/2000/gait_qa.htm#what) to obtain definitive scientific evidence for the efficacy of glucosamine and CS in the treatment of arthritis.

Glucosamine and CS are integral components of articular cartilage and are important to the physiologic and mechanical properties of this tissue. Glucosamine is involved in cartilage formation by acting as the precursor of the disaccharide unit in glycosaminoglycans (GAGs) (Baker and Ferguson, 2005; De los Reyes *et al.*, 2000; Scott *et al.*, 2005). Chondroitin sulfate is a GAG that is a component of the aggrecan structure that makes up articular cartilage (Freeman, 1979). It binds collagen fibrils and limits water content by cooperating with hyaluronan, which is also a GAG. Chondroitin sulfate plays a role in allowing the cartilage to resist tensile stresses during various loading conditions by giving the cartilage resistance and elasticity (Muir, 1986). Exogenously administered glucosamine and CS have been shown *in vitro* to have other physiological effects. Glucosamine stimulates chondrocytes to increase secretion of GAGs and proteoglycans (PGs) *in vitro* (Jimenez, 1996). There is also evidence of CS-based anti-inflammatory activity not related to prostaglandin metabolism, probably through a free radical scavenging effect (Raiss, 1985). Osteoarthritis is clinically characterized as the decomposition of cartilage by degradative enzymes. These enzymes are competitively inhibited by CS *in vitro* (Bartolucci *et al.*, 1991;

Bassleer *et al.*, 1992). Moreover, laboratory studies have demonstrated a synergistic effect when glucosamine and CS are administered together. Lippiello *et al.* (2000) noted that the coadministration of CS and glucosamine resulted in a greater increase of $^{35}SO_4$ incorporation into GAGs (97%) than demonstrated by either agent alone (glucosamine, 32%; CS, 32%). This synergistic effect was also observed in experiments on CS's antiprotease activity *in vitro* (Arner, 2002). However, the orally administered CS has to be absorbed through gastric/intestinal system into blood flow to show these effects in its intact form.

There are many arguments regarding whether or not orally administered CS is absorbed through gastric/intestinal system (Owens, 2004). We have found only very small amounts of relatively low-molecular weight CS chains (average molecular weight 15,000) in the blood over 24 h following oral administration to mice. The failure to observe significant bioavailability suggests a novel concept that CS might act in the absence of absorption, on the humoral immunosystem by stimulating the intestinal intraepithelial lymphocytes (IEL) through cytokine production (Akiyama *et al.*, 2004; Sakai *et al.*, 2002a). This chapter describes the effects of CS on immunosystem *in vivo* and *in vitro*.

III. Clinical Experience (David and Lynne, 2003) ───────

In an artificially induced cartilage injury model, Uebelhart *et al.* (1998) noted that treatment with CS resulted in a marked reduction in the loss of PSs as compared with controls. Lippiello *et al.* (1999) reported that the effect of CS given to normal dogs was an increase in the serum GAG levels. Using indirect assessments of cartilage metabolism, they found that serum from treated dogs increased biosynthetic activity (incorporation of radioactively labeled glucosamine) and decreased proteolytic degradation (release of ^{35}S) from prelabeled normal calf cartilage segments. Using a rabbit instability model created by transecting the anterior cruciate, Lippiello *et al.* (2000) found that the articular matrix was severely degraded in the untreated group while remaining essentially intact in the treated group. In a canine model of unilateral carpal synovitis, although no effect was observed if the treatment was started after the synovitis occurred, dogs pretreated with the combination of glucosamine and CS have shown less evidence of bone remodeling and lower lameness scores (Canapp *et al.*, 1999).

Glucosamine and CS are often used either separately or in combination for the treatment of arthritic ailments (Dechant *et al.*, 2005). The safety profile of these nutraceuticals has been reviewed (Hungerford and Valaik, 2003). When recommending a supplement to patients, the physicians should take into account the purity of the ingredients, reputation of the manufacturer, and the molecular weight of chondroitin supplied. An analysis of marketed products indicated that the amounts of glucosamine and CS present in the products sold often fell short of the declared values on the label (Adebowale *et al.*, 2000). Most of the commercially available supplements sold in Japan analyzed in our laboratory contained less CS than indicated on their label, and significant amounts of carrageenan was found in many of these products (data not published). These discrepancies may introduce the confusion underlying the potential benefits of these nutraceuticals in treating arthritic disease.

Several clinical trials exploring the efficacy of both glucosamine and CS in the treatment of OA have been performed over the past 30 years as indicated in an earlier section; the outcomes of these studies have also been reviewed (Leeb *et al.*, 2000; McAlindon *et al.*, 2000; Richy *et al.*, 2003). The goal of these reviews was to assess both the potential symptom-modifying (e.g., pain and functional efficacy) and structure-modifying (e.g., changes in joint space narrowing) activities of glucosamine and CS in alleviating symptoms of OA of the knee using outcome-oriented metaanalysis of these randomized clinical trials. The general conclusion from these reviews is that glucosamine ingestion shows efficacy in both narrowing joint space and some symptom-modifying parameters. However, although CS ingestion showed similar symptom-modifying effects, the structure-modifying benefits still need to be confirmed. Given this clinical evidence, there is clearly a need for more basic research aimed at elucidating the cellular and molecular mechanisms involved with these two interesting nutraceuticals.

IV. Metabolic Fate of Orally Administered Chondroitin Sulfates

The metabolic fate of orally administered CS is ambiguous (Ronca and Conte, 1993). Baici *et al.* (1993) investigated the ability of an oral dose of CS to impact the concentration of GAGs in humans. In this study, CS samples were administered to six healthy volunteers, six patients with rheumatoid arthritis, and six patients with OA. The concentration of GAGs in serum was reportedly unchanged following ingestion (Baici *et al.*, 1993). Morrison (1977) has indicated that the intact absorption of CS was extremely low, estimating the absorption rate to be between 0 and 8%. The complexity of this issue is based on the fact that CS is found in a wide range of molecular weights, chain lengths, charge distributions, with positional isomers of sulfo groups, and containing variable percentages of similar disaccharide residues comprised of sulfated glucuronic acid (GlcA) and *N*-acetylgalactosamine (GalNAc) as shown in Fig. 1. A further complication occurs because low-molecular weight derivatives of CS have also been pharmacologically produced and utilized in some of the pharmacokinetic and therapeutic studies and trials (Conte *et al.*, 1991; Ronca *et al.*, 1998). It is quite possible that the contrasting metabolic fates of orally administered CSs are a direct reflection

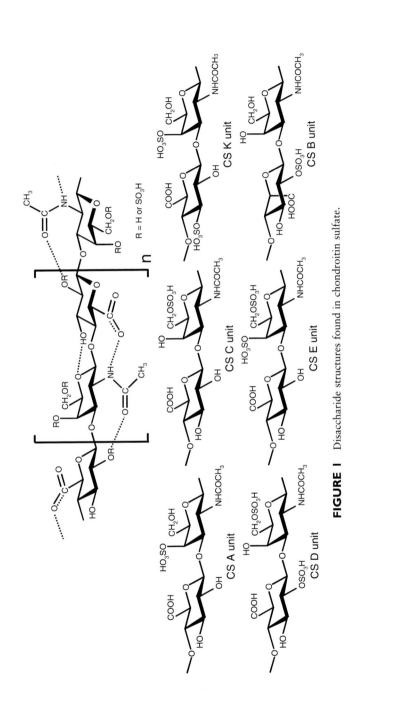

FIGURE 1 Disaccharide structures found in chondroitin sulfate.

of this dissimilarity in the primary structure and physical properties of these CS samples. The pharmacokinetic properties of a proprietary CS were investigated by Conte *et al.* (1995). Significant extraction procedures were utilized to generate a low-molecular weight product that could be characterized for structure, physiochemical properties, and purity. Only a fraction with a relative molecular weight of about 14 kDa was used in their experiments. This fraction showed a sulfate-to-carboxyl ratio of 0.95 due to the high percentage of monosulfated disaccharide sequences [55% CS-A (4-O-sulfonated GalNAc) and 38% CS-C (6-O-sulfonated GalNAc)], and a low amount of disulfated disaccharide sequences (1.1%). The purity of the preparation was greater than 97% CS. This sample was radioactively labeled and orally administered to the rats and dogs. Although more than 70% of the radioactivity was absorbed and was subsequently found in urine and tissues, the radioactivity associated with an intact molecule of CS corresponding to the molecular mass of the administered CS was relatively small (approximately 8.5%), and this percentage decreased rapidly over time. The majority of the radioactivity absorbed was actually associated with molecules with a molecular mass of less than or equal in size to GalNAc residues. This radioactivity increased over time and remained elevated. Radioactivity after 24 h was highest in the small intestine, liver, and kidneys (tissues responsible for the absorption, metabolism, degradation, and elimination of the compound); however, relatively high amounts of radioactivity were also found in tissues, which utilize amino sugars such as joint cartilage, synovial fluid, and trachea. This group also orally administered CS to healthy volunteers in either a single daily dose of 0.8 g or in two daily doses of 0.4 g. Although both dosing schedules increased plasma concentration of exogenous molecules associated with CS, the results have indicated that the oral administration of one dose of 0.8 g CS was the more effective regimen. Some physiological parameters associated with GAGs, such as hyaluronan, were also analyzed to investigate whether orally administered exogenous CS affects synovial fluid in patients with OA. The results indicated that the treatment with CS might also modify these parameters. Thus, despite all of these studies, the oral bioavailability and efficacy of CS remains controversial. However, the majority of physiological benefits subsequent to administration of CS appears to be a direct result of increased availability of the monosaccharide/disaccharide residues of CS produced by the action of enzymes found in the intestine (Hong *et al.*, 2002).

V. A New Concept for Explaining the Effect of Chondroitin Sulfate in Arthritis Treatment

Polysaccharides, such as CS, are clearly poorly absorbed through the digestive system. Moreover, we have shown that the half-life of CS in the circulatory system is 3–15 min, based on the pharmacokinetic study of intravenously administered CS (Sakai *et al.*, 2002b). Accordingly, it appears unlikely that orally administered CS is systemically distributed to connective tissues, such as cartilage and skin, and that exogenously administered CS directly stimulates chondrocyte synthesis of extracellular matrix components. This suggests that the mechanism of action of exogenously administered CS might be mediated from within the intestinal tract by other systems, such as the immunological system (Wrenshall *et al.*, 1999). Our laboratory has already shown that CS affects and upregulates the *in vitro* antigen-specific Th1 immune response on murine splenocytes sensitized with ovalbumin (OVA) and that CS suppresses the antigen-specific IgE responses (Sakai *et al.*, 2002a). These findings also suggest a therapeutic use of CS to control the IgE mediated allergic response. The number and position of O-sulfo groups varies among CS samples obtained from different sources (Alves *et al.*, 1997; Farias *et al.*, 2000; Santos *et al.*, 1992). We hypothesized that the immunological activity of orally administered CS might also be different among the several types of CS. Thus, it is important to determine the structure–activity relationship (SAR) of CS, particularly with respect to the number and position of O-sulfo groups in CS. Knowledge of the SAR of CS will be necessary to further explore its effective use as a therapeutic agent.

It is generally accepted that CD4+ T cells are subpopulations containing 2 cell types (Th1 and Th2), based on their different patterns of cytokine secretion (Mossmann and Coffman, 1989a,b). Th1 cells secrete IFN-γ, IL-2, and IL-12. Th2 cells produce IL-4, IL-5, and IL-10. IFN-γ and IL-12 induce the differentiation of Th0 cells to Th1 cells, whereas IL-4 induces the differentiation to Th2 cells (Fig. 2). Therefore, it is believed that an increase

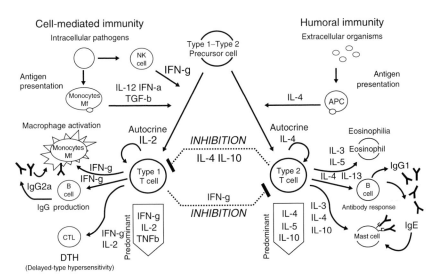

FIGURE 2   Overview of Th1/Th2 balance.

in IFN-γ and IL-12 shifts the Th1/Th2 cell balance to predominantly Th1, while an increase in IL-5 and IL-10 shifts the balance to predominantly Th2 (Akiyama *et al.*, 1999; Nagafuchi *et al.*, 2000). We have previously reported that CS induced Th1-type cytokine (IFN-γ, IL-2, and IL-12) secretion but suppressed Th2-type cytokine (IL-5 and IL-10) secretion by the OVA-sensitized splenocytes (Sakai *et al.*, 2002a). We have also already shown that both O-sulfo group content and position in CS is important for the Th1-promoted activity of murine splenocytes, in terms of the cytokine production and Th1/Th2 balance (Akiyama *et al.*, 2004). We first examined whether the activity was associated with the O-sulfo groups in CS and confirmed that the sulfation of a polysaccharide has played an important role in the activity. We have reported that CS induced the Th1-promoted activity while dextran, a neutral polysaccharide used as a control, did not (data not shown). In contrast, dextran sulfate also did not show significant effects on cytokine production by murine splenocytes (Fig. 3). These results indicate that the polysaccharide type and sulfation is critical for the Th1-promoted activity (Akiyama *et al.*, 2004). We subsequently showed the effect of the level of sulfation number and position of CS on the Th1-promoted activity (Akiyama *et al.*, 2004). While fully sulfonated CS exhibits Th1-promoted activity, intact CS-A and the partially O-sulfonated CS demonstrate higher activity CS (Fig. 1). These results strongly suggested that excess sulfo groups in CS could decrease the Th1-promoted and Th2-inhibitory activities of CS. Among the monosulfated CS, CS-A, -C, and -B, the CS-A sample showed highest activity (Figs. 1 and 3). This result suggested that the [-4)GlcA(β1–3)GalNAc4S(β1-]$_n$ sequence is more important for activity than the [-4)GlcA(β1–3)GalNAc6S (β1-]$_n$ or [-4)IdoA(β1–3)GalNAc4S(β1-]$_n$ sequences characteristic of CS-C and -B, respectively (Fig. 1). Chondroitin sulfate-B [dermatan sulfate (DS)], while nearly structurally identical to CS-A (it contains IdoA instead of GlcA), shows lower activity. This is surprising as the greater flexibility of the IdoA residue in CS-B is commonly used to explain the propensity of IdoA-containing GAGs to interact with proteins and display a large number of different biological activities (Kawashima *et al.*, 2002). Examination of the disulfated CS samples shows that the effects of CS-E on the Th2-inhibitory activity were higher than those of CS-D or -A (Fig. 3, also see structures shown in Fig. 1). These results suggested that the [-4)GlcA(β1–3) GalNAc4S6S(β1-]$_n$ sequence in CS-E is more important for high activity than the [-4)GlcA2S(β1–3)GalNAc6S(β1-]$_n$ sequence characteristically found in CS-D. Furthermore, these experiments demonstrate that the [-4)GlcA(β1–3) GalNAc4S(β1-]$_n$ and [-4)GlcA(β1–3)GalNAc4S6S(β1-]$_n$ sequences in CS are more critical for higher activity. Researchers have reported many biological activities for sulfated polysaccharides (Chaidedgumjorn *et al.*, 2002; Koyanagi *et al.*, 2003; Linhardt and Toida, 1997; Toida *et al.*, 1999). In most cases the number of sulfo groups in the polysaccharide directly correlates with the level of bioactivity (Chaidedgumjorn *et al.*, 2002; Koyanagi *et al.*, 2003; Toida *et al.*,

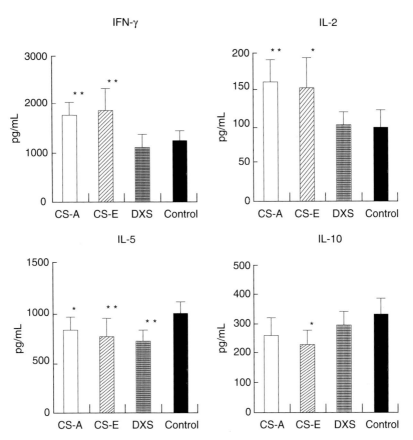

FIGURE 3 Effect of CS on the cytokine production of murine splenocyte *in vitro*. BALB/c mice ($n = 5$) were intraperitoneally injected on day 0 and 13 with 20 µg of ovalbumin (OVA) and 2 mg of $Al(OH)_2$ at a total volume of 400 µl. Spleen cells (5.0×10^6 cells/ml) were collected on day 14 and were cocultured with OVA (final 100 µg/ml). The amounts of cytokines in the supernatant were measured by ELISA. Asterisk indicates significance of difference from control value ($*p < 0.05$, $**p < 0.01$). Bars represent mean values ($\pm$S.D.) for six wells.

1999). Koyanagi *et al.* (2003), have shown that by increasing the number of sulfo groups in fucoidans (sulfonated fucans), its antiangiogenic and antitumor activities can be potentiated. Our laboratory has also reported the many biological activities of the chemically fully sulfated poly- and oligosaccharides (Chaidedgumjorn *et al.*, 2002; Suzuki *et al.*, 2001; Toida *et al.*, 1999, 2000). Chondroitin sulfate has been found in many tissues (Suzuki *et al.*, 1968) and cells (Ohhashi *et al.*, 1984; Petersen *et al.*, 1999; Stevens *et al.*, 1988), and has been reported to interact with various biologically important molecules and regulate their functions. We have demonstrated the importance of the content, position, and number of O-sulfo groups in

CS for immunological activity of the OVA-stimulated murine splenocytes *in vitro* (Akiyama *et al.*, 2004; Sakai *et al.*, 2002a). It was also shown that Th1-promoted and Th2-inhibitory activity of CS on murine splenocytes could be associated with binding to L-selectin. It has been reported that a large CS/DSPG interacts through its CS/DS chains with the adhesion molecules L- and P-selectin, CD44, and chemokines. Kawashima *et al.* (1999, 2000) and others (Capila and Linhardt, 2002; Hirose *et al.*, 2001) reported that oversulfated CS/DS, containing [-4)GlcA(β1-3)GalNAc4S6S (β1-]$_n$ sequences, interacts with L-selectin, P-selectin, and chemokines. Our findings may indicate that these same [-4)GlcA(β1-3)GalNAc4S6S(β1-]$_n$ sequences in CS would be associated with the strongest effects on the promotion of the Th1-type cytokine production and the inhibition of the Th2-type cytokine production. The present structural characterization of CS to Th1-promoted, and Th2-inhibitory activity is consistent with the high-affinity binding of CS, containing the [-4)GlcA(β1-3)-GalNAc4S(β1-]$_n$ and [-4) GlcA(β1-3)GalNAc4S6S(β1-]$_n$ sequences, to L-selectin (Kawashima *et al.*, 2002). These findings also may support our hypothesis that such an immunological activity could be associated with the binding of CS-A to L-selectin on T cell surface. These results also may indicate that differences in the content and position of O-sulfo groups in CS could markedly influence Th1-promoted and Th2-inhibitory activities, as do differences between GlcA and IdoA residues in CS. In these observations, however, the inhibition of CS binding to L-selectin could not be shown by FACS analysis using labeled antiL-selectin monoclonal antibody (Akiyama *et al.*, 2004). This result may suggest that the epitope region on L-selectin to antiL-selectin monoclonal antibody might not be located in the lectin region that binds to CS. We have not yet established the relationship between the various CS samples from natural products and the immunological activities. Thus, further studies are required on the relative L-selectin binding affinity of different types of CS to fully elucidate the importance of L-selectin-CS binding. The effect of heparin was also examined on Th1/Th2 balance and found to demonstrate the same level of activity as CS at identical doses (results not published). We are considering future studies to assess the effects of heparin and its derivatives on these activities to fully elucidate the SAR of GAG.

References

Adebowale, A. O., Cox, D. S., Liang, Z., and Eddington, N. D. (2000). Analysis of glucosamine and chondroitin sulfate content in marketed products and the Caco-2 permeability of chondroitin sulfate raw materials. *J. Am. Nutrac. Assoc.* **3**, 37–44.

Akiyama, H., Hoshino, K., Tokuzumi, M., Teshima, R., Mori, H., Inakuma, T., Ishiguro, Y., Goda, Y., Sawada, J., and Toyoda, M. (1999). The effect of feeding carrots on immunoglobulin E production and anaphylactic response in mice. *Biol. Pharm. Bull.* **22**, 551–555.

Akiyama, H., Sakai, S., Linhardt, R. J., Goda, Y., Toida, T., and Maitani, T. (2004). Chondroitin sulphate structure affects its immunological activities on murine splenocytes sensitized with ovalbumin. *Biochem. J.* **382**, 269–278.

Alves, A. P., Mulloy, B., Diniz, J. A., and Mourao, P. A. S. (1997). Sulphated polysaccharides from the egg jelly layer are species-specific inducers of acrosomal reaction in sperms of sea urchins. *J. Biol. Chem.* **272**, 6965–6971.

Arner, E. C. (2002). Aggrecanase-mediated cartilage degradation. *Curr. Opin. Pharmacol.* **2**, 322–329.

Baici, A., Horler, D., Moser, B., Hofer, H. O., Fehr, K., and Wagenhauser, F. J. (1993). Analysis of glycosaminoglycans in human serum after oral administration of chondroitin sulfate. *Rheumatol. Int.* **13**, 39–43.

Baker, C. L., Jr., and Ferguson, C. M. (2005). Future treatment of osteoarthritis. *Orthopedics* **28**(Suppl. 2), s227–s234.

Bartolucci, C., Cellai, L., Corradini, C., Corradini, D., Lamba, D., and Velona, I. (1991). Chondroprotective action of chondroitin sulfate: Competitive action of chondroitin sulfate on the digestion of hyaluronan by bovine testicular hyaluronidase. *Int. J. Tissue Reac.* **13**, 311–317.

Bassleer, C., Henrotin, Y., and Franchiment, P. (1992). *In-vitro* evaluation of drugs proposed as chondroprotective agents. *Int. J. Tissue Reac.* **14**, 231–241.

Canapp, S. O., McLaughlin, R. M., Jr., Hoskinson, J. J., Roush, J. K., and Butine, M. D. (1999). Scintigraphic evaluation of dogs with acute synovitis after treatment with glucosamine hydrochloride and chondroitin sulfate. *Am. J. Vet. Res.* **60**, 1552–1557.

Capila, I., and Linhardt, R. J. (2002). Heparin-protein interactions. *Angew. Chem.* **41**, 391–412.

Chaidedgumjorn, A., Toyoda, H., Woo, E. R., Lee, K. B., Kim, Y. S., Toida, T., and Imanari, T. (2002). Effect of (1-3)- and (1-4)-linkages of fully sulphated polysaccharides on their anticoagulant activity. *Carbohydr. Res.* **337**, 925–933.

Conte, A., Palmieri, L., Segnini, D., and Ronca, G. (1991). Metabolic fate of partially depolymerized chondroitin sulfate administered to the rat. *Drugs Exp. Clin. Res.* **17**, 27–33.

Conte, A., Volpi, N., Palmieri, L., Bahous, I., and Ronca, G. (1995). Biochemical and pharmacokinetic aspects of oral treatment with chondroitin sulfate. *Arzneim. Forsch.* **45**, 918–925.

David, S. H., and Lynne, C. J. (2003). Glucosamine and chondroitin sulfate are effective in the management of osteoarthritis. *J. Arthro.* **18**(Suppl. 1), 5–9.

De los Reyes, G. C., Koda, R. T., and Lien, E. J. (2000). Glucosamine and chondroitin sulfates in the treatment of osteoarthritis: A survey. *Prog. Drug Res.* **55**, 81–103.

Dechant, J. E., Baxter, G. M., Frisbie, D. D., Trotter, G. W., and McIlwraith, C. W. (2005). Effects of glucosamine hydrochloride and chondroitin sulphate, alone and in combination, on normal and interleukin-1 conditioned equine articular cartilage explant metabolism. *Equine Vet. J.* **37**, 227–231.

Farias, W. R., Valente, A., Pereira, M. S., and Mourao, P. A. S. (2000). Structure and anticoagulant activity of sulphated galactans. Isolation of a unique sulphated galactan from the red algae *Botryocladia occidentalis* and comparison of its anticoagulant action with that of sulphated galactans from invertebrates. *J. Biol. Chem.* **275**, 29299–29307.

Freeman, M. A. R. (Ed.) (1979). "Adult Articular Cartilage." Pitman Medical Publishing Company, London.

Jimenez, S. A. (1996). The effects of glucosamine on human chondrocyte gene expression. *In* "The Ninth Eular Symposium," p. 8. Madrid, European League Against Rheumatism, October 8–10.

Kawashima, H., Li, Y. F., Watanabe, N., Hirose, J., Hirose, M., and Miyasaka, M. (1999). Identification and characterization of ligands for L-selectin in the kidney. I. Versican, a large chondroitin sulphate proteoglycan, is a ligand for L-selectin. *Int. Immunol.* **11**, 393–405.

Kawashima, H., Hirose, M., Hirose, J., Nagakubo, D., Plaas, A. H. K., and Miyasaka, M. (2000). Binding of a large chondroitin sulphate/dermatan sulphate proteoglycan, versican, to L-selectin, P-selectin, and CD44. *J. Biol. Chem.* **275**, 35448–35456.

Kawashima, H., Atarashi, K., Hirose, M., Hirose, J., Yamada, S., Sugahara, K., and Miyasaka, M. (2002). Oversulphated chondroitin/dermatan sulphates containing GlcAβ1/IdoAα1-3GalNAc(4,6-O-disulphate) interact with L- and P-selectin and chemokines. *J. Biol. Chem.* **277**, 12921–12930.

Koyanagi, S., Tanigawa, N., Nakagawa, H., Soeda, S., and Shimeno, H. (2003). Oversulphation of fucoidan enhances its anti-angiogenic and antitumor activities. *Biochem. Pharmacol.* **65**, 173–179.

Hirose, J., Kawashima, H., Yoshie, O., Tashiro, K., and Miyasaka, M. (2001). Versican interacts with chemokines and modulates cellular responses. *J. Biol. Chem.* **276**, 5228–5234.

Hong, S. W., Kim, B. T., Shin, H. Y., Kim, W. S., Lee, K. S., Kim, Y. S., and Kim, D. H. (2002). Purification and characterization of novel chondroitin ABC and AC lyases from *Bacteroides stercoris* HJ-15, a human intestinal anaerobic bacterium. *Eur. J. Biochem.* **269**, 2934–2940.

Hungerford, M. W., and Valaik, D. (2003). Chondroprotective agents: Glucosamine and chondroitin. *Foot Ankle Clin.* **28**, 201–219.

Leeb, B. F., Schweitzer, H., Montag, K., and Smolen, J. S. (2000). A meta-analysis of chondroitin sulphate in the treatment of osteoarthritis. *J. Rheumatol.* **27**, 205–211.

Linhardt, R. J., and Toida, T. (1997). Heparin oligosaccharides: New analogs development and applications. *In* "Carbohydrates as Drugs" (Z. B. Witczak and K. A. Nieforth, Eds.), pp. 277–341. Marcel Dekker, New York.

Lippiello, L., Idouraine, A., McNamara, P. S., Barr, S. C., and McLaughlin, R. M. (1999). Cartilage stimulatory and antiproteolytic activity is present in sera of dogs treated with a chondroprotective agent. *Canine Prac.* **24**, 18–20.

Lippiello, L., Woodward, J., Karpman, R., and Hammad, T. A. (2000). *In vivo* chondroprotection and metabolic synergy of glucosamine and chondroitin sulfate. *Clin. Orthop. Relat. Res.* **381**, 229–240.

McAlindon, T. E., LaValley, M. P., Gulin, J. P., and Felson, D. T. (2000). Glucosamine and chondroitin for treatment of osteoarthritis. A systemic quality assessment and meta-analysis. *J. Am. Med. Assoc.* **283**, 1469–1475.

Morrison, M. (1977). Therapeutic applications of chondroitin-4-sulfate, appraisal of biological properties. *Folia Angiol.* **25**, 225–232.

Mossmann, R. T., and Coffman, L. R. (1989a). Th1 and Th2 cells: Different patterns of lymphokine secretion lead to different functional properties. *Annu. Rev. Immunol.* **7**, 145–173.

Mossmann, R. T., and Coffman, L. R. (1989b). Heterogeneity of cytokine secretion patterns and functions of helper T cells. *Adv. Immunol.* **46**, 111–147.

Muir, H. (1986). Current and future trends in articular cartilage research and osteoarthritis. *In* "Articular Cartilage and Osteoarthritis" (K. E. Kuettner, R. Schleyerbach, and V. C. Hascall, Eds.), p. 423. Raven Press, New York.

Nagafuchi, S., Hachimura, S., Totsuka, M., Takahashi, T., Goto, M., Yajima, T., Kuwata, T., Habu, S., and Kaminogawa, S. (2000). Dietary nucleotides can up-regulate antigen-specific Th1 immune responses and suppress antigen-specific IgE responses in mice. *Int. Arch. Allergy Immunol.* **122**, 33–41.

Ohhashi, Y., Hasumi, F., and Mori, Y. (1984). Comparative study on glycosaminoglycans synthesized in peripheral and peritoneal polymorphonuclear leucocytes from guinea pigs. *Biochem. J.* **217**, 199–207.

Owens, S., Wagner, P., and Vangsness, C. T., Jr. (2004). Recent advances in glucosamine and chondroitin supplementation. *J. Knee Surg.* **17**, 185–193.

Petersen, R. L., Brandt, E., Lindahl, U., and Spillmann, D. (1999). Characterization of a neutrophil cell surface glycosaminoglycan that mediates binding of platelet factor 4. *J. Biol. Chem.* **274**, 12376–12382.

Raiss, R. (1985). Einfluss von D-glucosamin sulfat auf experimenteil geschaedigten gelenkknorpel. *Fortschritte der Midizin* **103**, 658.

Richy, F., Bruyere, O., Ethgen, O., Cucherat, M., Henrotin, Y., and Reginster, J. Y. (2003). Structural and symptomatic efficacy of glucosamine and chondroitin in knee osteoarthritis: A comprehensive meta-analysis. *Arch. Int. Med.* **163**, 1514–1522.

Ronca, G., and Conte, A. (1993). Metabolic fate of partially depolymerized shark chondroitin sulfate in man. *Int. J. Clin. Pharmacol. Res.* **13**(Suppl.), 27–34.

Ronca, F., Palmieri, L., Panicucci, P., and Ronca, G. (1998). Anti-inflammatory activity of chondroitin sulfate. *Osteoarthritis Cartilage* **6**(Suppl. A), 14–21.

Sakai, S., Akiyama, H., Harikai, N., Toyoda, H., Toida, T., Maitani, T., and Imanari, T. (2002a). Effect of chondroitin sulfate on murine splenocytes sensitized with ovalbumin. *Immunol. Lett.* **84**, 211–216.

Sakai, S., Onose, J., Nakamura, N., Toyoda, H., Toida, T., Imanari, I., and Linhardt, R. J. (2002b). Pretreatment procedure for the microdetermination of chondroitin sulphate in plasma and urine. *Anal. Biochem.* **302**, 169–174.

Santos, J. A., Mulloy, B., and Mourao, P. A. S. (1992). Structural diversity among sulphated *a*-L-galactans from ascidians (tunicates). Studies on the species *Ciona intestinalis* and *Herdmania monus*. *Eur. J. Biochem.* **204**, 669–677.

Scott, D., Smith, C., Lohmander, S., and Chard, J. (2005). Osteoarthritis. *Clin. Evid.* **10**, 1402–1430.

Stevens, R. L., Fox, C. C., Lichtenstein, L. M., and Austen, K. F. (1988). Identification of chondroitin sulphate E proteoglycans and heparin proteoglycans in the secretory granules of human lung mast cells. *Proc. Natl. Acad. Sci. USA* **85**, 2284–2287.

Suzuki, S., Satio, H., Yamagata, T., Anno, K., Seno, N., Kawai, Y., and Furuhashi, T. (1968). Formation of three types of disulphated disaccharides from chondroitin sulphates by chondroitinase digestion. *J. Biol. Chem.* **243**, 1543–1550.

Suzuki, A., Toyoda, H., Toida, T., and Imanari, T. (2001). Preparation and inhibitory activity on hyaluronidase of fully O-sulfated hyaluro-oligosaccharides. *Glycobiology* **11**, 57–64.

Toida, T., Maruyama, T., Ogita, Y., Suzuki, A., Toyoda, H., Imanari, T., and Linhardt, R. J. (1999). Preparation and anticoagulant activity of fully O-sulphonated glycosaminoglycans. *Int. J. Biol. Macromol.* **26**, 233–241.

Toida, T., Suzuki, A., Nakajima, K., Chaidedgumjorn, A., and Imanari, T. (2000). Effect of 6-O-sulfonate hexosamine residue on anticoagulant activity of fully O-sulfonated glycosaminoglycans. *Glycoconj. J.* **17**, 393–399.

Uebelhart, D., Thonar, E. J., Zhang, J., and Williams, J. M. (1998). Protective effect of exogenous chondroitin 4,6-sulfate in the acute degradation of articular cartilage in the rabbit. *Osteoarthritis Cartilage* **6**, 39–46.

Web site. http://www.niams.nih.gov/ne/press/2000/gait_qa.htm#what.

Wrenshall, L. E., Stevens, R. B., Cerra, F. B., and Platt, J. L. (1999). Modulation of macrophage and B cell function by glycosaminoglycans. *J. Leukoc. Biol.* **66**, 391–400.

G. M. Campo, A. Avenoso, S. Campo, A. M. Ferlazzo, and A. Calatroni

Department of Biochemical, Physiological and Nutritional Sciences
School of Medicine, University of Messina
Policlinico Universitario
I-98125 Messina, Italy

Antioxidant Activity of Chondroitin Sulfate

I. Chapter Overview

Molecules in biological systems often perform more than one function. Many structures have the ability to scavenge free radicals, acting in living organisms as antioxidant, although their main biological function is different. During oxidative stress, the increase in concentration of these molecules seems to be a biological response that in synergism with the other antioxidant defense systems may protect cells from oxidation. Among these structures chondroitin sulfate (CS) has increasingly focused the interest of many research groups. This chapter briefly summarizes the action of CSs in reducing molecular damage caused by free radicals and associated oxygen reactants. The chondroitin-4-sulfate exerts higher antioxidant activity than chondroitin-6-sulfate. The specific sulfation pattern seems to play a central role in the inhibitory activity of these molecules on free radicals, since the suggested mechanism is entrapment by chelation of those metal cations, like

Advances in Pharmacology, Volume 53
Copyright 2006, Elsevier Inc. All rights reserved.

1054-3589/06 $35.00
DOI: 10.1016/S1054-3589(05)53020-5

Fe^{2+} and Cu^{2+}, that in turn, by Fenton's reaction, are responsible of reactive oxygen species (ROS) production. Chondroitin sulfate's protection on a wide variety of molecules (i.e., lipids, proteins, DNA, and so on) and in various cells from different organs is documented in several *in vitro* and *in vivo* experimental studies. Chondroitin-4-sulfate was shown to be able to reduce biological injury and free radical generation in several models of oxidative stress-induced damage in cellular cultures. Other investigations evaluated these antioxidant properties in experimental models of disease in animals and in human pathologies, especially arthritis. The antioxidant activity of CS could be used in the future as therapeutic agent in pathologies where free radicals are involved.

II. Background

It is widely known that the generation of free radicals and other ROS plays a key role in a large number of pathologies, including rheumatoid arthritis, liver disease, and atherosclerosis. These reactive molecules are formed during normal aerobic metabolism in cells and following phagocyte activation during infection/inflammation. A consequence of uncontrolled production of free radicals is damage to biomolecules leading to altered function and disease (Evans and Halliwell, 1999).

Free radicals can directly damage membrane lipids and other biological molecules such as proteins and nucleic acids. Oxidative injury occurs to some extent through the direct action of superoxide anions (O_2^-) and other ROS, but it is also partly secondarily derived from peroxide radicals, lipid hydroperoxides, and several lipid fragmentation products that behave as active oxidizing agents in various tissues such as the kidney, heart, liver, brain, lung, gut, skin, and so on (Halliwell *et al.*, 1992). A number of endogenous antioxidant defense mechanisms that limit the levels of potentially dangerous ROS, have been identified. Endogenous defenses are differentiated in enzymatic, superoxide dismutase (SOD), catalase (CAT), and glutathione peroxidase (GPx), and nonenzymatic systems that are able, in normal conditions, to neutralize free radicals.

The matrix metalloproteinases (MMPs) are a family of calcium-dependent zinc-containing endopeptidases, which are capable of degrading a wide variety of ECM components (Bode and Maskos, 2003). MMPs are known to play important roles in tissue remodeling during physiological processes, including tissue repair. The activity of MMPs is regulated by several types of inhibitors, of which the tissue inhibitors of metalloproteinases (TIMPs) are the most important (Nagase and Woessner, 1999). The balance between MMPs and TIMPs regulates tissue remodeling under normal conditions. A deregulation of this balance is characteristic feature of pathological conditions involving extensive tissue degradation and destruction, such as arthritis, diabetes, liver injury, and atherosclerosis. ROS are known to react with thiol groups, such as those involved in preserving MMP latency, so they could modulate the activity of MMPs (Wainwright, 2004).

Although oxidative stress is an unavoidable consequence of aerobic metabolism, the majority of four electron reduction of the O_2 molecule is of a rather low reactivity. However, trace amounts of unprotected transition metal ions, like Fe^{2+} and Cu^{2+}, can catalyze the Haber–Weiss reaction of the low-reactive O_2^- and H_2O_2 that gives rise to the highly toxic hydroxyl radical. O_2^- role in the iron or copper catalyzed Haber–Weiss reaction is the superoxide-assisted Fenton reaction (Halliwell and Gutteridge, 1999).

The catalytic effect of transition metal ions-induced OH˙ generation can be reduced by using molecules possessing chelating activity against these metal ions.

Glycosaminoglycans (GAGs) are a family of acid polysaccharides that display a variety of fundamental biological roles (Iozzo, 1998). The typical GAG structure consists of alternating units of uronic acid and hexosamine. Except for hyaluronic acid (HA), GAGs also contain sulfate groups and are covalently linked to proteins, to give proteoglycans (PGs). There are two major classes of sulfated GAGs—the glucosamine-containing family that includes heparan sulfates (HS) and heparin (Hep) and the galactosamine-containing family including CSs and dermatan sulfate (DS). A further GAG is keratan sulfate (KS), containing galactose and N-acetylglucosamine. In CS chains, the hexosamine residues usually carry sulfate esters at either carbon 4 or 6, with prevalence of 4 sulfation in C4S chain and of 6 sulfation in C6S chain. PGs function both as structural molecules and as scaffold structures binding a wide variety of protein ligands through GAG–protein and protein–protein interactions (Iozzo, 1998).

Several studies have shown antioxidant properties of GAGs, mainly for HA and C4S, probably due to their capacity to chelate transition metals like Cu^{2+} or Fe^{2+}.

III. The Ability of CS and HA to Chelate Metal Ions

The GAGs capacity to bind metal ions and other charged molecules is known since more than 50 years. Calcium ion environment in C4S has been elucidated by Cael et al. (1978)—the ion bridges carboxylate groups in separate chains and carboxylate and sulfate ester groups within a single chain.

Binding to CS of metal ions, such as Cu^{2+} and Na^+, investigated by using electron-spin resonance, viscometry, and ligand-field spectroscopy (Balt et al., 1983), was localized into the carboxylate group, and the sulfate group binds the ions with electrostatic interaction only. By X-ray absorption of CS–iron complexes, high-ordered state of the iron into the CS complex with respect to other iron complexes was shown (Yang *et al.*, 1986).

As already mentioned, calcium ion may bind both carboxylate and ester sulfate groups, in C4S. In C4S, all the major substituents of the disaccharide sugar rings are equatorial, except the axial sulfate ester group on position 4 of *N*-acetylgalactosamine. The position of the sulfate groups along the centerline of the polymer backbone gives high-negative charge density on the long axis of the molecule, and C4S does not self-aggregate. C6S, in which the sulfate groups are at the periphery of the molecule, can self-aggregate (Scott *et al.*, 1992). C4S displays a better antioxidant effect than C6S and than HA, which lacks sulfate ester group. In any case cations bind carboxylate groups—the higher antioxidant activity of C4S suggests that sulfate group at carbon 4 gives additional contribution to stabilize cation binding.

IV. *In Vitro* Studies

Many *in vitro* evidences that GAGs may protect endothelial cells by ROS were provided. In an experimental model of glutamate-induced neuronal toxicity, Okamoto *et al.* (1994) investigated the neuroprotective activity of CSPGs on excitotoxic cell death induced by excitatory amino acids. Albertini *et al.* (1996) showed that the antioxidant effect of PGs obtained from bovine cornea protected liposome from peroxidation and limited fragmentation induced by Fe^{2+}. Oxidation of low-density lipoprotein (LDL) in atherosclerosis is mediated by transition metals that in turn catalyze ROS production. Albertini *et al.* (1997) showed that C4S (and not C6S) inhibited copper-induced LDL oxidation. A possible initial key reaction in LDL oxidation, the reduction of copper(II) to copper(I) by LDL, was decreased in the presence of C4S, probably by masking copper-binding sites.

The effect of C4S and C6S on the oxidation of human HDL has been investigated by kinetic analysis (Albertini *et al.*, 1999). C4S increased the lag time and reduced the maximum rate of HDL oxidation induced by Cu^{2+}. On the contrary, C6S was ineffective. Since C4S was able to bind Cu^{2+}, authors suggested that this resulted in less Cu^{2+} available for HDL oxidation and likely represented the mechanism of the protective effect.

Volpi and Tarugi (1999a) investigated the antioxidant activity of CS, obtained from different sources, on Cu^{2+}-induced LDL oxidation, and the influence of CS charge (decreasing charge densities proved effective) and size (low-molecular masses were uneffective). Furthermore, Volpi and Tarugi (1999b) evaluated the antioxidant effect of various GAGs of different origin both on Cu^{2+}- and 2,2′-azobis(2-amidinopropane) hydrochloride (AAPH)-induced human LDL oxidation. HA had no effect. CS from beef trachea produced a very strong protective antioxidant effect.

Arai *et al.* (1999) studied the antioxidant activity of GAGs on Cu^{2+} and AAPH-induced oxidative modification of apolipoprotein E (apoE) in human very low-density lipoprotein (VLDL). The VLDL oxidation catalyzed by Cu^{2+} was suppressed by GAG, HS, Hep, and C4S, even though GAGs demonstrated no ability to scavenge α,α-diphenyl-β-picrylhydrazyl radical and no charge influence. An interaction between GAG and VLDL preserving the biological functions of apoE from oxidative stress was suggested.

On the contrary, Camejo *et al.* (1991) showed a prooxidant effect of GAGs on Cu^{2+}-induced LDL oxidation, with GAGs increasing Cu^{2+} affinity of apoprotein. Abuja (2002) also described a prooxidant action of C4S on LDL oxidation—aggregation of LDL in the presence of C4S, and not C6S, arises a complex, which can oxidize in the presence of ascorbate and urate and suggest entrapment of Cu^{2+} within.

Takahashi *et al.* (2002), by using electron-spin resonance to detect OH radicals, showed *in vitro* protective effect on eye tissues by a mixture of HA and CS (Viscoat) commonly used in phacoemulsification.

Morawski *et al.* (2004) reported that perineuronal nets, mainly consisting of large CSPGs interacting with HA and tenascin, which surround subpopulations of neurons, protect neurons against oxidative stress.

C4S showed antioxidant properties in reducing oxidative injury induced by different oxidizing agents in human skin fibroblast cultures (Campo *et al.*, 2004b). The treatment with commercial GAGs at different doses showed beneficial effects on cell growth, lipid peroxidation, reduced glutathione (GSH), SOD, and lactate dehydrogenase (LDH) levels in all oxidative models. HA and C4S exhibited the highest protection.

In fibroblast cultures exposed to $FeSO_4$ plus ascorbate (Campo *et al.*, 2004c), C4S and HA were able to limit cell death, DNA strand breaks, protein oxidation, OH generation, lipid peroxidation, and improved antioxidant defenses. The same beneficial effects were also obtained by adding purified human plasma GAGs to the same model of fibroblast cultures (Campo *et al.*, 2005a).

Oxidative stress induces MMPs/TIMPs imbalance (Wainwright, 2004). Purified human plasma C4S, by reducing ROS generation, was able to reduce MMPs/TIMPs imbalance caused in fibroblast cultures by $FeSO_4$ plus ascorbate (Campo *et al.*, 2005b).

V. *In Vivo* Studies

A. Animal Studies

Many *in vivo* laboratory works on antioxidant effect of GAG were carried out, which supported the findings of the *in vitro* researches.

CS was used complexed with iron as antianemic. The complex CS–Fe (Condrofer), given orally to rats in which severe experimental anemia had previously been induced, showed a more complete reversal of anemia than iron, probably due to the higher bioavailability of iron administered as complex (Barone *et al.*, 1988).

Supplementation in rats of the infused saline with CS reduced peroxidation of the peritoneum and prevented loss of ultrafiltration during peritoneal dialysis (Breborowicz *et al.*, 1994).

The contents of CS and HA in the surroundings of the bronchi were significantly increased after exposure to diesel exhaust particles (DEP), which have been shown to generate ROS, in the same areas in which cell damage and proliferating cell nuclear antigen-positive cells also increased (Sato *et al.*, 2001), suggesting that CS and HA in the lung contribute to cell process of recovery from injury caused by exposure to DEP.

CS antioxidant activity was exerted in rheumatoid arthritis (RA), in which ROS are thought to play an important role. Ronca *et al.* (1998) studied CS pharmacokinetics and tested its anti-inflammatory activity in rats. The results showed that compared with nonsteroidal anti-inflammatory drugs (NSAIDs), such as indomethacin or ibuprofen, CS appears to be more effective on cellular events of inflammation than on edema formation.

Beren *et al.* (2001) described an anti-inflammatory effect of a nutritional supplement consisting of a combination of glucosamine hydrochloride, purified sodium CS, and manganese ascorbate in a rat model of collagen-induced autoimmune arthritis (CIA).

Campo *et al.* (2003a) evaluated the antioxidant activity of HA and C4S in a rat model of CIA. Treatment with HA and C4S limited the erosive action in the articular joints of knee and paw, together with the possibly correlated synovial neutrophil infiltration and lipid peroxidation, while restored the endogenous antioxidants GSH and SOD. In Lewis rats with CIA, the treatment with HA and C4S again limited inflammation and the clinical signs in the knee and paw, reduced OH˙ production, decreased conjugated dienes (CD) levels, partially restored the endogenous antioxidants vitamin E (VE) and CAT, reduced MIP-2 serum levels and limited neutrophil infiltration (Campo *et al.*, 2003b). These data give further support to the possible role of endogenous GAGs to limit/control the progression of this detrimental disease, probably by working as metal chelators.

The hepatoprotective effect of CS on the antioxidant enzyme activity in total homogenate liver and mitochondria (Ha and Lee, 2003) and microsomal fractions of rats injected with CCl_4-induced liver injury was shown (Lee *et al.*, 2004).

Campo *et al.* (2004a) studied the effects of HA and C4S in a model of CCl_4-induced acute liver damage in rats. Several parameters were evaluated 24 h after CCl_4 administration, by intraperitoneal injection. Intraperitoneal treatment of rats with HA or C4S failed to exert any effect in the considered parameters, while the combination treatment with both GAGs decreased the serum levels of aminotransferases ALT and AST, inhibited lipid peroxidation by reducing hepatic MDA, reduced plasma TNF-α, restored the endogenous antioxidants, and decreased myeloperoxidase (MPO) activity, an index of neutrophil infiltration. These data suggest that HA and C4S could possess a different antioxidant mechanism, and consequently, the combined administration of both GAGs exerts a synergistic effect with respect to the single treatment.

HA or C4S intraperitoneally administered in a rat model of liver fibrosis induced by repeated injections of CCl$_4$ act successfully, especially when in combination, and reduced ALT and AST rise, lipid peroxidation, TIMPs activation and mRNA expression, partially restored SOD and GPx activities, and limited collagen deposition in the hepatic tissue (Campo et al., 2004d).

Campo et al. (2004e) also investigated the effect of the administration of C4S and HA in a cerulein-induced acute pancreatitis in rats. The results obtained showed that intraperitoneal pretreatment of rats with C4S, HA, or with both compounds ameliorated pancreatic cell conditions, restored the endogenous antioxidants GSH, CAT, and SOD, limited cell membrane peroxidation, and reduced neutrophil activation.

Finally, the treatment with CS was able to decrease MDA concentration and restore the SOD, CAT, and GPx activities in a dose-dependent manner in an experimental postmenopausal model in rats (Ha, 2004).

B. Human Studies

There are a multitude of positive clinical studies, involving different pathologies, in which CS acutely or chronically was administered.

Koch et al. (1993) showed that Viscoat (containing CS with HA) provided greater corneal endothelial protection than Healon (containing only HA) during iris-plane phacoemulsification. Kim and Joo (2004) concluded, by using the soft-shell technique, that Viscoat and Hyal-2000 (containing only HA) protected corneal endothelial cells during cataract surgery.

Shimamatsu (1998) reported that iron supplementation as i.v. iron–CS colloid may be a safely feasible ultimate way to rule out iron deficiency in hemodialysis patients with anemia resistant to recombinant human erythropoietin therapy i.v. A plausible explanation of these results is the iron chelating activity of CS preventing ROS formation.

Treatment with CS ameliorates symptoms and progression of osteoarthritis (OA). A large number of human studies have been performed with positive outcomes (Volpi, 2004). The exact role played by CS in limiting the effects of OA has not yet been elucidated. Fioravanti et al. (1991) and Rovetta (1991), by comparing in patients affected by OA the efficacy and the tolerance of galactosoaminoglucuronoglycan sulfate, by oral and/or intramuscular administration, with those of NSAIDs obtained good clinical results and good tolerance.

Morreale *et al.* (1996) assessed the clinical efficacy of CS, by intramuscular injection, in comparison with sodium diclofenac in a medium/long-term clinical study in patients with knee OA. Authors concluded that CS seems to have slow but gradually increasing clinical activity in OA and these benefits last for a long period after the end of treatment.

Coaccioli *et al.* (1998) evaluated the clinical efficacy and the tolerance of galactosaminoglucuronoglycan sulfate, administered both orally and intra-articularly, for the treatment of generalized and localized OA. Again a significant improvement of the articular function and excellent tolerance were observed.

Several other controlled clinical studies have been performed in osteoarthritic patients in order to evaluate the efficacy and tolerability against placebo (PBO) only. Uebelhart *et al.* (2004) investigated the efficacy and tolerability of a 3-month duration, twice a year, intermittent treatment with oral CS in knee OA patients, with positive results. The progression of erosion in the OA finger joints at 24 months resulted lower in patients treated with CS and naproxen than in patients taking naproxen only (Rovetta *et al.*, 2002). Improvement of the subjective symptoms was observed in patients with mono or bilateral knee OA treated for a period of 3 months with oral CS vs. PBO (Bourgeois *et al.*, 1998). Following a randomized, double-blind, PBO-controlled study by treating with CS patients with OA of the knee, Bucsi and Poor (1998) concluded that CS acts as a symptomatic slow-acting drug in knee OA.

Although in all these studies any possible mechanism of action played by CS or other GAGs was not investigated, and since in this pathology free radical attack seems to play a central role in cartilage degradation, it is plausible to suppose that, in part, the amelioration in OA symptoms could be due to a reduction in ROS activity.

VI. Antioxidant Mechanism

Several hypotheses about the antioxidant mechanism of CS and GAGs have been proposed. For example, Karlsson *et al.* (1988) suggested that the complex of GAGs with extracellular superoxide dismutase (E-SOD) may protect mammalian cells from free radical damage. Nevertheless, the most plausible explanation for CS, as well as for HA, is due to the presence of the carboxylic group of the glucuronic acid residue, always in the same spatial position, able to chelate metal ions, like Ca^{2+} (Cael *et al.*, 1978), and also like Cu^{2+} (Cu^{2+} ion binds CS more strongly that Ca^{2+} ion) (Dundstone, 1960) or Fe^{2+}, that are in turn responsible of the initiation of Fenton and Haber–Weiss reactions. The ability of these polysaccharides to chelate different ions and transition metals was extensively reported (Albertini *et al.*, 1997, 1999, 2000; Balogh *et al.*, 2003) and appears related to the antioxidant effect, since the metal entrapment could certainly decrease its availability for oxidation processes.

In C4S, sulfate group on the galactosamine residue may also interact with metal cation (Cael *et al.*, 1978). Albertini *et al.* (1999) suggested that a reasonable explanation for the different Cu^{2+} binding ability of C4S and C6S might be the distance between carboxylic and sulfate groups, which is shorter in C4S than in C6S. C6S may also positively reduce free radicals activity, although less than C4S (Campo *et al.*, 2004b). These data suggest that CS is differently able to bind iron and copper cations in solution. Albertini *et al.* (1997) suggested that the protective effect of C4S on Cu^{2+}-induced LDL oxidation depends upon electrostatic interactions masking some apoprotein copper-binding sites, which initiate oxidation process. C6S may be unable to realize a similar interaction, owing to the different position of the sulfate group. According to Volpi and Tarugi (1999b), the reversible GAG–LDL complex is based on hydrophobic interactions, as previously reported (Camejo *et al.*, 1991), introducing structural modifications that mask some copper-binding sites and decrease LDL susceptibility to copper-catalyzed oxidation. Arai *et al.* (1999) have supposed that the decomposition of GAGs by ROS produced neutralizing molecules that in turn may act as radical scavengers with consequent reduction in free radical activity.

Presti and Scott (1994) showed a direct scavenger action of HA on OH· generated by various oxidative systems.

A secondary activity of CS could be an anti-inflammatory effect exerted by chelating transition metals or by scavenging ROS.

VII. Pharmacological Strategies

CS administration orally or intravenously seems to be an interesting prospective of drug therapy to reduce free radical activity and the severity of diseases involving free radical generation, in particular OA. The antioxidants may act by reducing hydroperoxides and H_2O_2, by sequestering metal ions, by scavenging active free radicals, by repairing damage; or they may induce the biosynthesis of other antioxidants or defense enzymes.

The molecular characteristics of CS and its regulatory function on cell metabolism by binding growth factors, hormones, and other molecules of extracellular matrix, suggest that the mechanism of antioxidant action should be mainly expressed through both chelation activity and influence on antioxidants biosynthesis. The intravenously administration is the way in which a drug better does achieve target cells. Nevertheless, the oral route is more preferable because it is less invasive and easier for the patients,

TABLE I Conditions Showing Antioxidant Effects Following Treatment with Chondroitin Sulfate

Lipoproteins

Type of lipoprotein	Oxidative injury induced by	Reference
LDL	Cu^{2+}	Albertini et al., 1997; Volpi and Tarugi, 1999a
LDL	Cu^{2+} and AAPH	Volpi and Tarugi, 1999b
HDL	Cu^{2+}	Albertini et al., 1999
VLDL	Cu^{2+} and AAPH	Arai et al., 1999

Cell cultures

Type of added CS	Cell type	Oxidative injury induced by	Reference
Commercial	Rat cortical and hippocampal neurons	Excitatory amino acids	Okamoto et al., 1994
Commercial	Eye tissue	Phacoemulsification	Takahashi et al., 2002
Commercial	Human skin fibroblast	$CuSO_4$ plus ascorbate, $FeSO_4$ plus ascorbate or H_2O_2	Campo et al., 2004b
Commercial	Human skin fibroblast	$FeSO_4$ plus ascorbate	Campo et al., 2004c
From human plasma	Human skin fibroblast	$FeSO_4$ plus ascorbate	Campo et al., 2005a
			Campo et al., 2005b

Experimental animal model of diseases

Type of disease or injury	Animal	Oxidative injury induced by	Reference
Anemia	Rat	Iron-deficient diet	Barone et al., 1988
Inflammation	Rat	Zymosan and carrageenan	Ronca et al., 1998
Lung injury	Rat	Diesel exhaust particles	Sato et al., 2001
Autoimmune arthritis	Rat	CIA	Beren et al., 2001; Campo et al., 2003a,b
Acute liver injury	Rat	CCl_4	Campo et al., 2004a; Ha and Lee, 2003; Lee et al., 2004
Liver fibrosis	Rat	CCl_4	Campo et al., 2004d
Acute pancreatitis	Rat	Cerulein	Campo et al., 2004e
Menopause	Rat	Ovariectomy	Ha, 2004

Human diseases

Type of disease	Type of CS	Reference
Phacoemulsification	Viscoat	Kim and Joo, 2004; Koch et al., 1993
Osteoarthritis	Galactosoaminoglucuronoglycan sulfate	Coaccioli et al., 1998; Fioravanti et al., 1991; Rovetta, 1991
Hemodialysis	Iron–CS colloid	Shimamatsu, 1998
Osteoarthritis	Chondroitin sulfate	Bucsi and Poor, 1998; Bourgeois et al., 1998; Morreale et al., 1996; Rovetta et al., 2002; Uebelhart et al., 2004

although the amount of the active drug reaching the blood is controversial question.

Molecular size is another critical factor, which influences the rate of drug absorption. A study may be developed to identify and isolate the shortest CS chain able to chelate metal ions. In addition, CS could be chemically modified in order to better stabilize the chelation complex and to enhance direct free radical scavenger effect. However, the metabolic properties of chelating agents play a critical role in determining both their efficacy and toxicity, including inhibition of metal-containing enzymes.

VIII. Conclusions

Several basic science evidences, such as cell culture, or *in vitro* biochemical studies, suggest an antioxidant activity for CS that is able to reduce cell and tissue damage, due to free radical attack, mainly by sequestering transition metals that in turn catalyze ROS production. CS seems also to possess a slight radical scavenger activity. Cells from different tissue sources, such as endothelial cells, chondrocytes, neurons, and fibroblasts, obtained a beneficial antioxidant effect by CS treatment, as well as lipoproteins. To show the protective effect, several parameters were evaluated—inhibition of lipid peroxidation, restoring of endogenous antioxidants, such as SOD, CAT, GSH, GPx, VE, and so on, reduction of DNA damage, protein degradation and MMPs/TIMPs imbalance, and increased cell survival.

Using experimental animal models of diseases in which free radicals play an important role, CS was effective in the reduction of cartilage degradation and biochemical parameters amelioration in rats with induced arthritis, in rats with liver injury, and in models of lung intoxication and pancreatitis.

Some beneficial effects of CS in humans were also described, although mainly in the treatment of OA. Table I summarizes the antioxidant effects of CS.

References

Abuja, P. M. (2002). Aggregation of LDL with chondroitin-4-sulfate makes LDL oxidizable in the presence of water-soluble antioxidants. *FEBS Lett.* **512,** 245–248.

Albertini, R., Rindi, S., Passi, A., Bardoni, A., Salvini, R., Pallavicini, G., and De Luca, G. (1996). The effect of cornea proteoglycans on liposome peroxidation. *Arch. Biochem. Biophys.* **327,** 209–214.

Albertini, R., Ramos, P., Giessauf, A., Passi, A., and De Luca, G. (1997). Chondroitin 4-sulfate exhibits inhibitory effect durino Cu^{2+}-mediated LDL oxidation. *FEBS Lett.* **403,** 154–158.

Albertini, R., De Luca, G., Passi, A., Moratti, R., and Abuja, P. M. (1999). Chondroitin-4-sulfate protects high-density lipoprotein against copper-dependent oxidation. *Arch. Biochem. Biophys.* **365,** 143–149.

Albertini, R., Passi, A., Abuja, P. M., and De Luca, G. (2000). The effect of glycosaminoglycans and proteoglycans on lipid peroxidation. *Int. J. Mol. Med.* **6,** 129–136.

Arai, H., Kashiwagi, S., Nagasaka, Y., Uchida, K., Hoshii, Y., and Nakamura, K. (1999). Oxidative modification of apoliprotein E in human very-low-density lipoprotein and its inhibition by glycosaminoglycans. *Arch. Biochem. Biophys.* **367,** 1–8.

Balogh, G. T., Illes, J., Szekely, Z., Forrai, E., and Gere, A. (2003). Effect of different metal ions on the oxidative damage and antioxidant capacity of hyaluronic acid. *Arch. Biochem. Biophys.* **410,** 76–82.

Balt, S., de Boster, M. W., Booij, M., van Herk, A. M., and Visser-Luirink, G. (1983). Binding of metal ions to polysaccharides. Potentiometric, spectroscopic, and viscosimetric studies of the binding of cations to chondroitin sulfate and chondroitin in neutral and acidic aqueous media. *J. Inorg. Biochem.* **19,** 213–226.

Barone, D., Orlando, L., Vigna, E., Baroni, S., and Borghi, A. M. (1988). Ferric chondroitin 6-sulfate (Condrofer): A new potent antianemic agent with a favourable pharmacokinetic profile. *Drugs Exp. Clin. Res.* **14**(Suppl 1), 1–14.

Beren, J., Hill, S. L., Diener-West, M., and Rose, N. R. (2001). Effect of pre-loading oral glucosamine HCl/chondroitin sulfate/manganese ascorbate combination on experimental arthritis in rats. *Exp. Biol. Med.* **226,** 144–151.

Bode, W., and Maskos, K. (2003). Structural basis of the matrix metalloproteinases and their physiological inhibitors, the tissue inhibitors of metalloproteinases. *Biol. Chem.* **384,** 863–872.

Bourgeois, P., Chales, G., Dehais, J., Delcambre, B., Kuntz, J. L., and Rozenberg, S. (1998). Efficacy and tolerability of chondroitin sulfate 1200 mg/day vs chondroitin sulfate 3×400 mg/day vs placebo. *Osteoarthritis Cartilage* **6**(Suppl A), 25–30.

Breborowicz, A., Wieczorowska, K., Martis, L., and Oreopoulos, D. G. (1994). Glycosaminoglycan chondroitin sulfate prevents loss of ultrafiltration during peritoneal dialysis in rats. *Nephron* **67,** 346–350.

Bucsi, L., and Poor, G. (1998). Efficacy and tolerability of oral chondroitin sulfate as a symptomatic slow-acting drug for osteoarthritis (SYSADOA) in the treatment of knee osteoarthritis. *Osteoarthritis Cartilage* **6**(Suppl A), 31–36.

Cael, J. J., Winter, W. T., and Arnott, S. (1978). Calcium chondroitin 4-sulfate: Molecular conformation and organization of polysaccharide chains in a proteoglycan. *J. Mol. Biol.* **125,** 21–42.

Camejo, G., Camejo-Hurt, E., Rosengren, B., Wiklund, O., Lopez, F., and Bondjers, G. (1991). Modification of copper-catalyzed oxidation of low density lipoprotein by proteoglycans and glycosaminoglycans. *J. Lipid Res.* **32,** 1983–1991.

Campo, G. M., Avenoso, A., Campo, S., Ferlazzo, A. M., Altavilla, D., and Calatroni, A. (2003a). Efficacy of treatment with glycosaminoglycans on experimental collagen-induced arthritis in rats. *Arthr. Res. Ther.* **5,** R122–R131.

Campo, G. M., Avenoso, A., Campo, S., Ferlazzo, A. M., Altavilla, D., Micali, C., and Calatroni, A. (2003b). Aromatic trap analysis of free radicals production in experimental collagen-induced arthritis in the rat: Protective effect of glycosaminoglycans treatment. *Free Radic. Res.* **37,** 257–268.

Campo, G. M., Avenoso, A., Campo, S., Ferlazzo, A. M., Micali, C., Zanghì, L., and Calatroni, A. (2004a). Hyaluronic acid and chondroitin-4-sulphate treatment reduces damage in carbon tetrachloride-induced acute rat liver injury. *Life Sci.* **74,** 1289–1305.

Campo, G. M., D'Ascola, A., Avenoso, A., Campo, S., Ferlazzo, A. M., Micali, C., Zanghì, L., and Calatroni, A. (2004b). Glycosaminoglycans reduce oxidative damage induced by copper (Cu^{2+}), iron (Fe^{2+}) and hydrogen peroxide (H_2O_2) in human fibroblast cultures. *Glycoconj. J.* **20,** 133–141.

Campo, G. M., Avenoso, A., Campo, S., D'Ascola, A., Ferlazzo, A. M., and Calatroni, A. (2004c). Reduction of DNA fragmentation and hydroxyl radical production by hyaluronic acid and chondroitin-4-sulphate in iron plus ascorbate-induced oxidative stress in fibroblast cultures. *Free Radic. Res.* **38**, 601–611.

Campo, G. M., Avenoso, A., Campo, S., D'Ascola, A., Ferlazzo, A. M., and Calatroni, A. (2004d). The antioxidant and antifibrogenic effects of the glycosaminoglycans hyaluronic acid and chondroitin-4-sulphate in a subchronic rat model of carbon tetrachloride-induced liver fibrogenesis. *Chem. Biol. Interact.* **148**, 125–138.

Campo, G. M., Avenoso, A., Campo, S., Ferlazzo, A. M., and Calatroni, A. (2004e). Administration of hyaluronic acid and chondroitin-4-sulfate limits endogenous antioxidant depletion and reduces cell damage in experimental acute pancreatitis. *Pancreas* **28**, e45–e53.

Campo, G. M., Avenoso, A., D'Ascola, A., Campo, S., Ferlazzo, A. M., Samà, D., and Calatroni, A. (2005a). Purified human plasma glycosaminoglycans limit oxidative injury induced by iron plus ascorbate in skin fibroblast cultures. *Toxicol. In Vitro* **19**, 561–572.

Campo, G. M., Avenoso, A., Campo, S., D'Ascola, A., Ferlazzo, A. M., Samà, D., and Calatroni, A. (2005b). Purified human chondroitin-4-sulfate reduced MMPs/TIMPs imbalance induced by iron plus ascorbate in human fibroblast cultures. *Cell Biol. Intern.* **30**(1), 21–30.

Coaccioli, S., Allegra, A., Pennacchi, M., Mattioli, C., Ponteggia, F., Brunelli, A., Patucchi, E., and Puxeddu, A. (1998). Galactosaminoglucuronoglycan sulphate in the treatment of osteoarthritis: Clinical efficacy and tolerance of oral and intra-articular administrations. *Int. J. Clin. Pharmacol. Res.* **18**, 39–50.

Dunstone, J. R. (1960). Ion-exchange reactions between cartilage and various cations. *Biochem. J.* **77**, 164–170.

Evans, P., and Halliwell, B. (1999). Free radicals and hearing: Cause, consequence, and criteria. *Ann. NY Acad. Sci.* **884**, 19–40.

Fioravanti, A., Franci, A., Anselmi, F., Fattorini, L., and Marcolongo, R. (1991). Clinical efficacy and tolerance of galactosaminoglucuronoglycan sulfate in the treatment of osteoarthritis. *Drugs Exp. Clin. Res.* **17**, 41–44.

Ha, B. J. (2004). Oxidative stress in ovariectomy menopause and role of chondroitin sulfate. *Arch. Pharm. Res.* **27**, 867–872.

Ha, B. J., and Lee, J. Y. (2003). The effect of chondroitin sulphate against CCl_4-induced hepatotoxicity. *Biol. Pharm. Bull.* **26**, 622–626.

Halliwell, B., and Gutteridge, J. M. C. (1999). "Free Radicals in Medicine and Biology," 2nd Ed. Clarendon Press, Oxford.

Halliwell, B., Gutteridge, J. M., and Cross, C. E. (1992). Free radicals, antioxidants, and human disease: Where are we now? *J. Lab. Clin. Med.* **119**, 598–620.

Iozzo, R. V. (1998). Matrix proteoglycans: From molecular design to cellular function. *Ann. Rev. Biochem.* **67**, 609–652.

Karlsson, K., Lindahl, U., and Marklund, S. L. (1988). Binding of human extracellular superoxide dismutase C to sulphated glycosaminoglycans. *Biochem. J.* **256**, 29–33.

Kim, H., and Joo, C. K. (2004). Efficacy of the soft-shell technique using Viscoat and Hyal-2000. *J. Cataract Refract. Surg.* **30**, 2366–2370.

Koch, D. D., Liu, J. F., Glasser, D. B., Merin, L. M., and Haft, E. (1993). A comparison of corneal endhotelial changes after use of Healon or Viscoat during phacoemulsification. *Am. J. Ophthalmol.* **115**, 188–201.

Lee, J. Y., Lee, S. H., Kim, H. J., Ha, J. M., Lee, S. H., Lee, J. H., and Ha, B. J. (2004). The preventive inhibition of chondroitin sulfate against the CCl_4-induced oxidative stress of subcellular level. *Arch. Pharm. Res.* **27**, 340–345.

Morawski, M., Bruckner, M. K., Riederer, P., Bruckner, G., and Arendt, T. (2004). Perineuronal nets potentially protect against oxidative stress. *Exp. Neurol.* **188**, 309–315.

Morreale, P., Manopule, R., Galati, M., Boccanera, L., Saponati, G., and Bocchi, L. (1996). Comparison of the antiinflammatory efficacy of chondroitin sulfate and diclofenac sodium in patients with knee osteoarthritis. *J. Rheumatol.* **23**, 1385–1391.

Nagase, H., and Woessner, J. F., Jr. (1999). Matrix metalloproteinases. *J. Biol. Chem.* **274,** 21491–21494.

Okamoto, M., Mori, S., Ichimura, M., and Endo, H. (1994). Chondroitin sulfate proteoglycans protect cultured rat's cortical and hippocampal neurons from delayed cell death induced by excitatory amino acids. *Neurosci. Lett.* **172,** 51–54.

Presti, D., and Scott, J. E. (1994). Hyaluronan-mediated protective effect against cell damage caused by enzymatically produced hydroxyl (OH⁻) radicals is dependent on hyaluronan molecular mass. *Cell. Biochem. Funct.* **12,** 281–288.

Ronca, F., Palmieri, L., Panicucci, P., and Ronca, G. (1998). Anti-inflammatory activity of chondroitin sulfate. *Osteoarthritis Cartilage* **6**(Suppl A), 14–21.

Rovetta, G. (1991). Galactosaminoglycuronoglycan sulfate (matrix) in therapy of tibiofibular osteoarthritis of the knee. *Drugs Exp. Clin. Res.* **17,** 53–57.

Rovetta, G., Monforte, P., Molfetta, G., and Balestra, V. (2002). Chondroitin sulfate in erosive ostearthritis of the hands. *Int. J. Tissue React.* **24,** 29–32.

Sato, H., Onose, J., Toyoda, H., Toida, T., Imanari, T., Sagai, M., Nishimura, N., and Aoki, Y. (2001). Quantitative changes in glycosaminoglycans in the lungs of rats exposed to diesel exhaust. *Toxicology* **166,** 119–128.

Scott, J. E., Chen, Y., and Brass, A. (1992). Secondary and tertiary structures involving chondroitin and chondroitin sulphates in solution, investigated by rotary shadowing/electron microscopy and computer simulation. *Eur. J. Biochem.* **209,** 675–680.

Shimamatsu, K. (1998). Experience with i.v. iron chondroitin-sulphate colloid in Japanese haemodialysis patients. *Nephrol. Dial. Transplant* **13,** 1053.

Takahashi, H., Sakamoto, A., Takahashi, R., Ohmura, T., Shimmura, S., and Ohara, K. (2002). Free radicals in phacoemulsification and aspiration procedures. *Arch. Ophthalmol.* **120,** 1348–1352.

Uebelhart, D., Malaise, M., Marcolongo, R., De Vathaire, F., Piperno, M., Mailleux, E., Fioravanti, A., Matoso, L., and Vignon, E. (2004). Intermittent treatment of knee osteoarthritis with oral chondroitinsulfate: A one-year, randomized, double-blind, multicenter study versus placebo. *Osteoarthritis Cartilage* **12,** 269–276.

Volpi, N. (2004). The pathobiology of osteoarthritis and the rationale for using the chondroitin sulfate for its treatment. *Curr. Drug Targets Immune Endocr. Metabol. Disord.* **4,** 119–127.

Volpi, N., and Tarugi, P. (1999a). Influence of chondroitin sulfate charge density, sulfate group position, and molecular mass on Cu^{2+}-mediated oxidation of human low-density lipoproteins: Effect of normal human plasma-derived chondroitin sulfate. *J. Biochem.* **125,** 297–304.

Volpi, N., and Tarugi, P. (1999b). The protective effect on Cu^{2+}- and AAPH-mediated oxidation of human low-density lipoproteins depends on glycosaminoglycan structure. *Biochimie* **81,** 955–963.

Yang, C. Y., Bryan, A. M., Theil, E. C., Sayers, E. E., and Bowen, L. H. (1986). Structural variations in soluble iron complexes of models for ferritin: And x-ray absorption and Mossbauer spectroscopy comparison of horse spleen ferritin to Blutal (iron-chondroitin sulfate) and Imferon (iron-dextran). *J. Inorg. Biochem.* **28,** 393–405.

Wainwright, C. L. (2004). Matrix metalloproteinases, oxidative stress and the acute response to acute myocardial ischaemia and reperfusion. *Curr. Opin. Pharmacol.* **4,** 132–138.

N. Brandl*, J. Holzmann*, R. Schabus†, and M. Huettinger*

*Medical University Vienna
Center Physiology and Pathophysiology, 1090 Vienna
Währingerstrasse 10 Austria

†Department of Traumatology
University Hospital, 1090 Vienna
Währinger Gürtel 18–20, Austria

Effects of Chondroitin Sulfate on the Cellular Metabolism

I. Potential of the Versatile Molecule Chondroitin Sulfate to Interfere with Cellular Reactions

The vertebrate extracellular matrix (ECM) was for a long time believed to function mainly as a relative inert scaffolding to stabilize the physical structure of tissues. By now it is clear that the matrix plays a far more active and complex role in regulating the behavior of the cells that contact it—influencing their development, function, and metabolic manifestations. This chapter illustrates the evidence that pharmacological substitution of chondroitin sulfate (CS) functions by providing the source molecules for proper synthesis of aggrecan, the major cartilage matrix component. Furthermore, this chapter introduces the concept that it can be active in modulating the binding reactions that often form the basis for signaling events underlying proper matrix synthesis. The experimental evidence therefore is summarized.

Advances in Pharmacology, Volume 53
Copyright 2006, Elsevier Inc. All rights reserved.

1054-3589/06 $35.00
DOI: 10.1016/S1054-3589(05)53021-7

In this context, proteoglycans (PGs) are thought to play a major part in chemical signaling between cells. In a test tube, they bind various secreted signaling molecules such as certain protein growth factors, and it is likely that they do so in tissues. PGs also bind and regulate the activities of other types of secreted proteins such as proteolytic enzymes and protease inhibitors. Binding to a PG could control the activity of a protein in several ways: (1) it could immobilize the protein close to the site where it is produced, thereby restricting the range of action; (2) it could provide a reservoir of the protein for delayed release; (3) it could sterically alter or block the activity of the protein; (4) it could protect the protein from proteolytic degradation, thereby prolonging its action; and (5) it could alter or concentrate the protein for more effective presentation to cell-surface receptors. In addition, the glycosaminoglycan (GAG) portion can directly bind to cell surface receptors and transduce a signal. In some cases, the signaling molecules bind to the protein core of matrix PGs. As a prominent example, the ubiquitous growth regulatory protein transforming growth factor beta (TGFβ) binds to the core of decorin, what inhibits the activity of TGFβ. In most cases, however, the signaling molecules bind to the GAG chains of the PG. The GAG chains vary from type to type, what brings upon varying binding constants from tissue to tissue. In addition, the composition of the carbohydrate modifications can be adapted to metabolic situations, such as mechanical wear or inflammatory reactions, within each GAG type and provides adaptive modulation of the binding constant in addition to type specificity (Kim *et al.*, 1996; Plaas *et al.*, 1998, 2000). The range of diversity of the activities controlled by the binding is further expanded by this adaptive modification.

At the level of cell physiology, the concept of a beneficial effect of CS that is added externally in soluble form, includes that the earlier mentioned binding reactions of receptors, signal molecules, and proteases to the CSs linked to the plasma membrane or extracellular scaffold are competed by the soluble form created *in situ* by matrix degradation or by pharmacologic application. In the consequence the regulatory effects, such as immobilizing and restricting the range of action, steric alteration of the activity, protection from proteolytic degradation and concentration to form a reservoir or to allow for more effective presentation to cell-surface receptors, are all competed by the soluble form of orally substituted CS.

In the physiologic situation, binding of the respective molecules occurs to the static framework of the CS side chains in aggrecan, the predominant PG in cartilage. The dissociation equilibria of the bound molecules determine the contribution of this mechanism to the signals transmitted into chondrocytes. The equilibrium can be disturbed when aggrecan is degraded and soluble CS is set free, carrying the signal molecules away from the site of action. In addition, when externally added CS elevates the concentration within the cell matrix area, the soluble CSs compete with the matrix scaffold and exchange the signal molecules from the matrix what consequently leads to altered availability at the cell surface.

The details of this molecular concept are largely enigmatic, there is, however, considerable evidence from studies in neuronal and glia cells, which supports the assumption of a specific effectiveness of CSs in modifying the cell metabolism by signal transduction into the chondrocytes.

We are at the beginning of understanding the CS function at the cellular level, and although data are scarce, one cannot rule out one or more receptors for CS that transmit directly signals into cell.

II. Chondroitin Sulfate Functions in Nerve Tissue

A great deal of knowledge on the interaction of CS with cells was gathered in the last decade with brain cells, neurons as well as glia cells. The situation is somewhat similar to what can be seen in joint tissue, where chondrocytes are embedded in chondroitin sulfate proteoglycans (CSPGs) that create the environment in which differentiation and proliferation of the chondrocytes with assistance of cells from synovial tissue takes place. CSPGs are the most abundant subtype of PGs in the nerve tissue. They have a wide distribution in brain and are largely found in the ECM, where they interact with other proteins such as collagen, fibronectin, laminin, or vitronectin. These interactions are mediated in most cases by the GAG component of the PGs. A second class of PGs is found integrated in the plasma membrane of neurons and glia cells, either as transmembrane proteins or as glycosyl-phosphatidyl (GPI)–anchored molecules. These cell surface PGs are largely implicated in cell adhesion, process outgrowth, and synaptogenesis as well as in the binding of signal molecules like the growth factors of the Wnt family, fibroblast growth factor (FGF), and TGFβ.

Traditionally, the expression of heparan sulfate proteoglycans (HSPGs) can be associated with neuritogenesis, while CSPGs and dermatan sulfate proteoglycans (DSPGs) appear to provide inhibitory clues to growing neurites. However, the specificity seems largely to be determined by the type of neuron, as the opposite can be observed also. Mostly the effectiveness of the PGs is deduced from coincidence of axon guidance effects and positional expression of the PGs. There are only limited data on a molecular level, how these effects are brought upon. As found within retinal path finding in the *Xenopus* embryo, soluble HS interacts with native FGF-2 (Walz *et al.*, 1997). In studies with the *Xenopus* model, it was detected that addition of soluble GAGs altered the trajectory of different brain axon bundles in a rapid and reversible way. This effect was explained by a competitive interference of the soluble GAG with endogenous GAG-binding molecules (Walz *et al.*, 1997). As a result an imbalance of the growth cone adhesion to its surrounding environment can be observed.

As described by Rapp and Huettinger (2005), CS may compete with the uptake processes of lipoproteins mediated by low-density lipoprotein receptors. In other studies, GAG binding to neuronal surface was followed by internalization of the GAG itself. Binding was observed throughout the cell surface on the cell body, processes, and growth cone. Subsequently, accumulation into lysosomes, endoplasmic reticulum, and Golgi apparatus could be observed. Such mechanism is likely operative in chondrocytes also and would serve the purpose of delivering elements of matrix synthesis by catabolism of polymer CS in lysosomes and delivery of the products into endoplasmic reticulum and Golgi apparatus, where synthesis of aggrecan and other PGs is carried out. In addition, products of GAG degradation can take a different intracellular route and appear occasionally in the nucleus, resulting in some cell types in cell cycle arrest and trans-repressor activity on Fos and Jun/Ap-1 transcription (Busch *et al.*, 1992). Binding of CSPGs to surface receptors has been further shown to activate second messengers: raises in cytoplasmic calcium, cAMP levels, and activation of GTPase, PKc, and tyrosin kinase signaling pathways are among the effects reported upon binding of PGs— many of them of potential importance for chondrocytes. Although not all these effects were controlled with chondroitinase, to show the dependency on the GAG portion of the PGs, the role thereof is unquestionable.

The events occurring in a process that is called glial scarring, the central event presenting an obstacle for regrowing axons, uncover a pivotal role for the CSs. The noticeable outcome of these events, the growth cone collapse, is pungently induced by myelin components and more subtle by CSPGs. Treatment with chondroitinase and subsequent overcome of inhibition served as control for the relevance of the GAG component in the process. Here, a remarkable interaction of CSPGs with the Rho family of GTPases, which direct the formation of a wide range of cytoskeletal structuring processes, was uncovered. Neutralization of Rho activation allowed axons to cross CSPG barriers in cell culture models. Although in this report it was not possible to reverse the effect by chondroitinase treatment, a participation of the GAG portion is likely and is evident in other systems (Fawcett and Asher, 1999). Rho mediated signal transduction produce, for example, proliferation incentives only when a proper signal is given by integrins that there is adherence to ECM and prohibits transduction when the cell is liberated and suspended in medium. It will be interesting to find out whether soluble ECM components can imitate ECM or block the integrin related binding site.

Numerous reports point toward a versatile function of CS depending on the sulfation pattern.

Chondroitin sulfate proteoglycans and CSGAGs have been reported to inhibit neurite outgrowth *in vitro* (Bandtlow and Zimmermann, 2000; Davies *et al.*, 1997; Faissner and Steindler, 1995; McKeon *et al.*, 1991; Niederost *et al.*, 1999). This concept is consistent with findings that degradation of CS chains permitted the axonal regeneration after a spinal cord injury (Bradbury *et al.*, 2002). In contrast, DSD-1-PG, a PG that contains disulfated D disaccharide units [D-glucuronic acid-(2s)-N-acetyl-D-galactosamine (6s)] has been suggested to stimulate neurite outgrowth of cultured rat hippocampal neurons through its distinct CS side chain structure (Faissner *et al.*, 1994). Using a set of CSs with distinct sulfation percentage in the 4- and 6-position, we could demonstrate that the variation in the GAG chain exerts differential cellular effects. It was also of profound interest whether externally added CSs can compete with core protein bound CS to modulate the effects of tissue-synthesized matrix. In series of microscopic images three parameters of neuritic outgrowth activity, neurite length, number of neurites, and fasciculation (thickness of neurites) were analyzed at concentrations occurring in intact tissues. Fasciculation increased and number of neurites decreased with high di-sulfation. No significant differences on process length reduction were found between the CS isotypes. The data indicate that the soluble fragments from CS are actively modulating cell development. Besides dosage, sulfation density and position are relevant for effects of CS in neuronal regenerative activity (Rapp *et al.*, 2005).

Taken together, the underlying mechanisms by which CSPGs inhibit the cell machinery that coordinates neuronal growth are complex. In some cases, the inhibitory clues are attributed to the GAG portion of the molecule solely. In others, CSPGs cannot be made growth permissive after chondroitinase digest. The studies, however, provide rich information of what principal cellular events could contribute to changes in chondrocyte physiology mediated by provision of soluble CS. These are: (1) CS can be internalized and degraded, thus providing building blocks for matrix synthesis; (2) internalized CS can be transported to the nucleus and function there as a trans-activating gene expression regulator; (3) a complex interaction of CS within elements of the ECM that contacts integrins or transmembrane receptors plus; and (4) binding, exchange, and modulation of bound growth factors and proteases that all transmit to and activate intracellular distinct signal pathways. Many of these properties are tied to the modifications of sulfation. With all these data on the interaction of CS on neuronal growth, it seems possible to suggest a participation of CS in the pain reduction as found in studies of CS treatment of osteoarthritis (OA) (Leeb *et al.*, 2000). Nerve fibers can be found even in menisci, preferentially, alongside blood vessels. Delivery of soluble CS is ascertained by this anatomical situation (Mine *et al.*, 2000).

The following experimental evidence records what metabolic consequences relevant for OA pathology can be found in cells.

III. Biological and Pharmacological Changes in Chondroitin Sulfate Levels that Effect Metabolic Changes

There are numerous reports in which levels of CS in serum and synovial fluid were determined in normal and pathological conditions (Bautch *et al.*, 2000; Belcher *et al.*, 1997; Ettrich *et al.*, 1998; Fox and Cook, 2001; Hazell *et al.*, 1995; Heimer *et al.*, 1992; Ishimaru *et al.*, 2001; Kindblom and Angervall, 1975; Lewis *et al.*, 1999; Nakayama *et al.*, 2002; Saito *et al.*, 2002; Shinmei *et al.*, 1992; Smith *et al.*, 1980; Uesaka *et al.*, 2002; Yamada *et al.*, 1999). In view of the major risk factor for OA, age, the concomitant significant decrease of the C6S/C4S in synovial fluid is a remarkable discovery (Nakayama *et al.*, 2002). It is further corroborated by an examination of the levels of CS in synovial fluid of a collection of patients with staged OA (Kellgren and Lawrence scale I to IV) presenting a decline of C6S/C4S ratio from 5,6 at stage I to 2,7 at stage IV. The slow progressive form of OA within the ageing population seems different from the acute form of OA resulting from trauma, at least in terms of CS levels in synovial fluid (Shinmei *et al.*, 1992). Here, the ratios of C6S/C4S were found comparable to the healthy and age matched control group (approximately 27 years).

The levels of CS that can be achieved in serum by oral substitution were determined elaborately by several authors (Adebowale *et al.*, 2002; Conte *et al.*, 1995; Palmieri *et al.*, 1990; Volpi, 2002, 2003; Volpi and Maccari, 2005). By scintigraphic methods a tropism of CS for cartilaginous tissue in knee was found (Ronca *et al.*, 1998). Chondroitin sulfate that was labeled with Tc and injected was monitored for whole body distribution with a gamma camera. Although the intensity in the bloodstream was expected to be highest, a distinct area of very high intensity was seen over an area superimposable to the knee joint. Taken together, these results provide a basis for estimating the concentration that can be achieved in synovial fluid—approximately 10–50 μg/ml—to generate metabolic influences. In terms of reaction kinetics, the twofold to threefold elevation that was measured in serum could be even augmented by the tropism for joint space and thus influence high as well as low affinity binding processes. Thus, for all the hypothesized cellular mechanisms a sufficient change in concentration will be existent to produce a significant change in binding equilibrium.

IV. Effects of Soluble Chondroitin Sulfate on Chondrocytes _____

Cells building the body bearing tissue depend heavily on elements that confer mechanostability. The remarkable feature of cartilage is that local forces cause the elements involved in mechanostability to reorient and while loosing flexibility to gain stability. The reorientation is transduced into the cell and causes a number of reactions intracellularly, among others involved are actin-filaments (stress-fibers), microtubule, and intermediate filaments. They contact integrins located in the cell membrane and so couple to the extracellular components like fibronectin, collagen, and PGs over distance. At this point, a rich source of signaling is located, kinases and signal proteins tuning production of cytokines and proteinases that coordinate the cell metabolism. They all are complexed to the integrins receiving input of the level of mechanical stress. That this system is tangled by CS was probed by observing the effect of addition of CS on actin-filaments of fibroblasts after mechanical disruption of the monolayer. The induced reorientation of the monolayer, a situation comparable to wound healing, caused reorientation of stress fibers toward the wound area solely in cultures with CS added (Gschwentner and Huettinger, 1998).

We demonstrated by immunofluorescence microscopy that PGs have minor effects on the formation of stress fibers in confluent undisturbed fibroblast cultures. There was, however, a dramatic effect in regenerating fibroblast monolayers on the coordinated formation of stress fibers in the presence of CS but not other GAGs like HS (Fig. 1). The pictures demonstrate that CS in a regenerating fibroblast monolayer culture could induce stress fiber conformation concentrated toward the stressed area, indicating a mechanism likely to involve integrin signaling and stimulated actin turnover.

In OA, the chondrocytes lack anabolic effectiveness and catabolic reactions are dominating. Essentially the same signaling events are in effect in slow progressive OA, which is attributed to gene expression changes within ageing and acute forms that follow trauma (Aigner *et al.*, 2003, 2004; Hamerman, 1998).

For the elucidation of the metabolic effect of CS, it is of fundamental interest to pinpoint regulatory events tipping on either side of the balance, the inhibition of catabolic and the increase of anabolic reactions. There are solid reports on the interaction of ECM components including CSPGs with integrins and subsequent activation of signal transduction pathways (Gemba *et al.*, 2002; Makihira *et al.*, 1999; Midwood and Salter, 2001; Millward-Sadler *et al.*, 2000; Segat *et al.*, 2002). Mechanical stimulation of human

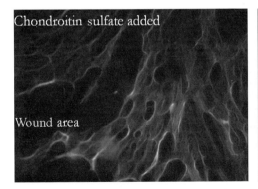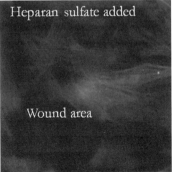

FIGURE I Stress fiber orientation at sites of laceration (wound area) is affected distinctly by CS but not other GAGs. Fibroblast were grown to 50% confluency and lacerated by scratching the monolayer. Cells were then grown with the indicated additions of GAGs (50 µg/ml) and the actin detected with fluorescent phalloidin and observed in a Zeiss Axiovert microscope.

articular chondrocytes *in vitro* results in increased levels of aggrecan mRNA and decreased levels of MMP-3 mRNA by a transduction process involving integrins and the focal adhesion kinases. The chondroprotective response is absent in chondrocytes from OA cartilage. Abnormalities of mechanotransduction leading to aberrant chondrocyte activity in diseased articular cartilage are therefore considered important in the progression of OA. As an example, HMPG is a CSPG, expressed by chondrocytes in fetal and in normal and osteoarthritic adult articular cartilage. HMPG is a receptor for ECM proteins, including type VI collagen, and regulates beta1 integrin binding to fibronectin in normal cells. In OA chondrocytes the function is impaired. Furthermore, analysis of mitogen-activated protein kinases (MAPKs) showed activation of extracellular signal-regulated kinase (ERK), c-Jun NH2-terminal kinase, and p38 MAPK in the consequence of activation of focal adhesion kinases. These data converge into the interpretation that focal adhesion kinase and MAPK mediate mechanotransduction, and activation of human articular chondrocytes and CSPGs are participating. Some reports extend the role for integrin subtypes to switch chondrocyte differentiation: one promotes chondrocyte differentiation, whereas another is necessary to stabilize the differentiated phenotype. It might serve as a working hypothesis that soluble CS interferes with these processes, but no experimental evidence exists yet. We have therefore started to substantiate the assumption by measuring the previously mentioned key signal events, p38 and ERK after adding CS in cell culture. Effects on these would bring insight into the cellular mechanisms driving the anabolic results found upon incubation of chondrocytes with CS (Bassleer *et al.*, 1998). Initially we found no alterations. However, when chondrocytes were provoked into a catabolic state with lipopolysaccharide (LPS), significant alterations came about. LPS is a bacterial cell wall component frequently associated with the induction of OA after bacterial infections (Benton *et al.*, 2002; Tiku *et al.*, 1992). LPS effects were profoundly modulated by TGFβ, CS, and both applied in combination. Most prominent, silencing of the LPS activated p38 stress signal by CS was superimposable to TGFβ mediated silencing. TGFβ also raised phospho-ERK1/2 levels threefold over LPS induced levels. In contrast, CS treatment alone or combined with TGFβ reduced phosphorylation significantly below LPS induced levels. Here, CS overrides the TGFβ effect (Fig. 2). Finally, LPS induced MMP-13 mRNA levels were further enhanced by TGFβ while inhibition resulted with CS. These results are the first direct linkage of interference of soluble CS with signal processes relevant in chondrocytes. In addition, they conform with *in vivo* findings that CS treatment proved to be more efficient in acute forms of cartilage degradation (Uebelhart *et al.*, 1998). That CS interferes with TGFβ signaling opens a variety of accomplishments for the tasks of CS. TGFβ is synthesized by human articular chondrocytes and stored in latent form in considerable amounts. Within inflammation, levels rise considerably, pointing toward a

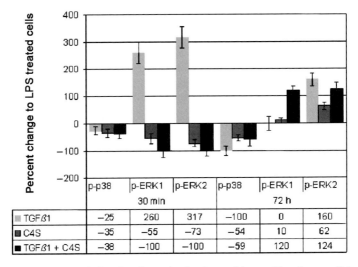

FIGURE 2   LPS induced phosphorylation levels of stress kinase p38 and extracellular signal related kinase (ERK1/2) are differentially regulated in human articular chondrocytes upon treatment with TGFβ, or CS, or both in combination. Cells were treated with LPS and the phosphorylation state of the signal proteins determined by immunoblotting with phospho-specific antibodies and the resulting densitometric values representing 0% change. Parallel incubations were performed with the additions indicated and the reduction in phosphorylation levels specified as negative and an increase as positive percentage.

crucial function (Glansbeek *et al.*, 1997, 1998; Lafeber *et al.*, 1997; Takahashi *et al.*, 2005; van Beuningen *et al.*, 1998; van den Berg, 1999; van der Kraan *et al.*, 1997). Application of TGFβ not only enhances inflammatory response but also decreases degradation of cartilage. Although, in common, TGFβ is considered to generate an anabolic state in human articular chondrocytes, opposite effects are reported not infrequently. This dichotomy of TGFβ seems to depend on the particular environmental, metabolic, and differentiation status of the chondrocyte receiving the TGFβ signal (Grimaud *et al.*, 2002; Selvamurugan *et al.*, 2004; van der Kraan *et al.*, 2002). From our experiments, it seems that CS has the effectiveness to participate in the decision making of the chondrocyte, how to execute a TGFβ signal. Such effectiveness will also confer to subsequent MMP expression control. TGFβ is known to exert a number of effects on MMPs (Grimaud *et al.*, 2002), most appealing in view of the dichotomic behavior, it was reported to downregulate MMP-1, -8, and -13 in chondrocytes near to cartilage lesions but to upregulate MMP-13 more distant to that lesion (Shlopov *et al.*, 2000).

The canonical TGFβ signaling via SMAD translocation to the cell nuclei (Heldin *et al.*, 1997), and subsequent regulation of transcription is modulated by signal cascades (Mengshol *et al.*, 2000), which are also target of soluble CS. The growth stimulation of human articular chondrocytes by TGFβ is partially influenced by activation of ERK, the extracellular signal related kinase (Yonekura *et al.*, 1999). ERK, on the other side can influence the expression of TGFβ receptor type I and II (Zhao and Buick, 1995), at least in certain cell types, and retard the translocation of SMAD complexes to the nucleus (Kretzschmar *et al.*, 1997). Furthermore, for MMP-13 induction by TGFβ, a certain level of p38 activation is a necessary prerequisite. This is evident from experiments where inhibitors of p38 abolish MMP-13 induction (Leivonen *et al.*, 2002, 2005). In summary, the complexity of the possible cellular effects promise a variety of stimulations for chondrocyte metabolism that are well controlled by cross talk with signal events and thus warrant biologically safe results. The precise knowledge of their meaning for the clinical outcome will certainly aid a precise application of the varieties of CS for specific types and stages of OA.

V. Concluding Statement

The chemical versatility of the CS molecule suggests a variety of options to interfere with metabolic and regulatory processes on the cellular level. Pivotal in these is certainly the influence on chondrocyte physiology, although interactions with cells composing the synovial tissue are not to be neglected. The concentration ranges that can be achieved with oral substitution of CS compounds suggest that high- and low-affinity interactions with the soluble CS can be influenced sufficiently to produce a cartilage maintenance effect. Tissue culture studies show that the sulfation pattern is of significance for the cellular processes invoked by CS. Clinical studies indicate that the sulfation pattern of CS in synovial fluid is specific for acute trauma associated OA and slow progressive OA as occurring with age. This suggests that future studies ought to include a differentiated evaluation of the effects of high C4S and C6S compounds in aged populations with slow progressive OA and such with acute OA resulting from trauma.

On the cellular level, we are beginning to nominate candidate mechanisms mediated by CS. Very plausibly, there are on one hand interactions of transmembrane proteins like integrins with ECM components, among them CSPGs. Thus, extracellular changes are connected to the cell membrane and transmitted into the chondrocyte. Any CSPG mediated contact may be influenced by elevation of soluble CS, with subsequent alteration of the transduced signal quantity. This type of interaction is in charge of regulating the adaptive cartilage construction in response to mechanical forces or change in the extracellular environment, a condition frequently found with increasing body weight within ageing and change of gait or after trauma. On the other hand, more direct interactions with extracellular receptors and ligands seem to generate cell-signaling events. Chondroitin sulfate interferes with TGFβ signaling, which opens a variety of accomplishments for the tasks of CS substitution.

In any case, regulation of stress kinase, p38, or ERK is up to now already found relevant. The influence on signal events can lead subsequently to MMP activity changes, which are crucial for cartilage maintenance. The regulatory capacity of CS can be projected from the initial hypothesis that is based on the manipulation of equilibria of binding events where one partner is CS, integral in ECM, and the soluble CS intercepting binding partners of the integral ECM component. So far this hypothesis was substantiated by documented influences on intracellular signal events. Although a number of hitherto unknown single events are likely, the chondrocyte, after interpretation of the cross talk, decides which metabolic action to take. The resulting evened out range of effect constitutes an advantage, as an on/off effect, as produced by acute intervention inhibitors in trial, could be of disadvantage when topic changes in mechanical stress necessitates cartilage degradation next to synthesis. The other consequence, a prolonged application to accumulate benefit, is acceptable as only rare-to-none side effects are reported with oral intake of CS.

References

Adebowale, A., Du, J., Liang, Z., Leslie, J. L., and Eddington, N. D. (2002). The bioavailability and pharmacokinetics of glucosamine hydrochloride and low molecular weight chondroitin sulfate after single and multiple doses to beagle dogs. *Biopharm. Drug Dispos.* **23**, 217–225.

Aigner, T., Zien, A., Hanisch, D., and Zimmer, R. (2003). Gene expression in chondrocytes assessed with use of microarrays. *J. Bone Joint Surg. Br.* **85**-A(Suppl 2), 117–123.

Aigner, T., Rose, J., Martin, J., and Buckwalter, J. (2004). Aging theories of primary osteoarthritis: From epidemiology to molecular biology. *Rejuvenation Res.* **7**, 134–145.

Bandtlow, C. E., and Zimmermann, D. R. (2000). Proteoglycans in the developing brain: New conceptual insights for old proteins. *Physiol. Rev.* **80**, 1267–1290.

Bassleer, C. T., Combal, J. P., Bougaret, S., and Malaise, M. (1998). Effects of chondroitin sulfate and interleukin-1[beta] on human articular chondrocytes cultivated in clusters. *Osteoarthritis Cartilage* **6**, 196–204.

Bautch, J. C., Clayton, M. K., Chu, Q., and Johnson, K. A. (2000). Synovial fluid chondroitin sulphate epitopes 3B3 and 7D4, and glycosaminoglycan in human knee osteoarthritis after exercise. *Ann. Rheum. Dis.* **59**, 887–891.

Belcher, C., Yaqub, R., Fawthrop, F., Bayliss, M., and Doherty, M. (1997). Synovial fluid chondroitin and keratan sulphate epitopes, glycosaminoglycans, and hyaluronan in arthritic and normal knees. *Ann. Rheum. Dis.* **56**, 299–307.

Benton, H. P., MacDonald, M. H., and Tesch, A. M. (2002). Effects of adenosine on bacterial lipopolysaccharide- and interleukin 1-induced nitric oxide release from equine articular chondrocytes. *Am. J. Vet. Res.* **63**, 204–210.

Bradbury, E. J., Moon, L. D., Popat, R. J., King, V. R., Bennett, G. S., Patel, P. N., Fawcett, J. W., and McMahon, S. B. (2002). Chondroitinase ABC promotes functional recovery after spinal cord injury. *Nature* **416**, 636–640.

Busch, S. J., Martin, G. A., Barnhart, R. L., Mano, M., Cardin, A. D., and Jackson, R. L. (1992). Trans-repressor activity of nuclear glycosaminoglycans on Fos and Jun/AP-1 oncoprotein-mediated transcription. *J. Cell Biol.* **116**, 31–42.

Conte, A., Volpi, N., Palmieri, L., Bahous, I., and Ronca, G. (1995). Biochemical and pharmacokinetic aspects of oral treatment with chondroitin sulfate. *Arzneimittelforschung* **45**, 918–925.

Davies, S. J. A., Fitch, M. T., Memberg, S. P., Hall, A. K., Raisman, G., and Silver, J. (1997). Regeneration of adult axons in white matter tracts of the central nervous system. *Nature* **390**, 680–683.

Ettrich, U., Fengler, H., Dressler, F., and Schulze, K. J. (1998). Uberblick uber den aktuellen Stand der messbaren Parameter des Knorpelstoffwechsels in verschiedenen Korperflussigkeiten. +AFs-Overview of the current status of measurable parameters of cartilage metabolism in various body fluids+AF0. *Z. Rheumatol.* **57**, 375–391.

Faissner, A., Clement, A., Lochter, A., Streit, A., Mandl, C., and Schachner, M. (1994). Isolation of a neural chondroitin sulfate proteoglycan with neurite outgrowth promoting properties. *J. Cell Biol.* **126**, 783–799.

Faissner, A., and Steindler, D. (1995). Boundaries and inhibitory molecules in developing neural tissues. *Glia* **13**, 233–254.

Fawcett, J. W., and Asher, R. A. (1999). The glial scar and central nervous system repair. *Brain Res. Bull.* **49**, 377–391.

Fox, D. B., and Cook, J. L. (2001). Synovial fluid markers of osteoarthritis in dogs. *J. Am. Vet. Med. Assoc.* **6**, 756–761.

Gemba, T., Valbracht, J., Alsalameh, S., and Lotz, M. (2002). Focal adhesion kinase and mitogen-activated protein kinases are involved in chondrocyte activation by the 29-kDa amino-terminal fibronectin fragment. *J. Biol. Chem.* **277**, 907–911.

Glansbeek, H. L., van der Kraan, P. M., Lafeber, F. P., Vitters, E. L., and van den Berg, W. B. (1997). Species-specific expression of type II TGF-beta receptor isoforms by articular chondrocytes: Effect of proteoglycan depletion and aging. *Cytokine* **9**, 347–351.

Glansbeek, H. L., van Beuningen, H. M., Vitters, E. L., van der Kraan, P. M., and van den Berg, W. B. (1998). Stimulation of articular cartilage repair in established arthritis by local administration of transforming growth factor-beta into murine knee joints. *Lab. Invest.* **78**, 133–142.

Grimaud, E., Heymann, D., and Redini, F. (2002). Recent advances in TGF-beta effects on chondrocyte metabolism: Potential therapeutic roles of TGF-beta in cartilage disorders. *Cytokine Growth Factor Rev.* **13**, 241–257.

Gschwentner, C., and Huettinger, M. (1998). Stress fiber analysis of fibroblasts grown on different proteoglycans. *Litera Rheumatol.* **24**, 9–13.

Hamerman, D. (1998). Biology of the aging joint. *Clin. Geriatr. Med.* **14**, 417–433.

Hazell, P. K., Dent, C., Fairclough, J. A., Bayliss, M. T., and Hardingham, T. E. (1995). Changes in glycosaminoglycan epitope levels in knee joint fluid following injury. *Arthritis Rheum.* **38**, 953–959.

Heimer, R., Sporer, R., Molinaro, L., Hansen, L., and Laposata, E. (1992). Normal human synovial fluid and articular cartilage contain similar intact proteoglycans. *Lab. Invest.* **66**, 701–707.

Heldin, C. H., Miyazono, K., and ten Dijke, P. (1997). TGF-[beta] signalling from cell membrane to nucleus through SMAD proteins. *Nature* **390**, 465–471.

Ishimaru, J. I., Ogi, N., Mizuno, S., and Goss, A. N. (2001). Quantitation of chondroitin-sulfates, disaccharides and hyaluronan in normal, early and advanced osteoarthritic sheep temporomandibular joints. *Osteoarthritis Cartilage* **9**, 365–370.

Kim, Y. J., Grodzinsky, A. J., and Plaas, A. H. (1996). Compression of cartilage results in differential effects on biosynthetic pathways for aggrecan, link protein, and hyaluronan. *Arch. Biochem. Biophys.* **328**, 331–340.

Kindblom, L. G., and Angervall, L. (1975). Histochemical characterization of mucosubstances in bone and soft tissue-tumors. *Cancer* **36**, 985–994.

Kretzschmar, M., Doody, J., and Massague, J. (1997). Opposing BMP and EGF signalling pathways converge on the TGF-beta family mediator Smad1. *Nature* **389**, 618–622.

Lafeber, F. P., van Roy, H. L., van der Kraan, P. M., van den Berg, W. B., and Bijlsma, J. W. (1997). Transforming growth factor-beta predominantly stimulates phenotypically changed chondrocytes in osteoarthritic human cartilage. *J. Rheumatol.* **24**, 536–542.

Leeb, B. F., Schweitzer, H., Montag, K., and Smolen, J. S. (2000). A meta-analysis of chondroitin sulfate in the treatment of osteoarthritis. *J. Rheumatol.* **27**, 205–211.

Leivonen, S. K., Chantry, A., Hakkinen, L., Han, J., and Kahari, V. M. (2002). Smad3 mediates transforming growth factor-beta-induced collagenase-3 (matrix metalloproteinase-13) expression in human gingival fibroblasts: Evidence for cross-talk between Smad3 and p38 signaling pathways. *J. Biol. Chem.* **277**, 46338–46346.

Leivonen, S. K., Hakkinen, L., Liu, D., and Kahari, V. M. (2005). Smad3 and extracellular signal-regulated kinase 1/2 coordinately mediate transforming growth factor-beta-induced expression of connective tissue growth factor in human fibroblasts. *J. Invest. Dermatol.* **124**, 1162–1169.

Lewis, S., Crossman, M., Flannelly, J., Belcher, C., Doherty, M., Bayliss, M. T., and Mason, R. M. (1999). Chondroitin sulphation patterns in synovial fluid in osteoarthritis subsets. *Ann. Rheum. Dis.* **58**, 441–445.

Makihira, S., Yan, W., Ohno, S., Kawamoto, T., Fujimoto, K., Okimura, A., Yoshida, E., Noshiro, M., Hamada, T., and Kato, Y. (1999). Enhancement of cell adhesion and spreading by a cartilage-specific noncollagenous protein, cartilage matrix protein (CMP/Matrilin-1), via integrin alpha1beta1. *J. Biol. Chem.* **274**, 11417–11423.

McKeon, R., Schreiber, R. C., Rudge, J. S., and Silver, J. (1991). Reduction of neurite outgrowth in a model of glial scarring following CNS injury is correlated with the expression of inhibitory molecules on reactive astrocytes. *J. Neurosci.* **11**, 3398–3411.

Mengshol, J. A., Vincenti, M. P., Coon, C. I., Barchowsky, A., and Brinckerhoff, C. E. (2000). Interleukin-1 induction of collagenase 3 (matrix metalloproteinase 13) gene expression in chondrocytes requires p38, c-Jun N-terminal kinase, and nuclear factor kappaB: Differential regulation of collagenase 1 and collagenase 3. *Arthritis Rheum.* **43**, 801–811.

Midwood, K. S., and Salter, D. M. (2001). NG2/HMPG modulation of human articular chondrocyte adhesion to type VI collagen is lost in osteoarthritis. *J. Pathol.* **195**, 631–635.

Millward-Sadler, M. O., Davies, L. W., Nuki, G., and Salter, D. M. (2000). Mechanotransduction via integrins and interleukin-4 results in altered aggrecan and matrix metalloproteinase 3 gene expression in normal, but not osteoarthritic, human articular chondrocytes. *Arthritis Rheum.* **43**, 2091–2099.

Mine, T., Kimura, M., Sakka, A., and Kawai, S. (2000). Innervation of nociceptors in the menisci of the knee joint: An immunohistochemical study. *Arch. Orthop. Trauma Surg.* **120**, 201–204.

Nakayama, Y., Narita, T., Mori, A., Uesaka, S., Miyazaki, K., and Ito, H. (2002). The effects of age and sex on chondroitin sulfates in normal synovial fluid. *Arthritis Rheum.* **46**, 2105–2108.

Niederost, B. P., Zimmermann, D. R., Schwab, M. E., and Bandtlow, C. E. (1999). Bovine CNS myelin contains neurite growth-inhibitory activity associated with chondroitin sulfate proteoglycans. *J. Neurosci.* **19**, 8979–8989.

Palmieri, L., Conte, A., Giovannini, L., Lualdi, P., and Ronca, G. (1990). Metabolic fate of exogenous chondroitin sulfate in the experimental animal. *Arzneimittelforschung* **40**, 319–323.

Plaas, A. H., West, L. A., Wong-Palms, S., and Nelson, F. R. (1998). Glycosaminoglycan sulfation in human osteoarthritis: Disease-related alterations at the non-reducing termini of chondroitin and dermatan sulfate. *J. Biol. Chem.* **273**, 12642–12649.

Plaas, A. H., Wong-Palms, S., Koob, T., Hernandez, D., Marchuk, L., and Frank, C. B. (2000). Proteoglycan metabolism during repair of the ruptured medial collateral ligament in skeletally mature rabbits. *Arch. Biochem. Biophys.* **374**, 35–41.

Rapp, A., and Huettinger, M. (2005). Role of chondroitin sulfate in the uptake of β-VLDL by brain cells. *Eur. J. Neurosci.* **96**, 37–43.

Rapp, A., Brandl, N., Volpi, N., and Huettinger, M. (2005). Evaluation of chondroitin sulfate bioactivity in hippocampal neurones and the astrocyte cell line u373: Influence of position of sulfate groups and charge density. *Basic Clin. Pharmacol. Toxicol.* **96**, 37–43.

Ronca, F., Palmieri, L., Panicucci, P., and Ronca, G. (1998). Anti-inflammatory activity of chondroitin sulfate. *Osteoarthritis Cartilage* **6**(Suppl A), 14–21.

Saito, T., Takeuchi, R., Mitsuhashi, S., Uesugi, M., Yoshida, T., and Koshino, T. (2002). Use of joint fluid analysis for determining cartilage damage in osteonecrosis of the knee. *Arthritis Rheum.* **46**, 1813–1819.

Segat, D., Comai, R., Di Marco, E., Strangio, A., Cancedda, R., Franzi, A. T., and Tacchetti, C. (2002). Integrins alpha-(6A)beta-1 and alpha-(6B)beta-1 promote different stages of chondrogenic cell differentiation. *J. Biol. Chem.* **277**, 31612–31622.

Selvamurugan, N., Kwok, S., Alliston, T., Reiss, M., and Partridge, N. C. (2004). Transforming growth factor-{beta}1 regulation of collagenase-3 expression in osteoblastic cells by cross-talk between the Smad and MAPK signaling pathways and their components, Smad2 and Runx2. *J. Biol. Chem.* **279**, 19327–19334.

Shinmei, M., Miyauchi, S., Machida, A., and Miyazaki, K. (1992). Quantitation of chondroitin 4-sulfate and chondroitin 6-sulfate in pathologic joint fluid. *Arthritis Rheum.* **35**, 1304–1308.

Shlopov, B. V., Gumanovskaya, M. L., and Hasty, K. A. (2000). Autocrine regulation of collagenase 3 (matrix metalloproteinase 13) during osteoarthritis. *Arthritis Rheum.* **43**, 195–205.

Smith, R. L., Gilkerson, E., Kohatsu, N., Merchant, T., and Schurman, D. J. (1980). Quantitative microanalysis of synovial fluid and articular cartilage glycosaminoglycans. *Anal. Biochem.* **103**, 191–200.

Takahashi, N., Rieneck, K., van der Kraan, P. M., van Beuningen, H. M., Vitters, E. L., Bendtzen, K., and van den Berg, W. B. (2005). Elucidation of IL-1/TGF-beta interactions in mouse chondrocyte cell line by genome-wide gene expression. *Osteoarthritis Cartilage* **13**, 426–438.

Tiku, K., Thakker-Varia, S., Ramachandrula, A., and Tiku, M. L. (1992). Articular Chondrocytes secrete Il-1 express membrane Il-1 and have Il-1 inhibitory activity. *Cell. Immunol.* **140**, 1–20.

Uebelhart, D., Thonar, E. J., Zhang, J., and Williams, J. M. (1998). Protective effect of exogenous chondroitin 4,6-sulfate in the acute degradation of articular cartilage in the rabbit. *Osteoarthritis Cartilage* **6**(Suppl A), 6–13.

Uesaka, S., Nakayama, Y., Yoshihara, K., and Ito, H. (2002). Significance of chondroitin sulfate isomers in the synovial fluid of osteoarthritis patients. *J. Orthop. Sci.* **7**, 232–237.

van Beuningen, H. M., Glansbeek, H. L., van der Kraan, P. M., and van den Berg, W. B. (1998). Differential effects of local application of BMP-2 or TGF-beta 1 on both articular cartilage composition and osteophyte formation. *Osteoarthritis Cartilage* **6**, 306–317.

van den Berg, W. B. (1999). The role of cytokines and growth factors in cartilage destruction in osteoarthritis and rheumatoid arthritis. *Z. Rheumatol.* **58**, 136–141.

van der Kraan, P. M., Glansbeek, H. L., Vitters, E. L., and van den Berg, W. B. (1997). Early elevation of transforming growth factor-beta, decorin, and biglycan mRNA levels during cartilage matrix restoration after mild proteoglycan depletion. *J. Rheumatol.* **24**, 543–549.

van der Kraan, P. M., Buma, P., van Kuppevelt, T., and van den Berg, W. B. (2002). Interaction of chondrocytes, extracellular matrix and growth factors: Relevance for articular cartilage tissue engineering. *Osteoarthritis Cartilage* **10**, 631–637.

Volpi, N. (2002). Oral bioavailability of chondroitin sulfate (Condrosulf) and its constituents in healthy male volunteers. *Osteoarthritis Cartilage* 10, 768–777.

Volpi, N. (2003). Oral absorption and bioavailability of ichthyic origin chondroitin sulfate in healthy male volunteers. *Osteoarthritis Cartilage* 11, 433–441.

Volpi, N., and Maccari, F. (2005). Microdetermination of chondroitin sulfate in normal human plasma by fluorophore-assisted carbohydrate electrophoresis (FACE). *Clin. Chim. Acta* 356, 125–133.

Yamada, H., Miyauchi, S., Hotta, H., Morita, M., Yoshihara, Y., Kikuchi, T., and Fujikawa, K. (1999). Levels of chondroitin sulfate isomers in synovial fluid of patients with hip osteoarthritis. *J. Orthop. Sci.* 4, 250–254.

Yonekura, A., Osaki, M., Hirota, Y., Tsukazaki, T., Miyazaki, Y., Matsumoto, T., Ohtsuru, A., Namba, H., Shindo, H., and Yamashita, S. (1999). Transforming growth factor-beta stimulates articular chondrocyte cell growth through p44/42 MAP kinase (ERK) activation. *Endocr. J.* 46, 545–553.

Walz, A., McFarlane, S., Brickman, Y. G., Nurcombe, V., Bartlett, P. F., and Holt, C. E. (1997). Essential role of heparan sulfates in axon navigation and targeting in the developing visual system. *Development* 124, 2421–2430.

Zhao, J., and Buick, R. N. (1995). Regulation of transforming growth factor beta receptors in H-ras oncogene-transformed rat intestinal epithelial cells. *Cancer Res.* 55, 6181–6188.

A. Fioravanti* and G. Collodel[†]

*Rheumatology Unit
Department of Clinical Medicine and Immunological Sciences
University of Siena
Siena, Italy

[†]Department of Pediatrics
Obstetrics and Reproductive Medicine
Biology Section
University of Siena
Siena, Italy

In Vitro Effects of Chondroitin Sulfate

I. Chapter Overview

Chondroitin sulfate (CS) is a glycosaminoglycan (GAG), which is naturally found in the extracellular matrix (ECM) of articular cartilage. It is composed of a long unbranched polysaccharide chain with a repeating disaccharide structure of N-acetylgalactosamine and glucuronic acid. CS is one of the symptomatic slow-acting drugs for OA (SYSADOA) used in Europe, and it has been shown to be effective for pain and functional symptoms. In addition, clinical trials have suggested a possible activity of CS as a structure-modifying drug for osteoarthritis (OA). The therapeutic effects of CS may be related to its *in vitro* action. In a model of human articular chondrocytes cultivated in clusters, CS (100–1000 μg/ml) increased the production of proteoglycans (PGs), with no detectable effects on collagen type 2 synthesis. In the presence of interleukin-1β (IL-1β), CS counteracted the effects of the cytokine on PG, collagen type 2,

1054-3589/06 $35.00
DOI: 10.1016/S1054-3589(05)53022-9

and prostaglandin E_2 (PGE_2) synthesis, suggesting that CS can reduce collagenolytic activity and increase matrix component production. In human articular OA chondrocytes cultivated in alginate bed, in the presence or absence of IL-1β for 10 days with and without pressurization cycles, CS (10–100 µg/ml) counteracts the negative effect of IL-1β on the concentration of PG measured in the culture medium. These metabolic evaluation results were confirmed by the morphologic findings obtained by transmission electron microscopy (TEM) and scanning electron microscopy (SEM). The obtained results have also shown that chondrocytes that have undergone a cycle of physiological pressurization are more responsive than cells that have not been subjected to this stimulus. Furthermore, CS inhibits the synthesis of stromelysin (MMP-3) induced by IL-1β by human osteoarthritic chondrocytes, and in articular chondrocytes isolated from rabbits, it decreased nitric oxide (NO)-induced apoptosis. Additional *in vitro* experiments have shown that CS inhibits leukocyte elastase, one of the mediators of cartilageneous degradation. CS reduces nuclear translocation of transcription factor nuclear factor kappa B (NF-κB) in rabbit chondrocytes stimulated with IL-1β. This evidence could partly explain the mechanism of action through which CS exerts its chondroprotective and anti-inflammatory effects.

II. Introduction

Current treatment of OA includes physical, pharmacological, and surgical approaches (Jordan *et al.*, 2003). In the past, pharmacological treatment of OA was largely confined to analgesic or nonsteroidal anti-inflammatory drugs (NSAIDs). These drugs are able to control pain symptoms, but their use is limited by the negative side effects on the gastrointestinal apparatus (Davies and Wallace, 1997) or on the articular cartilagineous metabolism (Huskisson *et al.*, 1995; Rashad *et al.*, 1989). Considerable interest has been shown in drugs able to prevent or delay/stabilize the pathological changes, which occur in OA joints, thereby limiting disease progression (Brandt, 1995). These drugs have been classified as disease-modifying OA drugs (DMOADs) (Lequesne *et al.*, 1994) or as structure-modifying drugs for OA (Group for the Respect of Ethics and Excellence in Science, GREES Osteoarthritis Section, 1996).

CS is a GAG, which is naturally found in the ECM of articular cartilage, and it is composed of a long unbranched polysaccharide chain with a repeating disaccharide structure of N-acetylgalactosamine and glucuronic acid.

CS is one of the SYSADOAs (Lequesne *et al.*, 1994) used in Europe, and it has been shown to be effective for pain and functional symptoms (Leeb *et al.*, 2000; Morreale *et al.*, 1996). Clinical trials suggest a possible activity of CS as a structure-modifying drug for OA (Michel *et al.*, 2005; Uebelhart *et al.*, 2004). The therapeutic effects of CS may be related to its *in vitro* action.

III. *In Vitro* Models for the Study of Structure-Modifying Drugs for OA

Articular cartilage is a highly specialized tissue that contains only one type of cell, that is, chondrocytes. Chondrocytes synthesize an ECM of PG, collagen, and other noncollagen proteins, which constitute a dense tissue that is able to support *in vivo* the effects of the mechanical load (Poole, 1993). Chondrocytes also have a rich enzymatic set (metalloproteases, cathepsins, and serine proteases) that is able to degrade the ECM components.

The metabolic activity of these cells is regulated by several mediators, such as cytokines, hormones, and growth factors, produced locally by the chondrocytes themselves and also by neighboring tissues (Poole, 1993). Chondrocyte functions are influenced by ECM composition and by the composition of the extracellular environment (O_2 tension, ionic concentration, pH, and so on) (Guilak *et al.*, 1997; Rajpurohit *et al.*, 1996; Urban *et al.*, 1993). The metabolic activity of chondrocytes is further influenced by mechanical factors, depending on the articular load (Guilak *et al.*, 1997).

Preclinical studies (*in vitro* and *in vivo* on animal models) are the starting point in research for drugs with potential structural activity in OA. These studies naturally have unquestionable scientific value, but they also bring with them a series of limits of which it is necessary to be aware of before extrapolating the obtained results in human pathology.

In vitro studies on chondrocytes or cartilage cultures are simplified biological systems that allow us to evaluate the effects and/or the mechanism of action of a drug with possible structural activity in OA. For *in vitro* experimentation, cartilage of human or animal origin, mono- or tridimensional chondrocytes, or cocultures of cartilage and synovia can be used. Each culture system presents advantages and disadvantages, and each is particularly suitable for exploring one particular aspect of chondrocyte metabolism (Guilak *et al.*, 1997; Vignon *et al.*, 1990). The studies using cartilage explants and three-dimensional cultures most closely replicate the *in vivo* situation with chondrocytes surrounded by a specialized pericellular matrix. On the other hand, if the study aims to investigate matrix deposition or the regulatory pathways of chondrocyte metabolism, an isolated cell culture system is recommended to avoid the presence of a preexisting matrix.

Using *in vitro* models, it is possible to evaluate the possible effects of a drug on cartilagineous anabolism through the study of chondrocytic proliferation and PG synthesis, collagen type 2, and of hyaluronic acid, always making certain that the products are biochemically normal (Henrotin and Reginster, 1999; Vignon *et al.*, 1990) (Table I). The anticatabolic activity of a substance can be expressed through the inhibition of the release or by the activity of chondrocytic metalloproteases (MMPs) (stromelysin, collagenases, gelatinases, and aggrecanases) of the activity of IL-1β or TNF-α or from other products of inflammation such as E$_2$ prostaglandin (PGE$_2$), free radicals of oxygen, and nitric oxide (NO) (Henrotin and Reginster, 1999; Vignon *et al.*, 1990) (Table I).

The chondroprotective action of a drug depends upon its capacity to shift the equilibrium between phenomena of degradation and that of repair, in favor of the last. From this premise, it is therefore logical that for each substance it is necessary to evaluate, *in vitro*, both the effects on the anabolic processes and the catabolic processes of the cartilagineous metabolism. Therefore, the importance of an isolated result does not allow for the immediate definition of a drug as a chondroprotective: a product can, for example, stimulate PG synthesis, but at the same time it can also induce a release of enzymes with lytic action, with a final balance that is not always in favor of reconstructive phenomena.

The *in vitro* models, which are the starting point for the evaluation of the effect and the mechanism of action of a drug with structural activity, also present an intuitive series of limits (Henrotin and Reginster, 1999; Vignon *et al.*, 1990). *In vitro* models only reproduce a small part of the physiopathology of chondrocytes and cartilage, as these cells and the ECM are removed from their natural environment and therefore are subtracted from a series of information and local and general interferences. The information and interferences are also mutable from one moment to the next and are

TABLE I *In Vitro* **Evaluation Effects of a Structure-Modifying Drug for OA**

Anabolic effects
Chondrocytes proliferation without cellular dedifferentiation
Proteoglycans synthesis
Collagen type 2 synthesis
Hyaluronic acid synthesis
Influence on local growth factors (TGF-β, EGF, FGF, PDGF)

Catabolic effects
Inhibition of the release or of the activity of chondrocitic metalloproteases
Inhibition of cytokines as IL-1β, TNFα, and so on
Inhibition of PGE$_2$
Inhibition of the release or of the activity of free radicals of oxygen
Inhibition of the release or of the activity of NO
Inhibition of lysosomal enzymes
Antiapoptotic activity

therefore difficult to reproduce *in vitro*. In fact, in *in vivo* conditions, there are influences of an imprecise number of hormonal substances and of local mediators, only partially understood, which can act on the level of the normal or pathological chondrocyte, modifying its functional aspects. Another limitation of *in vitro* experimentation is the lack of effects linked to movement and joint load that are very important for the modality of afflux and outflow of anabolic and catabolic material in the cartilagineous matrix and which therefore also fully condition the bioavailability of possible drugs. It has also been demonstrated that mechanical factors condition the metabolism and the morphology of chondrocytes (Fioravanti *et al.*, 2003; Guilak *et al.*, 1997; Parkkinen *et al.*, 1993; Sah *et al.*, 1992; Smith *et al.*, 2000; Urban, 1994). The biosynthetic response of chondrocytes to mechanical stimuli *in vitro* varies with the magnitude, frequency, and duration of loading (Fioravanti *et al.*, 2003; Parkkinen *et al.*, 1993; Sah *et al.*, 1992; Urban, 1994). The results of *in vitro* studies are then clearly influenced by some characteristics relative to the "material" utilized for preparing the culture, such as the origin (animal or human) of the cartilage and the age of the patient or the animal from which it was taken and, above all, the conditions (normal or pathological) of the tissue (Henrotin and Reginster, 1999). The diffusion of a drug is clearly superior in osteoarthritic cartilage compared to normal cartilage, and the chondrocytes of patients with OA are able to respond to more stimuli and with a greater intensity compared to less activated normal chondrocytes (Lafeber *et al.*, 1992). Another factor, which can affect the results of *in vitro* tests, is the concentration of the drug used in the culture medium. Theoretically, when a cartilagineous culture is used, it is best to consider concentrations of the drug near to those, which will be reached *in vivo* in synovial liquid; these concentrations should be further modified when cultures of isolated chondrocytes are used.

All of the considerations mentioned previously can explain the variability of the results obtained by different authors, and we must reflect upon the necessity of using more than one experimental model and on the opportunity to evaluate different parameters for the same type of drug before it can be defined with certainty as structure modifying for OA. *In vitro* tests always necessitate later confirmation *in vivo*, and we should not forget that a substance, which may be inactive *in vitro*, could demonstrate a structure-modifying action *in vivo*, for example, by acting on a level of some synthesized factors outside of joint cartilage.

IV. *In Vitro* Effects of CS

During the past 30 years, many authors have tested the effects of CS in diverse experimental conditions. Primarily, the interaction between human leukocyte elastase and CS has been studied (Baici and Bradamante, 1984).

Human leukocyte elastase, a serine proteinase from the azurophil granules of polymorphonuclear leukocytes, has been associated with different disorders, and it is also thought to participate in the pathophysiology of OA (Barrett, 1978) by degrading the two major constituents of ECM, collagen and PG. The interaction between elastase and CS occurs by the formation of electrostatic bonds between the negatively charged sulfate groups in the glycosaminogly-cans (GAGs) and positively charged groups on the enzyme. The interaction does not influence the active center of the enzyme but causes an indirect loss of its catalytic efficiency. The modulation of the extracellular activity of a potent mediator of cartilage breakdown, such as human leukocyte elastase by CS, may at least partly explain the chondroprotective action of this drug.

It was later confirmed (De Gennaro *et al.*, 1990) that treatment with CS significantly reduced the concentration of granulocyte elastase in the synovial liquid of patients with gonarthritis in the exudative phase.

Previous studies (Adeyemi *et al.*, 1986) had already demonstrated that the reduction in the concentration of elastases in synovial liquid after treatment with some NSAIDs was correlated with the reduction in the number of granulocytes in synovial liquid. In the case of treatment with CS, it is important to note how the levels of elastases are reduced, independently of possible variations in the number of granulocytes.

Besides CS, Bassleer *et al.* (1992) tested two other chondroprotective agents, glucosamine sulfate and GAG–peptide complex, on differentiated human articular chondrocytes cultured in clusters. Chondrocyte productions of PG, collagen type 2, PGE_2 were established by specific radioimmunoassays applied to the culture medium and in chondrocyte clusters. CS and glucosamine sulfate induced a stimulatory effect limited to PG production. None of these three substances affected basal PGE_2 production by human chondrocytes. Furthermore, collagenolytic activity was assayed in culture medium, showing the inhibition of this activity by CS.

IL-1β is widely accepted to be one of proinflammatory cytokines that plays a pivotal role in the pathophysiology of OA (Dinarello, 1988). It induces a cascade of catabolic events in chondrocytes, including the upregulation in genes of matrix MMPs, inducible nitric oxide synthase (iNOS), cyclooxygenase-2 (COX-2), and microsomal prostaglandin E synthase-1 (mPGEs1) and the release of NO and PGE_2. IL-1β also retards the anabolic activities of chondrocytes, leading to a decline in PG and collagen synthesis (Martel Pelletier, 2004).

For this reason, the next step by the Bassleer group (Bassleer *et al.*, 1998) was to test the effects of CS, in the presence or absence of IL-1β, on the metabolism of human articular chondrocytes cultivated in clusters *in vitro*.

Bassleer *et al.* (1986) have described a system of three-dimensional cultures of chondrocytes that allows enzimatically isolated human chondrocytes to aggregate and form a cluster. In the cluster, chondrocytes are morphologically and biosynthetically differentiated and two phases can be noted—when the cluster is formed with a large production of matrix components and when matrix surrounds the cells with a decrease in matrix component production.

In their long-term cluster culture model, Bassleer *et al.* (1998) confirmed that IL-1β induces a decrease in cartilage matrix element production, as collagen type 2 and PGs and an increase in PGE_2 synthesis. These effects of IL-1β are stronger at the beginning of the culture, which is probably why the access and fixation of IL-1β to its receptors is facilitated when the cells are surrounded by a flaky matrix, and when the cluster is constructed the IL-1β effects are weaker.

In the same study, Bassleer *et al.* demonstrated that CS counteracts the IL-1β induced effect, this effect has a stronger effect on PG production than on collagen type 2 production, and it is more potent at the beginning of culture. PG accumulation is slow in clusters, probably due to the effect of CS on PG synthesis processes and/or the integration of CS in aggrecan.

PGE_2, another catabolic mediator in the pathogenesis of OA, is formed from a series of enzymatic reactions called the arachidonic acid cascade, which mediates synoviocyte proliferation and is responsible for inflammatory and pain responses (Martel Pelletier, 2004).

Regarding PGE_2 production, Bassleer *et al.* (1998) noted that CS (at 500 or 1000 µg/ml) decreases total PGE_2 production and that CS (100–1000 µg/ml) inhibits the stimulating IL-1β effect on PGE_2 production during the first 16 days of culture.

A direct effect of chondroitin polysulfate on the production of aggrecans (Verbruggen *et al.*, 1999; Wang *et al.*, 2002) has been demonstrated by an increase of total ^{35}S incorporation rates. The same polysulfated polysaccharide increased the synthesis of high-molecular weight hyaluronan by chondrocyte derived fibroblast-like cells.

A new ultrastructural approach was carried out by Nerucci *et al.* (2000), investigating the *in vitro* effects of CS on human articular chondrocytes cultivated in the presence or in the absence of IL-1β during 10 days of culture with and without pressurization cycles. In this study, alginate was used as the support in the culturing of human chondrocytes, as it is considered to be a valid alternative to other culture techniques since it enables the chondrocyte to retain its 3D-structure and to maintain its characteristic cell shape, while preventing cell dedifferentiation. The effect of CS (10–100 µg/ml) with and without IL-1β was assessed in the culture medium of cells exposed to pressurization cycles in the form of sinusoidal waves (minimum pressure 1 MPa, maximum pressure 5 MPa) and at a frequency of 0.25 Hz for 3 h using the immunoenzymatic method for quantitative measurement of human PG (Figs. 1 and 2). On the 4th and 10th days of culture, the cells were used for morphological analysis by TEM (Fig. 3) and SEM (Fig. 4). They showed

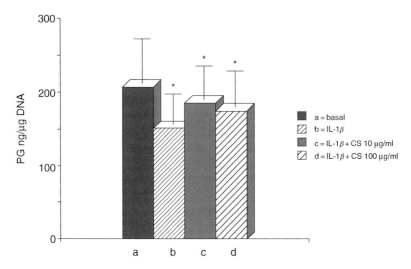

FIGURE 1   Total amount of PG measured in culture medium (ng/µg DNA) during 10 days of culture (pooled data) in basal conditions, in the presence of IL-1β, and in the presence of IL-1β and CS (10 and 100 µg/ml). Data are expressed as mean values ± SD. b vs. a; c vs. b; d vs. b: $p < 0.05$; *$p < 0.05$.

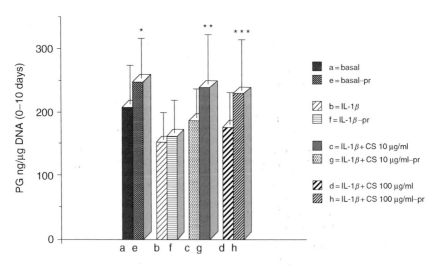

FIGURE 2   Total amount of PG measured in culture medium (ng/µg DNA) during 10 days of culture (pooled data) in basal conditions, in the presence of IL-1β, and in the presence of IL-1β and CS (10 and 100 µg/ml) with and without pressurization conditions. –pr = cyclic pressurization minimum pressure 1 MPa and maximum pressure 5 MPa at 0.25 Hz frequency. Data are expressed as mean values ± SD. e vs. a: *$p < 0.01$; g vs. c: **$p < 0.005$; h vs. d: ***$p < 0.003$.

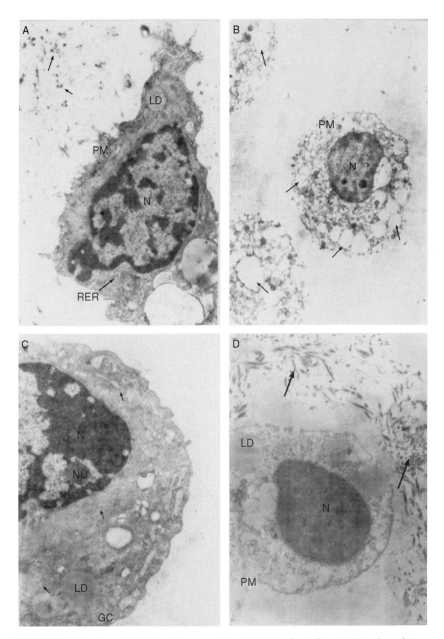

FIGURE 3   Sections of OA chondrocytes cultured *in vitro* for 4 days. (A) Basal conditions: the cell shows a euchromatic nucleus (N) and a cytoplasm abundant in endoplasmic rough reticulum (RER). The plasma membrane (PM) has a large number of processes in a matrix rich in collagen fibers and PG granules (arrows). Lipid droplets (LD); ×13,000. (B) Presence of IL-1β: the cell presents a very vacuolate cytoplasm (arrows). The matrix appears to be very poor.

that the addition of IL-1β determines a reduction in the concentration of PG in the culture medium (Fig. 1); this could be the result of the fact that cytokine induces an inhibition of PG synthesis by the chondrocytes, as shown in the morphological analysis. The morphological aspects show signs of cellular suffering with the presence of vacuoles (Figs. 3B and 4B) and the lack of cellular organelles typically responsible for the synthesis of the matrix glycoproteins (the endoplasmic reticulum, the Golgi apparatus, and mitochondria). When the cells were cultivated in the presence of IL-1β + CS, there was a restoration of PG concentration in the culture medium (Fig. 1). This fact confirms the protective role played by this substance, which counteracts the IL-1β induced effects and which might be used by the chondrocyte as a substratum for the synthesis of PG. The pressure values applied in this study were within the physiological range of human joints, as a pressure level of 5 MPa is most often encountered in the knee joint during normal gait (Hodge *et al.*, 1986; Parkkinen *et al.*, 1993). Chondrocytes undergoing physiological pressurization presented a greater metabolic activity, which was expressed in the increase of PG levels in the culture medium at basal conditions (Fig. 2). This fact was also confirmed in morphological analysis by TEM (Fig. 3D) and SEM (Fig. 4D–F). The increase in PG in the culture medium, which was also observed in basal conditions, could be determined by a stimulation activity induced by pressurization. The "stimulating" effect of the pressure did not, however, manage to counterbalance the negative effects determined by the addition of IL-1β ,which, in fact, induce a serious metabolic and morphological imbalance. The addition of CS created protection from the effects of IL-1β under the pressurization conditions used. The simultaneous use of pressurization with the presence of CS determined a highly significant increase in PG concentration, as though a synergism of action exists between the drug and the mechanical factor regarding IL-1β. The biochemical data was also supported by morphological analysis (Nerucci *et al.*, 2000).

Lippiello *et al.* (2003) tested the hypothesis that chondrocytes are more responsive to chondroprotective agents, glucosamine sulfate and CS, under *in vitro* conditions simulating *in vivo* joint stress. Synthetic and anticatabolic activities of bovine articular cartilage were assessed, and the response of cartilage to simulated conditions of *in vivo* stress varies, depending on the type of stress and age of the animal. Cartilage from older animals was more

---

Nucleus (N), plasma membrane (PM); ×6000. (C) Presence of IL-1β +CS100: the cell clearly recovers its good state of health. The nucleus (N) presents a nucleolus (NU). The cytoplasm contains rough and smooth endoplasmic reticuli (arrows); Golgi complex (GC) and lipid droplets (LD); ×14,000. (D) Basal condition and pressurization: the abundant presence of collagen fibers and PG granules (arrows) in the ECM is evident. Nucleus (N), lipid droplets (LD), and plasma membrane (PM); ×10,000.

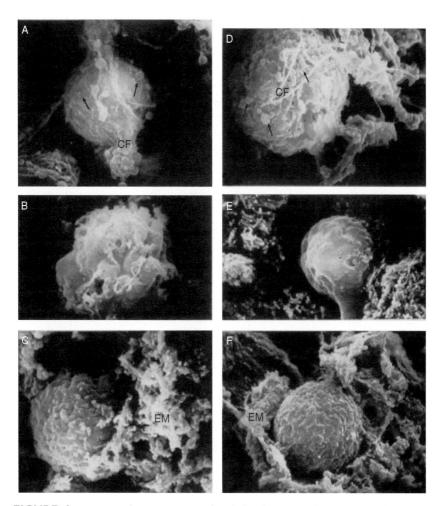

FIGURE 4   Scanning electron micrographs of chondrocytes cultured *in vitro* for 4 days. (A) Basal conditions: the cell exhibits a spherical shape and granules of secretion are evident on its surface (arrows). The network of collagenic fibrils (CFs) is also visible; ×3800. (B) Presence of IL-1β: the cellular damage is clear. The chondrocyte is devoid of granules and of matrix and the surface of the cells appears collapsed; ×4500. (C) Presence of IL-1β +CS100: the cell morphology has been partially restored. Newly formed elements of the extracellular matrix (ECM) have been secreted into the extracellular space; ×5000. (D–F) Chondrocytes subjected to pressurization. (D) Basal conditions: the cell shows a good state of health; granules of secretion (arrows) and collagenic fibrils (CFs) are evident; ×4500. (E) Presence of IL-1β: the cell is devoid of PG granules and of collagen fibers, but it does not appear collapsed; ×4500. (F) Presence of IL-1β +CS100: the cell shows a spherical shape and a rich extracellular matrix (ECM); ×3300.

responsive to stress and to glucosamine sulfate and CS. Pronase-induced matrix depletion and mechanical stress increased PG synthesis activity. Exposure to glucosamine sulfate and CS significantly enhanced this stress response from 85% to 91% and from 40% to 100%, respectively. Heat stress and stromelysin digestion decreased synthetic activity, which was reversed or normalized upon exposure to glucosamine sulfate and CS. Cartilage from young joints was somewhat refractory to the level of stress imposed and to treatment with glucosamine sulfate and CS. The differences observed may be a function of matrix mechanical properties between tissues and/or cell sensitivity to external factors. By enhancing the protective metabolic response of chondrocytes to stress, glucosamine sulfate and CS may improve their ability to repair and regenerate. These observations suggest that these compounds function as biological response modifiers (BRMs), agents that boost natural protective responses of tissues under adverse environmental conditions.

Chondrocytes in OA cartilage demonstrated morphologic changes that are characteristic features of apoptosis. This mechanism of cell death plays an important role in the pathogenesis of OA (Martel Pelletier, 2004).

The possibility that CS could have a protective role in apoptosis has been investigated (Reveliere et al., 1999). It was tested whether CS could reduce NO-induced apoptosis in vitro in articular rabbit chondrocytes, suggesting its protective effect by limiting cartilage degradation. Chondrocytes have been characterized as a major intra-articular cell source of NO, and NO appears to be one of the most potent inducers of chondrocyte apoptosis (Reveliere et al., 1999). In Reveliere's study, NO donors induced apoptosis of normal articular rabbit chondrocytes, and preincubation with CS (100 μg/ml) decreased the action of NO. It has been shown that CS is able to increase PG amounts in the matrix surrounding the cells, and the accumulation of matrix components around the cells may protect them against injury from IL-1β or NO.

A decrease in the number of apoptotic chondrocytes under CS sheds light on a new mechanism of the biological effect of this molecule that might exhibit disease- or structure-modifying properties.

Besides possessing the earlier mentioned anabolic effects, CS acts at different levels on the mediators of cartilage destruction such as MMPs.

Stromelysin-1 (metalloprotease-3, MMP-3) is a cartilage proteolytic enzyme, which induces cartilage destruction. The production of MMP-3 induced by IL-1β in chondrocyte cultures from patients with primary OA was inhibited by the addition of CS at different concentrations (Monfort et al., 2005).

It has been hypothesized (Vergés et al., 2004) that the clinical effect of CS could partially be due to a reduction in the activation of the NF-κB transcription factor in cultures of chondrocytes from rabbit knees stimulated by IL-1β.

NF-κB is an ubiquitous protein that specifically binds to DNA consensus sequences, activating its transcription. NF-κB exists in the cytoplasm in an inactive form (Fig. 5). When an extracellular stimulus induces the phosphorylation of an inhibitory subunit (a member of IkB family) and its subsequent degradation, the active complex becomes capable of migrating to the nucleus, where it recognizes the consensus sequences in DNA. NF-κB binding sites are present in the promoter regions of many genes (metalloproteases, iNOS, COX-2) involved in the pathophysiology of joint inflammation and tissue destruction (Tak and Firestein, 2001).

As already mentioned, the IL-1β cytokine plays a key role in the catabolic program of chondrocytes. Signal transduction starts with the interaction of IL-1β with its receptor (IL-1R), inducing the activation of different signaling pathways, among them that of mitogen-activated protein kinases (MAPKs), which increase the intracellular concentration of oxygen free radicals and the activation of transcription factor NF-κB followed by its nuclear translocation.

CS reduces nuclear translocation of transcription factor NF-κB in rabbit chondrocytes stimulated with IL-1β (Vergés *et al.*, 2004). This evidence

NF-κB activation pathway

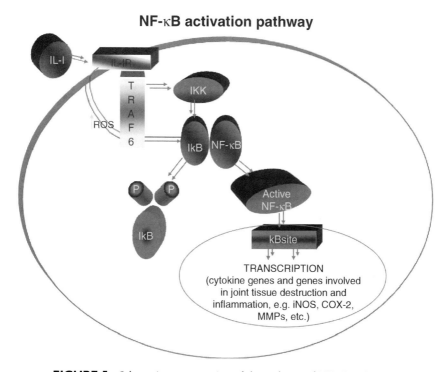

FIGURE 5   Schematic representation of the pathway of NF-κB activation.

could partly explain the mechanism of action through which CS exerts its chondroprotective and anti-inflammatory effects.

V. Conclusions

A number of *in vitro* studies have been performed to determine the mode of action of CS. It has been demonstrated that CS possesses both anabolic effects on cartilage metabolism and anticatabolic properties (Table II).

In various models of cartilage culture or of isolated chondrocytes, CS has demonstrated the capacity to stimulate the synthesis of PG, aggrecanases, and hyaluronic acid at a high-molecular weight. In cultures of human osteoarthritic chondrocytes, CS inhibits collagenolytic activity and the synthesis of stromelysin (MMP-3), and it counteracts the negative effects of IL-1β on PG, collagen type 2, and PGE_2 synthesis. CS is also able to prevent the apoptosis of chondrocytes induced *in vitro* by NO. Additional *in vitro* experiments have demonstrated that CS interacts with elastase of human leukocytes and that it determines a partial inhibition of activity (elastase is a potent mediator of cartilage degradation). The effects of CS on various mediators of inflammation and the degradation of cartilage can probably be explained on the basis of its capacity to reduce the nuclear translocation of transcription factor NF-κB induced by IL-1β.

In summary, although the mechanisms of action of CS on cartilage metabolism are not yet completely known, the data obtained from *in vitro* studies on cartilage or chondrocyte cultures certainly support the clinical findings describing CS as a symptom and structure-modifying drug in the treatment of OA.

TABLE II   *In Vitro* **Effects of CS**

Anabolic effects
Stimulation of proteoglycan synthesis (Bassleer *et al.*, 1992)
Stimulation of aggrecans synthesis and of high-molecular weight hyaluronan
(Verbruggen *et al.*, 1999; Wang *et al.*, 2002)

Anticatabolic and antiphlogistic effects
Inhibition of collagenolytic activity (Bassleer *et al.*, 1992)
Inhibition of the synthesis of stromelysin (Monfort *et al.*, 2005)
Inhibition of the effects of IL-1β on PG, collagen type 2, and PGE_2 synthesis
   (Bassleer *et al.*, 1998; Nerucci *et al.*, 2000)
Reduction of apoptosis of chondrocytes induced by NO (Hodge *et al.*, 1986)
Inhibition of leukocytic elastase activity (Baici and Bradamante, 1984)

References

Adeyemi, E. O., Hull, R. G., Chadwick, V. S., Hughes, G. R. V., and Hodgson, H. J. F. (1986). Circulating human leukocyte elastase in rheumatoid arthritis. *Rheumatol. Int.* **6**, 57–60.

Baici, A., and Bradamante, P. (1984). Interaction between human leukocyte elastase and chondroitin sulfate. *Chem. Biol. Interact.* **51**, 1–11.

Barrett, A. J. (1978). The possible role of neutrophil proteinases in damage to articular cartilage. *Agents Actions* **8**, 11–18.

Bassleer, C., Gysen, P., Foidart, J. M., Bassleer, R., and Franchimont, P. (1986). Human chondrocytes in tridimensional culture. *In Vitro Cell Dev. Biol.* **22**, 113–119.

Bassleer, C., Henrotin, Y., and Franchimont, P. (1992). *In-vitro* evaluation of drugs proposed as chondroprotective agents. *Int. J. Tissue React.* **14**, 231–241.

Bassleer, C., Combal, J. P., Bougaret, S., and Malaise, M. (1998). Effects of chondroitin sulfate and interleukin-1 beta on human articular chondrocytes cultivated in clusters. *Osteoarthritis Cartilage* **6**, 196–204.

Brandt, K. D. (1995). Towards pharmacologically modifying joint damage in osteoarthritis. *Ann. Intern. Med.* **122**, 874–875.

Davies, M. N., and Wallace, J. L. (1997). Nonsteroidal anti-inflammatory drug-induced gastrointestinal toxicity: New insight into an old problem. *J. Gastroenterol.* **32**, 127–133.

De Gennaro, F., Piccioni, P. D., Caporali, R., Luisetti, M., and Montecucco, C. (1990). Effetto del trattamento con galattosaminoglucuronoglicano solfato sulla elastasi granulocitaria sinoviale in pazienti con osteoartrosi. *Riv. It. Biol. Med.* **10**, 46–50.

Dinarello, C. A. (1988). Interleukin-1. *Ann. N.Y. Acad. Sci.* **546**, 122–132.

Fioravanti, A., Nerucci, F., Annefeld, M., Collodel, G., and Marcolongo, R. (2003). Morphological and cytoskeletal aspects of cultivated normal and osteoarthritic human articular chondrocytes after cyclical pressure: A pilot study. *Clin. Exp. Rheumatol.* **21**, 739–746.

Group for the Respect of Ethics and Excellence in Science (GREES Osteoarthritis Section) (1996). Recommendation for the registration of drugs used in the treatment of osteoarthritis. *Ann. Rheum. Dis.* **55**, 552–557.

Guilak, F., Sah, R., and Setton, L. A. (1997). Physical regulation of cartilage metabolism. *In* "Basic Orthopaedic Biomechanics" (V. C. Mow and W. C. Hayes, Eds.), pp. 179–207, 2nd ed. Lippincott-Raven, Philadelphia.

Henrotin, Y., and Reginster, J. Y. (1999). Experimental models of osteoarthritis. *In* "Osteoarthritis Clinical and Experimental Aspects" (J. Y. Reginster, J. P. Pelletier, J. Martel-Pelletier, and Y. Henrotin, Eds.), pp. 53–81. Springer-Verlag, Berlin.

Hodge, W. A., Fijan, R. S., Carlson, R. S., Burgess, R. G., Harris, W. H., and Mann, R. W. (1986). Contact pressures in the human hip joint measured *in vivo*. *Proc. Natl. Acad. Sci. USA* **83**, 2879–2883.

Huskisson, E. C., Bergg, H., Gilsen, P., Jubb, R. W., and Whitehead, J. (1995). Effects of antiinflammatory drugs on the progression of osteoarthritis of the knee. *J. Rheumatol.* **22**, 1941–1946.

Jordan, K. M., Arden, N. K., Doherty, M., Banwarth, B., Bijlsma, J. W. J., Dieppe, P., Gunther, K., Hauselmann, H., Herrero-Beaumont, G., Kaklamanis, P., Lohmander, S., Leeb, B., *et al.* (2003). EULAR recommendations 2003: An evidence based approach to the management of knee osteoarthritis: Report of a task force of the standing committee for international clinical studies including therapeutic trials (ESCISIT). *Ann. Rheum. Dis.* **62**, 1145–1155.

Lafeber, F. P., van der Kraan, P. M., van Roy, H. L., Vitters, E. L., Huber-Bruning, O., van den Berg, W. B., and Bijlsma, J. W. (1992). Local changes in proteoglycan synthesis during culture are different for normal and osteoarthritic cartilage. *Am. J. Pathol.* **140**, 1421–1429.

Leeb, B. F., Schweitzer, M., Montag, M., and Smolen, J. S. (2000). A metaanalysis of chondroitin sulfate in the treatment of osteoarthritis. *J. Rheumatol.* **27**, 205–211.

Lequesne, M., Brandt, K., Bellamy, N., Moskowitz, R., Menkès, C. J., Pelletier, J. P., and Altman, R. (1994). Guidelines for testing slow-acting and disease-modifying drugs in osteoarthritis. *J. Rheumatol.* **41**(Suppl.), 65–71.

Lippiello, L. (2003). Glucosamine and chondroitin sulfate: Biological response modifiers of chondrocytes under simulated conditions of joint stress. *Osteoarthritis Cartilage* **11**, 335–342.

Martel Pelletier, J. (2004). Pathophysiology of osteoarthritis. *Osteoarthritis Cartilage* **12** (Suppl. A), S31–S32.

Michel, B. A., Stucki, G., Frey, D., De Vathaire, F., Vignon, E., Bruchlmann, P., and Uebelhart, D. (2005). Chondroitins 4 and 6 sulfate in osteoarthritis of the knee: A randomized, controlled trial. *Arthritis Rheum.* **52**, 779–786.

Monfort, J., Nacher, M., Montell, E., Vila, J., Verges, J., and Benito, P. (2005). Chondroitin sulfate and hyaluronic acid (500–730 kDa) inhibit stromelysin-1 synthesis in human osteoarthritic chondrocytes. *Drugs Exp. Clin. Res.* **31**, 71–76.

Morreale, P., Manopulo, R., Galati, M., Boccanera, L., Saponati, G., and Bocchi, L. (1996). Comparison of the antiinflammatory efficacy of chondroitin sulfate and diclofenac sodium in patients with knee osteoarthritis. *J. Rheumatol.* **23**, 1385–1391.

Nerucci, F., Fioravanti, A., Cicero, M. R., Collodel, G., and Marcolongo, R. (2000). Effects of chondroitin sulfate and interleukin-1beta on human chondrocyte cultures exposed to pressurization: A biochemical and morphological study. *Osteoarthritis Cartilage* **8**, 279–287.

Parkkinen, J., Ikonen, J., Lammi, M. J., Laakkonen, J., Tammi, M., and Helminen, H. J. (1993). Effects of cyclic hydrostatic pressure on proteoglycan synthesis in cultured chondrocytes and articular cartilage explants. *Arch. Biochem. Biophys.* **300**, 458–465.

Poole, C. A. (1993). The structure and function of articular cartilage matrices. *In* "Joint Cartilage Degradation" (J. F. Woessner and D. S. Howell, Eds.), pp. 1–35. Dekker Mercel Inc., New York.

Rajpurohit, R., Koch, C., Tao, Z., Teixeira, C., and Shapiro, I. (1996). Adaptation of chondrocytes to low oxygen tension: Relationship between hypoxia and cellular metabolism. *J. Cell Physiol.* **168**, 424–434.

Rashad, S., Revel, P., Hemingway, A., Low, F., Rainsford, H., and Walker, F. (1989). Effects of nonsteroidal anti-inflammatory drugs on the course of osteoarthritis. *Lancet* **2**, 519–522.

Reveliere, D., Mentz, F., Merle-Beral, H., and Chevalier, X. (1999). Protective effect of chondroitin 4&6 sulfate on apoptosis of rabbit articular chondrocytes: Preliminary results. *Litera Rheumatol.* **24**, 15–20.

Sah, R. L. Y., Grodzinsky, A. J., Plaas, A. H. K., and Sandy, J. D. (1992). Effect of dynamic compression on matrix metabolism in cartilage explants. *In* "Articular Cartilage and Osteoarthritis" (K. E. Kuettner, R. Shleyerbach, J. C. Peyron, and V. C. Hascall, Eds.), pp. 373–392. Raven Press, New York.

Smith, R. L., Lin, J., Trindade, M. C. D., Shida, J., Kajiyama, G., Vu, T., Hoffman, A. R., van der Meulen, M. C., Goodman, S. B., Schurman, D. J., and Carter, D. R. (2000). Time-dependent effects of intermittent hydrostatic pressure on articular chondrocyte type II collagen and aggrecan mRNA expression. *J. Rehabil. Res. Dev.* **37**, 153–161.

Tak, P. P., and Firestein, G. S. (2001). NF-kappaB: A key role in inflammatory diseases. *J. Clin. Invest.* **107**, 7–111.

Uebelhart, D., Malaise, M., Marcolongo, R., DeVathairell, F., Piperno, M., Mailleux, E., Fioravanti, A., Matoso, L., and Vignon, E. (2004). Intermittent treatment of knee osteoarthritis with oral chondroitin sulfate: A one-year, randomized, double-blind, multicenter study versus placebo. *Osteoarthritis Cartilage* **12**, 269–276.

Urban, J., Hall, A., and Gehl, K. (1993). Regulation of matrix synthesis rates by the ionic and osmotic environment of articular chondrocytes. *J. Cell Physiol.* **154**, 262–270.

Urban, J. P. (1994). The chondrocyte: A cell under pressure. *Br. J. Rheumatol.* **33**, 901–908.

Verbruggen, G., Cornelissen, M., Elewaut, D., Broddelez, C., De Ridder, L., and Veys, E. M. (1999). Influence of polysulfated polysaccharides on aggrecans synthesized by differentiated human articular chondrocytes. *J. Rheumatol.* **26**, 1663–1671.

Vergés, J., Montell, E., Martinez, G., Heroux, L., and du Soulch, P. (2004). Chondroitin sulfate reduces nuclear translocation of transcription factor NF-kB and does not modify the activation state of activator protein-1 (AP1). EULAR Symposium, Berlin June, 9–12.

Vignon, E., Mazières, B., Richard, M., and Annefeld, M. (1990). Evaluation *in vitro* of a chondro-protector. *Rev. Rhum.* **9**(bis), 15S–18S.

Wang, L., Wang, J., Almqvist, K. F., Veys, E. M., and Verbruggen, G. (2002). Influence of polysulphated polysaccharides and hydrocortisone on the extracellular matrix metabolism of human articular chondrocytes *in vitro*. *Clin. Exp. Rheumatol.* **20**, 669–676.

Britta Dobenecker

Institute of Physiology
Physiological Chemistry and Animal Nutrition
Ludwig-Maximilians University Munich
Germany

Effect of Chondroitin Sulfate as Nutraceutical in Dogs with Arthropathies

I. Chapter Overview

Orthopedic problems in dogs that are degenerative or inflammatory arthropathies like osteoarthritis (OA) or also named degenerative joint disease (DJD) in middle-aged and geriatric patients are a main reason for consulting a veterinary practice or clinic. DJD is marked by a slow progressive degenerative process of synovial joints. The process is characterized by painful destruction of cartilage followed by bony reconstruction. The disease is often started by trauma or some predisposing stress through abnormalities of the limb axis, articular incongruity, synovial membrane inflammation, metabolic or idiopathic alterations leading to cartilage destruction. Often rupturing of tendons, such as the cruciate ligament, leads to the secondary form of DJD. Afflicted patients show lameness, immobility of different degree, and sometimes crepitation. In canine patients this often

Advances in Pharmacology, Volume 53
1054-3589/06 $35.00
DOI: 10.1016/S1054-3589(05)53023-0

results in gaining weight, what again causes a higher exposure of the afflicted joints.

II. Introduction

In dogs, secondary forms of DJD derived from congenital or acquired deformation of joints are more often seen than in man, where old-age arthrosis is the most frequently diagnosed form. Underlying processes are inflammation, instability of the joint, or trauma (Klee and Ungemach, 1998; Smith *et al.*, 1995), which can be found in dogs of all ages but is most commonly seen in young dogs of 4 years or less (Prieur *et al.*, 1994). Dysplastic joints are often seen in case of osteochondrosis or other developmental skeletal problems in dogs (Fox and Walker, 1993). The body weight of an adult dog as well as the weight curve of a puppy influences the progression of the OA, leading to a higher incidence in large breed dogs (Dobenecker *et al.*, 1998). But not only large and giant breed dogs that are known to be sensitive to nutritional and environmental influences on their skeletal development are often affected but also a number of medium and small breed dogs. Some breeds have a higher susceptibility to developmental skeletal diseases than others.

It can be hypothesized, that especially the belonging to a more chondrodystrophic breed increases the risk to develop skeletal problems throughout life (Dobenecker *et al.*, 2005; Laflamme, 2000).

Treatment of OA in dogs is based on surgery, weight reduction, exercise control, and administration of anti-inflammatory and analgesic agents (steroids, NSAIDs). The longing of owners and veterinarians for substances with disease-modifying, positive effects for a noninvasive treatment are great. These substances should be harmless, with lesser or no adverse side effects also in long-term use and easy to be administered by the owner. Chondroprotective substances or better named slow-acting drugs for OA (SADOA) are reported to have symptomatic effects and may protect cartilage from degeneration through stimulation of cartilage matrix formation and reducing the cartilage degradation. Therefore, they may maintain or even repair cartilage to stop progression of disease.

Forms of application are oral, intravenous, intra-articular, or intramuscular. The major advantage of oral administration is the easy way of application especially for long-term use in dogs. Often orally used chondroprotectives are named nutraceuticals, a neologism from nutrition and pharmaceuticals.

After oral administration of radioactive marked CS, 70% of the radioactivity was shown to be absorbed in dogs. A high concentration of the radioactivity was found in the synovial fluid and glycosaminoglycan-rich tissue like articular cartilage (Palmieri *et al.*, 1990).

CS together with mussel extract is a commonly used substance in prevention and management of DJD. These substances may act synergistically to reduce inflammation and degenerative symptoms in DJD patients. CS is a long-chain polymer of disaccharides found predominantly in cartilage. Sources of CS are cartilage tissue from shark, bovine, and whale. *In vitro* studies revealed increasing prostaglandin levels and decreasing activity of collagenolytic enzymes after adding CS.

Most of the *in vivo* studies were carried out in man, only few in horses and dogs. In the majority of cases, CS was employed in combination with other chondroprotective substances in these published trials (Table I). Moore (1996) found no effects in a case study with three dogs. In a large retrospective study of 2000 canine patients Anderson *et al.* (1999) had the same negative results. These dogs received CS, glycosaminoglycans, manganese, and ascorbic acid for different periods but at least for several weeks. On the other hand, significant amelioration of the symptoms of arthropathies was detectable after CS administration for 60 days in 110 dogs in a field study (Segal and Bousquet, 1999) and after a combined treatment with CS and Chitosan (Gerlach *et al.*, 2000; 30 dogs). None of these studies were placebo controlled or blinded. Therefore, the information about the effect of chondroprotective nutraceuticals, including CS in canine patients, derives often from anecdotal reports of owners and veterinarians or from studies in other species (Anderson *et al.*, 1999).

To verify the effects of the chondroprotective substance in ordinary canine patients with chronic DJD, a field study was conducted. In a placebo-controlled (group PL), double-blind study the effect of CS in comparison to another chondroprotective substance [New Zealand green-lipped mussel extract (group: ME)] was tested in dogs with joint diseases (Dobenecker *et al.*, 2002). The perceptions of the attending veterinarians and owners were evaluated.

III. Results and Conclusions

All attending dogs were patients of 12 veterinary clinics. In total 70 dogs of 21 different breeds, ages (CS 8.1 ± 4.3; ME 7.8 ± 3.8; PL 8.2 ± 3.9 year) and sexes (CS 10 males/11 females; ME 13 males/5 females; PL 13 males/ 6 females) were available for the study. Most of the dogs belonged to larger breeds; therefore the mean body weight was 34 ± 10 kg. In all groups, the relative deviation between actual and normal weight, defined as body weight at the age of 12 months, showed a tendency to overweight (CS $115 \pm 11\%$; ME $135 \pm 25\%$; PL $113 \pm 16\%$). No proband was younger than 1 year to ensure the termination of the main skeletal development; the mean age was 8 years. All of the attending dogs had a DJD of the shoulder, elbow, hip joint, and/or stifle. One major precondition was that no other medication was

TABLE I Studies with Oral Administered CS in Dogs and Horses

Author	Species	Number of probands	Substances	Period of administration	Study design	Result
Moore, 1996	Dog	3	CS, Gluc, Mn, As	1–2 months	Case report	–
Segal and Bousquet, 1999	Dog	110	CS	2 months	Field study	+
Anderson et al., 1999	Dog	>2000	CS, Gluc, Mn, As	Several weeks	Retrospective field study	–
Gerlach et al., 2000	Dog	30	CS, Chitosan	1 month	Field study	+
Dobenecker et al., 2002	Dog	58	CS, ME	3 months	Double-blind placebo controlled field study	–
Videla and Guerrero, 1998	Horse	15	CS	1 month	Placebo controlled trial	+
Hanson et al., 1997	Horse	25	CS, Gluc	2 months	Field study	Partly +

CS, Chondroitin sulfate; Gluc, glucosamine; Mn, manganese; As, ascorbic acid; +, significant improvement; –, no significant improvement.

necessary during the 12-week duration of supplementation as well as 2 weeks prior to the first examination. Especially the administration of steroidal or nonsteroidal antiphlogistics as well as other chondroprotective or homeopathic substances were reasons to exclude possible participants from the study. Seventy-one percent of the dogs had two joints affected with the highest prevalence for DJD in the hip joint. They were randomly allotted to the three test groups CS, ME, and PL.

The first group received a granulate with 5.6% CS, the second with 2.6% ME and 3% microcrystalline cellulose, and the third a granulate without active substances but 5.6% of the cellulose. All three products contained 55.5% malted and bruised wheat, 30% oatflakes, 5% herbarum, 2% honey, 1% soybean oil, 0.5% chicken meat extract, and 0.4% Aerosil® (inert fluxing material). All dogs received the same dosage of the granulate for 12 weeks together with the main repast of the day. With this the dogs of the CS group received 22 mg CS (Kraeber, Basel, Switzerland)/kg body weight per day.

At the beginning of the feeding trial a questionnaire had to be completed from both dog owners and treating veterinarian. For the owner a ranking of the symptoms with the criteria lameness, playing, recumbency, loading tolerance, gait, being blithe, and pain had to be made as well as statements about the duration of the disease and its progression. To access the degree of the arthropathy correctly, the owner should also specify the symptoms after respite and exposure, limitation of activity due to the arthropathy and total time of daily walks. The attending veterinarians had to answer questions about examination methods, hitherto treatment, characterization of kind, and degree of the arthropathy as well as the appraisal of pain, crepitation, and ability to compensate. After 12 weeks of feeding the test substances, the owner and veterinarians were asked to answer another questionnaire of same design. The examination of the patient in the clinic of the attending veterinarian should include X-rays and detailed diagnostics of the DJD.

Fifty-eight dogs (83%) finished the study, with 21 in the CS group, 18 in the ME, and 19 in the PL group. Twelve dogs had to be excluded from the analysis due to required appliance of painkiller or other medication as well as other reasons like refusal to ingest the supplement.

CS as well as ME administration did not lead to substantial ameliora-tion of the recorded symptoms or even total recovery. The evaluation of the questionnaires of the dog owners showed that they perceived the symptoms "lameness" and "pain" as the two, which most clearly changed to the better. In a range of 7 (1: much improved, 4: unchanged, 7: much worse) the mean values for both symptoms were not significantly different, whereas margin-ally lower values were obtained in the placebo group (Figs. 1 and 2). A high analogy was found between the perception of dog owners and attend-ing veterinarians. The latter also found a slight improvement in all three treatment groups, including the PL.

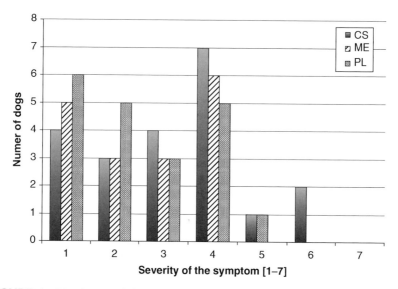

FIGURE 1   Distribution of the scaled answers concerning the symptom "lameness" (1: much improved and 4: unchanged to 7: much worse) in the chondroitin sulfate (CS), the mussel extract (ME) and the placebo group (PL). There were no significant differences between groups.

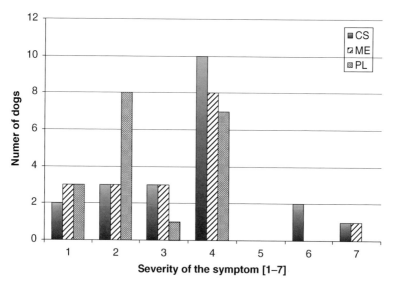

FIGURE 2   Distribution of the scaled answers concerning the symptom "pain" (1: much improved and 4: unchanged to 7: much worse) in the chondroitin sulfate (CS), the mussel extract (ME), and the placebo group (PL). There were no significant differences between groups.

The dog owners as well as the attending veterinarians, who generally had a high concordance in their statements, perceived only a slight improvement in all three groups including the placebo group. There were no significant differences between the effects in the CS and the other two groups. It has to be taken account of the large number of dogs with very good or good response (scaling 1, 2) in the placebo group. Reasons for these remarkable improvements of the symptoms in the group without use of effective substances may have been a coincidence of spontaneous transient improvement and the onset of treatment or rather an optimistic perception of the effects. This phenomenon is known as placebo effect. Another known effect to be considered in the field of veterinary medicine is the care effect (Löscher and Richter, 1999), for example, after more controlled training and exposure in periods of treatment. It clearly demonstrates how important it is to conduct a study designed with placebo control. The good agreement between the scoring of owners and veterinarians points to the relevance of carrying out a double blind study. Results from studies, which are not placebo controlled and double blinded, are therefore probably less significant. Referring to this, the results of Segal and Bousquet (1999) as well as Gerlach *et al.* (2000) concerning the effects of CS in dogs should be judged with caution. Besides, CS has been combined with glucosamin and chitosan (produced from crustaceans) in the latter study, probably influencing the effect of CS. Another point to be considered is the highly different material in a field study. The patients in our study (Dobenecker *et al.*, 2002) were selected under special conditions; the percentage of patients with inflammation in their affected degenerative joints, the formulation and dosage of the CS, or the feeding of the patients (interactions with medication) might have been different compared to other studies. In cases of acute arthropathies with inflammation and cellular conversions effects of CS may exist. A limitation of the significance of the own study might be the restricted duration of the study. The used time span of 12 weeks is possibly too short to show effects on a tissue with such a slow metabolism like articular-cartilage.

Results from studies in other species cannot be adopted for dogs under all circumstances. For example, quantitative differences in the pathophysiology of the articular-cartilage as well as species-specific differences in absorption, availability and metabolism of CS might exist. Results from studies, which are not placebo controlled or double blinded, should be judged considering the placebo and care effect.

References

Anderson, M. A., Slater, M. R., and Hammad, T. A. (1999). Results of a survey of small-animal-practitioners on the perceived clinical efficacy and safety of an oral nutraceutical. *Prev. Vet. Med.* 38, 65–73.

Daniel Uebelhart*,†, Ruud Knols*, Eling D de Bruin*,‡, and Gust Verbruggen§

*Department of Rheumatology and Institute of Physical Medicine
University Hospital
Zurich, Switzerland

†Department of Biochemistry
Rush Presbyterian-St. Luke's Medical Center
Chicago, Illinois

‡Institute for Human Movement Sciences
ETH Zurich, Switzerland

§Department of Rheumatology
Ghent University Hospital, Gent, Belgium

Chondroitin Sulfate as a Structure-Modifying Agent

I. Chapter Overview

The disease- or structure-modifying effects of chondroitin sulfate (CS) have been the focus of only a small number of studies performed *in vitro* or *in vivo* in animal models of osteoarthritis (OA) or joint degradation in the last decades. Some randomized controlled trials (RCTs) conducted on humans have integrated this feature as a primary or secondary evaluation outcome. The results of the survey conducted allowed the identification of a total of six RCTs performed in both knee OA and finger-joint OA. Only two groups, one in Belgium and one in Switzerland, have conducted these human studies. Based upon the results of these trials, it may be concluded that the daily oral administration of 800–1200 mg of chondroitin 4- and 6-sulfate appears to be able to limit or even stop the radiological progression of both femoro-tibial knee OA and interphalangeal finger OA in a time frame of a minimum of 1 year to up to 3 years of continuous or intermittent

Advances in Pharmacology, Volume 53
Copyright 2006, Elsevier Inc. All rights reserved.

1054-3589/06 $35.00
DOI: 10.1016/S1054-3589(05)53024-2

administration of the compound. The fundamental basis of this structure-modifying effect must certainly be originating from the *in vitro* demonstrated capacity of CS to inhibit some of the key enzymes and cytokines involved in both the development and the progression of OA disease. This point should clearly be further investigated *in vivo* as well as possible other modes of action of CS on the joint structures as articular cartilage might not be the only target element involved in OA. Nevertheless, the results available so far of published RCTs do already provide a strong support for a disease-modifying effect of CS.

II. Introduction

The first attempts at improving structure and function of the connective tissues of synovial joints, thereby alleviating the symptoms of degenerative joint disorders, were based on the vague assumptions that an exogenous administration of precursors of extracellular matrix (ECM) components would help articular cartilage cells to replace the lost environment. This presumption prompted physicians to use substances such as glucosamine and sulfated glycosaminoglycans (GAGs), that is, CS aimed at improving cartilage repair in degenerative joint disease. Likewise, the first intra-articular administration of chondroitin polysulfate (CPS) was based on the presumption that this heparinoid type of drug would replace hyaluronan as a lubricant and reduces fibrinogen levels in inflamed joints and that this would bring some therapeutical advantage (Eylau, 1959, 1960). Unexpectedly, some patients reported symptomatic relief after having undergone this therapeutic procedure, and some changes in the biochemical composition of synovial fluid could also be assessed (Momburg *et al.*, 1976).

Together with a profound search in those mechanisms, whereby tissues are modified and/or destroyed during the course of inflammatory or degenerative joint diseases, researchers began to think about biological agents capable of restoring damaged connective tissues in a more methodical manner. As articular cartilage is one of the principal target tissue affected as a consequence of rheumatic disorders, many investigations focused on the metabolic characteristics of the single cell homing in this tissue: the chondrocyte. Substances that were demonstrated to protect articular cartilage during the course of destructive joint disorders were therefore termed "chondroprotective agents." When this occurred *in vivo* in joints affected by OA, these agents were designed as "disease modifying osteoarthritis drugs" (DMOAD) (Altman *et al.*, 2000).

As the auto/paracrine growth factor and cytokine cascades behind development, homeostasis, and destruction of the ECM of articular cartilage were not known previously, the first investigations on biological agents capable of modifying the structure of connective tissues in a positive way concentrated mainly on the capability of these agents in improving the synthesis or impairing the degradation of ECM compounds, especially aggrecan and collagen. According to this definition, a number of substances could also be classified as connective tissue structure modifying agents (CTSMA). Among these, sulfated GAGs (chondroitin 4- and 6-sulfate and glucosamine), chemically modified tetracyclines, such as doxycycline and minocycline, and avocado/soybean unsaponifiables have been repeatedly cited.

A. Sulfated Polysaccharides and Chondroprotection

The so-called "chondromucoproteins" were among the first substances identified that were found to be able to improve the accumulation of ECM compounds (Kosher *et al.*, 1973; Nevo and Dorfman, 1972b; Nevo *et al.*, 1972a); they represent a mixture of proteoglycan (PG)-degradation products containing CS. It was then hypothesized that CS containing ECM-breakdown products somehow exerted a positive feedback on articular cartilage chondrocytes. The possibility of positively interfering with the *in vitro* connective tissue cell repair process using sulfated polysaccharides was first described in the mid 1970s (Schwartz and Dorfman, 1975; Verbruggen and Veys, 1977). A couple of years later, polysulfated CS was shown to improve the *in vivo* synthesis of hyaluronan in synovial joints of human subjects (Verbruggen and Veys, 1979). The same compound, as well as its naturally occurring analogue CS, was demonstrated to improve chondrocyte repair function *in vivo* in different experimental models of OA (Brennan *et al.*, 1987; Carreno *et al.*, 1986; Kalbhen, 1983; Uebelhart *et al.*, 1998a).

In addition, oral CS was also identified as a symptomatic slow-acting drug for OA (SYSADOA) as it was demonstrated in a couple of randomized, double-blind, placebo (PBO) controlled therapeutic trials (RCTs) that it was effective, with delayed onset of action, in alleviating the painful symptoms of OA (knee, finger, hip) and in improving the mobility of the OA joints as well as the overall mobility of the patient (see the corresponding chapter in this volume). For many years, CS was mostly documented as a SYSADOA but in some RCTs, with symptomatic efficacy as primary outcome, did also integrate the radiological progression as a secondary outcome. The quantitative radiological data provided by these studies supported further investigations regarding the structure-modifying effect of CS.

Therefore, RCTs provided results supporting that these CTSMA had DMOAD properties, as they were shown to retard the progression of human erosive OA in interphalangeal finger joints (Verbruggen and Veys, 1998a; Verbruggen *et al.*, 2002) and in knee joint as well (Uebelhart *et al.*, 1998b, 2004).

The objective of the present survey was to make a critical synthesis of the published literature available on RCTs regarding the structure- or disease-modifying effect of orally administered CS in patients suffering from OA. Based upon the literature available and taking into consideration that the *in vitro* studies and the *in vivo* animal trials were already mentioned earlier, only data originating from RCTs focusing on human OA disease and specifically addressing finger and knee OA are reported here; indeed, there are no data originating from structure-modifying RCTs available so far regarding other joints, for example, hip or spine.

III. Methods

A. Search Strategy

A computer-aided search was conducted (Dickersin *et al.*, 1994), integrating all publications between 1966 and 2005, and reported in MEDLINE (Ovid, PubMed, Gateway; 1966 to June 2005) and the Cochrane Database of Systematic Reviews (2005); the aim was to identify all studies that cover the topic of chondroprotective effects of CS in knee and/or finger OA. Additionally, we checked the citation lists to complete our selection.

The following generic search terms (according to the thesaurus of each individual database) were used: chondroitin, chondroitin sulfate or sulfate, finger OA, joint disease, knee OA, musculoskeletal diseases, OA, randomized or randomised, rheumatic diseases, and any combination of these search terms. Some restrictions were made regarding the language of the original publications; only papers in English, French, German, or Dutch language were included into the review process.

B. Inclusion Criteria and Data Collection

To be included in the review, all studies had to have examined the effects of CS on OA *in vivo* in human subjects. In addition, only randomized controlled trials (RCTs) were included in this review. Studies using at least one of the following types of outcome were included: joint space narrowing, minimum- and mean-joint space width, Kellgren- and Lawrence-radiological score, X-rays. Disagreement regarding inclusion of some of the studies was resolved by consensus between the coauthors. RCTs evaluating CS in combination with glucosamine or nonsteroidal anti-inflammatory drugs were excluded from the review process.

C. Data Abstraction

Two of the coauthors defined as reviewers (RK, EdB) independently assessed the predefined outcomes of the studies according to a standardized form. Variability presented for the outcome "chondroprotective effects of

CS" was reported. If necessary, means and measures of dispersion were approximated from the available data, tables, and figures directly from the published papers. A p value of 0.05 was used as the criterion for statistically significant results.

IV. Results

A. Study Characteristics

The literature search yielded a total of six reports, which met the basic eligibility criteria of being an RCT conducted *in vivo* with human subjects. All human studies included had in common that their primary or secondary outcome assessed the effect of oral CS as a drug able to modify the OA-disease activity and/or improve the structure of the OA joint (chrondropro-tection). A total of three RCTs included knee OA patients, whereas three RCTs included patients with finger joints OA.

B. Disease-Modifying Effects of CS on RCTs in Knee OA

A total or three RCTs were available including 462 knee OA patients. Of the three studies that evaluated the chondroprotective aspects of CS in human knee joint (as primary or secondary outcome), all of them were originating from Switzerland. One study was a one-center study (Michel *et al.*, 2005) whereas the two other studies (Uebelhart *et al.*, 1998b, 2004) were multicentric and included patients from various countries (France, Italy, Belgium) as well.

Two CS treatment modalities were used, which differed in their admin-istration sequence; one study (Uebelhart *et al.*, 2004) reported an intermit-tent treatment schedule of 2×3 months daily oral CS 800 mg treatment during 1 year; the two other studies used a treatment schedule of oral CS 800 mg daily given continuously for a total of 12 (Uebelhart *et al.*, 1998b) vs. 24 (Michel *et al.*, 2005) consecutive months.

At this point, it is important to say that disease-modifying effect of oral CS was the primary outcome of only one single RCT of 24-month duration (Michel *et al.*, 2005); regarding the two other 12-month duration studies mentioned, the chondroprotective effect of oral CS was only part of the secondary outcomes as these studies were primarily designed to test the symptomatic efficacy of the drug.

Uebelhart *et al.* (1998b and 2004) described that the radiological pro-gression after 12 months showed significant decreased joint space width in the PBO group ($p < 0.01$), meaning a narrowing of the joint space, whereas there was no change in the CS treated group. These results were provided in those two studies in which the radiological outcome was not the primary target of the study; in addition, the number of knee OA patients whose X-rays could be fully analyzed was relatively small, and the design of the studies was not identical in that the administration of CS was continuous (800 mg daily) in the first study (Uebelhart et al., 1998b) and in the second (Uebelhart et al., 2004), the administration of CS was intermittent (800 mg/day for two periods of 3 months each). The total duration was the same in both studies (12 months). Nevertheless, these initial exciting results provided the justification for the most recent clinical trial, which is the very first RCT with intention-to-treat analysis to be performed with structure-modifying effect as a primary outcome (Michel et al., 2005). Indeed, long-term treatment with continuous oral CS (800 mg daily) over 2 years did stop the radiographic progression of knee OA (Michel et al., 2005). Those patients who received a PBO ($n = 150$) experienced a significant decrease in their mean-joint width ($p = 0.04$) and their minimum joint space width ($p = 0.05$), whereas in sharp contrast, there was no joint space narrowing in the CS-treated group ($n = 150$). Therefore, the authors proposed that the clinical relevance of these positive results should be evaluated in further studies (Michel et al., 2005). A new international multicentric study aimed at confirming the chondroprotective effect of oral CS was already launched including significantly more patients and more careful selection of the patients upon entry on strict radiological criteria. The results are awaited in 2006. In addition, a large longitudinal multicenter trial is also ongoing in the USA under the supervision of the NIH in which some OA patients do receive CS alone or CS + glucosamine sulfate. The first results are available (Clegg et al., 2006). As the measurement of the progression of knee OA is based upon the radiological assessment of joint space narrowing in each of these RCTs, it appears important to discuss this major issue.

C. How to Measure the Structure or Disease-Modifying Activity of a Drug?

Based upon the European Agency for the Evaluation of Medicinal Products (EMEA) guidelines to test antiosteoarthritic drugs (CPMP, 1998), the best way to assess the chondroprotective activity of a drug would be to use the invasive arthroscopic procedure (Listrat et al., 1997), but for obvious ethical reasons, this diagnostic method is generally not well accepted and adopted for clinical trials. The EMEA guidelines did also approve the use of a noninvasive indirect method based upon the analysis of the actual joint space measured on high quality X-rays of the knee joint. A couple of groups have been working on various procedures to develop this quantitative radiological method because the qualitative evaluation of the progression of knee OA using the Kellgren and Lawrence scoring system (Kellgren and Lawrence, 1957) has been demonstrated not to be sensitive enough to evaluate the changes occurring in the OA joint and therefore might not be applicable in clinical trials. Considering the different methods of quantitative analysis of the X-rays proposed so far, Buckland-Wright and team developed an analysis of the joint space width using high-resolution plain film and double contrast macroradiographic investigation (Buckland-Wright, 1994; Buckland-Wright *et al.*, 1995), whereas Vignon and coworkers developed a system based on the digitalization of high-quality X-rays of the knee joint followed by an automatic or semiautomatic measurement of the joint space width (Fig. 1) with the assistance of a specific computer analysis software (Piperno *et al.*, 1998; Vignon *et al.*, 1999). In addition, based on the availability of high-quality X-rays, initially of the hip, later of the knee, Lequesne developed a method of analysis using a direct assessment of the joint width, called chondrometry, using a caliper (Lequesne, 1995). This method, which is certainly less sophisticated than the other two, nevertheless provided excellent results to assess the joint space loss in various types of OA, for instance in the rapid destructive type.

Considering the three RCTs taken into consideration in this survey, the quantitative assessment of joint space loss was performed by the original method of Vignon *et al.* (1999). More precisely, the measurement of the femoro-tibial joint space width was performed on standard weight-bearing antero-posterior X-rays of the knee joint in extension upon entry and after 12 months in the study of Uebelhart *et al.* (1998b), whereas standard antero-posterior X-rays of the knees were performed in weight-bearing monopodal position upon entry and after 12 months of follow-up in the CS intermittent administration study of Uebelhart *et al.* (2004). The only study with disease-modifying effect as primary outcome used standing, posteroanterior, weight-bearing X-rays of both left and right knees flexed to $\cong 20°$ with patients

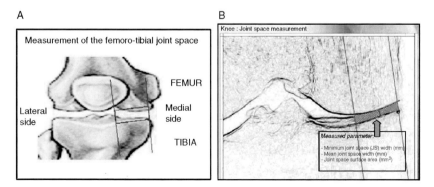

FIGURE 1   (A) Schematic view of the measurement of the femoro-tibial joint space. (B) After digitalization of the knee X-ray, definition of the zone of interest for automatic or semiautomatic measurement of the femoro-tibial joint space. (See Color Insert.)

positioned with the toes up, directly under the edge of the cassette and the knees bent to lie against the cassette. The X-ray beam was directed 5° downward at a site midway between the popliteal spaces. A foot map was drawn for each patient in order to reproduce the position when radiographed after 24 months at the end of the study.

From these details, it can be shown that both the positioning of the patients for the radiographic procedure did change and improve from the initial to the latest studies and most importantly that the X-rays procedure itself evolved from a classical antero-posterior view to a posteroanterior view with the X-ray beam ± parallel to the tibial plateau with a semiflexed position. In order to increase the precision of the measurement of the joint space, one could further add the exact positioning of the knee joint (X-ray beam angulation) with fluoroscopy, a procedure initially developed by Vignon and now applied in some recent clinical trials, for instance in testing the effects of doxycycline on progression of OA (Brandt *et al.*, 2005). The evolution of these radiological procedures allowed to reach a greater degree of precision in the measurement of the femoro-tibial joint space narrowing in the longitudinal follow-up of OA disease and also to increase the reproducibility of the method, as it has been recently demonstrated that some important pitfalls can interfere with the accuracy of the measurement (Mazzuca *et al.*, 2004).

D. Disease-Modifying Effects of CS in Finger Joint OA

A total of two RCTs regarding finger OA patients as the target population could be identified including a total of 284 patients. The two studies referred in this survey were performed at the Department of Rheumatology, University of Ghent in Belgium.

The first study referred in two papers was published in 1998 (Verbruggen and Veys, 1998a; Verbruggen *et al.*, 1998b) and was based on the use of a numerical scoring system for the anatomical evolution of finger joint OA developed by Verbruggen and Veys (1996). A total of 119 patients suffering from finger OA were included in this RCT with the primary outcome being structure- and disease-modifying effect of oral CS4 and -6 given as 3×400 mg/day over a period of 3 years. Standard posteroanterior X-rays of the interphalangeal (IP) joints were carried out upon entry and at yearly intervals up to completion of the study after 3 years. It was shown that the progression of OA in the IP finger joints in an individual patient can be determined by the evolution of this joint in various previously described anatomical phases: not affected (N), classical OA (S), loss of joint space (J), erosive OA (E), remodeled joint (R). The structure-modifying effect of oral CS was assessed for by the number of patients developing OA in previously normal IP joints (N > S) or progressing through the described anatomical phases of the disease (S > J; S > E, J > E, S > R, J > R; E > R). The results of this study showed that in the CS treated group of patients, there was a significant decrease in the number of patients with new erosive OA finger joints. The authors underlined this finding as being extremely relevant as it is known that finger OA becomes a clinical problem when pain and loss of function happen, which is when S joints progress to J and E joints. Indeed, during and after the E phase of anatomical progression, the finger joints will remodel and present with the nodular deformities characteristic of Heberden's and Bouchard's nodes.

Verbruggen *et al.* (2002) conducted two additional studies to assess the progression of finger OA and its modulation by two different DMOADs. Indeed, patients were included in two separate RCTs, but the results are reported and published in one single paper (Verbruggen *et al.*, 2002). A total of 45 patients received CPS (Arteparon®, Luitpold Werk, Munich, Germany), 50 mg intramuscularly twice weekly for 8 weeks every 4 months for a total duration of 3 years. A total of 34 patients received oral CS (Condrosulf®, IBSA, Lugano, Switzerland), 3×400 mg daily for a total duration of 3 years. Both the study with CPS and CS had a PBO group (total number of patients in the PBO group: $n = 85$). Standard posteroanterior X-rays of the IP finger joints were obtained at initiation of the trials and at yearly intervals up to completion of the studies after 3 years. Upon entry, almost 80% of the distal IP and 50% of the proximal IP joints were affected by OA. In a total of 40% of the patients, the classical picture of OA of the IP joints was complicated by manifest erosive OA changes. The two systems used to assess the progression of the anatomical lesions (Anatomical Lesion and Anatomical Phase Progression Score System) showed definite progression within 3 years, especially in the IP joints. When compared with the PBO controls, neither CPS nor CS was able to prevent the occurrence of OA in previously normal joints. However, when the classical OA associated anatomical lesions were considered, OA was less progressive in both CPS and CS groups. In addition, fewer patients treated with either CPS or CS developed erosive OA of the finger joints.

The authors conclude that the systems used to score the radiological progression of finger OA allowed to evaluate the structure-modifying effects of both DMOADs (CPS and CS), but they do also consider both studies as being pilot trials, which means that additional studies need to be performed in the future.

V. Discussion

Both *in vitro* and *in vivo* experiments made in various research centers regarding the effects on the metabolism of intercellular matrix molecules (collagens, PGs, aggrecan, hyaluronan) have shown that most (poly)-sulfated polysaccharides do influence connective tissue cells (chondrocytes, synoviocytes, fibroblasts) in a similar way (Francis *et al.*, 1993; Verbruggen and Veys, 1977, 1992; Verbruggen *et al.*, 1999). With the improvement of our insights in the auto/paracrine growth factor and cytokine pathways that control the homeostasis of healthy connective tissues, it became possible to study the mechanism of action of these CTSMAs. Investigations with sulfated polysaccharides showed that these agents operate in biological systems through a down modulation of important catabolic auto/paracrine cytokine pathways, such as IL-1, thereby improving the accumulation of ECM compounds in the cell-associated matrix of these cells. Experiments conducted with bovine chondrocytes obtained from macroscopically intact metacarpophalangeal joints showed that physiological concentrations of CPS were able to significantly reduce the downstream IL-1 effects and reduce collagenase, proteoglycanase, MMP-1, and MMP-3 activities (Sadowski and Steinmeyer, 2002).

Furthermore, CPS inhibited the IL-1-induced mRNA expression of tPA (Sadowski and Steinmeyer, 2002). Likewise, xylosan polysulfate and CPS restored the accumulation of aggrecan, hyaluronan, and type II collagen in the cell-associated matrix in IL-1β-treated human chondrocytes cultured in agarose. This effect probably resulted in part from the downregulation of the MMPs (Wang *et al.*, 2002). In cultured equine chondrocytes as well, CPS significantly reduced IL-1β-enhanced expression of iNOS that was paralleled by an increased release of NO. CPS downsized nitrite concentrations in the supernatants of these IL-1β-stimulated cultures (Tung *et al.*, 2002). Finally, a novel polysulfated polysaccharide cyclodextrin polysulfate showed cartilage structure-modifying effects *in vitro* as it improved the synthesis of aggrecan and the accumulation of cell-associated matrix macromolecules by human articular cartilage cells in alginate. Here, it was shown for the first time that this effect resulted in part from the direct repression of IL-1 as cyclodextrin polysulfate-treated cells expressed significantly lower amounts of intracellular IL-1α and -β levels (Verdonk *et al.*, 2005). The same β-cyclodextrin-treated chondrocytes released significantly less IL-6 in the supernatant culture media, an effect being known to result from auto/paracrine IL-1 stimulation. It is important to remind at this point that the concentrations of the culture supernatant polysaccharide of most of the reported *in vitro* experiments are in the same order of magnitude than plasma or cartilage tissue polysaccharide levels obtained in humans after per oral administration (Muller *et al.*, 1983; Volpi, 2002, 2003).

These basic science considerations might explain why natural compounds registered as drugs, such as chondroitin 4- and 6-sulfate, might have, in addition to their symptomatic efficacy, some chondroprotective effects in OA disease as they are able to modulate key cytokines and enzymes directly involved in the development and the progression of the OA disease. Indeed, OA disease is a chronic joint disease characterized by flares and periods of increased inflammatory activity; these periods are responsible for an increased degradation of matrix components and therefore the progression of the anatomical lesions.

As the results of our survey conducted to a small number of RCTs, which could be evaluated (total: $n = 6$), the present results should still be taken with some caution, and it seems important to wait for additional data regarding the structure-modifying effects of oral CS. In their meta-analysis of the structural and symptomatic efficacy of glucosamine and chondroitin in knee OA, Richy *et al.* (2003) reported positive results for glucosamine but no results for CS as of the time of this publication; there was no RCT available for CS with joint space narrowing as primary outcome.

In addition, an important question remains open, which is to know if drugs are always a suitable answer to disease modification in OA. As illustrated in a recent editorial of Dieppe (2005), there are still many unanswered questions regarding structural modification in OA, such as what is the clinical relevance of stopping the development of the OA process and if it really increases the quality of life of the patients, in addition to the difficult question of the price to pay to reach this goal.

VI. Conclusions

The results of this survey allowed the identification of a total of six RCTs in which some structure-modifying aspects have been evaluated as primary or secondary outcome. These studies focused on both knee OA and finger OA, but no data are available so far for other OA localizations such as hip and spine. On an evidence-based perspective, there are clearly not enough RCTs and data available so far to conclude that CS belongs to the category of the disease-modifying drugs for OA, but the available data in knee OA and finger OA provide a strong support to this hypothesis. Additional data from high-quality RCTs are awaited soon, which should allow an answer to this still open question.

Acknowledgments

The authors would like to thank Leanne Pobjoy for her excellent secretarial assistance.

References

Altman, R. D., Hochberg, M. C., Moskowitz, R. W., and Schnitzer, T. J. (2000). Recommendations for the medical management of osteoarthritis of the hip and knee. 2000 update. ACR subcommittee on osteoarthritis guidelines. *Arthritis Rheum.* **43**, 1905–1915.

Brandt, K. D., Mazzuca, S. A., Katz, B. P., Lane, K. A., Buckwalter, K. A., Yocum, D. E., Wolfe, F., Schnitzer, T. J., Moreland, L. W., Manzi, S., Bradley, J. D., Sharma, L., *et al.* (2005). Effects of doxycycline on progression of osteoarthritis: Results of a randomized, placebo-controlled, double-blind trial. *Arthritis Rheum.* **52,** 2015–2025.

Brennan, J. J., Aherne, F. X., and Nakano, T. (1987). Effects of glycosaminoglycan polysulfate treatment on soundness, hyaluronic acid content of synovial fluid and proteoglycan aggregate in articular cartilage of lame boars. *Can. J. Vet. Res.* **51,** 394–398.

Buckland-Wright, J. C. (1994). Quantitative radiography of osteoarthritis. *Ann. Rheum. Dis.* **53,** 268–275.

Buckland-Wright, J. C., MacFarlane, D. G., Lynch, J. A., Jasani, M. K., and Bradshaw, C. R. (1995). Joint space width measures cartilage thickness in osteoarthritis of the knee: High resolution plain film and double contrast macroradiographic investigation. *Ann. Rheum. Dis.* **54,** 263–268.

Carreno, M. R., Muniz, O. E., and Howell, D. S. (1986). The effect of glycosaminoglycan polysulfuric acid ester on articular cartilage in experimental osteoarthritis: Effects on morphological variables of disease severity. *J. Rheumatol.* **13,** 490–497.

Clegg, D. O, Reda, D. J., Harris, C. L., Klein, M. A., O'Dell, J. R., Hooper, M. M., Bradley, J. D., Bingham, C. O. 3rd, Weisman, M. H., Jackson, C. G., Lane, N. E., Crush, J. J., *et al.* (2006). Glucomine, chondroitin sulfate, and the two in combination for painful knee osteoarthritis. *N. Eng. J. Med.* **23,** 795–808.

Committee for Proprietary Medicinal Products (CPMP) (1998). Points to consider on clinical investigation of medicinal products used in the treatment of osteoarthritis. European Agency for the Evaluation of Medicinal Products, London.

Dickersin, K., Scherer, R., and Lefebvre, C. (1994). Identifying relevant studies for systematic reviews. *BMJ* **309,** 1286–1291.

Dieppe, P. (2005). Disease modification in osteoarthritis: Are drugs the answer? *Arthritis Rheum.* **52,** 1956–1959.

Eylau, O. (1959). Intra-articular heparin therapy of genuine arthrosis deformans of the knee joint. *Med. Klin.* **54,** 145.

Eylau, O. (1960). On the pathogenesis and causal treatment of arthrosis of the knee joint. *Med. Klin.* **55,** 2367–2370.

Francis, D. J., Hutadilok, N., Kongtawelert, P., and Ghosh, P. (1993). Pentosan polysulphate and glycosaminoglycan polysulphate stimulate the synthesis of hyaluronan *in vivo.* *Rheumatol. Int.* **13,** 61–64.

Kalbhen, D. A. (1983). Experimental confirmation of the antiarthritic activity of glycosamino-glycan polysulfate. *Z. Rheumatol.* **42,** 178–184.

Kellgren, J. H., and Lawrence, J. S. (1957). Radiological assessment of osteoarthritis. *Ann. Rheum. Dis.* **16,** 494–501.

Kosher, R. A., Lash, J. W., and Minor, R. R. (1973). Environmental enhancement of *in vitro* chondrogenesis. *Dev. Biol.* **35,** 210–220.

Lequesne, M. (1995). Chondrometry: Quantitative evaluation of joint space width and rate of joint space loss in osteoarthritis of the hip. *Rev. Rhum. Engl. Ed.* **62,** 155–158.

Listrat, V., Ayral, X., Paternello, F., Bonvarlet, J. P., Simonnet, J., Amor, B., and Dougados, M. (1997). Arthroscopic evaluation of potential structure modifying activity of hyaluronan (Hyalgan) in osteoarthritis of the knee. *Osteoarthritis Cartilage* **5,** 153–160.

Mazzuca, S. A., Brandt, K. D., Buckwalter, K. A., and Lequesne, M. (2004). Pitfalls in the accurate measurement of joint space narrowing in semiflexed, anteroposterior radio-graphic imaging of the knee. *Arthritis Rheum.* **50,** 2508–2515.

Michel, B. A., Stucki, G., Frey, D., De Valthaire, F., Vignon, E., Bruehlmann, P., and Uebelhart, D. (2005). Chondroitins 4 and 6 sulfate in osteoarthritis of the knee: A randomized, controlled trial. *Arthritis Rheum.* **52,** 779–786.

Momburg, M., Stuhlsatz, H. W., Vogeli, H., Vojtisek, O., Eylau, O., and Greiling, H. (1976). Clinical chemical changes in the synovial fluid following intra-articular injection of a glycosaminoglycan polysulfate. *Z. Rheumatol.* **35**(Suppl. 4), 389–390.

Muller, W., Panse, P., Brand, S., and Staubli, A. (1983). *In vivo* study of the distribution, affinity for cartilage and metabolism of glycosaminoglycan polysulphate (GAGPS, Arteparon). *Z. Rheumatol.* **42**, 355–361.

Nevo, Z., Horwitz, A. L., and Dorfman, A. (1972a). Synthesis of chondromucoprotein by chondrocytes in suspension culture. *Dev. Biol.* **28**, 219–228.

Nevo, Z., and Dorfman, A. (1972b). Stimulation of chondromucoprotein synthesis in chondrocytes by extracellular chondromucoprotein. *Proc. Natl. Acad. Sci. USA* **69**, 2069–2072.

Piperno, M., Hellio le Graverand, M. P., Conrozier, T., Conrozier, T., Bochu, M., Mathieu, P., and Vignon, E. (1998). Quantitative evaluation of joint space width in femorotibial osteoarthritis: Comparison of three radiographic views. *Osteoarthritis Cartilage* **6**, 252–259.

Richy, F., Bruyere, O., Ethgen, O., Cucherat, M., Henrotin, Y., and Reginster, J. Y. (2003). Structural and symptomatic efficacy of glucosamine and chondroitin in knee osteoarthritis: A comprehensive meta-analysis. *Arch. Intern. Med.* **163**, 1514–1522.

Sadowski, T., and Steinmeyer, J. (2002). Effects of polysulfated glycosaminoglycan and triamcinolone acetonid on the production of proteinases and their inhibitors by IL-1alpha treated articular chondrocytes. *Biochem. Pharmacol.* **64**, 217–227.

Schwartz, N. B., and Dorfman, A. (1975). Stimulation of chondroitin sulfate proteoglycan production of by chondrocytes in monolayer. *Connec. Tissue Res.* **3**, 115–122.

Tung, J. T., Venta, P. J., and Caron, J. P. (2002). Inducible nitric oxide expression in equine articular chondrocytes: Effects of antiinflammatory compounds. *Osteoarthritis Cartilage* **10**, 5–12.

Uebelhart, D., Thonar, E. J., Zhang, J., and Williams, J. M. (1998a). Protective effect of exogenous chondroitin 4,6-sulfate in the acute degradation of articular cartilage in the rabbit. *Osteoarthritis Cartilage* **6**(Suppl. A), 6–13.

Uebelhart, D., Thonar, E. J., Delmas, P. D., Chantraine, A., and Vignon, E. (1998b). Effects of oral chondroitin sulfate on the progression of knee osteoarthritis: A pilot study. *Osteoarthritis Cartilage* **6**(Suppl. A), 39–46.

Uebelhart, D., Malaise, M., Marcolongo, R., DeVathaire, F., Piperno, M., Mailleux, E., Fioravanti, A., Matoso, L., and Vignon, E. (2004). Intermittent treatment of knee osteoarthritis with oral chondroitin sulfate: A one-year, randomized, double-blind, multicenter study versus placebo. *Osteoarthritis Cartilage* **12**, 269–276.

Verbruggen, G., and Veys, E. M. (1977). Influence of sulphated glycosaminoglycans upon proteoglycan metabolism of the synovial lining cells. *Acta Rheumatol.* **1**, 75–92.

Verbruggen, G., and Veys, E. M. (1979). Influence of an oversulphated heparinoid upon hyaluronate metabolism of the human synovial cell *in vivo. J. Rheumatol.* **6**, 554–561.

Verbruggen, G., and Veys, E. M. (1992). Intra-articular injection of pentosanpolysulphate results in increased hyaluronan molecular weight in joint fluid. *Clin. Exp. Rheumatol.* **10**, 249–254.

Verbruggen, G., and Veys, E. M. (1996). Numerical scoring systems for the anatomical evolution of osteoarthritis of the finger joint. *Arthritis Rheum.* **39**, 308–320.

Verbruggen, G., and Veys, E. M. (1998a). Influence of chondroitin 4&6 sulfate on finger osteoarthrites in a double blind, controlled study versus placebo. *Litera Rheumatol.* **24**, 43–47.

Verbruggen, G., Goemaere, S., and Veys, E. M. (1998b). Chondroitin sulfate: S/DMOAD (structure/disease modifying anti-osteoarthritis drug) in the treatment of finger joint OA. *Osteoarthritis Cartilage* **6**(Suppl. A), 37–38.

Verbruggen, G., Cornelissen, M., Elewaut, D., Broddelez, C., De Ridder, L., and Veys, E. M. (1999). Influence of polysulfated polysaccharides on aggrecans synthesized by differentiated human articular chondrocytes. *J. Rheumatol.* **26**, 1663–1671.

Verbruggen, G., Goemaere, S., and Veys, E. M. (2002). Systems to assess the progression of finger joint osteoarthritis and the effects of disease modifying osteoarthritis drugs. *Clin. Rheumatol.* **21**, 231–243.

Verdonk, P., Wang, J., Elewaut, D., Broddelez, C., Veys, E. M., and Verbruggen, G. (2006). Cyclodextrin polysulphates enhance human chondrocyte extracellular matrix repair. *Osteoarthritis Cartilage* (In press).

Vignon, E., Conrozier, T., Piperno, M., Richard, S., Carrillon, Y., and Fantino, O. (1999). Radiographic assessment of hip and knee osteoarthritis. Recommendations: Recommended guidelines. *Osteoarthritis Cartilage* **7**, 434–436.

Volpi, N. (2002). Oral bioavailability of chondroitin sulfate (Condrosulf) and its constituents in healthy male volunteers. *Osteoarthritis Cartilage* **10**, 768–777.

Volpi, N. (2003). Oral absorption and bioavailability of ichthyic origin chondroitin sulfate in healthy male volunteers. *Osteoarthritis Cartilage* **11**, 433–441.

Wang, L., Wang, J., Almqvist, K. F., Veys, E. M., and Verbruggen, G. (2002). Influence of polysulphated polysaccharides and hydrocortisone on the extracellular matrix metabolism of human articular chondrocytes *in vitro*. *Clin. Exp. Rheumatol.* **20**, 669–676.

PART IV

Clinical Efficacy and Trials

Gust Verbruggen

Department of Rheumatology
Ghent University Hospital
Gent, Belgium

Chondroitin Sulfate in the Management of Erosive Osteoarthritis of the Interphalangeal Finger Joints

I. Chapter Overview

Interphalangeal (IP) finger joint osteoarthritis (OA) becomes symptom-atic during inflammatory episodes associated with the onset of "erosive" or "inflammatory" OA. The pathogenic mechanisms, which initiate the de-structive phases in the IP finger joints of these patients, are not known although catabolic cytokine pathways (e.g., TNF, IL-1, RANKL) most plau-sibly are involved. Polysulfated polysaccharides have been shown to inter-fere with these cytokines and their down-stream events. This observation may reveal how chondroitin sulfates (CSs) hold up the onset of the destruc-tive phases of erosive OA of the finger joints, and this probably explains the symptom-modifying properties of these drugs. When interfering with the onset of "inflammatory" or "erosive" OA, chondroitin sulfates obviously prevent the formation of nodosities in the finger joints of the patients. These properties allow classifying these agents among the "disease modifying

Advances in Pharmacology, Volume 53
1054-3589/06 $35.00
DOI: 10.1016/S1054-3589(05)53025-4

osteoarthritis drugs" (DMOAD) with "symptom-modifying osteoarthritis drug" (SMOAD) effects.

II. Introduction: The Pathology of Erosive Osteoarthritis _____

A. Osteoarthritis of the Finger Joints: The Clinics

Osteoarthritis becomes more generalized and progressive in women from their early 50s (Kellgren *et al.*, 1963; Moskowitz, 1972). Distal and proximal interphalangeal joints (DIP and PIP joints), and the first carpometacarpal (MCP) joints become more frequently involved (Kellgren *et al.*, 1963; Moskowitz, 1972). A 5-year observation period of patients with OA of the finger joints revealed that this group consisted almost exclusively of women who became symptomatic early in the fifth decade of life, and rapidly developed symmetrical involvement of the finger joints. Obviously, a considerable number of DIP and PIP joints became involved soon after the patients experienced their first inflammatory episodes or painful "nodules," and the patients continued to suffer symptoms for several years (Verbruggen and Veys, 1996). Incidence rates were consistent with previous reports (Ehrlich, 1972, 1975; Stecher, 1955). The roentgenograms of the affected joints showed a rather aggressive evolution in half of the patients, and the appearance was that of an inflammatory disease. These patients experienced more inflammatory symptoms and occasionally needed NSAID or analgesic treatment. The MCP joints were less frequently affected, and the frequency of involvement of the different MCP joints pointed to mechanical factors as the main initiators of OA. These observations confirm that in women in the fifth decade of life, factors other than mechanical ones play a role in the pathogenesis of OA of IP finger joints. Hormonal changes are known to affect the clinical outcome of OA in experimental animals (Rosner *et al.*, 1982; Silberberg and Silberberg, 1963; Silberberg *et al.*, 1958). The mechanisms through which changes in sex steroid levels increase the incidence or severity of OA are not understood. Rather than through direct effects on the cartilage cell, female hormones may influence the pathology of OA by acting on inflammatory cells, thereby increasing the risk of inflammatory processes in synovial joints. Osteoarthritic PIP and DIP joints can become severely inflamed in the perimenopausal period (Cecil and Archer, 1926; Crain, 1961; Ehrlich, 1972, 1975; Peter *et al.*, 1966; Stecher, 1955; Stecher and Hauser, 1948) and in women, rheumatoid arthritis (RA) also shows a peak incidence around the menopause (Goemaere *et al.*, 1990).

B. The Pathology of Erosive Osteoarthritis: The Roentgen Picture

Conventional roentgenograms remain the best available method to follow OA patients in daily practice. Single bilateral posteroanterior hand radiographs are considered sensitive enough to assess finger joint OA (Altman *et al.*, 1990; Kallman *et al.*, 1989). The anatomical evolution of OA of the DIP and PIP joints in women of menopausal age has been documented and was shown to progress through predictable phases. During a 5 years' observation period, a substantial number of patients had been found to show erosive changes in the DIP and PIP joints. These changes were characterized by complete loss of the joint space preceding or coinciding with the appearance of subchondral cysts eroding the entire subchondral plate. These erosive episodes subsided spontaneously and were followed by processes of repair, as appeared from the follow-up. The MCP joints did not show this erosive evolution. This observation has allowed scoring systems to be designed to quantify the anatomical progression of finger joint OA (Verbruggen and Veys, 1996).

The anatomical phases in the evolution of OA of the finger joints are the following (Fig. 1):

1. Normal ("N") joints: no signs of OA.

2. Stationary ("S") phase: classical appearance of OA. Small ossification centers and osteophytes are present at the joint margins. Narrowing of the joint space can occur (Fig. 1A).

3. Loss of joint space ("J" phase): after remaining for a variable time in the stationary phase, some joints (almost exclusively PIP or DIP) become destroyed. The joint space completely disappears within a relatively short period of time (Fig. 1B).

4. Erosive ("E") phase: concurrently with or shortly after the disappearance of the articular cartilage (J phase), the subchondral plate becomes eroded. The appearance is that of a pseudo-enlargement of an irregular joint space (Fig. 1B–D). Roentgenograms obtained at yearly intervals showed that changes in phases from "S" over "J" to "E" could occur within 1 year. This destructive episode ("J" and "E" phases) is always followed by repair or remodeling.

5. Remodeling ("R") phase: new irregular sclerotic subchondral plates are formed, and in between these a new joint space becomes visible. Huge osteophytes are formed during this phase (Fig. 1C and D).

Contrary to what is seen in most chronically progressive rheumatic disorders, the inflammatory episodes spontaneously subsided, and most of the joints in the "J" or "E" phases remodeled during the observation period (R phase). "R" joints no longer showed any evolution. On the roentgen picture, the erosive lesions are identical to those described earlier in so-called "erosive osteoarthritis" of the finger joints (Cecil and Archer, 1926; Crain, 1961; Stecher and Hauser, 1948). The R joint is the final stage of the disease and clinically appears as a Heberden (DIP) or Bouchard (PIP) node.

Scores were attributed to the distinct consecutive anatomical phases recognized in the course of the disease, and this scoring system allowed the

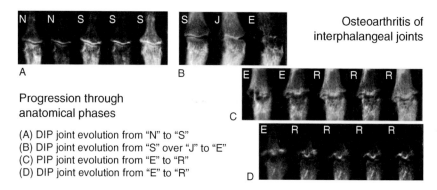

Osteoarthritis of
interphalangeal joints

Progression through
anatomical phases

(A) DIP joint evolution from "N" to "S"
(B) DIP joint evolution from "S" over "J" to "E"
(C) PIP joint evolution from "E" to "R"
(D) DIP joint evolution from "E" to "R"

FIGURE I   Anatomical phases in the progression of OA of the finger joints. "N": nonaffected joints; "S": stationary OA phase: classical appearance of nonerosive OA; "J": loss of joint space phase; "E": erosive phase; "R": remodeling phase. The progression through these phases in four different IP joints is shown. Roentgenograms were taken with 1-year intervals.

anatomical changes in OA joints to be scored. The anatomical phase progression (APP) score was obtained by comparing the anatomical scores at entry with those at the end of a study period. The APP score enabled clinicians to define the rate of OA progression in joints.

C. Inflammatory Cytokines in the Pathology of Erosive OA

The roentgen picture of an IP joint in the erosive phase of OA with the prominent erosion of the subchondral plate is suggestive for an uncontrolled aggressive osteoclastic activity, which is known to occur as a consequence of a unidirectional TNF/IL-1/RANKLigand cascade.

A similar unidirectional TNF/IL-1 cascade is operational in RA and in the spondylarthropathy (SPA)-associated forms of destructive arthritis. TNF-α, derived from an inflamed synovial membrane, has been shown to trigger an IL-1-induced destruction of the extracellular environment of articular cartilage (Brennan *et al.*, 1989). Neutralizing TNF-α, in these disorders has led to a complete halting of the destructive processes and eventually resulted in obvious repair in the affected joints (Lipsky *et al.*, 2000). Interference with TNF-α or IL-1 pathways could thus be of use when chondroprotective therapy in patients with erosive OA of the IP joints is considered.

D. Connective Tissue Structure-Modifying Agents and DMOADs

The first intra-articular administration of chondroitin polysulfate (CPS) in humans was based on the presumption that this heparinoid type of drug would replace hyaluronan as a lubricant and reduces fibrinogen levels in inflamed joints and that this would bring on a therapeutical advantage (Eylau, 1959, 1969). Unexpectedly, some patients reported symptomatic relief after having undergone this procedure, and even some changes in synovial fluid chemistry were reported (Momburg et al., 1976). Therefore, the first attempts at improving structure and function of the connective tissues of synovial joints, thereby alleviating the symptoms of degenerative joint disorders, were based on vague assumptions that an abundant administration of precursors of extracellular matrix (ECM) components would help articular cartilage cells to replace the lost environment.

Together with a profound search on mechanisms whereby joint tissues are destroyed in the course of inflammatory or degenerative joint diseases, searchers more methodically sought for biological agents capable of restoring damaged connective tissues. As articular cartilage is one of the principal target tissues affected in the course of rheumatic joint disorders, many investigations focused on the metabolic characteristics of the single cell homing in this tissue—the chondrocyte. Substances that protected articular cartilage during the course of destructive joint disorders were termed chondroprotective agents. When this occurred *in vivo* in joints with OA these agents were termed DMOAD (Altman et al., 2000).

As the auto/paracrine growth factor and cytokine cascades behind development, homeostasis, and destruction of the ECM of articular cartilage were not known previously, the first investigations on biological agents capable of modifying the structure of connective tissues in a positive way mainly concentrated on the capability of these agents of improving synthesis, or impairing the degradation of ECM compounds, that is, aggrecan and collagen. According to this definition, a number of substances could be classified as connective tissue structure-modifying agents (CTSMA). Among these, sulfated glycosaminoglycans, such as chondroitin sulfate and chondroitin polysulfate, have been repeatedly cited.

III. Chondroitin Sulfates and the Management of Erosive Osteoarthritis of the Finger Joints

A. Chondroprotective or DMOAD Effects of Chondroitin Sulfates

Data on chondroprotection in hand OA are scarce. The DMOAD effects of chondroitin sulfates on erosive OA of the IP finger joints have been appraised in two randomized, double blind, placebo-controlled studies (Verbruggen et al., 1998, 2002). Especially systems, allowing the anatomical changes in OA joints to be scored, enabled clinicians to define the rate of OA progression in joints. These scoring systems were based on the consecutive and predictable anatomical phases recognized in the course of the disease (Verbruggen and Veys, 1996).

Two chondroitin sulfates with possible DMOAD effects—naturally occurring chondroitin sulfate of bovine origin (CS) and a chemically poly-sulfated chondroitin sulfate (CPS) were used in two series of patients with OA of the finger joints (Verbruggen et al., 1998, 2002). The patients were included in two separate randomized, double-blind, placebo-controlled trials. Posteroanterior roentgenograms of the metacarpophalangeal and IP finger joints were obtained at the start of this prospective study and at yearly intervals. Almost 80% of the distal IP and 50% of the proximal IP were affected at study entry. In approximately 40% of the patients, the classic picture of OA of the IP joints was complicated by manifest erosive OA changes. One hundred and sixty-five patients were followed during 3 years.

The following variables were used to compare the study populations at entry (the CPS- and CS-treated patients and both placebo groups):

1. The numbers of IP joints affected in each patient
2. The numbers of patients presenting at least one IP joint in a destructive (J, E) or remodeling (R) phase
3. The anatomical phase scores of the 16 IP joints.

As the evaluation of these three variables on the roentgenograms at entry allowed to conclude that both placebo groups were not different, the 85 patients of the two studies that had received placebo were combined in one group—the "placebo" group. Forty-six of the patients received CPS and 34 received CS.

At entry, the placebo and the CS group were not different when the previously mentioned variables were considered. The CPS-treated patients, however, were less affected at start than the patients of the placebo group (Verbruggen et al., 2002).

When the therapeutic results obtained were analyzed, the APP scores of the IP joints over 3 years appeared to be significantly lower in the CPS-treated patients, whereas CS treatment showed a tendency to retard disease progression (Fig. 2). The individual patient's risk of developing erosive OA was assessed. This risk of developing the erosive type of OA was determined by assessing the number of patients presenting exclusively nonerosive OA joints (N or S phases) at study entry, of which at least one IP joint progressed to a destructive phase ("J" to "E") over a 3-year period. Seven of these "nonerosive" patients out of 46 from the placebo group, progressed through destructive phases ("J" to "E") and became "erosive" in one or more IP joints. Only 1 patient out of 35, and 2 patients from the 34 with exclusively "stationary" OA joints in CPS and CS groups, respectively, developed the destructive phases. Although an interesting observation, these differences were not significant (Verbruggen et al., 2002) (Table I).

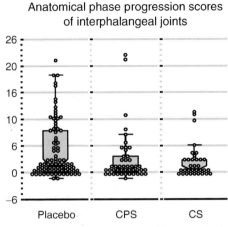

Anatomical phase progression scores
of interphalangeal joints

diff. vs. placebo: $p = 0.033$, $p < 0.075$

FIGURE 2   Anatomical phase progression scores over 3 years of follow-up of the interphalangeal (DIP and PIP) joints of each patient. Notched Box-and-Whisker plots represent median values, upper and lower quartiles. Differences (p-values) in progression scores between the placebo group (Tot-Pl) and the CPS- and CS-treated groups are given.

TABLE I   Number of "Nonerosive" OA Patients Developing "Erosive" Interphalangeal Joint OA

	Number	Nonerosive OA at start	Erosive OA during follow-up	Difference	
Tot-Pl	85	46	7		
CPS	46	35	1	$\chi^2 = 2.164$	$p > 0.050$
CS	34	24	2	$\chi^2 = 0.194$	$p > 0.050$

χ^2 test; p-values are given.

Additionally, the individual patient's risk to worsen their "erosive OA" was evaluated by looking at the number of subjects whose joints showed further progression through the destructive phases during follow-up (Fig. 3).

Progression to the erosive (E) phase in patients whose joints previously showed stationary OA or loss of the joint space (S or J phases) was significantly haltened. 29.4% of the placebo-treated subjects developed frank "erosive" OA in previously stationary OA joints (S/J→E). In CS- and CPS-treated groups, development of "erosive" OA occurred in 8.8% out of 34, and in 8.7% out of 46 patients, respectively. An "S" to "E" or a "J" to "E" phase type of evolution occurred in 20.0% and 22.4% of the 85 placebo-treated patients, respectively. One (2.9%) and two (5.9%) of the CS-treated

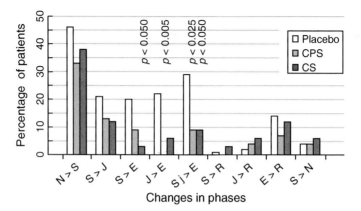

FIGURE 3 Proportions of patients in the placebo group and in the CPS- and CS-treated groups presenting a change in anatomical phase in an interphalangeal joint during the 3 years of follow-up. Differences (*p*-values) in the proportions of patients in the respective groups (placebo vs. CPS or CS) presenting a particular change are given. N: nonaffected; S: stationary nonerosive OA; J: OA joint with disappeared joint space; E: erosive OA joint; R: remodeled OA joint.

patients progressed through these phases. Four out of 46 (8.7%), and none of the 46 (0.0%) CPS-treated patients showed this "S" to "E" or a "J" to "E" phase type of evolution. Once in one of the destructive phases, proportions of patients whose IP joints showed remodeling were not affected by either treatment (Verbruggen *et al.*, 1998, 2002). These differences were statistically significant. When compared with the placebo controls, none of the chondroitin sulfates prevented OA from occurring in previously normal finger joints.

B. "SMOAD" or "SYSADOA" Effects of Chondroitin Sulfates

The results of two randomized, double-blind, placebo-controlled studies on clinical responses of patients with erosive hand OA on CS therapy have been reported (Goemaere *et al.*, 1997; Malaise *et al.*, 1996). The outcomes of these studies remarkably agreed. Malaise *et al.* (1996) followed a cohort of 37 patients of which 20 were kept on CS and 17 were on placebo for 3 years. Although the patients experienced marked placebo effects, significant intragroup differences were noticed for global spontaneous pain in the CS group from the 12th month on. Intergroup differences became significant in favor of CS after 6 months of treatment. Grip strength measurements improved significantly after 6 months in the CS-treated patients. Intergroup differences became significant for this item in favor of CS after 12 months. Other parameters (e.g., DIP) circumference did not change. Goemaere *et al.*

TABLE II Global Efficacy and Toxicity of Chondroitin Sulfate in the Treatment of Osteoarthritis of the Interpahalangeal Finger Joints

	Global efficacy		Global toxicity	
	Patient	Doctor	Patient	Doctor
0–4 months	NA	NA	NA	NA
4–8 months	$p = 0.223$	$p = 0.094$	$p = 0.524$	$p = 0.381$
8–12 months	$p = 0.064$	$p = 0.052$	$p = 0.317$	$p = 0.273$

Intragroup changes in global efficacy and global toxicity reported by patients and doctors; endpoint analysis; χ^2 test; p-values are given; NA: not applicable.

(1997) reported the outcomes in a 101 patients cohort that was followed during 1 year). Forty-nine of them received 1200 mg of CS daily and 52 were kept on placebo. A borderline significant change of the global impression of efficacy by patient and physician, which were chosen as the primary outcome measures, was recorded after an 8–12 months treatment period (Table II). Other variables (e.g., VA pain scale, use of analgesics/NSAIDs, pain on pressure, grip strength, and an in-house functional index) did not change significantly during follow-up. Both studies thus disclosed a weak and late onset effect, and this type of effect seemed to have been confirmed in two open label trials in which a smaller number of patients were included (Leeb *et al.*, 1996; Rovetta *et al.*, 2004).

IV. Discussion

A 3-year follow-up of the 165 patients with finger joint OA enabled to investigate the DMOAD effects of two chondroitin sulfates. Chondroitin sulfate and chondroitin polysulfate have an identical polysaccharide backbone. Their degree of sulfating is different. Both these sulfated polysaccharides have profound and similar effects on the synthesis and turnover of the structural ECM compounds of human connective tissues (e.g., articular cartilage and synovial membrane) (Francis *et al.*, 1993; Schwartz and Dorfman, 1975; Uebelhart *et al.*, 1998b; Verbruggen and Veys, 1977, 1979, 1982; Wiebkin and Muir, 1973) and may thus affect connective tissue repair. These polysaccharide (poly)sulfates have a "tropism" for connective tissues, such as cartilage (Conte *et al.*, 1995; Dupuy *et al.*, 1976; Gallacchi and Muller, 1982; Panse *et al.*, 1976; Ronca and Conte, 1993), and at least chondroitin polysulfate was shown to have "structure modifying" properties *in vivo* (Howell *et al.*, 1986; Verbruggen and Veys, 1979). This study did not allow concluding that chondroitin sulfate or chondroitin polysulfate treatment prevented patients with OA of the finger joints to develop OA in previously unaffected joints. New OA joints were seen in the same proportions of the patients in control and treated groups. The high proportions of joints involved at study entry, and the fact that changes in the anatomy of finger joints that become osteoarthritic during follow-up are often subtle, may render this variable less efficient to assess the effects of drugs on the progression of hand OA. However, the morbidity of the disease was significantly reduced in both treated populations. Evolution through the destructive anatomical phases, characteristic of "erosive" or "inflammatory" OA of the finger joints, was significantly reduced in the CPS treatment group. CS-treated subjects showed a tendency to progress at a slower rate. Similar results were suggested in an open label study on patients with erosive OA of the finger joints where 12 patients were treated with 800 mg/day of orally administered chondroitin sulfate plus naproxen, and 12 others received naproxen only. Radiological hand examinations were performed at baseline and again after 12 and 24 months. The anatomical progression of the disease after 24 months seemed somewhat reduced in patients treated with chondroitin sulfate (Rovetta et al., 2002). The reduction of the proportion of subjects developing frank "erosive" OA in previously stationary OA joints in CS- and CPS-treated groups is of clinical interest.

It is admitted that fewer IP joints of the CPS-treated patients, when enrolled in the study, were affected. In addition, these IP joints scored lower in the anatomical phase score system. Lower numbers of patients of this group had their IP joints in destructive phases. It is speculative to argue that these patients belonged to a less aggressive population not at risk to develop "erosive" OA. By no means, however, proportionally less erosive finger joints at the time of inclusion indicate a lower risk for the CPS-treated patients to develop erosive OA in previously nonerosive OA joints. Otherwise, development of "erosive" OA during follow-up might have been expected to occur more frequently in a population with higher proportions of "nonerosive" OA patients. Possibly, retardation of OA progression is related to the effects of these drugs on catabolic activity and/or repair function of connective tissue cells (e.g., articular cartilage chondrocytes and synovial lining cells) (Francis et al., 1993; Mcfarlane et al., 1991; Schwartz and Dorfman, 1975; Verbruggen and Veys, 1977, 1979, 1982; Wiebkin and Muir, 1973). These anticatabolic and anti-inflammatory effects may also have been responsible for the modest clinical improvement these patients experienced during follow-up.

The roentgen picture of an IP joint in the erosive phase of OA with the prominent erosion of the subchondral plate is suggestive for an uncontrolled aggressive osteoclastic activity, which is known to occur as a consequence of a unidirectional TNF/IL-1/RANKLigand cascade (Wei et al., 2005; Zhang et al., 2001). A similar unidirectional TNF/IL-1 cascade is operational in RA and in the SPA-associated forms of destructive arthritis. TNF-α, derived from an inflamed synovial membrane, has been shown to trigger an IL-1-induced destruction of the extracellular environment of articular cartilage (Brennan *et al.*, 1989). Neutralizing TNF-α, in these disorders has led to a complete halting of the destructive processes and eventually resulted in obvious repair in the affected joints (Lipsky *et al.*, 2000). Interference with TNF-α or IL-1 pathways could thus be of use when chondroprotective therapy in patients with erosive OA of the IP joints is considered.

The possibility of interfering with connective tissue cell repair processes *in vitro* by sulfated polysaccharides was first described in the mid-1970s (Schwartz and Dorfman, 1975; Verbruggen and Veys, 1977). Later, poly-sulfated chondroitin sulfate was shown to improve the synthesis of hyaluronan in synovial joints *in vivo* in human subjects (Verbruggen and Veys, 1979). The same drug, as well as its naturally occurring analog chondroitin sulfate, improved chondrocyte repair function *in vivo* in different experimental models of OA (Brennan *et al.*, 1987; Carreno *et al.*, 1986; Kalbhen, 1983; Uebelhart *et al.*, 1998b). Randomized, double-blind, placebo-controlled therapeutic trials allowed to conclude that these CTSMA had DMOAD properties as they were shown to retard the progression of erosive OA in IP finger joints (Verbruggen *et al.*, 1998, 2002) and of OA of the knee in human beings (Uebelhart *et al.*, 1998a, 2004).

In vitro and *in vivo* experiments in various research centers concerning the effects on the metabolism of intercellular matrix molecules (proteoglycans, aggrecans, hyaluran) have shown that most (poly)sulfated polysaccharides influence connective tissue cells (cartilage cells, synovial cells, fibroblasts) in a similar way (Francis *et al.*, 1993; Verbruggen and Veys, 1977, 1992, 1999). When our insights in the auto/paracrine growth factor and cytokine pathways that control the homeostasis of healthy connective tissues had improved, it became possible to study the mechanism of action of these CTSMA. Investigations with sulfated polysaccharides showed that these agents operate in biological systems through a down-modulation of important catabolic auto/paracrine cytokine pathways, such as IL-1, thereby improving the accumulation of ECM compounds in the cell-associated matrix of these cells. Experiments with bovine cartilage cells obtained from macroscopically intact metacarpophalangeal joints showed physiological concentrations of chondroitin polysulfate to significantly reduce downstream IL-1 effects such as collagenase, proteoglycanase, and MMP-1 and MMP-3 activities (Sadowski and Steinmeyer, 2002). Likewise, xylosan polysulfate and chondroitin polysulfate restored the accumulation of aggrecan, hyaluronan and type II collagen in the cell-associated matrix in IL-1β-treated human chondrocytes cultured in agarose. This effect probably resulted in part from the downregulation of MMPs (Wang *et al.*, 2002). Also, in cultured equine chondrocytes chondroitin polysulfate significantly reduced IL-1β-enhanced expression of iNOS that was paralleled by an increased release of NO. Chondroitin polysulfate downsized nitrite concentrations in the supernatants of these IL-1β-stimulated cultures (Tung *et al.*,

2002). Finally, a novel polysulfated polysaccharide cyclodextrin polysulfate showed cartilage structure-modifying effects *in vitro* as it improved the synthesis of aggrecan and the accumulation of cell-associated matrix macromolecules by human articular cartilage cells in alginate. Here, it was shown for the first time that this effect resulted in part from the direct repression of IL-1 as cyclodextrin polysulfate-treated cells expressed significantly lower amounts of intracellular IL-1α and -β levels (Verdonk *et al.*, 2005).

In summary, finger joint OA becomes symptomatic during inflammatory episodes associated with the onset of "erosive" or "inflammatory" OA. The pathogenic mechanisms, which initiate the destructive phases in the IP finger joints of these patients, are not known although catabolic cytokine pathways (e.g., TNF, IL-1, RANKL) most plausibly are involved. Polysulfated polysaccharides have been shown to interfere with these cytokines and their down-stream events. This observation may reveal how chondroitin sulfates hold up the onset of the destructive phases of erosive OA of the finger joints, and this probably explains the symptom-modifying properties of these drugs. When interfering with the onset of "inflammatory" or "erosive" OA, chondroitin sulfates obviously prevent the formation of nodosities in the finger joints of the patients. These properties allow classifying these agents among the DMOAD (Howell *et al.*, 1995; Lequesne *et al.*, 1994) with SMOAD effects.

References

Altman, R., Alarcon, G., Appelrouth, D., Bloch, D., Borenstein, D., Brandt, K., Brown, C., Cooke, T. D., Daniel, W., Gray, R., Greenwald, M., Hochberg, M., *et al.* (1990). The American college of rheumatology criteria for the classification and reporting of osteoarthritis of the hand. *Arthritis Rheum.* 33, 1601–1610.

Altman, R. D., Hochberg, M. C., Moskowitz, R. W., and Schnitzer, T. J. (2000). Recommendations for the medical management of osteoarthritis of the hip and knee. 2000 update. ACR subcommittee on osteoarthritis guidelines. *Arthritis Rheum.* 43, 1905–1915.

Brennan, F. M., Chantry, D., Jackson, A., Maini, R., and Feldmann, M. (1989). Inhibitory effect of TNF alpha antibodies on synovial cell interleukin-1 production in rheumatoid arthritis. *Lancet* 2, 244–247.

Brennan, J. J., Aherne, F. X., and Nakano, T. (1987). Effects of glycosaminoglycan polysulfate treatment on soundness, hyaluronic acid content of synovial fluid and proteoglycan aggregate in articular cartilage of lame boars. *Can. J. Vet. Res.* 51, 394–398.

Carreno, M. R., Muniz, O. E., and Howell, D. S. (1986). The effect of glycosaminoglycan polysulfuric acid ester on articular cartilage in experimental osteoarthritis: Effects on morphological variables of disease severity. *J. Rheumatol.* 13, 490–497.

Cecil, R. L., and Archer, B. H. (1926). Classification and treatment of chronic arthritis. *JAMA* 87, 741–746.

Conte, A., Volpi, N., Palmieri, L., Bahous, I., and Ronca, G. (1995). Biochemical and pharmacological aspects of oral treatment with chondroitin sulfate. *Drug Res.* 45, 918–925.

Crain, D. C. (1961). Interphalangeal osteoarthritis. Characterized by painful, inflammatory episodes resulting in deformity of the proximal and distal articulations. *JAMA* 175, 1049–1053.

Dupuy, J. C., Harmand, M. F., and Blanquet, P. (1976). ACS marqué au 99mTc et scintigraphie du cartilage. *Isotopes radioactifs en clinique et recherche* 12, 183.

Ehrlich, G. E. (1972). Inflammatory osteoarthritis: I. The clinical syndrome. *J. Chron. Dis.* 25, 317–328.

Ehrlich, G. E. (1975). Osteoarthritis beginning with inflammation. Definitions and correlations. *J. Am. Med. Assoc.* 232, 157–159.

Eylau, O. (1959). Intra-articular heparin therapy of genuine arthrosis deformans of the knee joint. *Med. Klin.* 54, 145.

Eylau, O. (1969). On the pathogenesis and causal treatment of arthrosis of the knee joint. *Med. Klin.* 55, 2367–2370.

Francis, D. J., Hutadilok, N., Kongtawelert, P., and Ghosh, P. (1993). Pentosanpolysulphate and glycosaminoglycan polysulphate stimulate the synthesis of hyaluronan *in vivo*. *Rheumatol. Int.* 13, 61–64.

Gallacchi, G., and Muller, W. (1982). Incorporation of intramuscularly injected glycosaminoglycan polysulfate in human joint cartilage. *In* "International Drug Symposium Arteparon[R]" (N. Dettmer and H. Greiling, Eds.), pp. 99–102. EULAR Publishers, Basel.

Goemaere, S., Ackerman, C., Goethals, K., De Keyser, F., Van der Straeten, C., Verbruggen, G., Mielants, H., and Veys, E. M. (1990). Onset of symptoms of rheumatoid arthritis in relation to age, sex and menopausal transition. *J. Rheumatol.* 17, 1620–1622.

Goemaere, S., Verbruggen, G., and Veys, E. M. (1997). Per oral administration of chondroitinsulfate in patients with osteoarthritis of the finger joints. Results of a double-blind placebo-controlled trial. *Clin. Rheumatol.* 16, 529.

Howell, D. S., Muniz, O. E., and Carreno, M. R. (1986). Effect of glucosaminoglycan polysulfate ester on proteoglycan-degrading enzyme activity in an animal model of osteoarthritis. *In* "Advances of Inflammation Research" (I. Otterness, A. Lewis, and R. Capetola, Eds.), pp. 197–206. Raven Press, New York.

Howell, D. S., Altman, R. D., Pelletier, J.-P., Martel-Pelletier, J., and Dean, D. D. (1995). Disease modifying antirheumatic drugs: Current status of their application in experimental animal models of osteoarthritis. *In* "Osteoarthritic Disorders" (E. Kuettner and V. Goldberg, Eds.), pp. 365–377. American Academy of Orthopedic Surgeons, Rosemont, IL.

Kalbhen, D. A. (1983). Experimental confirmation of the antiarthritic activity of glycosaminoglycan polysulfate. *Z. Rheumatol.* 42, 178–184.

Kallman, D. A., Wigley, F. M., Scott, W. W., Hochberg, M. C., and Tobin, J. D. (1989). New radiographic grading scales for osteoarthritis of the hand. *Arthritis Rheum.* 32, 1584–1591.

Kellgren, J. H., Lawrence, J. S., and Bier, F. (1963). Genetic factors in generalized osteoarthrosis. *Ann. Rheum. Dis.* 22, 237–245.

Leeb, B. F., Petera, P., and Neumann, K. (1996). Results of a multicenter study of chondroitin sulfate (Condrosulf) use in arthroses of the finger, knee and hip joints. *Wien Med. Wochenschr.* 146, 609–614.

Lequesne, M., Brandt, K., Bellamy, N., Moskowitz, R., Menkes, C. J., Pelletier, J. P., and Altman, R. (1994). Guidelines for testing slow acting drugs in osteoarthritis. *J. Rheumatol.* 21(Suppl 41), 65–71.

Lipsky, P. E., van der Heijde, D. M., St Clair, E. W., Furst, D. E., Breedveld, F. C., Kalden, J. R., Smolen, J. S., Weisman, M., Emery, P., Feldmann, M., Harriman, G. R., and Maini, R. N. (2000). Infliximab and methotrexate in the treatment of rheumatoid arthritis. Anti-tumor necrosis factor trial in rheumatoid arthritis with concomitant therapy study group. *N. Engl. J. Med.* 343, 1594–1602.

Malaise, M. G., Wang, F., and Bassleer, C. (1996). A three-year double-blind study with oral chondroitin sulfate 4&6 in patients suffering from Heberden's and Bouchard's osteoarthritis. *Clin. Rheumatol.* **15**, 551.

Mcfarlane, D. G., Buckland-Wright, J. C., Emery, P., Fogelman, I., Clark, B., and Lynch, J. (1991). Comparison of clinical, radionuclide, and radiographic features of osteoarthritis of the hands. *Ann. Rheum. Dis.* **50**, 623–626.

Momburg, M., Stuhlsatz, H. W., Vogeli, H., Vojtisek, O., Eylau, O., and Greiling, H. (1976). Clinical chemical changes in the synovial fluid following intra-articular injection of a glycosaminoglycan polysulfate. *Z. Rheumatol.* **35**(Suppl 4), 389–390.

Moskowitz, R. W. (1972). Clinical and laboratory findings in osteoarthritis. *In* "Arthritis and Allied Conditions" (J. L. Hollander and D. J., McCarty Jr., Eds.), Lea & Febiger, Philadelphia.

Panse, P., Zeiller, P., and Sensch, K. H. (1976). Distribution and excretion of a glyco-saminopolysulfate in the rabbit after parenteral application. *Drug Res.* **26**, 2024–2029.

Peter, J. B., Pearson, C. M., and Marmor, L. (1966). Erosive arthritis of the hands. *Arthritis Rheum.* **9**, 365–388.

Ronca, G., and Conte, A. (1993). Metabolic fate of partially depolymerized shark chondroitin sulfate in man. *Int. J. Clin. Pharm. Res.* **13**(Suppl), 27–34.

Rosner, I. A., Malemud, C. J., Goldberg, V. M., Papay, R. S., Getzy, L., and Moskowitz, R. W. (1982). Pathologic and metabolic responses of experimental osteoarthritis to estradiol and estradiol antagonist. *Clin. Orthop.* **167**, 280–286.

Rovetta, G., Monteforte, P., Molfetta, G., and Balestra, V. (2002). Chondroitin sulfate in erosive osteoarthritis of the hands. *Int. J. Tissue React.* **24**, 29–32.

Rovetta, G., Monteforte, P., Molfetta, G., and Balestra, V. (2004). A two-year study of chondroitin sulfate in erosive osteoarthritis of the hands: Behavior of erosions, osteophytes, pain and hand dysfunction. *Drugs Exp. Clin. Res.* **30**, 11–16.

Sadowski, T., and Steinmeyer, J. (2002). Effects of polysulfated glycosaminoglycan and triamcinolone acetonid on the production of proteinases and their inhibitors by IL-1alpha treated articular chondrocytes. *Biochem. Pharmacol.* **64**, 217–227.

Schwartz, N. B., and Dorfman, A. (1975). Stimulation of chondroitin sulfate proteoglycan production by chondrocytes in monolayer. *Connect. Tissue Res.* **3**, 115–122.

Silberberg, R., Thomasson, R., and Silberberg, M. (1958). Degenerative joint disease in castrate mice. 2. Effects of orchiectomy at various ages. *AMA Arch. Pathol.* **65**, 442–444.

Silberberg, M., and Silberberg, R. (1963). Modifying actions of estrogen on the evolution of osteoarthrosis in mice of different ages. *Endocrinology* **72**, 449–451.

Stecher, R. M., and Hauser, H. (1948). Heberden's nodes. VII. The roentgenological and clinical appearance of degenerartive joint disease of the fingers. *Am. J. Roentgenol.* **59**, 326–337.

Stecher, R. M. (1955). Heberden's nodes: A clinical description of osteoarthritis of the finger joints. *Ann. Rheum. Dis.* **14**, 1–10.

Tung, J. T., Venta, P. J., and Caron, J. P. (2002). Inducible nitric oxide expression in equine articular chondrocytes: Effects of antiinflammatory compounds. *Osteoarthritis Cartilage* **10**, 5–12.

Uebelhart, D., Thonar, E. J., Zhang, J., and Williams, J. M. (1998a). Protective effect of exogenous chondroitin 4,6-sulfate in the acute degradation of articular cartilage in the rabbit. *Osteoarthritis Cartilage* **6**(Suppl), 6–13.

Uebelhart, D., Thonar, E. J., Delmas, P. D., Chantraine, A., and Vignon, E. (1998b). Effects of oral chondroitin sulfate on the progression of knee osteoarthritis: A pilot study. *Osteoarthritis Cartilage* **6**(Suppl A), 39–46.

Uebelhart, D., Malaise, M., Marcolongo, R., DeVathaire, F., Piperno, M., Mailleux, E., Fioravanti, A., Matoso, L., and Vignon, E. (2004). Intermittent treatment of knee osteoarthritis with oral chondroitin sulfate: A one-year, randomized, double-blind, multicenter study versus placebo. *Osteoarthritis Cartilage* 12, 269–276.

Verbruggen, G., and Veys, E. M. (1977). Influence of sulphated glycosaminoglycans upon proteoglycan metabolism of the synovial lining cells. *Acta Rheumatol.* 1, 75–92.

Verbruggen, G., and Veys, E. M. (1979). Influence of an oversulphated heparinoid upon hyaluronate metabolism of the human synovial cell *in vivo*. *J. Rheumatol.* 6, 554–561.

Verbruggen, G., and Veys, E. M. (1982). Proteoglycan metabolism of connective tissue cells. An *in vitro* technique and its relevance to *in vivo* conditions. *In* "Degenerative Joints" (G. Verbruggen and E. M. Veys, Eds.), pp. 113–129. Excerpta Medica, Amsterdam.

Verbruggen, G., and Veys, E. M. (1996). Numerical scoring systems for the anatomic evolution of osteoarthritis of the finger joints. *Arthritis Rheum.* 39, 308–320.

Verbruggen, G., Goemaere, S., and Veys, E. M. (1998). Chondroitin sulfate: S/DMOAD (structure/disease modifying anti-osteoarthritis drug) in the treatment of finger joint OA. *Osteoarthritis Cartilage* 6(Suppl A), 37–38.

Verbruggen, G., and Veys, E. M. (1992). Intra-articular injection of pentosanpolysulphate results in increased hyaluronan molecular weight in joint fluid. *Clin. Exp. Rheumatol.* 10, 249–254.

Verbruggen, G., Cornelissen, M., Elewaut, D., Broddelez, C., De Ridder, L., and Veys, E. M. (1999). Influence of polysulfated polysaccharides on aggrecans synthesized by differentiated human articular chondrocytes. *J. Rheumatol.* 26, 1663–1671.

Verbruggen, G., Goemaere, S., and Veys, E. M. (2002). Systems to assess the progression of finger joint osteoarthritis and the effects of disease modifying osteoarthritis drugs. *Clin. Rheumatol.* 21, 231–243.

Verdonk, P., Wang, J., Elewaut, D., Broddelez, C., Veys, E. M., and Verbruggen, G. (2005). Cyclodextrin polysulphates enhance human chondrocyte extracellular matrix repair. *Osteoarthritis Cartilage* 13, 887–895.

Wang, L., Wang, J., Almqvist, K. F., Veys, E. M., and Verbruggen, G. (2002). Influence of polysulphated polysaccharides and hydrocortisone on the extracellular matrix metabolism of human articular chondrocytes *in vitro*. *Clin. Exp. Rheumatol.* 20, 669–676.

Wei, S., Kitaura, H., Zhou, P., Ross, F. P., and Teitelbaum, S. L. (2005). IL-1 mediates TNF-induced osteoclastogenesis. *J. Clin. Invest.* 115, 282–290.

Wiebkin, O. W., and Muir, H. (1973). Factors affecting the biosynthesis of sulphated glycosaminoglycans by chondrocytes in short-time maintenance culture isolated from adult tissue. *In* "Biology of Fibroblast" (E. Kulonen and J. Pikkaraininen, Eds.), pp. 231–252. Academic Press, London.

Zhang, Y. H., Heulsmann, A., Tondravi, M. M., Mukherjee, A., and Abu-Amer, Y. (2001). Tumor necrosis factor-alpha (TNF) stimulates RANKL-induced osteoclastogenesis via coupling of TNF type 1 receptor and RANK signaling pathways. *J. Biol. Chem.* 276, 563–568.

Géraldine Bana*, Bénédicte Jamard[†],
Evelyne Verrouil[†], and Bernard Mazières[‡]

*Paul-Sabatier University, Faculty of Pharmacy
Toulouse, France

[†]Rangueil University Hospital
Toulouse, France

[‡]Paul-Sabatier University
Faculty of Medicine and Rangueil University Hospital
Toulouse, France

Chondroitin Sulfate in the Management of Hip and Knee Osteoarthritis: An Overview

I. Chapter Overview

The aim of this chapter is to evaluate the symptomatic/structural efficacy and the tolerance of the chondroitin sulfate (CS) in the treatment of knee and hip osteoarthritis (OA) through a meta-analysis of randomized clinical trials. A search for any randomized, double-blind, placebo (PBO)-controlled, prospective trial whose aim was to assess the symptomatic and/or structural activity of oral CS in the treatment of knee or hip OA was performed through data sources and then through a manual search of the reference section of all articles retrieved by the primary search. This search was limited to articles published *in extenso* in peer-reviewed journals between 1980 and 2005, in English or French languages, presenting sufficient data and lasting more than 4 weeks. We found a modest effect of the CS on the relief of pain and on the improvement of the joint function (pooled effect sizes 0.60 ± 0.34 and 0.57 ± 0.31, respectively). The risk of being a

Advances in Pharmacology, Volume 53
1054-3589/06 $35.00
DOI: 10.1016/S1054-3589(05)53026-6

responder was 1.83 ± 0.34, and the mean number of patients needed to treat was about 9.2 ± 5.4. We could also put in evidence a delay in CS's action and a carry-over effect of this drug after the end of the treatment. A small structural efficacy was demonstrated, but further studies are needed to confirm these results. The tolerance to the CS was excellent. Chondroitin sulfate could be a useful tool in the treatment of OA but still subsist the question of which OA-patients could take the best advantage of it. Moreover, further investigation on CS's structural efficacy and long-term tolerance are needed.

II. Introduction

Osteoarthritis is the most common form of arthritis, affecting the knee in 30% and the hip in 4–10% of people aged 65 and over (Nevitt *et al.*, 1995; Van Sasse *et al.*, 1989). Even if roughly 50% of them only have signs and symptoms, the number of adults clinically affected by this disease is considerable especially in the elderly and is increasing with the increasing average age in the populations.

Current treatments for OA include pharmacological modalities (pain relief with analgesics, nonsteroidal anti-inflammatory drugs, steroid injections) and nonpharmacological modalities (including exercises, patient education, diet when required, and total joint replacement). The recommendations from the European League Against Rheumatism (Jordan *et al.*, 2003) and the guidelines of the American College of Rheumatology (American College of Rheumatology Subcommittee on Osteoarthritis Guidelines, 2000) include these treatment options. The EULAR recommendations also included the so-called "symptomatic slow acting drugs for treating osteoarthritis" (SYSADOA) in the 10 final bullets for the management of the disease.

The need to define new classes of drugs for treating OA was an emerging concept in France, in the early 1990s, to try to correctly classify old drugs that were in the market but whose assessment was poor (Group for Management of Osteoarthritis, 1990). Each year, in Giens, near Toulon, on the Côte d'Azur, a meeting was held including representatives of the pharmaceutical industry, of the faculty, and of the registration authorities. In 1992, one of the topics addressed at this annual meeting was the classification of the so-called "antiarthritic drugs." The concept of SYSADOA was proposed (Avouac and Dropsy, 1993) and officially presented as an editorial in the *French Journal of Rheumatology* by Michel Lequesne (Lequesne, 1994). Then it was adopted at the international level during the 5th Joint World Health Organization and International League of Association for Rheumatology Task Force Meeting, held in Geneva from June 29–July 2, 1993 (Lequesne *et al.*, 1994). These SYSADOA are defined on several pragmatic observations: they have a 1-month delay of action after onset, a

1–2-month carry-over activity after discontinuation, they are well tolerated (particularly at the gastrointestinal level) with few and minor adverse events opposite to nonsteroidal anti-inflammatory drugs. This therapeutic class includes five compounds: chondroitin and glucosamine sulfates, diacerein, avocado–soybean extracts, and hyaluronic acid. The latter is locally delivered by intra-articular route. All these drugs have randomized controlled trials vs. PBO. Fifteen years after the emerging concept of SYSADOA and after three meta-analyses (Leeb *et al.*, 2000; MacAlindon *et al.*, 2000; Richy *et al.*, 2003), time is coming to attempt and overview on one of these drugs, the CS.

Chondroitin sulfates are glycosaminoglycans (GAGs) naturally present in the matrix of mammalians' cartilages. They are a major component of the aggrecan that is responsible for most of the properties of joint cartilage. Chondroitin sulfates are prescribed as SYSADOA but also are highly suspected to have disease-modifying capacities.

III. Methods

Our main objective was to have a general view of the different clinical trials dealing with CS in the treatment of OA of knee and hip. We focused more precisely on the efficacy and tolerance aspects.

A. Selection of Papers

We searched for any randomized, double-blind, PBO-controlled, prospective trial whose aim was to assess the symptomatic and/or structural activity of oral CS in the treatment of knee or hip OA. To do so, we went through several data sources (Medline/PubMed, Cochrane Controlled Trial Register), and then we conducted a manual search of the reference section of each of the articles retrieved by the primary search. *Osteoarthritis* and *chondroitin sulfate* were entered as medical subject headings and as textwords. We limited the search to articles published *in extenso* in peer-reviewed journals between 1980 and 2005, in English or French languages. To increase the homogeneity of the analysis, all studies lasting less than 4 weeks or not presenting sufficient data were excluded.

Any of the publications selected for the meta-analysis had to contain data on the efficacy variables proposed by EULAR, FDA, or EMEA guidelines (Committee for Proprietary Medicinal Products, 1998; Food and Drug Administration, 1999; Lequesne *et al.*, 1994; WHO, 1995):

Variables demonstrating a symptomatic efficacy: Algo-functional Lequesne index (LI) (Lequesne, 1997), Western Ontario and MacMaster

Universities (Bellamy *et al.*, 1988) (WOMAC), investigator's or patient's global assessment, evaluation of pain on a visual analog scale (VAS) (Huskisson, 1982), walking time, nonsteroidal anti-inflammatory drug (NSAID), or analgesic consumption.

Variable(s) demonstrating a structural efficacy: Evolution of the mean joint space width (MJSW), joint surface area (JSA), and minimum joint space narrowing (MJSN) (Vignon *et al.*, 2003).

The tolerance was assessed by comparing the adverse events observed in patients treated by CS and in patients treated by PBO.

The studied populations appeared to be highly homogeneous, certainly because of the very similar inclusion criteria. Thus, when possible, the outcomes were pooled in order to emerge general remarks on CS actions.

B. Quality Assessment

The different studies selected were scored for quality by two reviewers using an instrument that have been developed and tested (Chalmers *et al.*, 1981; MacAlindon *et al.*, 2000; Rochon *et al.*, 1994). Any differences were resolved by consensus.

The scale scores the different publications regarding their compliance to 14 points (control appearance, allocation concealment, patient blinding, observer blinding to treatment, observer blinding to results, prior estimation of the number of patients to involve, compliance testing, inclusion of pre-treatment variables in analysis, presentation of statistical end points, statistical evaluation of type II error, presentation of confidence limits, quality of statistical analysis, withdrawals, side effects discussion).

C. Data Extraction

We took interest in the effect size reported on the main criteria by the study: pain, assessed on VAS and algo-functional LI. This effect size is the difference between the treatment and the PBO arms at the end of the trial, divided by the pooled SD (Cohen, 1988). The effect size is a unitless value centered at zero:

At zero, the efficacy of the treatment is considered as equal to the PBO's one.

A negative effect size suggests that the treatment is less efficient than PBO.

A positive effect size suggests that the treatment is more efficient than PBO.

Cohen's scale (Cohen, 1988) states that 0.8 reflects a clinically large effect, 0.5 a moderate effect, and 0.2 a small effect.

Finally, we determined the percentage of the population that could be defined as responder on the basis of investigators' global assessment: patients judged improved or very good and good results were considered as responders.

Then, we could calculate the number of patients to treat to improve one patient [number needed to treat (NNT)]. A value >1 for the NNT means the treatment is more beneficial than control whereas a value <1 for the NNT means the treatment is less beneficial than control.

IV. Results

Twenty-six randomized controlled clinical trials were identified by the search strategy. Of these primary hits, we selected 7 studies that fulfilled all the criteria. They were listed for the study design, number of patient included, inclusion criteria, CS dosage, study duration, outcome measures chosen, results of the intention-to-treat (ITT) analysis. The reasons for not selecting the other publications are presented in Table I.

TABLE I   Reasons for Not Including Studies in the Meta-Analysis

RCTs *reviewed for* *inclusion criteria*	*Number of* *studies* 26	*References*
Insufficient data	−7	Anonymous, 2000; Conrozier, 1998; Kerzberg *et al.*, 1987; Mathieu, 2002; Morreale *et al.*, 1996; Pavelka *et al.*, 1999; Rovetta, 1991
Other language than French or English (Russian, Hebrew)	−5	Aleekseeva *et al.*, 1999, 2003; Debi *et al.*, 2000; Nasonova *et al.*, 2001; Tsvetkova *et al.*, 1992
No peer review	−1	L'Hirondel, 1992
Neither knee or hip OA treatment (temporo-mandibular, spine, finger)	−3	Nguyen *et al.*, 2001; Verbruggen *et al.*, 1998, 2002;
Administration paths not *per os* (cream)	−1	Cohen *et al.*, 2003
CS used in combination (manganese ascorbate, glucosamine)	−2	Das and Hammad, 2000; Leffler *et al.*, 1999
RCTs matching inclusion criteria	7	Bourgeois *et al.*, 1998; Bucsi and Poor, 1998; Mazières *et al.*, 2001, 1992; Michel *et al.*, 2005; Uebelhart *et al.*, 1998, 2004

A total number of 909 patients (468 treated with CS and 441 treated with PBO) were enrolled in the meta-analyses. The number of patients entering the study was relatively balanced between PBO and CS branches [except one study (Bourgeois *et al.*, 1998) designed with three arms]. The rates of drop out may be considered as low, with a mean around 11.5% (range from 1.6% to 27.0%).

Demographic baselines were well matched in each study and no statistical differences between the groups were observed for age (mean: 62.7 years), sex, body mass index (mean: 27.8 kg/m^2), and radiological score (mean Kellgren-Lawrence: 1.81) at inclusion. The dosages of CS used varied from one study to another, with a minimum daily dose from 800 mg to 2 g, in 1–3 takes.

The selected studies were mainly dedicated to CS efficacy choosing several primary criteria: pain release (VAS), algo-functional indexes (LI and WOMAC), decrease of anti-inflammatory drug, or analgesics consumption and structural modifying activity (mean joint space width) (Table II).

A. Symptomatic Efficacy on Pain

Data for the VAS pain were available and valuable in six publications (Bourgeois *et al.*, 1998; Bucsi and Poor, 1998; Mazières *et al.*, 1992, 2001; Uebelhart *et al.*, 1998, 2004). The studies showed a difference between the decrease of pain obtained in patients treated with CS and the decrease obtained in patients treated with PBO. This difference reaches the statistical significance at the latest 3 months and at the earliest 14 days after the beginning of the treatments, except for the study by Mazières (Mazières *et al.*, 2001) in which a significant difference was only obtained in the completer population.

A total of 609 patients were followed for pain evaluation. As presented in the Fig. 1, CS was found to have a small to large effect in relief of the pain (polled effect size = 0.60; 95% CI: 0.26–0.94). The mean decrease of pain after 3 months of treatment was 22.2 mm on the VAS scale with CS while it was 10.5 mm with PBO (Fig. 2). After 6 months of treatment, the difference is even higher with a mean decrease of 40 mm with CS vs. 15 mm with PBO. After a latency period, the CS became more and more efficient as the treatment lasted, compared to the PBO.

The pain evaluation is biased as in most of the studies, the use of concomitant antalgic or anti-inflammatory therapeutics (acetaminophen, NSAID) as rescue drug, was allowed for ethic reasons. Even if the intake of these drugs is generally stopped 48 h (for NSAIDs) or 12–24 h (for acetaminophen) before the assessment visits, such practices could level down the difference between the two groups of treatment and penalize the study.

Thus, when studying the pain evolution, it is really important to follow in parallel the consumption of analgesics or NSAID taken by the patient.

TABLE II Data from the 7 Selected Studies

Author (year)	Study design	Number of patients	Inclusion criteria	CS dosage	Study duration	Variables	Results	ITT	Quality score
Mazières et al. (1992)	R, DB, C vs. Pl, multic.	120	>45, idiopathic KOA or HOA (ACR), Kellgren I-III, daily pain > 3 years, VAS ≥ 40 mm, LI ≥ 4	2 g/d (2 × 1g) p.o.	3 months treatment + 2 months follow-up	1: NSAIDs consumption 2: Pain (VAS) LI overall patient and investigator judgement	↓ S since M1 to M5 ↓ S since M3 to M5 ↓ S since M4 ↓ S since M3 (M4 for investigator) and to M5	Yes?	9
Bourgeois et al. (1998)	R, DB, C vs. Pl, multic.	127	>45, KOA (ACR), Kellgren I-III, conservation of articular joint space, stable daily administration of NSAIDs for at least 1 month	1,2 g/d (A) or 3 × 400 mg/d (B) p.o.	3 months	1: LI 2: Pain (VAS) NSAIDs consumption Overall patient and investigator judgement	↓ S since D14 (A), D42 (B) ↓ S since D14 (A), D42 (B) NS S in favor of CS	Yes	6
Busci and Poor (1998)	R, DB, C vs. Pl, multic.	85	Idiopathic or secondary clinically symptomatic KOA for >6 months, Kellgren I-III	800 mg/d p.o.	6 months	Spontaneous joint pain (VAS) Paracetamol consumption Walking time LI Global efficacy and tolerability judgement by patient and investigator	↓ S since M3 Trend in favour of CS NS ↓ S since M6 ↓ S since M1 S in favor of CS	?	7
Uebelhart (1998)	R, DB, C vs. Pl, monoc.	46	35–78, clinically symptomatic KOA, at least 25% remaining joint space	800 mg/d (2 × 400) p.o.	12 months	1: Pain (VAS) overall mobility capacity 2: MJSW JSA MJSN biochemical markers	↓ S since M3 ↑ S since M6 ↓ S with Pl/stable with CS Same trend (NS) No change ↓ S for OC, KS, D-pyr and pyr	?	7

(continues)

TABLE II (continued)

Author (year)	Study design	Number of patients	Inclusion criteria	CS dosage	Study duration	Variables	Results	ITT	Quality score
Mazières (2001)	R, DB, C vs. Pl, multic.	130	>50, clinically and radiographically confirmed KOA (ACR), $4 \leq LI \leq 11$, VAS activity ≥ 30 mm, regular consumption of NSAIDs for 3 months, Kellgren I-III	1 g/d p.o.	3 months treatment + 3 months follow-up	1: LI 2: Pain quality of life Patient and investigator judgement Acet. and NSAID consumption	Trend in favor of CS NS Trend in favor of CS NS Trend in favor of CS NS Trend in favor of CS NS Trend in favor of CS NS	Yes	13
Uebelhart et al. (2004)	R, DB, C vs. Pl, multic.	110	>40, clinically symptomatic idiopathic KOA (ACR), Kellgren I-III	800 mg/d p.o.	12 months: 3 months treatment + 3 months follow-up + 3 months treatment + 3 months follow-up	1: LI 2: Pain (VAS) Walking time Global patient and investigator judgement	↓ S since M9 ↓ S since M9 ↓ S since M6 Always in favor of CS	Yes	11
Michel et al. (2005)	R, DB, C vs. Pl, monoc.	300	40-85, clinically symptomatic KOA (ACR), Kellgren I-III	800 mg/d p.o.	24 months	1: Joint space loss 2: Pain and function (WOMAC)	↓ S with Pl/ stable with CS NS difference	Yes	11

R, randomized; DB, double-blind; C, controlled; CS, chondroitin sulphate; Pl, placebo; 1, main criteria; 2, secondary criteria; S, statistically significant difference; NS, nonstatistically significant difference; ITT, intention to treat; PP, per protocol; LI, Lequesne index; MJSW, mean joint space width; JSA, joint surface area; MJSN, minimum joint space narrowing; VAS, visual analogue scale; OC, serum osteocalcin; KS, serum antigenic keratan sulphate; pyr, total urinary pyridinoline; D-pyr, total urinary deoxy-pyridinoline.

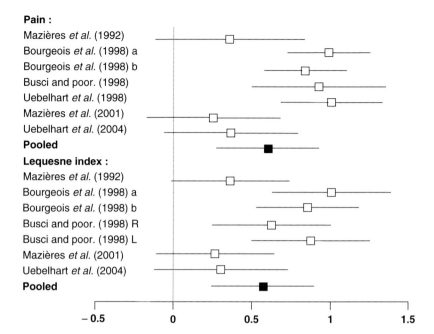

FIGURE 1   Effect sizes of symptomatic outcomes: Pain and Lequesne index (R: right knee; L:left knee).

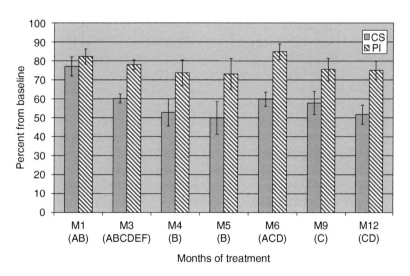

FIGURE 2   Pooled data on pain (assessed by VAS) reported after months of treatment, expressed in percent from baseline (A: Bucsi and Poor,. 1998; B: Mazieres *et al.*, 1992; C: Uebelhart *et al.*, 2004; D: Uebelhart *et al.*, 1998; E: Bourgeois *et al.*, 1998; F: Mazieres *et al.*, 2001).

Four studies (Bourgeois *et al.*, 1998; Bucsi and Poor, 1998; Mazières *et al.*, 1992; 2001) reported information on this aspect with a general trend in favor of CS; a significant difference between CS and PBO groups was obtained after 1 month of treatment in two studies (Mazières *et al.*, 1992; Uebelhart *et al.*, 2004), and the rescue drug consumption in PBO group appeared to be double than in the CS group after 12 months of treatment (Uebelhart *et al.*, 2004).

B. Symptomatic Efficacy on Function

Data for algo-functional LI were available and valuable in five publications (Bourgeois *et al.*, 1998; Bucsi and Poor, 1998; Mazières *et al.*, 1992, 2001; Uebelhart *et al.*, 2004) and in one publication (Michel *et al.*, 2005) for WOMAC.

Regarding LI, a statistically significant difference was found between outcomes of patients treated with CS and treated with PBO at the latest after 9 months of daily treatment, except for the study by Mazières *et al.* (2001) in which significance is reached only in completer population.

When pooling the results of the five studies (Bourgeois *et al.*, 1998; Bucsi and Poor, 1998; Mazières *et al.*, 1992, 2001; Uebelhart *et al.*, 2004) (total of 563 patients: 295 under CS and 268 under PBO), the effect size is found to be about 0.57 (95% CI: 0.26–0.88) what corresponds to a moderate efficacy. The mean decrease of the LI after 3 months of daily treatment was 3.4 with CS (32.2% from baseline) and only 1.4 with PBO (13.9% from baseline) (Fig. 3). This difference remained constant during the following months and so until 12 months of treatment.

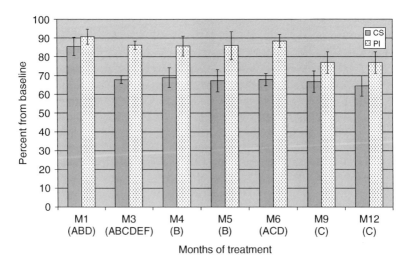

FIGURE 3   Pooled data on LI reported after months of treatment, expressed in percent from baseline (A: Bucsi and Poor(R), 1998; B: Mazieres *et al.*, 1992; C: Uebelhart *et al.*, 2004; D: Bucsi and Poor(L), 1998; E: Bourgeois *et al.*, 1998; F: Mazieres *et al.*, 2001).

C. Delay of Onset

All selected studies show evidence of a delay in the action of the drug. The outcomes reported during the first months of treatment are generally similar between treated group and PBO group. This latency period can be remarked on pain relief as well as on LI improvement and lasts about 1 month.

D. Carry-Over Effect

In three studies (Mazières *et al.*, 1992, 2001; Uebelhart *et al.*, 2004), follow-up period allowed to show a continuous activity of the CS along the time, even after the end of the administration schedule of the drug; these results suggest a persistent action of the CS that could be seen both in pain and function outcomes.

The follow-up period is unfortunately too short to assess the real duration of the persistent action, but data permit to show that it lasts at least 3 months after 3 months of treatment (Mazières *et al.*, 2001; Uebelhart *et al.*, 2004).

E. Assessment by the Patient/Physician

In all studies (Bourgeois *et al.*, 1998; Mazières *et al.*, 2001; Uebelhart *et al.*, 1998, 2004), mentioning the overall assessment of the treatment efficacy by the patient or the physician, a common trend in favor of CS was reported. A statistically significant difference was reached after 42, 90, or 180 days of treatment (depending on the study) but was reached only with the completer population in one trial (Mazières *et al.*, 2001).

As shown in the Table III, the mean relative risk of being responder to the treatment for a patient is 1.83 ± 0.34 and the mean number of patient needed to treat is about 9.2 ± 5.4.

F. Structure-Modifying Efficacy

The structure-modifying efficacy of the CS was part of the evaluation criteria in three studies (Michel *et al.*, 2005; Uebelhart *et al.*, 1998, 2004) and was the main criteria in one (Michel *et al.*, 2005).

According to the study by Michel *et al.* (2005), the patients who received PBO once a day during 2 years, experienced significant reduction in mean joint space width (-0.14 ± 0.61 mm, $p = 0.001$) and minimum joint space width (-0.07 ± 0.56 mm, $p = 0.05$) while patients who received CS remained unchanged. The corresponding effect size is about 0.25. These results reinforced the trend already suggested by the two previous studies by Uebelhart *et al.* (1998 and 2004), performed during 1 year in a small number of patients ($n = 46$).

TABLE III Relative Risk of Being a Responder for Patients Treated with CS and NNT

Study	Risk of being a responder	NNT
Bourgeois *et al.* (1998) 1200 mg	2.03	6.65
Bourgeois *et al.* (1998) 3 × 400 mg	2.09	5.6
Bucsi and Poor (1998)	2.23	6.8
Mazières *et al.* (2001)	1.35	18.1
Uebelhart *et al.* (2004)	1.82	5.3
Combined	1.83 ± 0.34	9.2 ± 5.4

Nevertheless, no difference was reported regarding the WOMAC score in Michel *et al.*'s (2005) study, raising the question of the interest of a radiographic improvement without any clinical relief.

G. Tolerance

All the studies concluded on a good to excellent tolerability of the CS. Neither the nature nor the frequency of the adverse events was reported to be significantly different to the PBO arm. In some cases, CS was even better tolerated than PBO (Uebelhart *et al.*, 2004).

Nevertheless, it has to be noticed that several studies put in evidence intestinal disorders (abdominal pain, nausea, epigastralgia, constipation, diarrhea, pyrosis). The prevalence of these side effects occurred to be significantly higher in the CS group in the study by Mazières *et al.* (2001), but this significant difference was not confirmed in the six other studies.

Other side effects were occasionally reported in patients under CS treatment but were not considered as drug-related: respiratory disorder, headache, vertigo, allergic episode, eyelid edema, cutaneous manifestations (pruritus, pruriginous eruption), ankle edema, cardiac problem, urinary tract infection, and falling hair.

Clinical laboratory evaluation did not detect any changes in the blood, renal, or liver biological parameters.

V. Discussion

According to the results analyzed, we can conclude to a true but modest effect of the CS on the relief of pain and on the improvement of the joint function in patients treated. Good evidence is now available that this symptomatic slow acting drug is a valuable therapeutic tool for OA (Jordan *et al.*, 2003).

Nevertheless, this evaluation must be biased as only few methodologically correct papers are available. Only few papers are dealing with CS activity, among which rare studies report proof of an obvious efficacy. If the symptomatic effect of this drug is discussed for about 30 years, we observe a growing interest in the utility that may have a daily long-term treatment in the slow down of the worsening of the disease. The study by Michel *et al.* (2005) is the first one using a structural end point as main criteria, even if structural change is a secondary criteria in several other studies.

Regarding structural aspects, further studies with high number of subjects and lasting at least 2 years are needed to find any evidence of a consistent safe of joint space width. In this respect, the National Center for Complementary and Alternative Medicine (NCCAM) along with the National Institute of Arthritis and Musculoskeletal and Skin Diseases (NIAMS) launched in 2000 a large scale study including about 1600 patients with knee OA (GAIT: Glucosamine Chondroitin Arthritis Intervention Trial). This study is PBO-controlled, parallel, double-blind, five-arm clinical trial (glucosamine sulfate alone, CS alone, combination of glucosamine and CS, celecoxib and PBO), and the main criteria is the narrowing of joint space (http://nccam.nih.gov/news/19972000/121100/qa.htm#1). The results of this study must be published in November 2005. Since this time, the symptomatic efficacy of the GAIT study was published (Clegg *et al.*, 2006).

The CS provides a relatively slow variation in the symptoms, with a delay of action of about 1 month, however, the therapeutic effects lasted longer even after the suspension of treatment, that is, 3 months of carry-over effect after 3 months of treatment, what could be justified as a sequential therapeutic schedule of 3 months of treatment cycles spaced with 3 months without treatment as assessed in one trial (Uebelhart *et al.*, 2004).

The tolerance of CS can be considered as excellent, which provides a great advantage with regard to NSAID, especially on the gastrointestinal tract.

The still open question concerning CS, as the other SYSADOA, is to which OA patients these drugs are useful? It seems logical to assume that the best patients should be those with mild to moderate symptomatic disease, to decrease NSAID intake and their side effects, and patients with mild to moderate structural damages to preserve the cartilage loss; but today, there is no data in the literature to ascertain such conclusions.

References

Aleekseeva, L. I., Benevolenskaia, L. I., Nasonov, E. L., Chichasova, N. V., and Kariakin, A. N. (1999). Structum (chondroitin sulfate): A new agent for the treatment of osteoarthritis. *Ter. Arkh.* **71**, 51–53.

Alekseeva, L. I., Arkhangel'skaia, G. S., Davydova, A. F., Karmil'tseva, E. A., Kogan, K. M., Mazurov, V. I., Rebrov, A. P., Riabitseva, O. F., Shemerovskaia, T. G., and Lakushin, S. S. (2003). Long-term effects of structum administration (according to data from multicenter trial). *Ter. Arkh.* **75**, 82–86.

American College of Rheumatology Subcommittee on Osteoarthritis Guidelines (2000). Recommendations for the medical management of osteoarthritis of the hip and knee: 2000 update. *Arthritis Rheum.* **43**, 1905–1915.

Anonymous (2002). European multicenter study on effectiveness of chondroitin sulfate in gonarthrosis: A new look at biochemical and radiologic result. *Presse Med.* **29**(Suppl. 27), 15–18.

Avouac, B., and Dropsy, R. (1993). Méthodologie des essais thérapeutiques des médicaments de base de l'arthrose. *Thérapie* **48**, 315–319.

Bellamy, N., Buchanan, W. W., Goldsmith, C. H., Campbell, J., and Stitt, L. W. (1988). Validation of WOMAC: A health status instrument for measuring clinically important patent relevant outcomes to antirheumatic drug therapy in patients with osteoarthritis of the hip or the knee. *J. Rheumatol.* **15**, 1833–1840.

Bourgeois, P., Chales, G., Dehais, J., Delcambre, B., Kuntz, J. L., and Rozemberg, S. (1998). Efficacy and tolerability of chondroitin sulfate 1200 mg/day vs chondroitin sulfate 3 × 400 mg/day vs placebo. *Osteoarthritis Cartilage* **6**(Suppl. A), 25–30.

Bucsi, L., and Poor, G. (1998). Efficacy and tolerability of oral chondroitin sulfate as a symptomatic slow-acting drug for osteoarthritis (SYSDOA) in the treatment of knee osteoarthritis. *Osteoarthritis Cartilage* **6**(Suppl. A), 31–36.

Chalmers, T. C., Smith, H., Jr., Blackburn, B., Silverman, B., Schroeder, B., Reitman, D., and Ambroz, A. (1981). A method for assessing the quality of a randomized control trial. *Control Clin. Trials* **2**, 31–49.

Clegg, D. O., Reda, D. J., Harris, C. L., Klein, M. A., O'Dell, J. R., Hooper, M. M., Bradley, J. D., Bingham, C. O., 3rd, Weisman, M. H., Jackson, C. G., Lane, N. E., Cush, J. J., *et al.* (2006). Glucosamine, chondroitin sulfate, and the two in combination for painful knee osteoarthritis. *N. Engl. J. Med.* **354**, 795–808.

Cohen, J. (1988). "Statistical Power Analysis for the Behavioral Sciences," 2nd Ed. Lawrence Erlbaum Association, Hillsdale, NJ.

Cohen, M., Wolfe, R., Mai, T., and Lewis, D. (2003). A randomized, double blind, placebo controlled trial of the topical cream containing glucosamine sulfate, chondroitin sulfate, and camphor for osteoarthritis of the knee. *J. Rheumatol.* **30**, 523–528.

Committee for Proprietary Medicinal Products (1998). "Points to Consider on Clinical Investigation of Medicinal Products Used in the Treatment of Osteoarthritis." European Agency for the Evaluation of Medicinal Products, London, UK.

Conrozier, T. (1998). Anti-arthrosis treatments: Efficacy and tolerance of chondroitin sulfate (CS 4 & 6). *Presse Med.* **27**, 1862–1865.

Das, A., Jr., and Hammad, T. A. (2000). Efficacy of a combination of FCHG49 glucosamine hydrochloride, TRH122 low molecular weight sodium chondroitin sulfate and manganese ascorbate in the management of the knee osteoarthritis. *Osteoarthritis Cartilage* **8**, 343–350.

Debi, R., Robinson, D., Agar, G., and Halperin, N. (2000). GAG for osteoarthritis of the knee: A prospective study. *Harefuah* **138**, 451–453.

Food and Drug Administration (1999). Guidance for Industry: Clinical Development Programs for Drugs, Devices, and Biological Products Intended for the Treatment of Osteoarthritis. FDA document 07/1999. Food and Drug Administration, Washington, DC.

Group for Management of Osteoarthritis (1990). Special meeting on osteoarthritis. *Rev. Rhum. Mal. Osteoartic.* **57**(9bis), 1S–50S.

Huskisson, E. C. (1982). Measurement of pain. *J. Rheumatol.* **9**, 768–769. http://nccam.nih. gov/news/19972000/121100/qa.htm#1.

Jordan, K. M., Arden, N. K., Doherty, M., Bannwarth, B., Bijlsma, J. W. J., Dieppe, P., Gunther, K., Hauselmann, H., Herrero-Beaumont, G., Kaklamanis, P., Lohmander, S., Leeb, B., *et al.* (2003). EULAR recommendations 2003, an evidence based approach to the management of knee osteoarthritis: Report of a task force of the Standing Committee for International Clinical Studies Including Therapeutic Trials ESCISIT. *Ann. Rheum. Dis.* **62**, 1145–1155.

Kerzberg, E. M., Roldan, E. J. A., Castelli, G., and Hubermann, E. D. (1987). Combination of a glycosaminoglycans and acetylsalicylic acid in knee osteoarthritis. *Scand. J. Rheumatol.* **16**, 377–380.

L'Hirondel, J. L. (1992). Etude clinique en double insu du sulfate de chondroïtine per os versus placebo dans la gonarthrose fémoro-tibiale (125 patients). *Litera Rheumatol.* **14**, 77–85.

Leeb, B., Schweitzer, H., Montag, K., and Smolen, J. (2000). A metaanalysis of chondroïtine sulphate in the treatment of osteoarthritis. *J. Rheumatol.* **27**(1), 205–211.

Leffler, C. T., Philippi, A. F., Leffler, S. G., Mosure, J. C., and Kim, P. D. (1999). Glucosamine, chondroitin, and manganese ascorbate for degenerative joint desease of the knee or low back: A randomized, double-blind, placebo-controlled pilot study. *Mil. Med.* **164**, 85–91.

Lequesne, M. (1994). Les antiarthrosiques symptomatiques d'action lente: Un nouveau concept thérapeutique? *Rev. Rhum. Mal. Osteoartic.* **61**, 75–79.

Lequesne, M., Brandt, K., Bellamy, N., Moskowitz, R., Menkes, C. J., and Pelletier, J. P. (1994). Guidelines for testing slow acting drugs in osteoarthritis. *J. Rheumatol.* **21**(Suppl), 65–73.

Lequesne, M. G. (1997). The algofunctional indices for hip and knee osteoarthritis. *J. Rheumatol.* **24**, 779–781.

MacAlindon, T. E., La Valley, M. P., Gulin, J. P., and Felson, D. T. (2000). Glucosamine adn chondroitin for treatment of osteoarthrtis: A systematic quality assessment and meta-analysis. *JAMA* **15**, 1469–1475.

Mathieu, P. (2002). Radiological progression of internal femoro-tibial osteoarthritis in gonarthrosis. Chondro-protective effect of chondroitin sulfates ACS4-ACS6. *Presse Med.* **31**(29), 1386–1390.

Mazières, B., Loyau, G., Menkes, C. J., Valat, J. P., Dreiser, R. L., Charlot, J., and Masounabe-Puyanne, A. (1992). Chondroitin sulfate for the treatment of coxarthrosis and gonarthrosis: A prospective, multicenter, placebo-controlled, double-blind trial with five months follow-up. *Rev. Rhum. Mal. Osteoarthric.* **59**, 466–472.

Mazières, B., Combe, B., Phan Van, A., Tondut, J., and Grynfeltt, M. (2001). Chondroitin sulfate in osteoarthritis of the knee: A prospective, double blind, placebo controlled multicenter clinical study. *J. Rheumatol.* **28**, 173–181.

Michel, B. A., Stucki, G., Frey, D., DeVathaire, F., Vignon, E., Bruehlmann, P., and Uebelhart, D. (2005). Chondroitin 4 and 6 sulfate in osteoarthritis of the knee: A randomized, controlled trial. *Arthritis Rheum.* **52**(3), 779–786.

Morreale, P., Manopulo, R., Galati, M., Boccanera, L., Saponati, G., and Bocchi, L. (1996). Comparison between the anti-inflammatory efficacy of chondroitin sulfate and diclofenac sodium in patients with knee osteoarthritis. *J. Rheumatol.* **23**, 1358–1391.

Nasonova, V. A., Alekseeva, L. I., Arkhangel'skaia, G. S., Davydova, A. F., Karmil'tseva, E. A., Kogan, K. M., Mazurov, V. I., Rebrov, A. P., Riabitseva, O. F., Shemerovskaia, T. G., Shmidt, E. I., Iakushin, S. S., *et al.* (2001). Result of the multicenter clinical trial of Structum preparation in Russia. *Ter. Arkh.* **73**, 84–87.

Nevitt, M. C., Lane, N. C., Scott, J. C., Hochberg, M. C., Pressman, A. R., Genant, H. K., and Cummings, S. R. (1995). Radiographic osteoarthritis of the hip and bone mineral density. *Arthritis Rheum.* **38**, 907–916.

Nguyen, P., Mohamed, S. E., Gardiner, D., and Salinas, T. (2001). A randomized double-blind clinical trial of the effect of chondroitin sulfate and glucosamine hydrochloride on temporomandibular joint disorders: A pilot study. *Cranio* **19**, 130–139.

Pavelka, K., Bucsi, L., and Manopulo, R. (1999). Double-blind, dose effect study of oral CS 4&6 1200 mg, 800 mg, 200 mg, against placebo in the treatment of femoro-tibial osteoarthritis. *Litera Rheumatol.* **24**, 21–30.

Richy, F., Bruyere, O., Ethgen, O., and Cucherat, M. (2003). Structural and symptomatic efficacy of glucosamine and chondroïtin in knee osteoarthritis. *Arch. Intern. Med.* **163**, 1514–1522.

Rochon, P. A., Gurwitz, J. H., Cheung, C. M., Hayes, J. A., and Chalmers, T. C. (1994). Evaluating the quality of articles published in journal supplements compared with the quality of those publish in the parent journal. *JAMA* **272**, 108–113.

Rovetta, G. (1991). Galactosaminoglycuronoglycan sulfate (matrix) in therapy of tibiofibular osteoarthritis of the knee. *Drugs Exp. Clin. Res.* **17**, 53–57.

Tsvetkova, E. S., Agababova, E. R., and Bogomolova, N. A. (1992). Cartilage-protective preparations in the therapy of osteoarthritis. *Ter. Arkh.* **64**(5), 59–60.

Uebelhart, D., Thonar, E. J., Delmas, P. D., Chantraine, A., and Vignon, E. (1998). Effects of oral chondroitin sulfate on the progression of knee osteoarthritis: A pilot study. *Osteoarthritis Cartilage* **6**(Suppl A), 39–46.

Uebelhart, D., Malaise, M., Marcolongo, R., DeVathaire, F., Piperno, M., Mailleux, E., Fioravanti, A., Matoso, L., and Vignon, E. (2004). Intermittent treatment of the knee osteoarthritis with oral chondroitin sulfate: A one-year, randomized, double-blind, multicenter study versus placebo. *Osteoarthritis Cartilage* **12**, 269–276.

Van Sasse, J. L. C. M., Van Romunde, L. K. J., Cats, A., Vandenbroucke, J. P., and Valkenburg, H. A. (1989). Epidemiology of osteoarthritis: Zoertermeer survey. Comparison of radiologic osteoarthritis in a Dutch population with that in 10 other populations. *Ann. Rheum. Dis.* **48**, 271–280.

Verbruggen, G., Goemaere, S., and Veys, E. M. (1998). Chondroitin sulfate: S/DMOAD (structure/disease modifying anti-osteoarthritis drug) in the treatment of finger joint OA. *Osteoarthritis Cartilage* **6**(Suppl A), 37–38.

Verbruggen, G., Goemaere, S., and Veys, E. M. (2002). Systems to assess the progression of finger joint osteoarthritis and the effect of disease modifying osteoarthritis drugs. *Clin. Rheumatol.* **21**, 231–243.

Vignon, E., Piperno, M., Hellio le Graverand, M. P., Mazzuca, S. A., Brandt, K. D., Mathieu, P., Favret, H., Vignon, M., Merle-Vincent, F., and Conrozier, T. (2003). Measurements of radiographic joint space width in the tibiofemoral compartment of the osteoarthritis knee: Comparison of standing anteroposterior and Lyon Schuss views. *Arthritis Rheum.* **48**, 378–384.

World Health Organization (1995). "Guidelines for the Clinical Investigation of Drugs Used in Rheumatic Diseases," pp. 7–24. European Drug Guidelines, Series 5. World Health Organization, Regional Office for Europe. European League Against Rheumatism, Copenhaguen.

Daniel Uebelhart*,†, Ruud Knols*, Eling D de Bruin*,‡, and Gust Verbruggen§

*Department of Rheumatology and Institute of Physical Medicine
University Hospital Zurich, Switzerland

†Department of Biochemistry, Rush Presbyterian-St. Luke's Medical Center
Chicago, Illinois

‡Institute for Human Movement Sciences, ETH Zurich, Switzerland

§Department of Rheumatology, Ghent University Hospital, Gent, Belgium

Treatment of Knee Osteoarthritis with Oral Chondroitin Sulfate

I. Chapter Overview

Knee osteoarthritis (OA) is a frequent chronic musculoskeletal condition, encountered mostly in elderly people. The therapeutic approaches of knee OA is based on both nonpharmacological and pharmacological therapies. Regarding the pharmacological therapies, there is now a large panel of evidence to support the use of symptomatic slow-acting drugs for OA (SYSADOA), which is a generic term used for those medications for OA acting on the symptoms of the disease with delayed onset, reducing pain and improving both the joint function and the overall mobility of the patients, and having, in addition, a remanent effect when the administration is stopped. Among them, orally administered chondroitin sulfate (CS) is of special interest in the indication of knee OA, a condition in which a couple of randomized controlled trials (RCTs) have been performed in the last 20 years. Our survey could identify a total of 11 RCTs including 1443

Advances in Pharmacology, Volume 53
1054-3589/06 $35.00
DOI: 10.1016/S1054-3589(05)53027-8

knee OA patients, where oral CS was administered daily vs. placebo (PBO) from a couple of months to up to 2 years continuously or intermittently. Based upon the methodological quality of the studies incorporated in the survey, it can be concluded so far that the oral administration of CS in knee OA does significantly reduce pain and improve the joint function and mobility, as well as the overall mobility of the patients with a level of tolerability and safety, which can be qualified as excellent. As a consequence, most of the patients can significantly reduce their intake of analgesics and NSAIDs, drugs known to predispose to some major side effects. Therefore, the authors would suggest the systematic introduction of oral CS, based on its demon-strated efficacy and excellent tolerability, as a ground therapy for knee OA. Our own recommendation fits well with the most recent EULAR guide-lines for the treatment of knee OA and the conclusions of three published meta-analyses.

II. Introduction

Osteoarthritis is the most common form of arthritis in Western popu-lations, and its prevalence increases with age. Due to an overall trend of aging in our population, this disease condition is already known to be a major contributor to the increase in health costs, and it represents a serious social and economical burden for the coming generations (Cooper, 1998). OA of the knee, also known as gonarthrosis, is the form of OA targeting the knee joint, which is the principal large joint to be affected. The increased incidence with the advance of age is well known, and patients affected will present with pain, decreased mobility, and various degrees of disability, consequently also with a significantly decreased quality of life. The costs attributable to knee OA are huge, especially taking into account surgical procedures, such as osteotomy, but especially total or partial knee replace-ment. The gender repartition is in favor of women as compared to men with a ratio of about 2:1; therefore, significantly more women are being affected by knee OA (Cooper, 1998). Nevertheless, in many cases the original diag-nosis of knee OA is based upon X-rays, and it is worth noting that in about 30% of the aged population over 65, the diagnosis is positive even if some patients do not report symptoms of pain and/or restriction of mobility (Cooper *et al.*, 2000). The cause of knee OA is generally unknown, but in many cases it is considered to be of multifactorial origin. Clear evidence of a link between an identified causative factor and the development of knee OA are known in some well-identified general conditions, such as aging, gender, overweight, and some local factors such as trauma, occupation, and align-ment (Cooper *et al.*, 2000). In minority of the cases, the cause can be genetic, for instance, in some families affected by mutations in type II collagen or procollagen (Spector *et al.*, 1996). Patients affected by knee OA complain of pain and functional disability, and these two symptoms represent most of the reasons why patients with this condition will refer to their physician. Of course, when the symptoms become more important and consequently the patient can barely move, this does also mean an increased risk of further morbidity and even mortality, especially considering an elderly population. In addition, the decreased quality of life is also a very important negative consequence to be taken into account as the reduction of mobility will also impair social and personal contacts (Murray and Lopez, 1997).

This is why knee OA should absolutely be taken as a very serious chronic health condition generally affecting elderly people and definitively not as a normal physiological condition affecting the knee joints of the aging population. A direct consequence of this recognition is that both basic and clinical sciences have focused on this disease condition since many years in order to better understand its etiology and mode of progression and try to develop strategies to prevent the disease and/or limit its progression.

A. Therapeutic Options for Knee Osteoarthritis: Drugs, No Drugs, or Both?

For many years, physicians did only treat the actual symptoms of knee OA using both nonpharmacological and pharmacological treatments. Among the nonpharmacological options, the list includes education (Mazzuca *et al.*, 1997), exercise (Messier *et al.*, 2000), insoles, orthotic devices, weight loss, spa, laser, and many other ones. The most relevant therapeutic options were reviewed in the Eular Recommendations 2003 for the management of knee OA (Jordan *et al.*, 2003). For information, the same type of guidelines were published for the management of hip OA (Zhang *et al.*, 2005). Taking into account these guidelines, most of the nonpharmacological treatments did have a level of evidence of 1B (meaning that the evidence came from at least one RCT) with various effect sizes and a strength of recommendation of category B (meaning a category 2 evidence or extrapolated recommendation from category 1 evidence). On the other hand, pharmacological treatments are intended to alleviate the symptoms of pain, facilitate the mobilization of the affected joint(s), and therefore ameliorate the overall mobility of the patient. Most of the substances used in this category do directly reduce pain and/or control the inflammatory process that occurs at some stages of knee OA. For instance, among the large choice of substances or procedures that are currently used for the treatment of knee OA, some are applied locally at the level of the affected joint, such as topical capsaicin or nonsteroidal anti-inflammatory drugs (NSAIDs), some can be injected into the joint cavity such as steroids or hyaluronan (HA) and HA derivatives. Additionally, joint lavage can also be used in some cases. The other pattern of administration of symptomatic-active substances is of course the oral way that is convenient, well known regarding pharmacocinetics and also very well accepted by both OA patients and their physicians. The generic list of orally taken drugs involved in the treatment of knee OA is relatively short and includes antalgics, NSAIDs, opioid analgesics, psychotropic drugs, sex hormones, and SYSADOA.

B. Symptomatic Slow-Acting Drugs for OA

This latest category is of special interest in the context of the present chapter as it includes CS. It should be mentioned at this point that SYSA-DOA can both be administered orally (most frequently) or intra-articularly (less frequently) with substances such as HA and HA derivatives.

A general characteristic of the SYSADOA is their delayed mode of action (this is why they are called "slow-acting drugs") on the painful symptoms of knee OA. Indeed, most of these drugs will begin to be active and modulate pain between 2 and 3 weeks after the beginning of their intake, whereas analgesics or NSAIDs are rapidly acting agents on knee OA symptoms. Another important feature of SYSADOA is their remanent activity. In fact, after an overall period of daily intake of about 3 months for the oral formulations or 3–5 weekly intra-articular injections of HA or HA derivatives, the administration of the drug can be stopped, and most of the patients will continue to benefit from the treatment for a period extending from 3 to 6 months for the oral formulations and 6–12 months for the intra-articular formulations.

In sharp contrast with these effects, the patients taking analgesics or NSAIDs will rapidly escape and present pain again once the treatment is stopped.

These two aspects, delayed mode of action and remanence of the thera-peutic effect once the treatment is stopped, are the typical features and characteristics of the SYSADOA and are not shared by any other class of therapeutic agents used for the treatment of knee OA.

In addition, regarding the safety of these compounds, it can be said that their tolerability profile (oral formulations) is generally good to excellent with a few gastrointestinal side effects reported at the initiation of the therapy, which stop after a couple of days. No serious life-threatening side effects have ever been reported with this class of drugs, some introduced to the market in 1960s, which means that the data available from pharmacovigilance cover a period of more than 40 years.

One important comment must be made at this stage as some of the SYSADOA are sold as prescription free and over-the-counter (OTC) sub-stances in all drugstores in the USA since many years, whereas they are registered and were sold as prescription drugs in Europe from the very beginning. The point is that the European SYSADOA oral preparations have to be fully registered as drugs by the European and/or national regu-latory agencies, which means that they have to fulfill severe criteria of quality and safety and that they have been fully analyzed regarding their pharmacotoxicologic characteristics and industrial processing. These requirements are not applied to the SYSADOA sold as OTCs in the American market, which means that their actual content in active substance and as well as its quality are not prerequisite to being sold to the American patients. Some analyses have been performed, for instance for CS, and it was not a big surprise to find major differences in terms of quality or quantity in different brands sold as OTCs, most of them not even having the effective concentration of CS in each pill as mentioned in the accompanying documentation. A direct consequence of this major difference between the European and the American SYSADOA market is that the studies performed on the other side of the Atlantic provide results, which can be considered as nonreliable in assessing the efficacy and tolerability of these substances. This might also explain why some of these drugs are just mentioned but not recommended by the American College of Rheumatology (ACR) subcommittee on OA (ACR, 2000). A real effort in terms of quality controls and regulations should certainly be undertaken by the American agencies responsible for the drug market, such as the FDA, in order to ensure that the American patients receive the proper treatment for their knee OA and that what they take has reasonable chances to positively affect their health condition.

Coming back to the EULAR recommendations 2003 for the management of knee OA (Jordan *et al.*, 2003), these substances and procedures have also been evidence-based checked and the results included in the report of the Task Force of the Standing Committee for International Clinical Studies Including Therapeutic Trials (ESCISIT). The levels of evidence and the strength of recommendation of these various therapies are summarized in Table I.

In order to perform this survey of the available studies to assess the clinical efficacy and tolerability of oral CS, we used a specific methodological approach, which is explained in detail underneath. The problem with SYSADOA drugs is that a large number of the original trials were open and nonrandomized; only few trials were RCTs, which does mean that they reached a level of evidence that can be considered as good. In addition, due to the small number of RCTs, only a few meta-analyses were published so far, and their conclusions are clearly restricted to the limited material they had access to. This is the reason why we chose to review the evidence on the basis of the published literature, which was critically analyzed.

III. Methods

A. Search Strategy

A computer-aided search of MEDLINE was conducted (Dickersin *et al.*, 1994) from 1966 up to 2005 (Ovid, PubMed, Gateway; 1966 to June 2005) and the Cochrane Database of Systematic Reviews (June 2005), to identify

TABLE I   **EULAR-Recommendations 2003 (Knee Osteoarthritis)**

Type	Intervention	Evidence	Recommendation
Noninvasive	Acetaminophen Paracetamol	1B	A
Drugs	Conventional NSAIDs	1A	A
	Coxibs	1B	A
	Chondroitine sulfate	1A	A
	Glucosamine sulfate	1A	A
	Topical NSAIDs	1A	A
	Topical capsaicin	1A	A
Noninvasive, non drugs	Patient education	1A	A
	Active physiotherapy	1B	A
Invasive, intra-articular	Steroids	1B	A

1A, Level of evidence—Best mark: Highest level of the evidence. A, Strength of recommendation—Best mark: Highest level of strength of recommendation.

all studies that cover the use of oral CS in knee OA. Additionally, we checked the citation lists to complete our selection.

The following generic search terms (according to the thesaurus of each individual database) were used: Chondroitin, chondroitin sulfate or sulfate, joint disease, knee, musculoskeletal diseases, OA, randomized or randomised, rheumatic diseases, and combinations of these search terms. Restrictions were made regarding the language of the publications, and only papers in English, French, German, or Dutch language were included into this review process.

B. Inclusion Criteria and Data Collection

To be included in the review, all studies had to have examined the effects of oral CS on OA. For the effect of CS in human beings, only randomized controlled trials (RCTs) were included in this review. Studies using at least one of the following types of outcome were included: Lequesne algofunctional index (AFI), pain, walking time, and the Womac questionnaire. Disagreement regarding inclusion of the studies was resolved by consensus between authors. RCTs evaluating chondroitin in combination with glucosamine, NSAIDs, as well as RCTs evaluating other forms than oral CS were excluded from the review process.

C. Assessment of Methodological Quality

Two reviewers (RK and EdB) independently assessed the methodological quality of the studies according to the Delphi Criteria List (Verhagen *et al.*, 1998), a set of nine criteria for quality assessment: (1) use of randomization;

(2) concealment of treatment allocation (i.e., concealing the group-assignment sequence until a potential-study participant has been approached and has provided informed consent); (3) equivalence (or similarity) of groups at baseline regarding the most important prognostic indicators; (4) specification of the eligibility criteria; (5) blinding of the outcome assessors; (6) blinding of the care providers; (7) blinding of the patients; (8) reporting of point estimates and measures of variability for the primary outcome measures; and (9) use of an intention-to-treat analysis.

For each quality criterion, three rating categories were available: "yes, met criteria"; "no, did not meet criteria"; and "don't know." The results of the methodological quality of the reports are presented in Table I.

Percentage agreement and Cohen's Kappa statistic were calculated with GRAPHPAD? Software (Version 2002) and were interpreted in accordance with Landis and Koch's benchmarks for assessing the agreement between raters: poor (<0), slight (0.0–0.20), fair (0.21–0.40), moderate (0.41–0.60), substantial (0.61–0.80), and almost perfect (0.81–1.0) (Landis and Koch, 1977).

D. Data Abstraction

Two of the coauthors (RK, EdB) independently assessed the predefined outcomes of each study according to a standardized form. Variability presented for the outcome effectiveness of CS to alleviating symptoms of pain and functions was reported. If necessary, means and measures of dispersion were approximated from figures in the papers. A p value of 0.05 was used as the criterion for statistically significant results.

IV. Results

A. Study Design and Characteristics

The literature search yielded 11 reports that met the basic eligibility criteria of being an RCT that examined the effects of oral CS on knee OA.

A total of 1443 patients were included in these 11 studies. Four studies were originating from France: Mazieres *et al.* (2001), Bourgeois *et al.* (1998), Conrozier (1998), and L'Hirondel (1992); four from Switzerland: Michel *et al.* (2005), Uebelhart *et al.* (1998), Uebelhart *et al.* (2004), and Uebelhart *et al.* (unpublished); one from Belgium: Malaise *et al.* (1999); one from Hungary: Bucsi and Poor (1998); and one from the Tschech Republic: Pavelka *et al.* (1999).

Several varieties of CS modalities were used, which differed in dosage and treatment time; the daily dosage differed from 500 to 1200 mg CS. Two reports compared the effectiveness of different dosages of CS in knee OA

(Bourgeois et al., 1998; Pavelka et al., 1999). The effective treatment time and administration differed from 2×3 months intermittent (Conrozier, 1998; Malaise et al., 1998; Uebelhart et al., 2004) to 3 months continuously (Bourgeois et al., 1998; Mazieres et al., 2001; Pavelka et al., 1999), 6 months continuously (Bucsi and Poor, 1998; L'Hirondel, 1992; Uebelhart et al., unpublished), 12 months continuously (Uebelhart et al., 1998), and 24 consecutive months (Michel et al., 2005).

B. Effect of Oral CS on the Lequesne's Algofunctional Index

A total of seven reports described a decrease of the Lequesne's AFI, which is an integrated score (Lequesne et al., 1987) combining pain and function as a result of the administration of oral CS (Bourgeois et al., 1998; Bucsi and Poor, 1998; Conrozier, 1998; L'Hirondel, 1992; Malaise et al., 1998; Pavelka et al., 1999; Uebelhart et al., 2004). Significant differences between CS and PBO groups regarding the reduction of the AFI score appeared at different time points in the treatment schedule. One report (L'Hirondel, 1992) described significant results between the CS and the PBO group after 2 months, and all the time points thereafter toward 1 year. Significant differences between the CS and the PBO group were found at respectively 3 ($p < 0.05$) and 6 months ($p < 0.01$) after the beginning of the CS treatment (Bucsi and Poor, 1998). Two reports by Uebelhart et al. (2004) and Malaise et al. (1998) described significant differences between the CS and the PBO group at 9 (both $p < 0.05$) and 12 months (both $p < 0.01$), respectively, but in this case the administration of CS or PBO was sequential and not daily continuous with two periods of treatment of 3 months each (month 0–3 and 6–9) over 1 year. A significant effect after 1 year between the CS and PBO group was described in one study (Conrozier, 1998) ($p < 0.05$). Two studies compared different dosages of oral CS as compared to PBO (Bourgeois et al., 1998; Pavelka et al., 1999). Three times CS 400 mg/day was compared with 1200 mg/day taken as a single daily dose. After 3 months, the reduction of the AFI was significant in both CS groups ($p < 0.0001$). An additional result of this study was that a single dose of CS 1200 mg/day did not differ from a dosage of CS 3×400 mg/day (Bourgeois et al., 1998). One study described the results of CS 1200 and 800 mg/day. Both dosages were more effective than a dosage of CS 200 mg/day or a PBO 3 months after the beginning of the treatment (Pavelka et al., 1999).

In contrast with the previous positive studies, the authors also retained the findings from two reports (Mazieres et al., 2001; Uebelhart et al., unpublished) with good methodological quality. These publications only observed a trend toward the efficacy of CS in knee OA, however, no significant differences between CS intervention and the PBO group could be observed.

C. Effect of Oral CS on the Huskisson's Visual Analog Scale for Pain

Seven reports described a significant decrease of the Huskisson's visual analog scale for pain (Huskisson, 1976) as a result of a treatment with oral CS (Bourgeois *et al.*, 1998; Bucsi and Poor, 1998; Conrozier, 1998; L'Hirondel, 1992; Malaise *et al.*, 1998; Pavelka *et al.*, 1999; Uebelhart *et al.*, 1998). A significant difference was reported after 6 weeks ($p = 0.0009$) on the VAS pain scale in two groups of patients taking CS 3×400 mg/day and 1200 mg/day, respectively, as compared to the PBO group. This effect remained after 3 months for both CS dosages (Bourgeois *et al.*, 1998). A dosage of CS 1200 mg/day taken at once was significantly more effective than the PBO ($p = 0.0075$) or CS 200 mg at day 14 ($p = 0.0001$). CS 1200 mg/day was also more effective than the PBO ($p = 0.000$), CS 200 mg ($p = 0.000$), or CS 800 mg ($p = 0.0064$) at day 42 after the beginning of the study. One-thousand-two-hundred mg CS/day was even more effective than a PBO or 200 mg CS at day 90 (both $p = 0.0000$) (Pavelka *et al.*, 1999). One report (L'Hirondel, 1992) described significant results ($p < 0.05$) between the CS and the PBO group after 2 months, and all the time points thereafter up to 1 year. Significant differences between the CS and PBO group were found at 3 and 6 months, respectively (both $p < 0.05$), after the beginning of the CS treatment (Bucsi and Poor, 1998). Two reports (Malaise *et al.*, 1998; Uebelhart *et al.*, 2004) described significant differences for the VAS pain between both CS and the PBO group at 9 and 12 months (both $p < 0.05$). Both Conrozier (1998) and Uebelhart *et al.* (1998) found significant differences compared to the PBO group for VAS pain 12 months after the beginning of the treatment.

On the contrary, in two recent studies with good methodological quality (Mazieres *et al.*, 2001; Uebelhart *et al.*, unpublished), the VAS pain scale showed greater, however, nonsignificant improvement as compared to PBO.

D. Effect of Oral CS on the Walking Time

Three research groups reported on the outcome walking time evaluated as the minimum time in seconds necessary to perform a well-defined walk on a flat track course (Bucsi and Poor, 1998; Malaise *et al.*, 1998; Uebelhart *et al.*, 2004). The mean walking time showed a significant improvement after 3 and 6 months of intervention in the CS group in the study of Bucsi and Poor (1998). The PBO group did not improve over this time period. These results were mirrored in the study of Malaise *et al.* (1998). This group reported a significant reduction in walking time from month 3 onward ($p < 0.05$; -12.7%), which improved with time (-17.9% after 12 months). No variations in measured walking time were shown in the PBO group. After 6 months of intervention, the improvement in the CS group was such that the groups differed significantly from each other ($p < 0.05$). In contrast to the former two studies, Uebelhart *et al.* (2004) showed an increase in walking time after 6 months of intervention only, but in this case, CS or PBO were administered sequentially over 2×3-month periods. Three months of intervention did not result in a change. However, after 12 months, this group found an 18% overall reduction in the walking time of the CS group vs. only 0.5% reduction in the PBO group.

E. Effects of Oral CS on the WOMAC Score

Two reports estimated treatment effects on the WOMAC Score (Bellamy *et al.*, 1988), a health-status instrument integrating pain, stiffness, and physical function in knee and hip OA patients (Michel *et al.*, 2005; Uebelhart *et al.*, unpublished). During the 2-year study period reported by Michel *et al.* (2005), the total WOMAC score did not show a significant improvement, neither for study completers analysis (PP) nor for the intention-to-treat analysis. There was neither statistically significant difference between the two study groups at baseline nor at the end of the study. In this study, patients were not originally enrolled for the intensity of their symptoms, and the study was designed to assess the structure-modifying effect of CS, which might well explain these results. Similar results were also reported by Uebelhart *et al.* (unpublished). In the case of this study, knee OA patients received a daily treatment of CS of avian origin, considered since then as less effective as the classical shark or bovine CS classically used in all the other studies reported here.

F. Safety and Tolerability of Oral CS

Oral CS is used as a drug for the treatment of OA since the early 1960s in many European countries, and all data from pharmacovigilance do confirm that the drug is safe and does not represent any kind of health hazard for the patients. Regarding its tolerability profile, some minor gastrointestinal discomfort has been related at the initiation of therapy in a small number of sensitive patients, mostly with the higher daily doses (800–1200 mg), but these symptoms disappeared spontaneously after a couple of days or with a reduction of the daily dosage for a short period of time. This excellent safety and tolerability profile makes the drug especially well indicated by elderly patients. These aspects were fully documented in each of the reported RCTs and confirm the above comments.

G. Assessment of the Methodological Quality of the Analyzed Studies

The reviewers agreed on 88 out of 99 methodological ratings (88.89%). The remaining disagreements were resolved after discussion between the two reviewers. The inter-reviewer k-statistic was 0.8, 95% confidence interval 0.66–0.89. The median criteria score on the Delphi list (range: 1–9) is 6 (Table II). Both Michel *et al.* (2005) and Uebelhart *et al.* (2004) were rated positively on 8 of 9 methodological criteria. Seven of 11 trials avoided potential selection bias by using an appropriate method to random the allocation sequence (Bourgeois *et al.*, 1998; Bucsi and Poor, 1998; Malaise *et al.*, 1998; Mazieres *et al.*, 2001; Pavelka *et al.*, 1999; Uebelhart *et al.*, 2004, unpublished). All trials reported group similarity at baseline regarding the most important prognostic factors, stated the eligibility criteria, and blinded the patient to treatment (Bourgeois *et al.*, 1998; Bucsi and Poor, 1998; Conrozier, 1998; L'Hirondel, 1992; Malaise *et al.*, 1998; Mazieres *et al.*, 2001; Michel *et al.*, 2005; Pavelka *et al.*, 1999; Uebelhart *et al.*, 1998, 2004, unpublished). The outcome assessors were blinded in 6 of 11 trials (Malaise *et al.*, 1998; Mazieres *et al.*, 2001; Michel *et al.*, 2005; Uebelhart *et al.*, 1998, 2004, unpublished). The care providers were blinded in 3 of 11 trials (Uebelhart *et al.*, 1998, 2004, unpublished). One out of 11 trials stated point estimates and measures of variability, that is, the 95% CI level for primary outcomes (Michel *et al.*, 2005). An intention-to-treat analysis was performed in 7 out of 11 trials (Conrozier, 1998; Malaise *et al.*, 1998; Mazieres *et al.*, 2001; Michel *et al.*, 2005; Pavelka *et al.*, 1999; Uebelhart *et al.*, 2004, unpublished).

V. Discussion

The authors did analyze the available literature (published and not published) regarding the clinical efficacy and tolerability of oral CS assessed in good quality RCTs. A large number of open, nonrandomized studies were therefore not considered to fulfill the level of entry of the database used and were excluded from this work. Finally, a total of 11 studies whose results are reported here did meet the basic criteria of eligibility to enter this survey.

A. About Bias and Confounders in Knee OA Studies

Analyzing the results of these RCTs, it is necessary to consider the fact that knee OA is a chronic disease that takes time to develop, and it is considered that from pre-OA, in which only minor metabolic events could possibly be assessed but are generally not known from both the patient and the physician, to clinical knee OA, in which the characteristic symptoms of pain and limitation of mobility are manifest, the time frame can extend from years to many decades. This feature makes the study of knee OA very difficult and quite challenging. Only some patients do present with rapidly progressing knee OA whose origin is generally unknown but which can be associated with crystal arthropathies such as calcium pyrophosphate disease also called chondrocalcinosis. In those cases, the progression of OA is rapid

TABLE II Characteristics of Eligible Clinical Trials of Chondroitin Sulfate Prescription

Source, year	No. of subjects (N baseline; ♂♀; N endpoint)	Type of study	Mode of administration	Dose of administration (mg)	Methodological score
Michel et al., 2005	300; 146/154; –	RCT	Daily tablet oral	800	8
Uebelhart et al., 2004	110; 21/89; –	RCT	1 sachet/day	800	8
Mazieres et al., 2001	131; 33/97; –	RCT	Gelcap	500	6
Uebelhart et al., 1998	46; 22/24; 42	RCT	2 sachets/day	2×400	6
Malaise et al., 1998	120; 21/89; 110	RCT	1 sachet/day	800	6
Uebelhart et al., unpublished material	143; 41/102; –	RCT	2 capsules/day	2×500	7
Bucsi and Poor, 1998	85; 34/51; 80	Two-center RCT	Not reported	800	4
Bourgeois et al., 1998	127; 31/97; 127	RCT	Sachets of oral gel	1200	4
Pavelka, et al., 1999	140; 36/104; 137	RCT	1 sachet/day	1200/800/200	5
Conrozier, 1998	104; –/–; 68	RCT	1 sachet/day	800	5
L'Hirondel, 1992	129; 87/42; 125	RCT	3 sachets/day	3×400	4

and the destruction of the joint can happen as fast as in 1 year, but as stated, this is not the "normal" progression of knee OA, and therefore the real time frame of the natural progression of the disease must be accounted for rather in terms of decades. In sharp contrast with these features, all the performed studies, even good quality RCTs did only last a couple of months up to a maximum of 2 years of follow-up, which remains a short time frame to study such a chronic disease and the actual impact of drugs or even nonpharmacological procedures. It must also be considered that the patients entering these trials are at various stages of the progression of their disease, and even if the pain level at entry or a combined score such as the AFI or the WOMAC are used as inclusion criteria, this does only partially reflect the effective stage of the disease for any individual patient. An additional relevant problem originates from the fact that most of the studies do report results regarding the evolution of the symptomatology at the level of one knee joint but do not consider the contralateral knee joint, which is very often also having some grade of OA, or if normal, suffers from a major redistribution of the body weight affecting the lower extremities of patients having a unilateral knee OA. In order to take this point into account and to consider that each patient has two knees that can only function when they are coupled, some special analyses of the data can be made using GEEM statistics (May and Johnson, 1996; Zeger and Liang, 1986); this type of analysis was applied only in one of the studies included (Uebelhart *et al.*, 2004). In the nonpublished study reported in this survey (Uebelhart *et al.*), the inclusion criteria based on pain and functional impairment level assessed by the AFI, but the setting point upon entry was certainly not high enough to ensure any significant changes with a 6-month progression between both CS and PBO treated groups.

In addition, this study could also illustrate the important finding that the origin of CS, which is used clinically in the every day practice and in the various clinical trials performed so far, might not have the same efficacy, depending on its origin. It is a matter of fact that, until now, no synthetic preparation of CS has ever been used and that all the CS is extracted and purified from the aggrecan fraction of the glycosaminoglycans (GAGs). For instance, fish CS is mostly extracted from the cartilaginous skeleton of the shark, whereas porcine or bovine CS is extracted from the trachea of both species (NB. bovine CS requires a special preparation procedure recognized by the FDA to insure the material is BSE free) and avian CS from the chicken sternum. The physicochemical and biochemical features of these various CS are not exactly the same, for instance considering the ratio between their actual content in $\Delta 4$ and $\Delta 6$ dissacharides. There are some preliminary *in vitro* indications that this ratio could affect the capacity of CS to inhibit some key enzymes, such as stromelysin (MMP3), which are involved in the development and/or the progression of OA disease. This might also explain in part why the only RCT using an avian formulation of CS to treat knee OA patients (Uebelhart *et al.*, unpublished) did not perform as well as compared to all other RCTs that used shark or bovine CS in the same indication and for an equivalent treatment duration (6 months).

As stated earlier, there are clearly a large number of possible bias and confounders that might be encountered in clinical studies dealing with knee OA patients, and therefore, even the results originating from the best RCTs should be considered critically and applied with some caution.

B. CS is an Effective SYSADOA for the Treatment of Knee OA

Nevertheless, the results of this survey, taking into account only the RCTs (10 studies published in peer-reviewed journals and one study not published so far) having the highest methodological quality, can be qualified in the overall as very positive for CS as an oral SYSADOA useful for the treatment of knee OA and significantly alleviating the symptoms of the patients.

The outcomes selected by the investigators of these studies are sound and widely recognized by the international community (Altman *et al.*, 1986) and the European (CPMP, 1998) and national regulatory authorities as well.

C. Practical Clinical Considerations and Recommendations

Regarding the effect of oral CS on both pain and function assessed by AFI, WOMAC, Huskisson's VAS, overall mobility, and walking time, it has been demonstrated that the most effective dosage in knee OA was the continuous intake of CS 800 mg/day taken orally over 1 year; the sequential administration over twice a 3-month period over 1 year did also provide good clinical results due to the remanent action of the drug but should certainly not be proposed to highly symptomatic patients. In order to reach a better control of pain, it was demonstrated that CS 1200 mg/day given for 2 weeks at initiation of therapy instead of CS 800 mg/day provided even better results. The optimal length of therapy with oral CS is still debated, and there is definitely no good answer to this point as the maximum trial duration was 2 years as of now. Considering the chronicity of knee OA and the excellent tolerability profile of CS, the clinical recommendation would be certainly to administer the drug for a couple of years if the symptoms, the overall mobility, and the quality of life of the patient are clearly ameliorated under treatment. As stated in the most recent EULAR recommendations for the management of knee OA (Jordan *et al.*, 2003), oral CS had a level of evidence classified 1A with an effect size range of 1.23–1.50 and a strength of recommendation of level A, which is clearly a strong support to our own clinical recommendations.

D. Comparison of Our Survey with the Published Meta-Analyses

A total of three meta-analyses have been published so far on oral CS (Leeb *et al.*, 2000; McAlindon *et al.*, 2000; Richy *et al.*, 2003). All did define oral CS as a good and well indicated SYSADOA for the symptomatic treatment of knee OA with a tolerability profile that makes this treatment well indicated for OA patients.

VI. Conclusions

Based upon our own survey of 11 RCTs, the data available from three published meta-analyses and the latest EULAR recommendations for the management of knee OA, it can be concluded that the long-term administration of oral CS is safe, well tolerated, and well indicated to control the symptoms of pain and increase the overall mobility of patients suffering from knee OA.

Acknowledgments

The authors would like to thank Leanne Pobjoy for her excellent secretarial assistance.

References

Altman, R., Asch, E., Bloch, D., Bole, G., Borenstein, D., Brandt, K., Christy, W., Cooke, T. D., Greenwald, R., and Hochberg, M. (1986). Development of criteria for the classification and reporting of osteoarthritis: Classification of osteoarthritis of the knee. *Arthritis Rheum.* **29**, 1039–1049.

American College of Rheumatology Subcommittee on Osteoarthritis Guidelines (ACR). (2000). Recommendations for the medical management of osteoarthritis of the hip and the knee. *Arthritis Rheum.* **43**, 1905–1915.

Bellamy, N., Buchanan, W. W., Goldsmith, C. H., Campbell, J., and Stitt, L. W. (1988). Validation study of WOMAC: A health status instrument for measuring clinically important patient relevant outcomes to antirheumatic drug therapy in patients with osteoarthritis of the hip or knee. *J. Rheumatol.* **15**, 1833–1840.

Bourgeois, P., Chales, G., Dehais, J., Delcambre, B., Kuntz, J. L., and Rozenberg, S. (1998). Efficacy and tolerability of chondroitin sulfate 1200 mg/day vs chondroitin sulfate 3 × 400 mg/day vs placebo. *Osteoarthritis Cartilage* **6A**, 25–30.

Bucsi, L., and Poor, G. (1998). Efficacy and tolerability of oral chondroitin sulfate as a symptomatic slow-acting drug for osteoarthritis (SYSADOA) in the treatment of knee osteoarthritis. *Osteoarthritis Cartilage* **6A**, 31–36.

Committee for Proprietary Medicinal Products (CPMP). (1998). "Points to consider on clinical investigation of medicinal products used in the treatment of osteoarthritis." European Agency for the Evaluation of Medicinal Products, London.

Conrozier, T. (1998). Anti-arthrosis treatments: Efficacy and tolerance of chondroitin sulfates (CS 4&6). *Presse Med.* **27**, 1862–1865.

Cooper, C. (1998). Epidemiology of osteoarthritis. *In* "Rheumatology" (J. H. Klippel and P. A. Dieppe, Eds.), pp. 1–20. Mosby, London.

Cooper, C., Snow, S., McAlindon, T. E., Kellingray, S., Stuart, B., Coggon, D., and Dieppe, P. A. (2000). Risk factors for the incidence and progression of radiographic knee osteoarthritis. *Arthritis Rheum.* **43**, 995–1000.

Dickersin, K., Scherer, R., and Lefebvre, C. (1994). Identifying relevant studies for systematic reviews. *BMJ* **309**, 1286–1291.

Huskisson, E. C. (1976). Assessment for clinical trials. *Clin. Rheum. Dis.* **2**, 37–49.

Jordan, K. M., Arden, N. K., Doherty, M., Bannwarth, B., Bijlsma, J. W., Dieppe, P., Gunther, K., Hauselmann, H., Herrero-Beaumont, G., Kaklamanis, P., Lohmander, S., Leeb, B., *et al.* (2003). EULAR recommendations 2003: An evidence based approach to the management of knee osteoarthritis. *Ann. Rheum. Dis.* **62**, 1145–1155.

Landis, J., and Koch, G. (1977). The measurement of observer agreement for categorical data. *Biometrics* **33**, 159–174.

Leeb, B. F., Schweitzer, H., Montag, K., and Smolen, J. S. (2000). A meta-analysis of chondroitin sulfate in the treatment of osteoarthritis. *J. Rheumatol.* **27**, 205–211.

Lequesne, M. G., Mery, C., Samson, M., and Gerard, P. (1987). Indexes of severity for osteoarthritis of the hip and knee. *Scand. J. Rheumatol.* **65**, S85–S89.

L'Hirondel, J. L. (1992). Klinische Doppelblindstudie mit oral verabreichtem Chrondointin-sulphat gegen Placebo bei der tibiofemoralen Gonarthrose. *Litera Rheumatol.* **14**, 77–85.

Malaise, M., Marcolongo, R., Uebelhart, D., and Vignon, E. (1999). Efficacy and tolerability of 800 mg oral chrondroitin 4&6 sulfate in the treatment of knee osteoarthritis: A randomised, double blind, multicentre study versus placebo. *Litera Rheumatol.* **24**, 31–42.

May, W. L., and Johnson, W. D. (1996). Generalized estimating equations for multivariate response with the variates having different distributions. *J. Biopharm. Stat.* **6**, 139–153.

Mazieres, B., Combe, B., Phan Van, A., Tondut, J., and Grynfeltt, M. (2001). Chondroitin sulfate in osteoarthritis of the knee: A prospective, double blind, placebo controlled multicenter clinical study. *J. Rheumatol.* **28**, 173–181.

Mazzuca, S. A., Brandt, K. D., Katz, B. P., Chambers, M., Byrd, D., and Hanna, M. (1997). Effects of self-care education on the health status of inner-city patients with osteoarthritis of the knee. *Arthritis Rheum.* **40**, 1466–1474.

McAlindon, T. E., LaValley, M. P., Gulin, J. P., and Felson, D. T. (2000). Glucosamine and chondroitin for the treatment of osteoarthritis: A systematic quality assessment and meta-analysis. *JAMA* **283**, 1469–1475.

Messier, S. P., Loeser, R. F., Mitchell, M. N., Valle, G., Morgan, T. P., Rejeski, W. J., and Ettinger, W. H. (2000). Exercise and weight loss in obese older adults with knee osteoarthritis: A preliminary study. *J. Am. Geriatr. Soc.* **48**, 1062–1072.

Michel, B. A., Stucki, G., Frey, D., De Vathaire, F., Vignon, E., Bruehlmann, P., and Uebelhart, D. (2005). Chondroitins 4 and 6 sulfate in osteoarthritis of the knee: A randomized controlled trial. *Arthritis Rheum.* **52**, 779–786.

Murray, C. J. L., and Lopez, A. D. (1997). "The Global Burden of Disease" World Health Organisation, Geneva.

Pavelka, K., Manopulo, R., and Bucsi, L. (1999). Double-blind, dose-effect study of oral chondroitin 4&6 sulfate 1200 mg, 800 mg, 200 mg and placebo in the treatment of knee osteoarthritis. *Litera Rheumatol.* **24**, 21–30.

Richy, F., Bruyere, O., Ethgen, O., Cucherat, M., Henrotin, Y., and Reginster, J. Y. (2003). Structural and symptomatic efficacy of glucosamine and chondroitin in knee osteoarthritis: A comprehensive meta-analysis. *Arch. Int. Med.* **163**, 1514–1522.

Spector, T. D., Cicuttini, F., Baker, J., Loughlin, J., and Hart, D. (1996). Genetic influences in women: A twin study. *BMJ* **312**, 940–943.

Uebelhart, D., Knüsel, O., Osterkorn, K., Berz, S., Przybylski, C., and Theiler, R. Oral chondroitin sulfate in patients with femorotibeal osteoarthritis: A six-month multicentre, randomised double-blind, placebo-controlled, parallel-group study. Unpublished (personal communication).

Uebelhart, D., Thonar, E. J., Delmas, P. D., Chantraine, A., and Vignon, E. (1998). Effects of oral chondroitin sulfate on the progression of knee osteoarthritis: A pilot study. *Osteoarthritis Cartilage* **6A**, 39–46.

Uebelhart, D., Malaise, M., Marcolongo, R., De Vathaire, F., Piperno, M., Mailleux, E., Fioravanti, A., Matoso, L., and Vignon, E. (2004). Intermittent treatment of knee osteoarthritis with oral chondroitin sulfate: A one-year, randomized, double-blind, multicenter study versus placebo. *Osteoarthritis Cartilage* **12**, 269–276.

Verhagen, A., de Vet, H., de Bie, R., Kessels, A. G., Boers, M., Bouter, L. M., and Knipschild, P. G. (1998). The Delphi list: A criteria list for quality assessment of randomized clinical trials for conducting systematic reviews developed by Delphi consensus. *J. Clin. Epidemiol.* **51**, 1235–1241.

Zeger, S., and Liang, L. (1986). Longitudinal data analysis using generalized linear models. *Biometrics* **73**, 13–22.

Zhang, W., Doherty, M., Arden, N., Bannwarth, B., Bijlsma, J., Gunther, K. P., Hauselmann, H. J., Herrero-Beaumont, G., Jordan, K., Kaklamanis, P., Leeb, B., Lequesne, M., *et al.* (2005). EULAR evidence based recommendations for the management of hip osteoarthritis: Report of a task force of the EULAR Standing Committee for International Clinical Studies Including Therapeutics (ESCISIT). *Ann. Rheum. Dis.* **64**, 669–681.

Index

Contents of Previous Volumes

Liver Slices as a Model in Drug Metabolism
James L. Ferrero and Klaus Brendel

Use of cDNA-Expressed Human Cytochrome P450 Enzymes to Study Potential Drug–Drug Interactions
Charles L. Crespi and Bruce W. Penman

Pharmacokinetics of Drug Interactions
Gregory L. Kedderis

Experimental Models for Evaluating Enzyme Induction Potential of New Drug Candidates in Animals and Humans and a Strategy for Their Use
Thomas N. Thompson

Metabolic Drug–Drug Interactions: Perspective from FDA Medical and Clinical Pharmacology Reviewers
John Dikran Balian and Atiqur Rahman

Drug Interactions: Perspectives of the Canadian Drugs Directorate
Malle Jurima-Romet

Overview of Experimental Approaches for Study of Drug Metabolism and Drug–Drug Interactions
Frank J. Gonzalez

Volume 44

Drug Therapy: The Impact of Managed Care
Joseph Hopkins, Shirley Siu, Maureen Cawley, and Peter Rudd

The Role of Phosphodiesterase Enzymes in Allergy and Asthma
D. Spina, L. J. Landells, and C. P. Page

Modulating Protein Kinase C Signal Transduction
Daria Mochly-Rosen and Lawrence M. Kauvar

Preventive Role of Renal Kallikrein—Kinin System in the Early Phase of Hypertension and Development of New Antihypertensive Drugs
Makoto Kartori and Masataka Majima

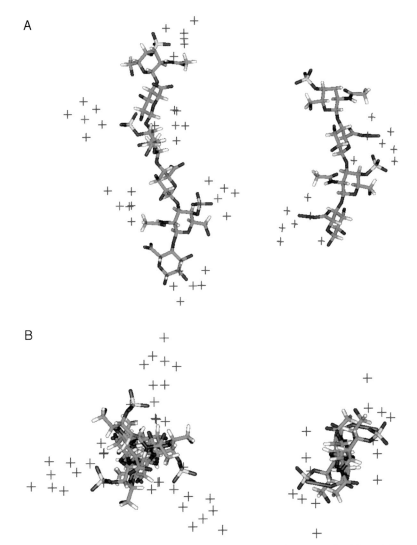

CHAPTER 4, FIGURE 2 X-ray diffraction structures of C4S, in (A) side and (B) end views, shown in stick representation with carbon green, oxygen red, nitrogen blue, and cation purple. Water in the crystal structure and sodium ions are shown as star shapes. On the left of each panel is the structure 1C4S (in which the cation is sodium) and on the right is 2C4S (in which the cation is closely coordinated calcium). In 1C4S the helix makes a complete turn every three disaccharides, whereas in 2C4S the polysaccharide is more extended, making a complete turn every two disaccharides.

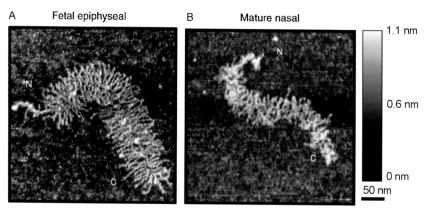

CHAPTER 4, FIGURE 4 Atomic force microscopy images: (A) Fetal epiphyseal aggrecan; (B): Adult nasal aggrecan. The N-terminal globular domains, as well as the heavily glycosylated CS domains, can clearly be seen. The closely packed chondroitin side-chains are shorter and perhaps have a wider length distribution, in the adult PG. Reproduced with permission from Ng *et al.* (2003).

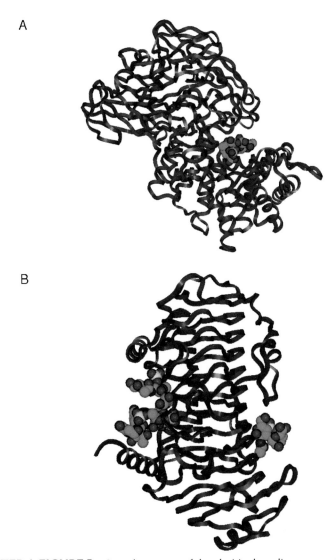

CHAPTER 4, FIGURE 5 Crystal structures of chondroitin-degrading enzymes in complex with oligosaccharides. The proteins are shown as ribbons that follow the backbone atoms, and the oligosaccharides are shown in a space-filling representation colored as in Fig. 2. (A) Chondroitin AC lyase, with a C4S tetrasaccharide in the active site (Huang *et al.*, 2001). (B) Chondroitin B lyase, with a DS hexasaccharide degraded into three disaccharides in the binding site (on the left of the image) (Michel *et al.*, 2004). These two enzymes are unrelated in structure, in the way they bind to the substrate and in their mechanism of action. Chondroitin B lyase displays a dermatan binding site distant from the active site, occupied in this structure by a DS disaccharide (on the right of the image).

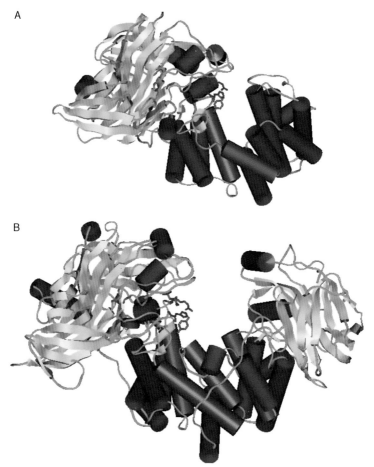

CHAPTER 5, FIGURE 6 Structural comparison of cAC and cABC I. (A) Structure of chondroitinase AC from *Pedobacter heparinus* based on the crystal structure of Fethière *et al.* (1999) and Huang *et al.* (2001). (B) Structure of chondroitinase ABC I from *Proteus vulgaris* based on the crystal structure by Huang *et al.* (2003). The similarities in the domains of both enzymes are evident. On a closer inspection, the middle domain of cABC I has very little sequence identity with the catalytic domain of cAC (and bacterial hyaluronidases). However, the residues that are implicated to play important roles in catalysis are conserved in both enzymes (Prabhakar *et al.*, 2005). These catalytic residues are shown in full (purple). The more open cleft of cABC I is possibly suggestive of this enzyme's ability to accommodate a variety of oligosaccharide geometries and thus its wider substrate specificity.

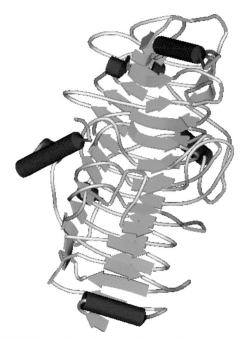

CHAPTER 5, FIGURE 7 Chondroitinase B from *Pedobacter heparinus*. Structure of chondroitinase B based on the crystal structure of Huang *et al.* (1999) and Michel *et al.* (2004). Chondroitinase B is the only known enzyme that cleaves dermatan sulfate as its sole substrate. The structure shows the right-handed parallel β-helix fold representative in chondroitinase B and pectate lyases. The authors thank Dr Rahul Raman for support in preparing this schematic.

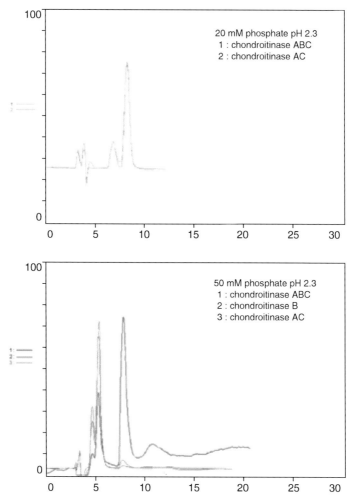

CHAPTER 7, FIGURE 3 HPLC analysis of CS/DS for the identification of low IdoA-containing chains. GAGs were isolated from laryngeal cartilage and then digested with the various chondroitinases and subjected to HPLC eluted with either 20 mM or 50 mM phosphate buffer to identify IdoA-containing structures, other than disaccharides (D. H. Vynios, unpublished results).

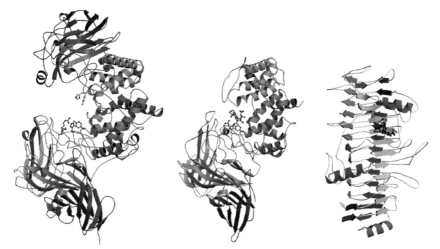

CHAPTER 9, FIGURE 3 Comparison of crystal structures of chondroitinases PvulABCI (left), FlavoAC (center), and FlavoB (right).

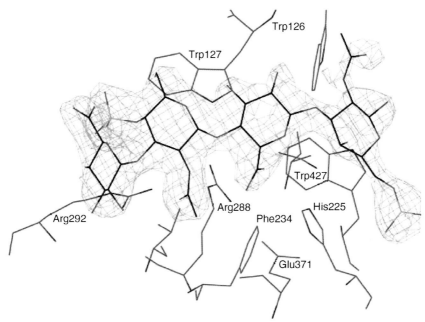

CHAPTER 9, FIGURE 4 Chondroitin-4,6-sulfate tetrasaccharide in the active site of FlavoAC Tyr234Phe mutant.

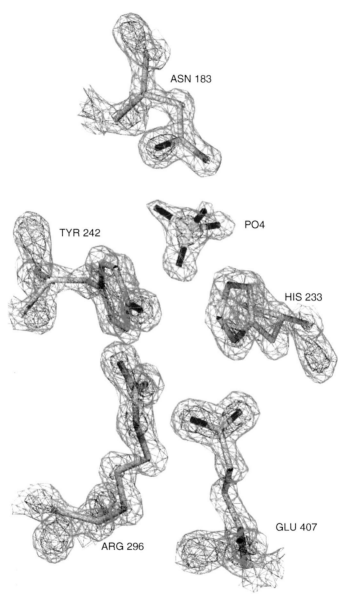

CHAPTER 9, FIGURE 5 Experimental electron density map of the active site region of ArthroAC. Green contours are drawn at 3σlevel, red contours at 5σ level. In the native structure, there is a phosphate ion in the active site. Nitrogen atoms are blue, oxygens are red, carbons are gray, and phosphorus is yellow.

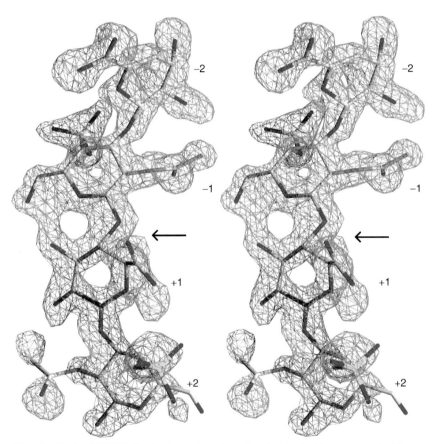

CHAPTER 9, FIGURE 6 Conformation of the chondroitin-4-sulfate tetrasaccharide substrate bound in the active site of ArthroAC. Omit electron density map is drawn at the 3σ level.

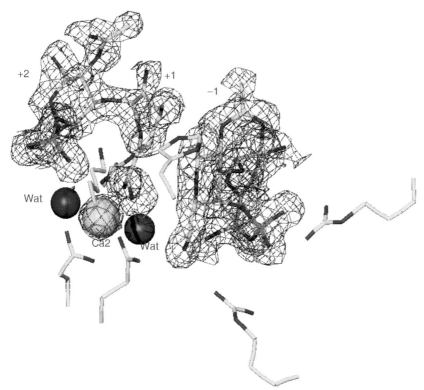

CHAPTER 9, FIGURE 8 Three disaccharide products bound in the active site of chondroitinase B. Bound calcium atom is shown as a yellow sphere, two water molecules as red spheres.

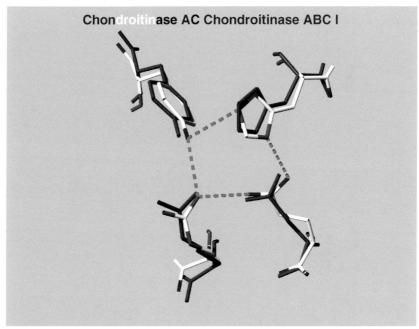

CHAPTER 9, FIGURE 9 The superposition of the active-site tetrad of FlavoAC and PvulABCI. The Asn175 of FlavoAC and Arg500 of PvulABCI are also shown.

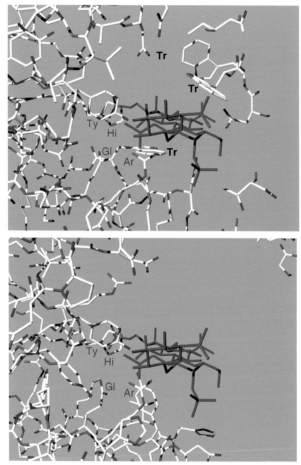

CHAPTER 9, FIGURE 10 The disposition of the substrate in FlavoAC (left) was transferred to PvulABCI (right) based on the superposition of the active site tetrad. In this open form of PvulABCI are very few contacts between the enzyme and its substrate.

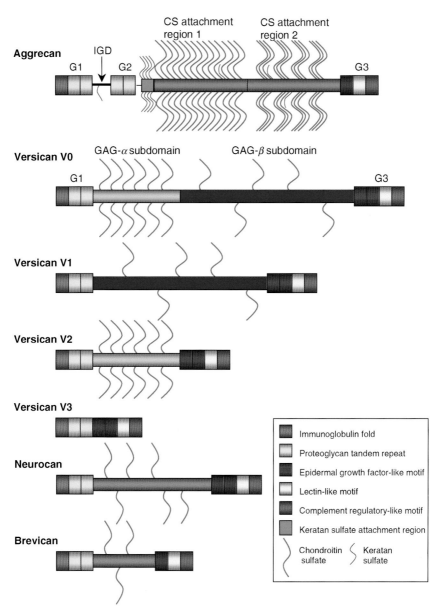

CHAPTER 10, FIGURE 2 Schematic diagrams of the major large CS containing PGs that form aggregates with hyaluronan (hyalectins). CS, chondroitin sulfate; IGD, interglobular domain.

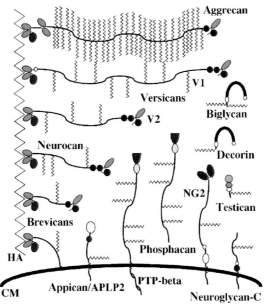

Modules:

● Immunglobulin	● Immunglobulin	⬭ C-type lectin
⬭ Link	○ Fibronectin III	● Laminin-G
● EGF	▼ Carboanhydrase	○ Follistatin
● Sushi	• Kunitz prot. inh.	◉ Ca²⁺-binding

CHAPTER 16, FIGURE 1 Secreted and cell surface CSPGs, which have been observed in the central nervous system. Schematic presentation of the PGs with common ECM modules represented in color. The interactions of the N-terminal domains of the lecticans with haluronan (HA) are indicated at the left side. The anchorage of cell surface bound PGs to the cell membrane (CM) via GPI moieties (brevican) or transmembrane domains is indicated at the bottom. Protein parts, which contain cysteins and may represent less established extracellular protein modules, are indicated as white globules. Regions lacking cysteins, which might have a mucine-like character, are indicated as black lines. Bolder lines in decorin and biglycan represent leucine rich repeats. Zigzag-lines represent transmembrane domains (small), CS chains (medium), and HA (big).

A

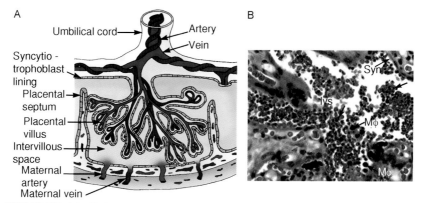

CHAPTER 18, FIGURE 1 (A) Schematic diagram of a portion of human placenta. (B) Photograph of a tissue section of *P. falciparum*-infected placenta fixed with 10% formaldehyde and stained with hemotoxylin and eosin. IVS, intervillous space; Syn, syncytiotrophoblast lining; Mφ, macrophage/mococytes; arrows, IRBCs.

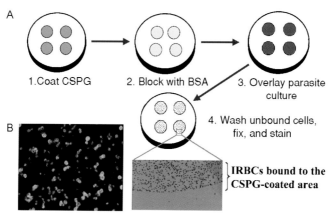

CHAPTER 18, FIGURE 2 (A) Schematic diagram illustrating the various steps of *in vitro* cytoadherence assay used for assessing the binding of IRBCs to CSPG coated onto plastic Petri dishes. The CSPG solutions (10–15 μl at 10–400 ng/ml in PBS) are spotted as 4 mm spots, blocked with 2% BSA in PBS, overlaid with parasite culture. The unbound cells washed off with PBS, and bound cells are fixed, stained with Giemsa, and photographed under a microscope. (B) Photograph under a microscope, showing the binding of IRBCs prestained with SYBR Green to CSPG-coated plates.

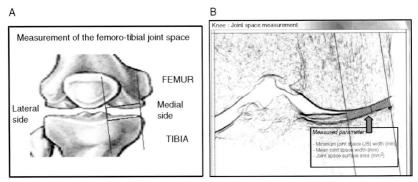

CHAPTER 24, FIGURE 1 (A) Schematic view of the measurement of the femoro-tibial joint space. (B) After digitalization of the knee X-ray, definition of the zone of interest for automatic or semiautomatic measurement of the femoro-tibial joint space.